THE SEX ATLAS

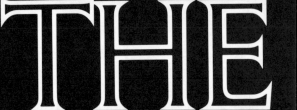
THE

SEX ATLAS

A NEW ILLUSTRATED GUIDE

ERWIN J. HAEBERLE, Ph. D., D. A.

A CONTINUUM BOOK · THE SEABURY PRESS · NEW YORK

1978
The Seabury Press
815 Second Avenue, New York, New York 10017

Special acknowledgement is made to Liz Green for the technical illustrations, and to these photographers whose work appears on the following pages: Coni Beeson (pp. 147, 148, 149, 167, 172, 173, 479); Tee A. Corinne (p. 40); Honey Lee Cottrell (pp. 100, 191); Dr. Vincent DeFeo (p. 44 left); Linda Fredrickson (pp. 14, 15, 17, 18, 19, 150, 162); Tom Sikes (pp. 82, 83). Complete acknowledgments and credits for photographs reproduced by permission in this book appear on page 509, which constitutes an extension of this copyright page.

Library of Congress Cataloging in Publication Data
Haeberle, Erwin.   The sex atlas.
(A Continuum book)
Bibliography: p. 495. Includes index.
1. Sex.   2. Sex (Psychology).   3. Sex role.   4. Sexual deviation.   5. Sexism.   I. Title.
HQ12.H33   301.41   77-13513   ISBN 0-8164-9160-7

CONTENTS

INTRODUCTION

This book offers a critical summary of current sexual knowledge. It is written for readers of any age who are interested in human sexuality and who want to know more about its history and social implications.

It can, of course, hardly be said that there is a lack of printed material on the subject. The list of pertinent publications already seems endless and is still growing. There are now so many studies, surveys, reports, guides, manuals, journals, newsletters, and magazine articles devoted to "sex" in all of its aspects that only a few full-time specialists can hope to keep track of them. Indeed, even these specialists have to specialize further if they want to remain up-to-date. Thus, most of them concentrate on selected areas of research, such as sexual anatomy, the physiology of sexual responses, reproduction and contraception, sex therapy, sex education, gender identity problems, sexual minorities, the history of sexual customs, sex legislation, erotic art, sexual ethics, etc. This special research is being conducted in many countries by countless individuals with a variety of goals and methods working from very different assumptions. The results are therefore often uncertain, contradictory, and confusing. Moreover, they are constantly being revised. Under the circumstances, many ordinary citizens may find it as hard as ever to be well informed and to reach any firm conclusions that could help them in their own lives. In the end they may come to feel that the more they read about sex, the less they know.

However, there is no need to give up and to leave the matter entirely to the "experts." We may still be very far from understanding human sexuality, but there are a few basic insights which are no longer disputed and which deserve to be shared as widely as possible. Especially in the United States recent research has produced a certain professional consensus on many formerly obscure and disputed issues, and this is already reflected in some of the newer textbooks, college courses, and educational television programs. In other words, while many areas of sex research remain controversial, it has now become possible to offer the general public a first integrated, if still somewhat limited view.

The Sex Atlas represents another attempt in this direction. It does not contain any fresh speculations or sensational findings. Nor does it want to scandalize, radicalize, or otherwise upset anyone. It deliberately refrains from presenting any research of its own. Instead, it merely repeats what has been said many times by the best contemporary scholars and scientists. In short, it is nothing more and nothing less than a piece of popularization. It is not trying to say anything new, but rather to state the well-known as clearly as possible in a coherent and methodical fashion.

This does not mean that the text is entirely factual and free of value judgments. On the contrary, even the casual reader will quickly discover that value judgments are openly expressed or at least implied in many parts of the book. After all, the very concept of research itself implies an attack on conventional wisdom and, if necessary, a breaking of taboos. No responsible sex researcher has ever pretended complete neutrality. A moral commitment is unavoidable whenever one deals with social issues, and, as everyone knows, sex can be and often is a source of intense human conflicts. To the extent, therefore, that sex research deals with these conflicts, it has always been forced to "take sides" and to plead for some social change. From Havelock Ellis and Freud to Kinsey and Masters and Johnson, sex researchers have never hesitated to ask for new sexual values and attitudes. Any summary of their work would be incomplete if it did not reflect this concern.

On the other hand, *The Sex Atlas* does not try to record every interest or belief of every scientist who has ever studied sexual problems. Instead, the text is rather discriminating and selective. It gives preference to the most widely accepted current views and does not dwell on certain traditional arguments that have long proved to be unproductive. It further examines, wherever possible, the underlying assumptions of past and present research and tries to simplify the professional language. Thus, in many instances, the theories, theses, claims, and conclusions of a particular writer have been rephrased or translated from scientific jargon into plain English. Where esoteric or foreign expressions had to be retained, short definitions have been provided in brackets.

A special effort has also been made to be systematic, i.e. to organize the various bits of information into a unified whole and to present the reader with a practical frame of reference. *The Sex Atlas* therefore emphasizes certain important facts over and over again and repeatedly mentions the same historical personalities and historical dates. For the same reason, it also refers to the same classical authors and even the same great books in different chapters.

The text itself does not assume any prior knowledge on the reader's part, but begins "from scratch," as it were, building its case in successive stages and explaining every new piece of information as it is introduced. Therefore, the book will be best appreciated by those who read it straight through from beginning to end. This procedure also recommends itself to teachers and students who use the work as a textbook.

However, the individual parts, chapters, sections, and paragraphs can also be studied separately, since they are firmly embedded in a larger framework. Frequent cross-references and the very structure of the book itself will quickly establish the appropriate context, and thus there is little danger of getting lost in meaningless details. The over-all picture always remains clear. Again for the purpose of greater clarity, corresponding sections (such as those dealing with male and female anatomy or heterosexual and homosexual intercourse, for example) follow the same basic pattern and, where appropriate, even use identical language. This again makes for a certain amount of repetition, but it can also help in pointing out parallels that might otherwise be overlooked.

The fact that the discussion of the male here always precedes that of the female also reflects a didactic purpose. From a strictly biological point of view, it would perhaps make more sense to put the female sex first, but when it comes to practical problems, such as contraception, infertility, and sexual dysfunction, it is more useful to go against the current habits of thought and to begin with the male.

Finally, a word about the illustrations: The American public has long been accustomed to lavishly illustrated coffee table books on anything from sea shells to wrought iron gates, the history of warfare, and the various breeds of domestic cat, but books on human sexuality have rarely been known to make generous use of pictures. Textbooks dealing with sexual matters have, as a rule, used anatomical drawings, graphs, charts, and statistics, and occasionally even reproductions of work of art, but almost never photographs of human beings and human sexual behavior. Such photographs have hitherto been mainly restricted to so-called pornographic books and magazines. As a result, many readers have been left with the impression that there is something "dirty" or shameful about sex.

However, it seems that the time has finally come to bring the subject completely into the open and to end the embarrassment once and for all. *The Sex Atlas* therefore simply ignores the traditional fears and restraints and treats human sexuality like any other subject matter: Illustrations are offered wherever they can contribute to understanding the text.

At the same time, it is assumed that such understanding cannot be confined to mere technicalities. The readers are also given an opportunity to test (and perhaps change) their general sexual attitude. Indeed, for some such "Sexual Attitude Restructuring" may well be the greatest benefit they derive from this book. In any case, it is hoped that both the text and the illustrations will give many people a new appreciation of their sexual capacities and thus also help them to be more tolerant toward their fellow human beings. Accurate information can alleviate or even eliminate much of our present needless sexual misery.

ACKNOWLEDGMENTS

As I have explained in the introduction, the present book, as any textbook of this kind, is essentially a summary of work done by others. I therefore gladly discharge my duty of acknowledging my debt to those great scholars and scientists on whose writings I have relied in my effort. Their research, not my own, has provided the real substance of the following text. The most important of my sources have been the well-known publications of Alfred C. Kinsey and his associates and of Clellan S. Ford and Frank A. Beach, Lester A. Kirkendall, John Money, and William E. Masters and Virginia Johnson. In addition, I have made use of the work of several, hitherto untranslated, Middle-European cultural historians, especially Jos van Ussel (*Sexualunterdrückung*, Reinbeck b. Hamburg 1970) and Annemarie and Werner Leibbrand (*Formen des Eros*, 2 vols., Freiburg Br./München 1973). Of course, these and the many other original researchers to whom I am indebted are also repeatedly listed throughout the text, in the reference notes, and in the bibliography.

My own work of compiling, evaluating, and synthesizing the abundant source material has been immensely helped by several friends and colleagues without whom I would have lost my perspective. They have offered much useful advice and constructive criticism. I especially thank Professor Dr. Vincent J. DeFeo of the Department of Anatomy and Reproductive Biology, John A. Burns School of Medicine, University of Hawaii, Honolulu, who checked the first section of my book for basic accuracy and gave me a number of practical hints for its improvement. I have followed most of his suggestions. Any possibly remaining errors or omissions are, of course, my own. I am also deeply grateful to Professor Dr. Harvey L. Gochros of the School of Social Work, University of Hawaii, for his active interest in this project. His experienced eye focused mainly on the pedagogical aspect of my text, and from him I have learned a great deal about the effective presentation of research material in the classroom. He was also the first to call my attention to the problems of the sexually oppressed. My visits with him and his students have always been profitable and enlightening. I would further like to thank Professor Dr. Ronald J. Pion of the Department of Obstetrics and Gynecology, John A. Burns School of Medicine, University of Hawaii for some valuable material and information. In addition, I have received much-appreciated help and advice from Professor Dr. Charlotte Armster Gebhardt and Dr. Jerold Wikoff of the Department of German, Dartmouth College, from Professor Dr. Paul McCarthy of the Department of East Asian Languages, University of Minnesota, Minneapolis, and from Professor Dr. John R. Clarke, Department of the History of Art, Yale University. Special thanks are also due to Gene G. Bernal of the ESL program of the Modesto City Schools, Modesto, California, for his assistance at crucial moments and for organizing some of my often expansive files.

Finally, it is my particular pleasure to acknowledge my debt to Dr. Robert Theodore McIlvenna and his colleagues of the National Sex Forum, San Francisco, California. For several years they have given me the most generous encouragement. Indeed, without them this book might never have seen the light of day. I especially appreciate the competence and patience of Dr. Laird Sutton who shot most of the photographs for this book. At the same time I thank Salli Rasberry and Dr. Phyllis Lyon for their critical support and their help in my efforts to avoid the bias of male chauvinism. If I should not have fully succeeded it is certainly not their fault. I have also gratefully followed some helpful recommendations from Dr. Richard L. Bennett, Director of the Akron Sex Forum, Akron Ohio. Last, but not least, I thank Drs. Eberhard and Phyllis Kronhausen for permission to reproduce some material from their famous collection of erotic art.

ERWIN J. HAEBERLE

San Francisco, 1977

THE SEX ATLAS

THE HUMAN BODY

There are many ways of looking at the human body. We can admire it as the noblest of God's creations, despise it as the prison of the soul, worship it as the temple of love, fear it as the source of temptation, or study it as a scientific object. Only this much is certain: Whatever we see in it will reflect our own attitudes and intentions.

Most modern societies take a rather negative attitude toward the human body and especially toward its sexual functions. This manifests itself, for example, in the great moral concern about "indecent" clothing, "dirty" books and films, and sex education in public schools. In fact, there is a widespread conviction that the world is being inundated by a flood of sex and nudity which threatens the very foundations of our civilization.

However, our Western civilization, which is now several thousand years old, has not always worried about such problems. For the ancient Greeks and Romans, the nude human body was a familiar sight. Athletes practiced and performed in the nude at the gymnasium (Greek *gymnos:* nude). The participants at the original Olympic games (and at all other sports events) were nude. Public and private buildings were decorated with sculptures and paintings of nude men and women. The sexual aspect of nudity was openly recognized. Statues of certain deities, such as Hermes and Priapus, displayed an erect penis as the symbol of strength and fertility. Artistic representations of sex organs were worn in the form of jewelry as a good luck charm. The actors of the comic stage wore monstrous penises as part of their costume. In short, there was an open and joyful acceptance of the human body and human sexuality. The contrast to our modern world could hardly be more striking.

Many people today believe that the rise of Christianity is responsible for this unfortunate change. Indeed, some Christian writers are willing to concede as much to their secular critics. However, such a view is far too simplistic. Many supposedly Christian attitudes toward the human body are only a few hundred years old and would have been incomprehensible to the church of earlier ages. For example, the moral obsession with masturbation, or the notion that children are "innocent" and should be kept ignorant about sex, were all but unheard of before the 18th century. In the early 16th century, the great humanist Erasmus of Rotterdam was still able to write popular texts for children dealing with such topics as sexual intercourse before, in, and outside of marriage, pregnancy, birth, prostitution, aphrodisiacs, castration, and venereal disease (Erasmus, *Colloquia Familiaria*). A few hundred years later these texts were considered too outspoken even for adults.

The sense of shame or indignation at the sight of the nude human body which today pervades so much of our culture is also of relatively recent origin. In medieval Europe, nudity was not considered a moral issue. Families slept in the nude together in the same room, often in the same bed. Inns and hostels expected their guests to sleep together with strangers of both sexes. A person refusing to share his bed or to take off his clothes would have been suspected of being diseased or disfigured. Public nudity was common in bathhouses, which were favorite social gathering places for men and women of all ages. At special holidays, pretty nude girls could be seen in civic parades. Occasionally, even men of the church appeared completely nude in religious processions.

It was not until after the epidemic spread of syphilis during the 16th and 17th centuries and the rise of the middle classes that nudity began to be viewed as obscene. The whole attitude toward the human physical functions changed. The former intimacy was now rejected as disgusting and unhealthy. People no longer ate from the same dish or drank from the common mug. Instead of their fingers they began to use knives and forks. The wealthy started to wear special sleeping clothes or nightgowns. Privacy became a growing concern. The bed was removed from the living room and hidden in a separate bedroom. The bathhouses were closed, recreational swimming in lakes and rivers became sexually segregated until finally public nude bathing as such was prohibited altogether. In other words, the open acceptance of the body and its functions gradually turned into prudery. By the 19th century, society had become so sensitive about bodily functions that the mere mention of sex, reproduction, digestion, or perspiration was considered offensive. Indeed, even simple words like "thigh" and "breast" could no longer be used in polite conversation. The entire human body was taboo.

As modern Western civilization conquered the world, this prudery was then often imposed by force on uncomprehending and reluctant peoples for whom complete or partial nudity had always been a way of life. Even today, certain struggling Asian and African nations are engaged in an effort to "civilize" their citizens by asking them to wear clothes to which they have never been accustomed. Ironically, in the meantime, some of the richest and most advanced Western nations have begun to revert to the less prudish standards of former historical periods. (For a more detailed discussion of these developments, see the third part of this book, "Sex and Society.")

While our modern culture has subjected us to a great deal of sexual repression, it has nevertheless made an important contribution toward a more humane life for all of mankind—the scientific exploration of the human body and its functions.

Our ancient and medieval ancestors possessed very little exact biological and medical knowledge. When they were sick, they depended largely on folk remedies, superstitions, or outright magic. Magical and mystical beliefs also governed their sexual and reproductive lives. For example, most men and women were convinced that the right "love potion" could win the heart of even the most unwilling partner. There was also a belief that certain experiences of a pregnant woman could "mark" her baby, and that coitus during the night would lead to the conception of blind children. People knew nothing about the circulation of blood, hormones, the male and female sex cells (sperm and egg), and other modern discoveries. In the opinion of the most respected scholars, not only men but also women produced some seminal fluid, and it was generally assumed that the mixing of these fluids inside the womb was essential for procreation. It was further assumed that the fetus came to life only during the fifth month of pregnancy at the time of the so-called quickening (i.e., the moment when the mother first feels the fetal movements).

These and similar misconceptions were finally laid to rest by modern science. However, the facts as we see them today did not emerge quickly and easily. Some biological laws and the causes of certain diseases were discovered only after centuries of patient observation. Occasionally, scientific research led to such unexpected results that, for a long time, people simply refused to accept them. Indeed, to this very day science continues to challenge our traditional way of thinking and sometimes even our way of life.

A recent striking example is the scientific observation of human sexual responses in the laboratory. The findings disproved many widely held assumptions. It was shown, for instance, that the sexual capacity of women is at least as great as that of men and, in some respects, even greater. Obviously, such a realization cannot remain without consequences for the overall relationship between the sexes. In this, as in other cases, scientific insight may well lead to profound social changes.

Such changes, although perhaps necessary, are not always welcome. It is therefore hardly surprising that, throughout its history, science has met with a great deal of resistance. Whenever scientists questioned the conventional wisdom they were attacked and ridiculed, and sometimes their discoveries were suppressed and ignored. Very often, however, society objected not only to specific discoveries, but to the very idea of science itself. Even today, many people feel a kind of instinctive revulsion at the humorless, merciless, shameless way in which scientists seem to "take all the mystery out of life."

Indeed, it cannot be denied that there is something sacrilegious about the scientific approach to problems. In their pursuit of knowledge, scientists not only disregard God, but also show little respect for hallowed human traditions. Questions of morality, legality, or even of good taste do not concern them. Nothing is too sacred for their curiosity, and they view everything with the same neutral detachment.

This characteristic detachment of science requires a particular emotional and intellectual discipline, a special frame of mind which is typically "modern." In Greek and Roman antiquity and in the Middle Ages, man considered himself an integral part of the world and would not have wanted or dared to detach himself from it. He was not used to suppressing his feelings or moral concerns, but reacted to everything with his whole personality. He believed not only that he lived at the center of the universe, with the sun, the moon, and all the stars revolving around him, but also that everything in this universe had some personal meaning for him and was somehow related to his fate. Something happened because the gods or God made it happen in order to reward or punish him. For example, health was seen as the reward of righteousness; death and disease were the wages of sin. There was no differentiation between causal and normative laws. The law of nature was divine will. Explanation and justification were one and the same.

The beginning of modern science can be described as that moment in history when explanation and justification were first separated. As long as health and sickness, sunshine and rain, good and bad harvests were regarded as reward or punishment for man's conduct, factual cause and moral end were always seen together. Science became possible only when man began to disregard all supernatural influences and their meaning. From then on, he studied "nature as such," without any reference to divine intentions and human concerns.

The scientist looks at the human body "objectively," i.e., he regards it strictly as an object to be observed, weighed, and measured. He is not interested in its beauty, sinfulness, or even in its health. His only aim is to understand its functions, not to pronounce them good or bad. He does not make value judgments, but judgments of fact. In other words, the scientist tries to describe what is, not prescribe what should be. If he should find the body to be diseased, he may list the symptoms of the disease and search for its causes, but as a scientist he would make no attempt at healing. That is basically a moral enterprise, and it is undertaken by people who use scientific knowledge to help their fellow human beings. It is true that today the role of the scientist and that of the healer are often played by one and the same person, a physician, for example. Nevertheless, a good physician knows that he does, in fact, perform two separate functions and that, on occasion, he may have to keep them separate. For instance, he may know as a scientist that continued heavy smoking will kill a certain patient. As a healer, he may suggest to the patient that he give up his cigarettes. This suggestion would, of course, be based on the moral (not scientific) judgment that the value of life is higher than that of smoking pleasure. However, if the patient held the opposite values and preferred to die rather than stop smoking, the physician would find himself restricted to his role as a scientist who simply observes the effects of smoking on a dying man. (A dramatic example is the case of Sigmund Freud. As a scientist, he knew that his smoking would kill him. As a healer, he could have acted upon this knowledge and given up his cigars. As a patient, he refused to do so and died of cancer of the jaw.)

Nonscientists often find it difficult to appreciate the scientific point of view. Particularly in the early days of modern science, the majority of people mistook the scientist's suspension of moral judgment for callousness and indifference, if not frivolity. For example, when in the 16th and 17th centuries scientists first dissected human corpses for the sake of anatomical knowledge, their contemporaries were horrified. It would never have occurred to them to "donate their bodies to science." On the contrary, they often prohibited this kind of research altogether. As a result, many anatomists had to keep their work secret and pay criminal "body snatchers" to steal corpses from the cemetery or even right from the gallows. (In our own time, some sex researchers have also had to begin their work in secrecy and to pay prostitutes to serve as objects of study.)

Nevertheless, over the centuries people realized that the objective investigation of the human body and its functions could bring them great benefits. Although the essence of science itself is moral neutrality, scientific knowledge can very well be used for moral purposes. The healing and prevention of diseases is only the most obvious example. Equally important is man's liberation from needless fears and narrow superstitions which prevent him from realizing his full potential. Thanks to science, man has made great progress toward that goal. Indeed, every new scientific discovery adds to his ability to master his own fate.

In recent decades, the advance of sex research has been especially dramatic. Almost every day scientists add to our understanding of the human sexual and reproductive functions. In the past, these functions were firmly linked, and people had little control over them. Sexual intercourse led to reproduction, and reproduction was impossible without sexual intercourse. Unless they were abstinent, sexual partners were unable to limit the number of their children, and many women died of exhaustion after too many births. On the other hand, those couples who remained childless had to accept their infertility as the will of "nature." In the meantime, reproduction has become a matter of conscious choice. Scientific insight into the reproductive process has made it possible to develop effective methods of contraception, and today unwanted pregnancies can easily be avoided. Furthermore, many formerly hopeless cases of infertility can now be treated successfully, sometimes by means of artificial insemination, i.e., without any direct sexual contact. Now for the first time in human history, the sexual and reproductive functions can be completely separated.

These modern developments have far-reaching social consequences as they lend support to the growing demand for full sexual equality. Traditionally, the biological differences between the sexes have always been used as a justification for forcing men and women into different social roles. Thus, men chose to believe that "nature" had destined women for motherhood, and that this "natural" calling made them unfit for any other task. (For some unexplained reason, fatherhood was not considered to have the same crippling effect.) However, now that women have become free to embrace or reject motherhood as they please, such notions are difficult to maintain. Indeed, the belief in the "natural" inferiority of women is now being exposed as nothing more than the ideology of men who want to justify their position of privilege.

We can be certain that continued scientific research will eventually also disprove many of our present beliefs, no matter how self-evident they might seem. Especially when it comes to sex we are not always as detached and objective as we think we are. Very often our observations are colored by unrecognized prejudices and unquestioned moral assumptions, and thus we are still in danger of confusing value judgments with judgments of fact. In short, where our own interests are involved we are as likely as ever to mistake convention for "nature." However, we can learn from the history of modern science that, in the long run, our self-interest is best served by strict objectivity. Science began when man started to disregard the divine and human aspects of everything he studied. Paradoxically, this very disregard then opened the door to deeper understanding. Only if we are prepared to transcend our narrow personal concerns, can we hope to find out the truth about ourselves and thus become really free.

Thanks to the mass media, new scientific insights into the human bodily functions can now be shared by a greater number of people than ever before. Most men and women today know more about anatomy and physiology than any ancient or medieval doctor. Yet in spite of all their theoretical knowledge, many of them are ill at ease with themselves. Unlike their ancestors, they feel alienated from their own bodies, i.e., they experience them as unfamiliar and strange. Indeed, it seems that the very same historical developments that enabled modern man to look at himself with scientific detachment also robbed him of his former self-acceptance.

Our technological society imposes a great deal of discipline on all of us. We are usually not allowed to express our emotions, follow our impulses, or devote our energies to the pursuit of pleasure. On the contrary, in the interest of our work we have to adjust to fixed timetables for activity and relaxation, always appear even-tempered, suppress any sign of spontaneity, and deliberately dull our senses. In short, we are forced to transform ourselves into well-functioning instruments of labor. As a result, we have become used to treating the human body as a machine, and our increased understanding of its functions is mainly used to add to its "efficiency."

Many people also carry this attitude over into their sexual relationships. This becomes apparent, for example, in their great concern with youth and physical vigor. Thus, they are often quite eager to try any new diet, experiment with any new drug, use any new gadget or device, and train themselves in any new technique that promises to strengthen their erotic capacities. Furthermore, there are now countless sex guides, love books, and marriage manuals which discuss the technical aspects of sex in great detail and thereby hope to turn the reader into an expert lover.

There is no doubt that such books can indeed be very helpful. After centuries of repression, a frank description of human sexual functioning and the possible variations of sexual intercourse can free men and women from unnecessary inhibitions. Unfortunately, some of them also gain the false impression that sexual happiness is a matter of great expertise and athletic ability, and since they themselves seem to lack either talent or practice, they end up feeling inadequate. In fact, even many of those who succeed in mastering all erotic skills discover that the mere mechanics of sex leave them unsatisfied. Eventually, they realize that the desire to control and manipulate their bodies for the sake of performance cripples them as human beings. It depersonalizes all their relationships, and finally renders them incapable of true enjoyment.

It is for this reason that, in recent years, more and more people (especially the young) have abandoned the mechanistic approach to sex and have developed a less demanding attitude toward the human body. They are beginning to understand that the modern world of discipline and competition has distorted their perceptions, and they try to regain the sensual awareness of former historical periods through "sensitivity training." Thus, they literally get back in touch with themselves and arrive at a point where they can accept and appreciate their own bodies without exploiting them.

At the same time, most young men and women today have again become able to look at the nude human body without embarrassment. Indeed, for many of them nudity is now once more a familiar sight to which they do not attach any exaggerated significance. However, it is unfortunate that there also continues to be widespread and persistent ignorance about the bodily functions, especially those that have to do with sex. Indeed, there remain not only some prudish members of the older generation, but also a few of the new one who are uninformed or even seriously misinformed about the physiological processes underlying their behavior. It therefore seems both justified and necessary to take advantage of the welcome new climate of sexual candor and to offer an unobstructed, if somewhat limited, view of the subject.

The following pages provide some basic information about the sexual aspect of the human body, especially the male and female sex organs, the human sexual response, reproduction, contraception, and abortion. In addition, there is a brief discussion of some physical disorders that can impair normal sexual functioning. The psychological aspects of human sexual behavior are discussed in the second part of this book, "Human Sexual Behavior."

1. THE PROCESS OF SEXUAL DIFFERENTIATION

The sex of a human being is determined at the time of fertilization. However, for the first few weeks of their lives the unborn males and females are indistinguishable. Their maleness or femaleness manifests itself only gradually over a period of time.

We are all used to identifying newborn children as either boys or girls according to their different external sex organs. Still, apart from these organs, they look very much alike. The typical male or female appearance of men or women results from developments that do not begin until many years later. The full extent of human sexual differences appears only after both males and females have reached sexual maturity, i.e., when they can have children of their own.

Most of us think of sex as the simplest and most fundamental of all human distinctions. Indeed, this very assumption is implied in our language. The word "sex" is derived from the Latin *sexus* which, in turn, has its roots in the verb *secare:* to cut, separate, or divide. In the strict sense of the term, therefore, "sex" simply refers to that which divides the human race (and most higher animal and some plant life) into two distinct groups—males and females. Every individual belongs to either one of these groups, i.e., to one of the two sexes. A person is either of male or female sex.

All of this seems plain enough. However, recent scientific research has shown that the traditional simple definitions of maleness and femaleness are quite inadequate and that, in some cases, the matter can actually be very complicated. When a modern scientist is asked to identify a person as either male or female, he takes at least seven different factors into account:

1. Chromosomal Sex
The cells of the male body contain one X and one Y chromosome, while those of the female body contain two X chromosomes. However, recently several other chromosomal combinations have been discovered.

2. Gonadal Sex
The male has testicles (male gonads); the female has ovaries (female gonads). However, in rare cases both testicular and ovarian tissue may be present in the same body.

3. Hormonal Sex
The hormones secreted by the testicles or ovaries play an important part in developing the male or female body before birth and during puberty. A lack, imbalance, or oversupply of these hormones has a decisive influence on a person's anatomy and physiology.

4. Internal Accessory Reproductive Structures

The male has sperm ducts, seminal vesicles, a prostate gland, etc., while the female has Fallopian tubes, a uterus, a vagina, etc. In rare cases, some or all of these organs may be underdeveloped or missing.

5. External Sex Organs

The male has a penis and a scrotum; the female has a clitoris, major and minor lips, etc. In rare cases, some or all of these organs may be underdeveloped or missing.

6. Sex of Assignment and Rearing

A child with a male body will usually be raised as a male. However, it is possible to raise such a child as a female, and vice versa.

7. Sexual Self-identification

A child with a male body who is taught to assume the role of a male will usually learn to consider himself male. However, it is possible that in spite of parental suggestions he nevertheless ends up identifying himself as female. Conversely, a child with a female body who is taught to assume the role of a female may nevertheless identify herself as male.

Scientists now realize that these seven variables may be independent of each other. For example, a newborn child may have the internal sex organs of a female while the external sex organs appear to be those of a "sexually unfinished" male. On the basis of this deceptive appearance, the child may then be declared a boy and raised as such. (See also "Sexual Malformations.") Another example is a person whose sexual self-identification is at odds with the sex that has been assigned to him. (See "Transsexualism.") Such possible incongruities can, of course, create many medical and social problems. Fortunately, most people are clearly male or female by all seven criteria and therefore require no special professional help during their sexual development.

However, even where maleness and femaleness are not in doubt, there still may be some uncertainty about the proper social roles of males and females. Thus, in the past men and women were often assumed to have very little in common. They were not only expected to look different, but also to behave differently. Based on this expectation, most societies developed different social roles and different moral standards for the two sexes.

Modern research has raised a great deal of doubt about these traditional assumptions, although one major difference between males and females remains undisputable: that which concerns their reproductive functions. While both sexes are needed to make the creation of new human life possible, only women actually conceive, bear, and nurse children. In most other respects, however, the sexual differences are not as fundamental as it might seem. Indeed, many male and female characteristics that were formerly considered inborn and unchangeable have been shown to be inbred, i.e., the result of cultural influences. It is, of course, not always easy to draw a dividing line between biological inheritance and social conditioning. The scientific study of these matters is still in its beginnings. In the meantime, it seems useful to remember the many similarities between the sexes. Generally speaking, men and women would far better understand each other if they realized that they are alike in their basic anatomy and physiology.

The following pages summarize the physical differences between the sexes as they emerge during the process of sexual maturation. For sexual differences in behavior and social status, see "The Development of Sexual Behavior" and "The Social Roles of Men and Women."

MALE AND FEMALE ANATOMICAL DEVELOPMENT

The anatomical difference between men and women is not very great. Even their sexual systems are quite similar and, indeed, in their first stages of development they are indistinguishable. Later structural modifications make the male and female sex organs complementary to each other, but even then one can still recognize their common origin. In other words, while the sexual differences (just as all other physical features of the future human being) are already programmed into every fertilized egg, they materialize only slowly over a period of time. In some isolated instances, the development may even be thwarted and remain incomplete. (See "Sexual Malformations.")

As mentioned earlier, in some cases it may be difficult to identify a particular individual as male or female. However, in our everyday lives we are usually content with determining a person's sex on the basis of certain obvious characteristic physical and psychological traits. Traditionally, these traits have been known as sexual characteristics, and they can be divided into three different categories:

1. **The primary sexual characteristics** are the external sex organs. They are already present at birth and thus make it possible to determine whether a newborn child is a boy or a girl.
2. **The secondary sexual characteristics** are those physical features that develop during puberty and which further accentuate the anatomical difference between males and females.
3. **The tertiary sexual characteristics** are those psychological qualities that are nurtured in one sex and discouraged in the other.

The primary and secondary sexual characteristics are biologically determined, and they constitute a person's maleness or femaleness. The tertiary sexual characteristics are culturally determined, and they constitute a person's masculinity or femininity.

The following paragraphs restrict themselves to the physical characteristics. For the psychological aspects of sexual differentiation, see "The Development of Sexual Behavior" and "The Social Roles of Men and Women."

THE PRIMARY SEXUAL CHARACTERISTICS

The sex organs are the most obvious sexual characteristic. They are also the only external sign of whether a newborn baby is a boy or a girl. However, while the male and female sex organs are very different in appearance, they are similar in origin and structure. In fact, they develop from the same embryonic cell mass. The difference comes about only gradually during the baby's growth before birth. (Also see "Pregnancy.") The sex organs do not become fully functional until after puberty when, under the influence of certain hormones, they finally complete their growth. (Also see "The Role of Hormones.")

The Male

In the first weeks after conception, the male as well as the female embryo is a tiny organism without recognizable human features. However, it does have a primitive head and limb buds which begin to grow into real arms and legs. The embryo further possesses a ridge of tissue which is destined to develop into sex organs. Indeed, the first beginnings of sex glands or gonads can already be found, but, at this point they are still sexually undifferentiated, i.e., they are the same for both sexes. Externally, a hump (suggestive of the male) with a groove (suggestive of the female) can be observed at the spot where the future sex organs will grow. As the male embryo slowly begins to look more human toward the end of the third month of its life, the hitherto undifferentiated gonads develop into testicles. The external hump assumes the shape of a penis, and the groove closes. (As evidence of this original groove, each male retains a pink scar line running down the underside of his penis all the way from the glans to the anus.) Two patches of skin on either side of the hump begin to form the scrotum. (In the female, they become the major lips to the vulva.)

As the embryo grows into the fetus, the sex organs continue to develop together with the entire body. Between the seventh and ninth months the testicles normally descend into the scrotum.

In the period between birth and puberty, the sex organs do not show any dramatic further development. However, during the ages of 12 to 17 boys normally experience a noticeable growth of their sex organs and eventually their first ejaculation of semen. They will also notice that some hair (called pubic hair) begins to grow at the base of the penis. All of this indicates that the sex organs are completing their maturation. (For further details, see "The Male Sex Organs.")

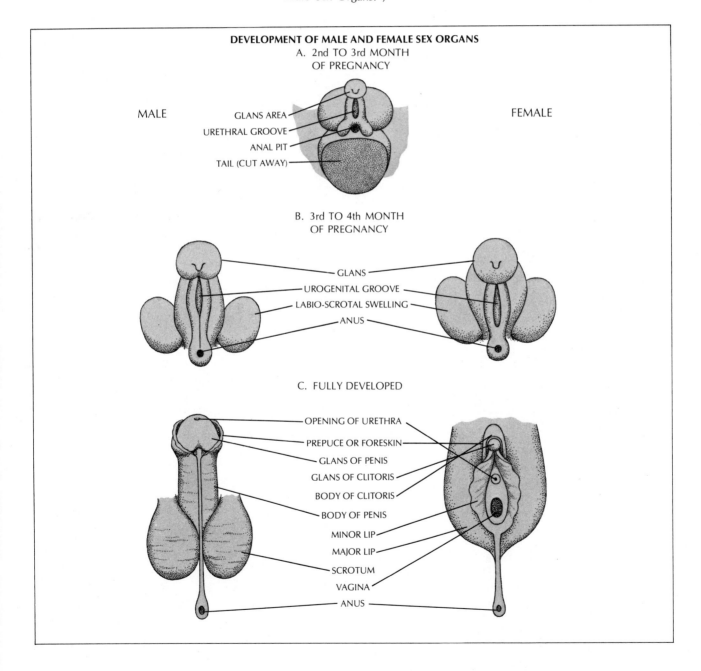

DEVELOPMENT OF MALE AND FEMALE SEX ORGANS

MALE   FEMALE

A. 2nd TO 3rd MONTH
OF PREGNANCY

GLANS AREA
URETHRAL GROOVE
ANAL PIT
TAIL (CUT AWAY)

B. 3rd TO 4th MONTH
OF PREGNANCY

GLANS
UROGENITAL GROOVE
LABIO-SCROTAL SWELLING
ANUS

C. FULLY DEVELOPED

OPENING OF URETHRA
PREPUCE OR FORESKIN
GLANS OF PENIS
GLANS OF CLITORIS
BODY OF CLITORIS
BODY OF PENIS
MINOR LIP
MAJOR LIP
SCROTUM
VAGINA
ANUS

The Female
Both the female and the male embryo remain sexually undifferentiated for the first few weeks of their lives. They do possess the beginnings of sex glands or gonads, but these beginnings are the same for both sexes. Just as the male, the female also shows a hump and a groove at the spot where the future external sex organs will develop. However, in her case the hump develops into the clitoris while the groove remains open, forming the minor lips and the vestibule of the vulva. Two patches of skin on either side develop into the major lips. (In the male, they develop into the scrotum.) The original gonadal structures which develop into testicles in the male evolve into ovaries in the female.

Between her birth and puberty, a girl's sex organs do not undergo any dramatic further development. However, during the ages of 11 to 13 some hair (pubic hair) will begin to grow on her vulva, and her first menstruation can normally be expected at that time. These signs indicate that she is close to sexual maturation. (For further details, see "The Female Sex Organs.")

The secondary sexual characteristics begin to appear during puberty as a result of hormonal stimulation. They become apparent first in females, a little later in males. By the time their physical growth is completed, the bodies of men and women show several marked differences. (See also "The Role of Hormones.")

The following paragraphs summarize the physical changes of puberty. These changes may occur very slowly and extend over a period of more than a decade, or they may appear rather suddenly and be completed within one or two years. While general social conditions, diet, and climate may affect the development, much of it is also determined by heredity. For example, Asian men usually remain less muscular and develop less facial and body hair than European men.

THE SECONDARY SEXUAL CHARACTERISTICS

The Male
In the male, the first body changes of puberty are the growth of the testicles, the appearance of pubic hair at the base of the penis, and an enlargement of the penis. These changes indicate that the body is reaching sexual maturity, and sometime thereafter the first ejaculation can occur. However, at first the ejaculate may not contain any sperm cells, but consist mainly of fluid from the prostate gland. (The first ejaculation may occur during masturbation or spontaneously while the boy is asleep. In the latter case, he is said to have a "wet dream.")

During puberty, the body grows rapidly in size. The shoulders become wider than the hips, the chest enlarges in every dimension, and the muscles in the arms, legs, and shoulders grow stronger and more obvious. The pubic hair becomes more dense and rather kinky, gradually forming a triangle that points upward toward the navel. Some hair also develops in the armpits (called axillary hair) and, in some males, on the chest. Generally, the male is hairier than the female. Eventually, he also develops facial hair which will grow into a beard unless it is shaved off regularly. As the male sex organs grow in size, the larynx (voice box or "Adam's apple") also enlarges. As a result, men generally have a deeper voice than women.

The Female
Females experience the physical changes of puberty in the following order: First, the breasts begin to enlarge. Then some straight and later kinky or curly hair appears on the vulva. This pubic hair forms a triangle pointing downward. Eventually, some hair will also appear in the armpits (called axillary hair). During this time, the body grows in height, and the hips become wider than the shoulders. Fatty tissue in and around the breasts, shoulders, hips, and buttocks gives the female body its generally rounder appearance. The first menstruation (also known as menarche) indicates approaching sexual

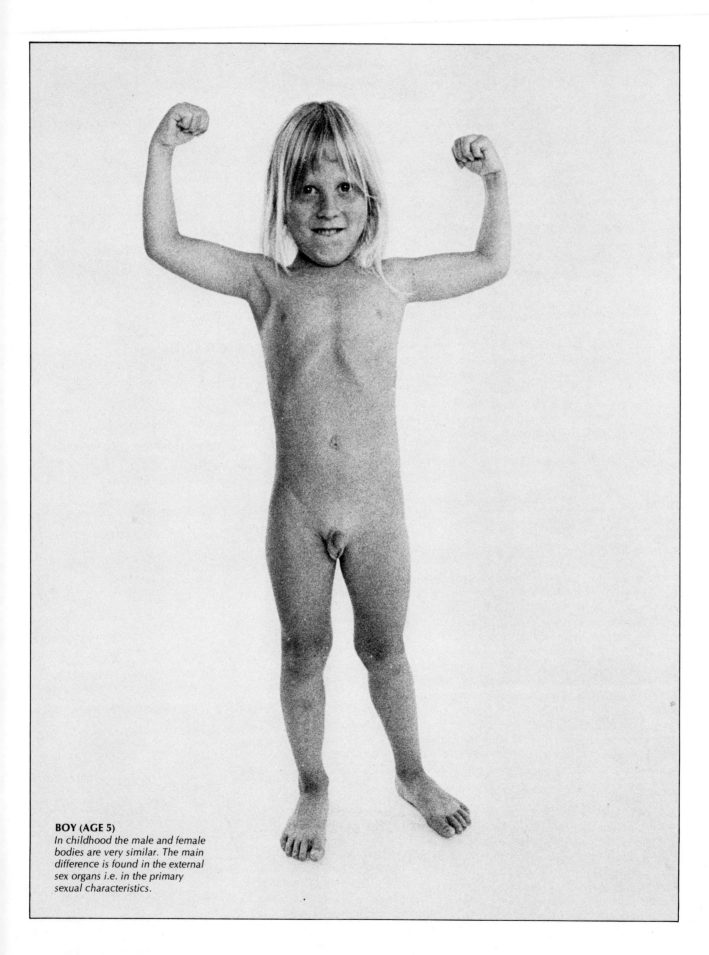

BOY (AGE 5)
In childhood the male and female bodies are very similar. The main difference is found in the external sex organs i.e. in the primary sexual characteristics.

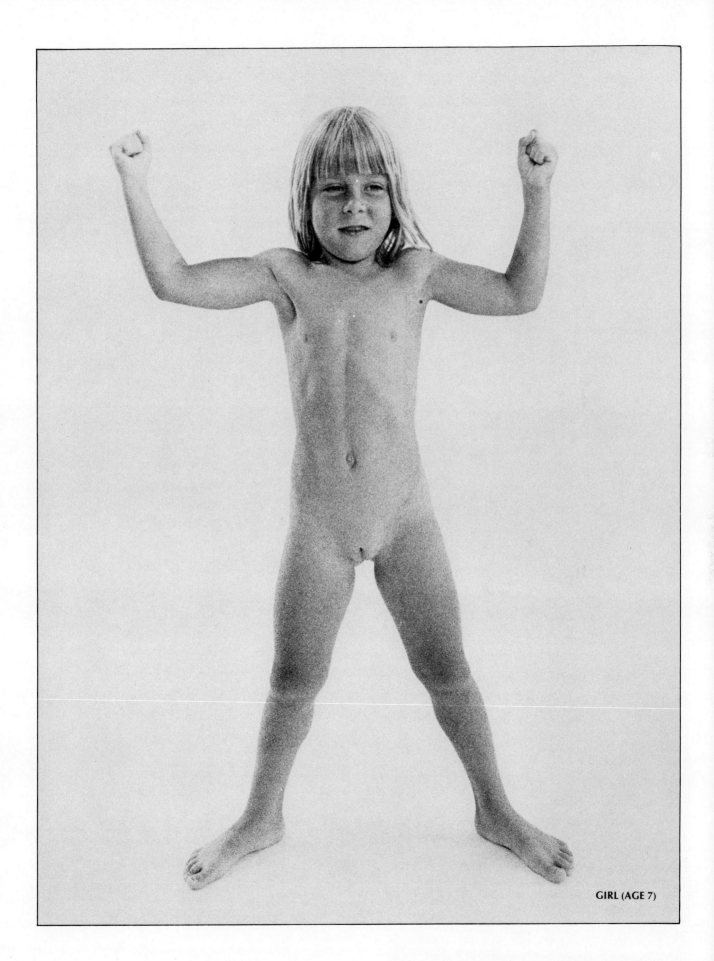

GIRL (AGE 7)

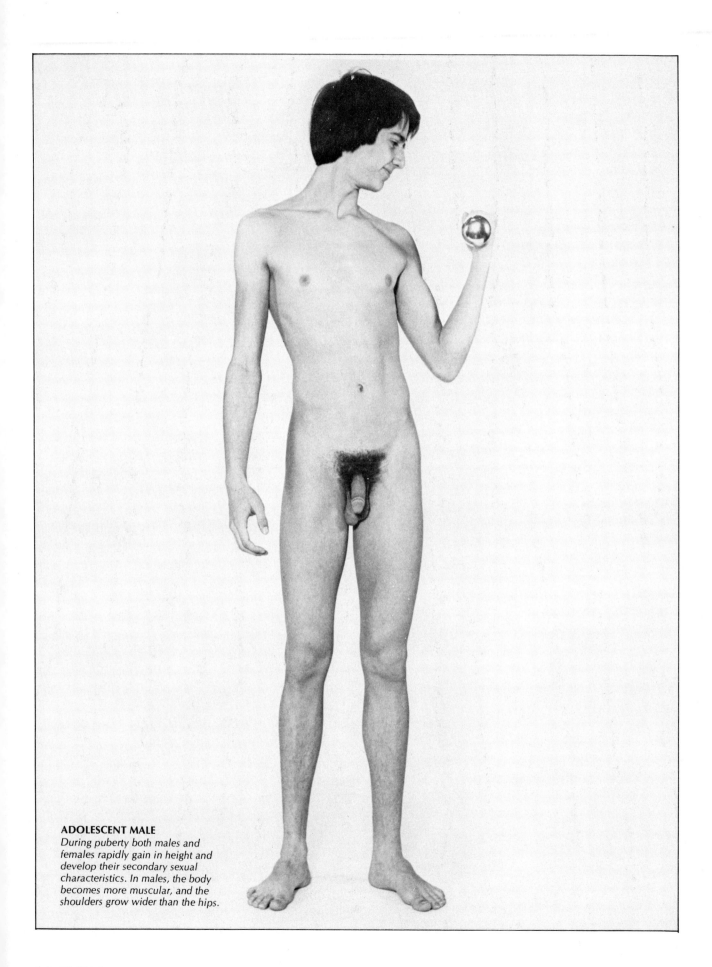

ADOLESCENT MALE
During puberty both males and females rapidly gain in height and develop their secondary sexual characteristics. In males, the body becomes more muscular, and the shoulders grow wider than the hips.

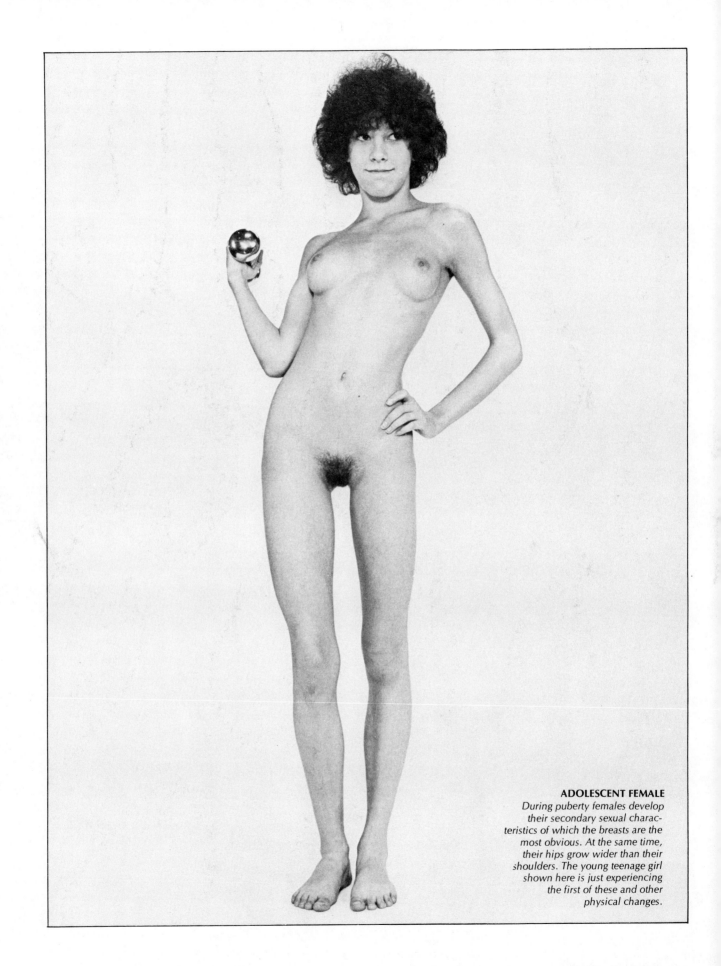

ADOLESCENT FEMALE
During puberty females develop their secondary sexual characteristics of which the breasts are the most obvious. At the same time, their hips grow wider than their shoulders. The young teenage girl shown here is just experiencing the first of these and other physical changes.

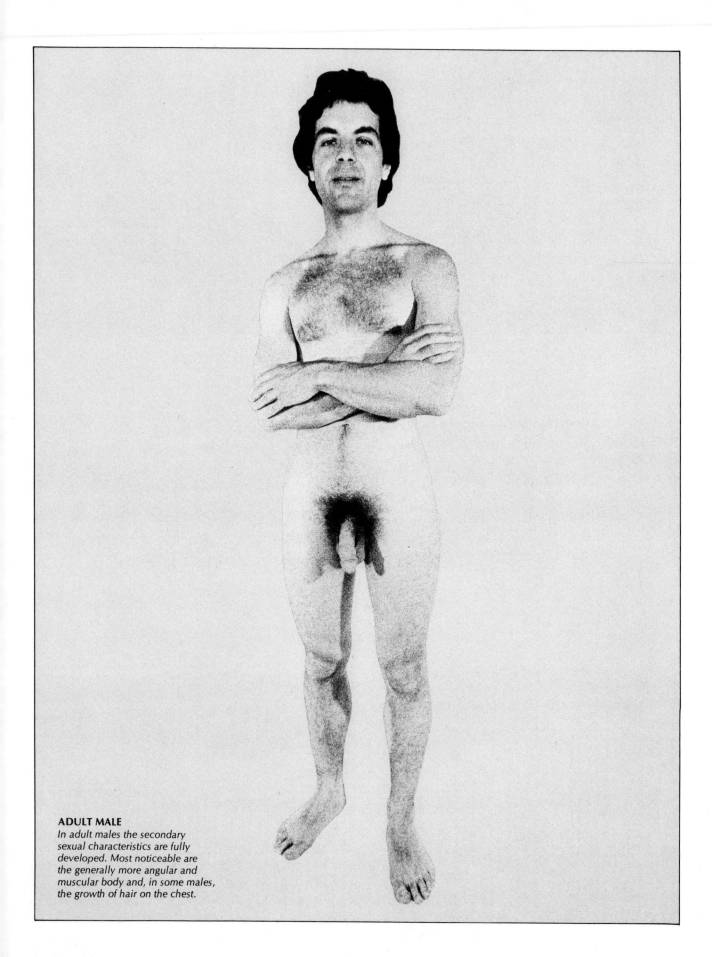

ADULT MALE
In adult males the secondary sexual characteristics are fully developed. Most noticeable are the generally more angular and muscular body and, in some males, the growth of hair on the chest.

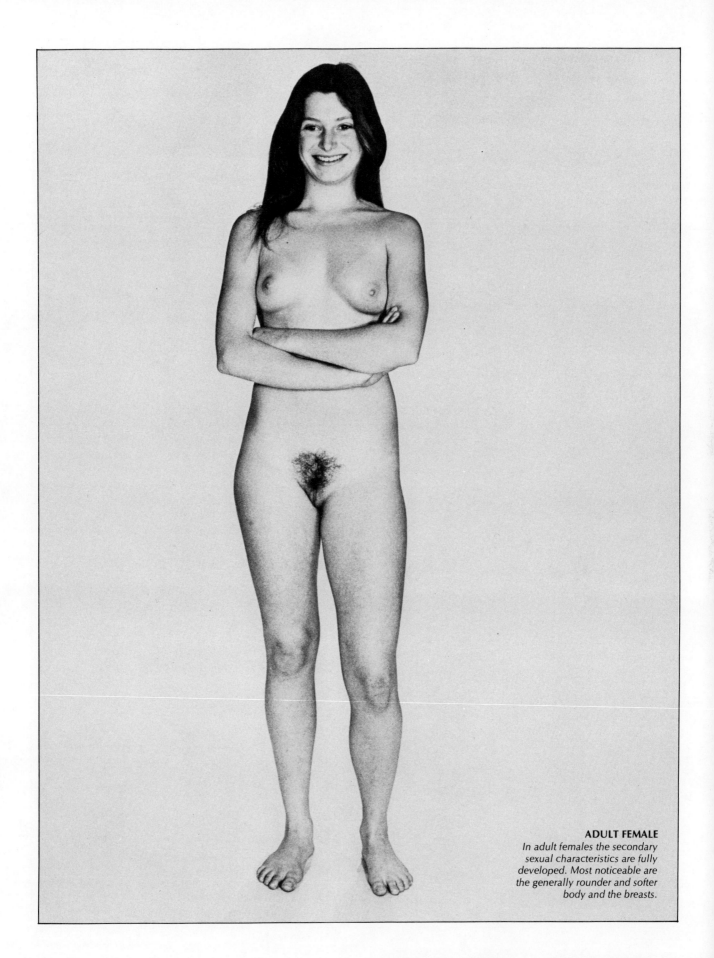

ADULT FEMALE
In adult females the secondary sexual characteristics are fully developed. Most noticeable are the generally rounder and softer body and the breasts.

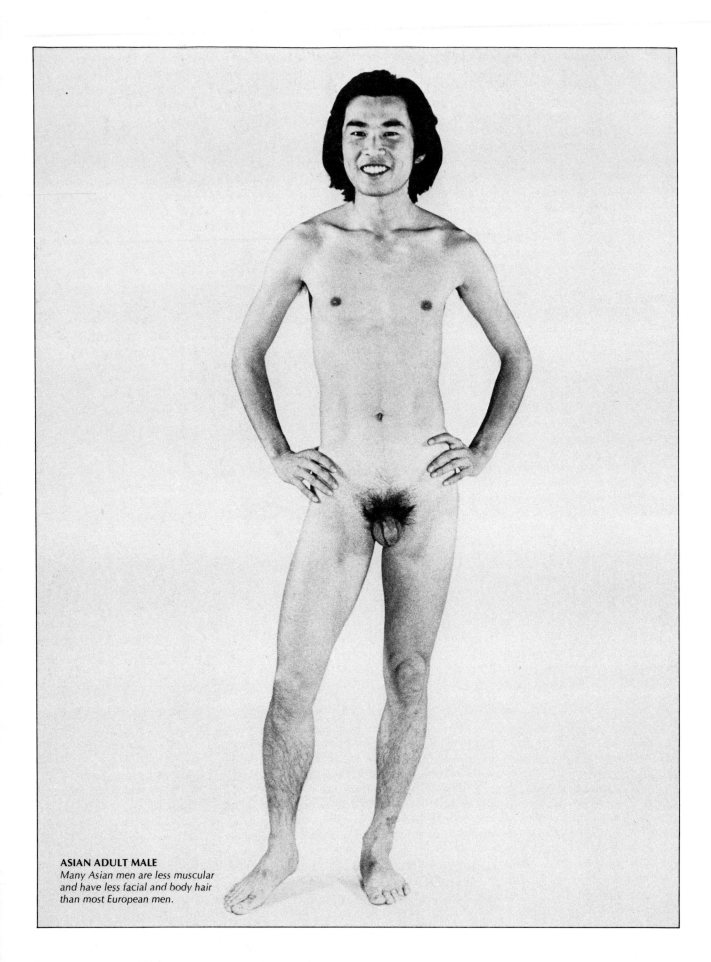

ASIAN ADULT MALE
*Many Asian men are less muscular
and have less facial and body hair
than most European men.*

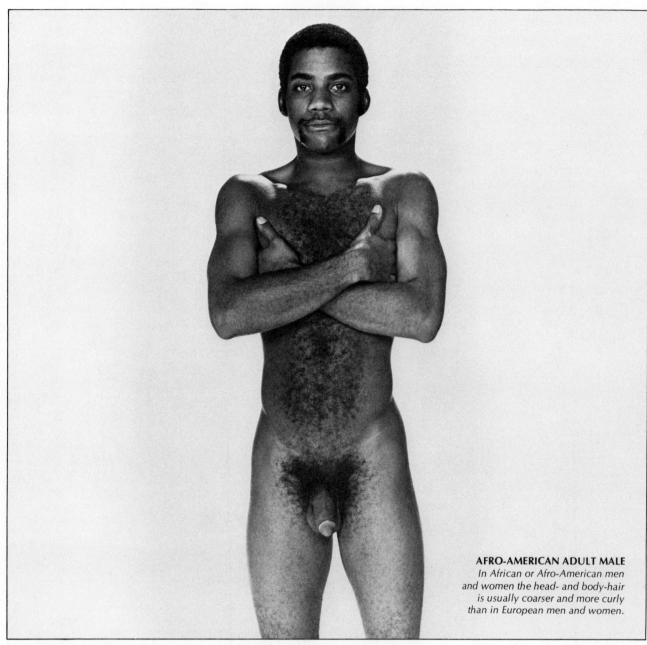

AFRO-AMERICAN ADULT MALE
In African or Afro-American men and women the head- and body-hair is usually coarser and more curly than in European men and women.

Not all secondary sexual characteristics are present or equally pronounced in all human beings. There is some slight variation between groups in different parts of the globe and even between different individuals within each group. Most often, this is more obvious in males than in females.

maturity. In the beginning, the menstrual cycles are still irregular, and in some of them there may be no ovulation. In other words, for a while a girl may menstruate and still be largely infertile. Indeed, a woman usually gains her full reproductive capacity only one or two years after her first menstruation.

In females, there is no decisive enlargement of the larynx and therefore no voice change comparable to the one taking place in males. In general, women are also less muscular and slightly shorter than men.

At the end of puberty, the breasts have developed their typical rounded shape and thus become the most obvious female secondary sexual characteristic. However, they do not produce milk until after pregnancy. (See "Birth.")

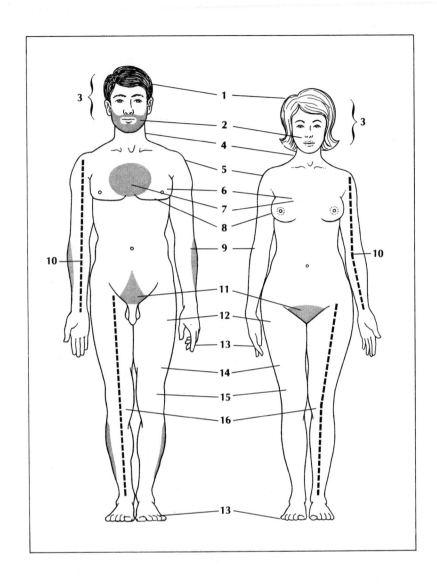

THE SECONDARY SEXUAL CHARACTERISTICS

The Male: On the average, taller and heavier than the female.
1. *Head hair:* may fall out with age. **2.** *Facial hair:* grows throughout adult life.
3. *Features:* more pronounced, face longer, head (front to back) longer. **4.** *Neck:* thicker, longer, larynx one-third larger. **5.** *Shoulders:* broader, squarer. **6.** *Chest:* larger in every dimension. **7.** *Body hair:* more evident, especially on chest and arms. **8.** *Breasts:* rudimentary in size. **9.** *Muscles:* bigger, more obvious. **10.** *Arms:* longer, thicker, "carrying angle" straight. **11.** *Pubic hair:* growing up to a point, forming triangle. **12.** *Hips:* narrower. **13.** *Hands and feet:* larger, fingers and toes stronger and blunter. **14.** *Thighs:* more cylindrical with bulge of muscles. **15.** *Legs:* longer, bulging calves. **16.** *Angle of thigh and leg:* as with "carrying angle" of arm, forming straight line, thigh to ankle.

The Female: On the average, shorter and lighter than the male.
1. *Head hair:* more lasting. **2.** *Facial hair:* very faint, usually noticeable only in later years. **3.** *Features:* more delicate, face rounder, head smaller, rounder (from top). **4.** *Neck:* shorter, more rounded, larynx smaller. **5.** *Shoulders:* more rounded, sloping. **6.** *Chest:* smaller, narrower. **7.** *Body Hair:* very light and faint. **8.** *Breasts:* prominent, also well-developed nipples with large surrounding rings. **9.** *Muscles:* largely hidden under layers of fat. **10.** *Arms:* "carrying angle" bent. **11.** *Pubic hair:* forming straight line across at top. **12.** *Hips:* wider, more rounded. **13.** *Hands and feet:* smaller and narrower. **14.** *Thighs:* wider at top and shorter in length. **15.** *Legs:* shorter with smoother contours. **16.** *Angle of thigh and leg:* as with "carrying angle" of arm, slightly bent, forming an angle at the knee.

THE ROLE OF HORMONES

The proper anatomical development of males and females as well as their ability to reproduce depend on the functioning of special glands in their bodies. The scientific study of these glands and their secretions is still in progress and much remains to be learned about them.

People have, of course, long been familiar with some of the more complex glands (such as those in the mouth, skin, or female breast) which release their particular secretions (saliva, sweat, milk) onto a surface through their own ducts. Such secretions are easily detected, traced, and measured, and they serve an obvious localized function. However, the human body also possesses ductless glands which release their secretions directly into the bloodstream. These glands are called endocrine (Greek: internally secreting) glands. Their secretions, which may stimulate or regulate the functioning of various other, often remote organs, are known as hormones (from the Greek *hormaein*: to arouse). Every human body contains a number of endocrine glands and many different hormones which serve a great variety of purposes. The following paragraphs restrict themselves to a discussion of those hormones that affect a person's sexual and reproductive capacities.

In regard to sex and reproduction, the most important endocrine glands are the pituitary gland and the male and female gonads or sex glands. The pituitary gland is located at the base of the brain. It is sometimes called the "master gland" because its hormones stimulate and coordinate the other endocrine glands. Among the pituitary hormones that are of particular interest here are FSH (follicle-stimulating hormone) and LH (luteinizing hormone). They stimulate the male and female gonads to produce hormones of their own. (In males, LH is usually referred to as ICSH [interstitial-cell-stimulating hormone] because it acts upon the interstitial cells, the producers of hormone in the testicles.

The gonads or sex glands are the testicles in the male and the ovaries in the female. (See "The Male Sex Organs" and "The Female Sex Organs.") The hormones produced by the gonads are called gonadal hormones, and they can be divided into clearly distinct groups. One group of hormones that are particularly prominent in mature males are known as androgens. Another group of hormones particularly prominent in mature females are known as estrogens. (The female gonads also produce still another hormone called progesterone, which is important for a woman's reproductive life.) However, while there is a preponderance of androgens in men and of estrogens in women, both groups of hormones are present in every individual. The gonadal hormones play an important role in a person's sexual maturation. Their first decisive influence appears even before birth.

The human embryo is sexually undifferentiated during the first few weeks of its life. The primitive beginnings of its gonads are the same for both sexes. At the spot where the future external sex organs are destined to grow, there is a hump (suggestive of the male) and a groove (suggestive of the female). A clear differentiation begins only toward the end of the second month after conception. In the case of a male embryo, the production of the hormone testosterone (one of the androgens) is started, which slowly transforms the embryonic genital hump into a penis. The groove running down its underside closes, forming a single internal tube: the urethra. The gonads become identifiable as testicles, and, in the last weeks before birth, they descend into the scrotum. Without this prenatal production of testosterone in males, their proper anatomical development is impossible.

In the case of a female embryo, nothing special or additional is needed because the external and internal sex organs differentiate "automatically." (In a sense, therefore, the female sex might be called the "basic" or "primary" one.) In the absence of a specific stimulation by androgens, the originally undifferentiated gonads are transformed into ovaries. The embryonic genital hump grows into the clitoris. (Compared to the penis, the clitoris remains much smaller because of a lack of testosterone to stimulate its growth.) The genital groove, on the other hand, remains open and deepens, forming the minor lips and the vestibule of the vulva.

In the period between birth and puberty, there are no further dramatic changes in a person's sexual development. The levels of androgen and estrogen remain rather low and are nearly equal in both sexes. At about the age of eight, a gradual buildup of hormone levels begins. By about ten or eleven, this increase becomes very substantial, especially in females. The pituitary gland releases great quantities of FSH and LH (called ICSH in males) which stimulate the secretion of gonadal hormones as well as the production of sperm in the testicles and of eggs in the ovaries. In males, the androgens rise to a slightly higher level than the estrogens, and, in females, the estrogens rise to a much higher level than the androgens. As a result of this intensified hormonal bombardment, the male and female bodies develop their secondary sexual characteristics. This general physical maturation also fully develops the capacities of the nervous system, and thus creates the basis for the complete male and female sexual response.

In those rare cases where boys or girls lose or fail to develop their gonads, their overall physical development is affected. Their ability to respond sexually remains limited and, of course, the secondary sexual characteristics never become pronounced. For example, a boy whose testicles fail to descend or who is castrated before puberty retains a rather juvenile general appearance and never experiences the typically male enlargement of the larynx and the resulting voice change. In 18th-century Europe music lovers took advantage of this fact when they provided the opera stage with a very special type of human voice—that of the *castrato*. A great number of young boys with promising voices were castrated in order to preserve their tonal clarity and high pitch. At the same time they received a rigorous musical training. Eventually some of them developed into adult male sopranos or contraltos of incomparable vocal force and virtuosity who could look forward to a life of fame and fortune. The greatest composers, such as Handel, Gluck, and Mozart, wrote major parts in their operas for castrated males. Since today this type of voice is no longer available, these operas have to be rearranged for modern voices, or they are simply no longer performed.

The castration of adults does not have the same obvious result as that of children. This has long been known in many Asian and Middle Eastern countries where, in the past, adult male slaves or servants were castrated for the sake of obtaining harem guards who would be unable to impregnate their master's wives. (Actually, a sterilization would have been sufficient for this purpose.) Apart from their infertility these so-called eunuchs did not necessarily show any other physical deficiencies. The modern stereotype of the eunuch as a falsetto-voiced, bald, fat weakling is false. Again, the public of 18th-century Europe seems to have had a remarkable and very realistic appreciation of the biological facts. For example, in Mozart's popular opera, *The Abduction from the Seraglio*, the part of the harem guard is, quite appropriately, written for a deep bass voice (moreover, he is portrayed as quite lecherous). As a rule the adult human body is capable of adjusting to a lack of gonadal hormones within a few months, although in some instances there may be some premature physical deterioration over the years. In any case today the effects of castration, such as they are, can be almost completely corrected by hormonal treatment.

As mentioned earlier, the scientific study of hormones continues as many important questions about their effects are still unanswered. Nevertheless there is now some general, if vague, knowledge of these problems among the public at large. Indeed, many men and women today discuss hormonal influences as readily and casually as their diets. Unfortunately many popular notions about the role of hormones are quite mistaken, especially in regard to sex.

Part of the confusion can be explained by the history of endocrinology (the study of endocrine glands and their secretions). Among the first hormones to be discovered were those secreted by the gonads or sex glands. Since the gonads were known to produce male and female gametes or sex cells, the gonadal hormones were soon simply referred to as sex hormones, and they were also divided into male and female sex hormones. However, this all too convenient analogy is faulty. While the male sex cells (sperm) are produced only in the male (and are therefore properly named), the so-called male sex hormones (androgens) are produced in both males and females. Correspondingly, the female sex cell (egg) is produced only in females (and is therefore properly named), whereas the so-called female sex hormones (estrogens) are produced in both sexes. The distinction between "male" and "female" sex hormones is therefore misleading. In fact, it is regrettable that the gonadal hormones were ever called "sex hormones" in the first place, because this term has led to the misconception that they somehow determine sexual behavior. For example, some people believe that the sex hormones are the direct cause of sexual desire, and that an increase in these hormones will increase the desire just as effectively as their reduction will reduce it. Indeed, there is a widely held false opinion that one can prevent a man from engaging in any sexual activity at all by depriving him of his sex glands and thus his "sex hormones." In some countries sex offenders are being castrated under the assumption that this will put an end to their offensive behavior. However, modern scientific studies clearly show that, for a grown man, the removal or loss of the testicles may have little or no immediate effect on his sexual capacities. (Except, of course, that he becomes infertile. The same is true for a woman whose ovaries become inactive after menopause. Her sexual responsiveness remains undiminished.) Still, the indignity of a forced castration may cause severe psychological damage to someone who shares the common sexual superstitions. In this indirect way his sexual abilities may very well become impaired. The lack of androgens alone does not necessarily diminish sexual interest or inhibit sexual expression. It often decreases the level of sexual performance somewhat, but drastic changes may not become obvious until many years later.

Among the general public it is still not always understood that, in human beings, the ability to reproduce and the ability to respond sexually are two different matters. While the sex glands are indispensable for a young person's physical maturation and human reproduction, they are not essential for the sexual responsiveness of adults. In other words, there can be no reproduction without sex cells (sperm and egg), but there can very well be sexual activity without "sex hormones" (androgens and estrogens).

Reference and Recommended Reading

Money, John, and Ehrhardt, Anke A. *Man & Woman, Boy & Girl: Differentiation & Dimorphism of Gender Identity.* Baltimore and London: Johns Hopkins University Press, 1973 (cloth); 1976 (paper).

Money, John, and Tucker, Patricia. *Sexual Signatures: On Being a Man or a Woman.* Boston: Little, Brown & Company, 1975 (cloth); 1976 (paper).

Sex Information and Education Council of the U.S. (SIECUS), *Sexuality and Man*, New York: Charles Scribner's Sons, 1970.

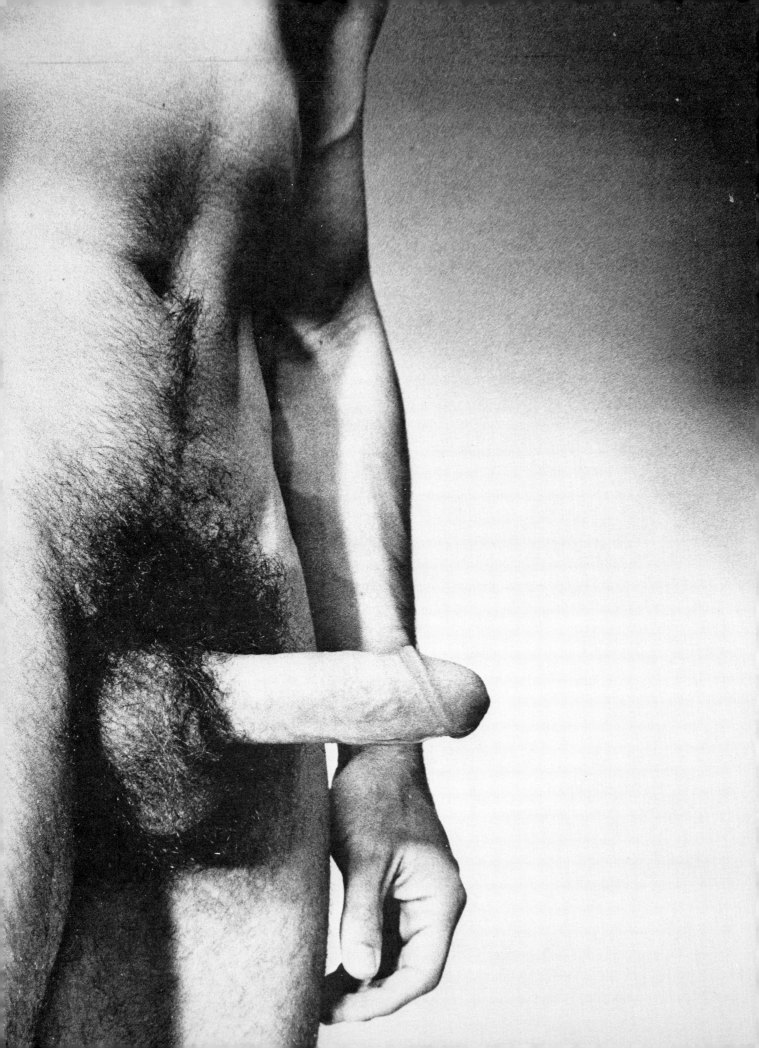

Many young people today also find little need for prudery. As a rule they are neither awed nor disgusted by any part of the human anatomy. Instead they are simply curious. For them sex is just another part of life with which they have to become familiar. Particularly during puberty, when they observe their own sexual maturation, they often feel alienated from their bodies. They demand objective information as a means to get back in touch with themselves. As such information becomes generally available in the future, the sex organs are likely to lose much of their former mystery and fascination. On the other hand, a realistic understanding of their own sexual anatomy may very well help many people to lead healthier and more productive lives.

The following pages present a detailed description of the male sex organs beginning with those that are visible outside the body. In a young person these external sex organs usually create the greatest initial interest. However, in order to understand their function, one also has to consider the internal sex organs of which many people never become aware at all.

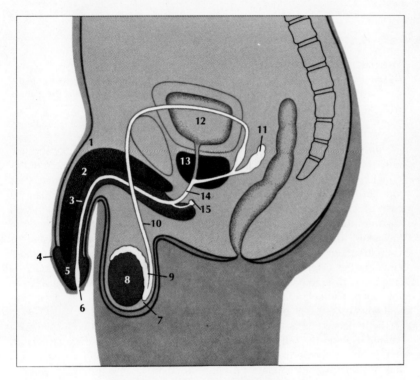

THE MALE SEX ORGANS

1. *Penis*
2. *Corpus cavernosum (one of a pair)*
3. *Corpus spongiosum*
4. *Foreskin*
5. *Glans*
6. *Opening of urethra*
7. *Scrotum*
8. *Testicle (one of a pair)*
9. *Epididymis (one of a pair)*
10. *Vas deferens (one of a pair)*
11. *Seminal vesicle (one of a pair)*
12. *Urinary bladder*
13. *Prostate gland*
14. *Urethra*
15. *Bulbourethral (Cowper's) gland (one of a pair)*

The male external sex organs consist of the penis and the scrotum. The testicles and their attachments, which are contained in the scrotum, are usually considered internal organs, although they are outside the abdominal cavity.

THE EXTERNAL SEX ORGANS

The Penis

The penis (Latin: tail) is a cylindrical organ which contains erectile tissue. To be more precise, there are three elongated spongy bodies inside the penis which extend through its entire length—two running parallel on top (the two *corpora cavernosa*) and one running along the underside (the *corpus spongiosum*). This latter body contains the urethra (the duct through which urine and semen are released). Heavy arteries can quickly fill these spongy bodies with blood, thus causing them to stiffen. As a result, the penis becomes erect. Conversely, when the blood leaves the spongy tissue the erection subsides. Erections of the penis are usually triggered by sexual excitement, but they can also occur for other reasons. (For details, see "The Male Sexual Response.")

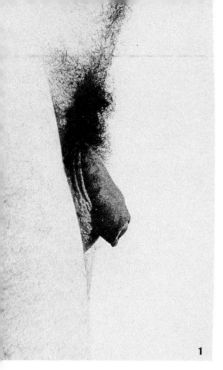
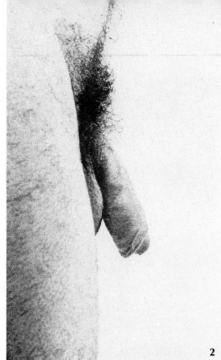
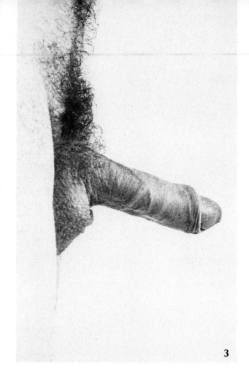

1 2 3

THE UNCIRCUMCIZED PENIS
(1) Foreskin covering the glans of the unexcited penis. (2) With a beginning erection, the glans begins to protrude from the foreskin. (3) With the erection complete, the glans is fully exposed.

During an erection the penis increases in size. This is possible because the skin covering it is very loose. In fact, toward the end of the penis some of this skin forms a freely hanging fold known as the foreskin or prepuce. This foreskin normally covers the tip or head of the penis called the glans. In the case of an erection, however, the glans protrudes from the foreskin and becomes fully exposed. The glans is usually slightly thicker than the body of the penis, and its shape has been compared to that of an acorn. (Glans is Latin for acorn.) Actually it is the extension of the *corpus spongiosum,* and it contains the external opening of the urethra. Since its smooth surface is studded with innumerable nerve endings, the glans is extremely sensitive to the touch, particularly around its rim. By the same token it.is also an important source of sexual pleasure for the male.

The underside of the glans is attached to the foreskin by a thin tissue called frenum. Behind the rim of the glans and under the foreskin there are glands that secrete a cheese-like substance known as smegma. If the foreskin is tight this smegma may accumulate and cause irritation. In any case, good personal hygiene demands daily washing of the glans and removal of the smegma. For this the foreskin has to be pulled back.

Tightness of foreskin (also called phimosis) is one of the reasons for a popular operation called circumcision. It consists of the surgical removal of the foreskin. This practice has a long tradition among Jews and Moslems, for whom it also has a religious significance. However, in the meantime circumcision has found wide general acceptance, and in the United States today most males are circumcised as a matter of course right after birth regardless of their religion. Circumcision has no effect on a man's sexual abilities.

The average length of a grown man's penis is between 3 and 4 inches when flaccid and between 5 and 7 inches when erect. However, there may be great variations in size from one individual to the next. Contrary to some widely accepted myths, the size of the penis is not related to a man's body build, skin color, or sexual prowess. A very short man may have a larger penis than a tall one (and vice versa), a white man may have a larger penis than a black man (and vice versa), and a man with a small penis may have more orgasms than a man with a large penis (and vice versa). Furthermore, some penises which greatly differ in size when they are flaccid may be of identical size when they are erect.

For reasons that are not entirely clear, many men in our culture seem concerned about the size of their penises. However, such concern is completely unwarranted. Even a penis that remains relatively small during an erection serves every function of a larger penis. A woman's vagina, for instance, adjusts to any penis, no matter what its size, and since the vaginal walls contain few nerve endings, any difference in the woman's sensations depends on the firmness of her muscles surrounding the vaginal barrel as well as psychological factors. (For details, see "The Female Sexual Response.") The latter is also true for sensations inside the rectum during anal intercourse. There is practically no feeling at all beyond the anal sphincter muscles. (This, incidentally, is the reason why some people who introduce long and hard objects into their rectum may seriously hurt themselves without realizing it.)

The Scrotum

The scrotum is a bag or pouch of skin which contains the testicles, and which hangs between the thighs at the base of the penis. The skin of the scrotum is comparatively dark and contains many sweat glands. Inside the scrotum there are two separate compartments, each of which contains one testicle and its spermatic cord which leads upward into the abdominal cavity. Part of this spermatic cord is a thin tube through which the sperm travels—the *vas deferens*. It is this *vas deferens* that is cut in a vasectomy. (For details, see "Contraception.") The spermatic cord also contains blood vessels, nerves, and muscles. In response to certain stimuli, especially cold temperatures, these muscles contract and pull the testicle closer to the abdomen. At the same time, the skin of the scrotum will also contract and appear thick and wrinkled. Ordinarily, however, the scrotum hangs loose, and its skin looks thin and smooth. In a way the scrotum acts like a thermostat, trying to provide an even temperature for the continuous production of sperm which is taking place inside the testicles. This temperature has to be slightly lower than that of the rest of the body.

The male internal sex organs consist of the testicles which produce hormones and sperm, a system of ducts which transport and store the sperm, and some accessory organs whose secretions become part of the ejaculated semen.

THE INTERNAL SEX ORGANS

The Testicles

The testicles (the male sex glands or gonads) are formed within the abdomen during the development of the embryo. However, before the birth of a baby boy they normally descend into his scrotum. In the mature male the testicles are two oval-shaped bodies of about 1½ inches in length which are suspended in two separate sacs inside the scrotum outside the abdominal cavity. Although both testicles are of about the same size, the left one usually hangs a little lower and thus may give the appearance of being larger.

The testicles serve a double function:

- They produce sperm which may be ejaculated through a system of genital ducts.
- They produce hormones which are secreted directly into the bloodstream.

The Production of Sperm

A testicle is composed of hundreds of small compartments which contain tightly coiled tubes not much thicker than a hair. Inside these tubes (called seminiferous tubules) the process of sperm production (called spermatogenesis) takes place. This process begins when the male reaches puberty and continues without interruption throughout his life. The production of sperm proceeds in three steps:

1. The first step begins with the cells that lie closest to the outer edge of the tube. These cells are called primitive spermatogonia and, like any other

cell in the body, they have 46 chromosomes, including an X chromosome and a Y chromosome. By means of cell division a single primitive spermatogonium forms two new identical daughter cells. One of these takes the place of the original cell, while the other moves toward the center of the tube. This latter cell is called the primary spermatocyte.

2. The primary spermatocyte does not duplicate itself the way all other cells do, but divides in a unique way: It splits in half, as it were, allotting 22 chromosomes plus 1 X chromosome to one of the new cells, and 22 chromosomes plus 1 Y chromosome to the other. The two new cells are called secondary spermatocytes, and each of them contains only half as many chromosomes (23) as all other body cells.

3. The two secondary spermatocytes move even closer to the center of the tube, and each divides again in the ordinary fashion, duplicating itself exactly. The four new cells are called spermatids. These spermatids now change their shape, develop a tail, and thus grow into mature sperm cells called spermatozoa. The entire process through all three stages of development takes about 64 days. As is obvious from their origin and development, spermatozoa come in two varieties: those containing an X chromosome (and 22 other chromosomes), and those containing a Y chromosome (and 22 other chromosomes). In case of a fertilization the X-bearing spermatozoa will help to produce girls; the Y-bearing spermatozoa will help to produce boys. (For details, see "Conception.")

The Production of Hormones

As described in a previous section, the male and female gonads (testicles and ovaries) also produce certain hormones. These gonadal hormones have been divided into male hormones (androgens) and female hormones (estrogens). However, these terms are somewhat misleading because both "male" and "female" hormones can be found in every male and female body. It is only the quantity of these hormones that differs. Before puberty, the androgen and estrogen levels in boys and girls are nearly equal. Then, during adolescence, the balance begins to shift. In the male body the androgens rise to a slightly higher level than the estrogens, and in the female body the estrogens rise to a much higher level than the androgens.

In the male the increase of androgens during puberty helps to produce the secondary male sexual characteristics. In the female the increase of estrogens helps to produce the secondary female sexual characteristics. There is still much to be learned about the role of hormones in the human body. Nevertheless, a few basic facts have already been established:

While the gonadal hormones are necessary for a young person's physical maturation, they are not essential for the continued sexual activity of adults. In other words, males and females need the gonadal hormones during adolescence to develop their full sexual potential. However, once the potential has been attained they can function sexually without these hormones. This has long been recognized in the case of women whose gonads (the ovaries) cease functioning after menopause without diminishing their sexual responsiveness. Many people are less willing to concede that the same is also true for men who might be deprived of their gonadal hormones (by castration, for example). Indeed, in many countries adult males are still being castrated in the belief that this will eliminate their sexual capacities. However, this belief is erroneous. (For details, see "The Role of Hormones.")

THE SYSTEM OF GENITAL DUCTS

The sperm cells produced in the testicles are transported to their point of discharge from the body by a system of genital ducts. These ducts, which consist of matched pairs (in sequence: epididymides, vasa deferentia, ejaculatory ducts), lead from the testicles into the abdominal cavity where they eventually join the urethra, a single tube which discharges sperm as well as urine.

The Epididymides

The sperm cells which are constantly being produced in the seminiferous tubules are moved into collection tubes which lie on the surface of each testicle. Such a collection tube is called epididymis (plural: epididymides), and it is about 20 feet long. However, it is so twisted and convoluted that it seems no longer than the testicle itself. A sperm cell needs several weeks to traverse the collection tube. During this time it develops a limited ability to move by itself.

The Vasa Deferentia

Once the sperm cells have emerged from the collection tube, they enter a shorter and rather straight tube called vas deferens (plural: vasa deferentia). This tube leads from the scrotum into the abdomen. The lower portion of the vas deferens can be felt through the scrotal skin. Since it is so easily located, it can also easily be cut in a sterilization operation known as a vasectomy. (For details, see "Contraception.")

Inside the abdomen the two vasa deferentia (one associated with each testicle) bend in a long curve and lead up to a point behind the urinary bladder where they become enlarged, each forming a sort of sac or storage compartment called ampulla (plural: ampullae). The sperm cells are moved to these storage compartments to await ejaculation. The ampullae join the ducts of two other sac-like organs, the seminal vesicles, to form short and straight tubes called ejaculatory ducts. These ejaculatory ducts run inside the prostate gland and there join the urethra. (For details, see below.) Before entering the ejaculatory ducts, the sperm cells have only a limited capacity of moving by themselves. Instead, they are transported mainly by the movement of tiny hair-like structures inside the tubes and by muscular contractions. However, immediately upon ejaculation they begin to move very vigorously. This dramatic change is produced by several fluids from various sources which together make up the semen. Swimming in the semen, the sperm cells gain their full energy.

The Urethra

The urethra is a single tube which leads from the bladder to the tip of the penis. (The urethra should not be confused with the two ureters which lead from the kidneys to the bladder.) In the male, the urethra serves two important functions: to release either urine or semen. (Because of certain muscles, urine and semen cannot be released together.) While the urine enters the urethra directly from the bladder, the semen is composed of several different fluids which enter through special openings in the urethral wall mainly in the region of the prostate gland.

ACCESSORY ORGANS

In order to survive after their ejaculation, the sperm cells need to swim in a thick, nourishing, protective fluid called semen. Actually, the semen is composed of several different fluids which come together at various points in the urethra. The most important of these fluids are produced by the organs described below.

The Seminal Vesicles

The seminal vesicles are two sacs which lie next to the ampullae (the enlarged endings of the vasa deferentia) behind the bladder and near the top of the prostate gland. It was formerly believed that the seminal vesicles just served as storage space for accumulated sperm. However, today the opinion prevails that their main function is to provide a fluid which, together with that of the prostate gland, activates the vigorous movement of the sperm cells after ejaculation.

The Prostate Gland

The prostate gland is a firm, round body about the size of a chestnut, and it lies directly below the bladder. It is traversed by the urethra as well as the two ejaculatory ducts described earlier. The prostate constantly produces secretions. Some of these are passed off with the urine. Others make up the greater portion of the semen.

In some older men, the prostate gland enlarges, causing pressure on the enclosed part of the urethra and thus making urination difficult. In these cases, the removal of the prostate by surgery may become necessary.

The Bulbourethral Glands (Cowper's Glands)

Below the prostate gland, there are two small glands about pea size which during sexual excitement secrete a clear, alkaline fluid into the urethra. Often a small drop of this fluid can be seen at the opening of the penis well in advance of an actual ejaculation. It is not entirely impossible for the drop to contain some stray sperm cells. (This could account for the rare cases of pregnancy without ejaculation of semen.)

The semen discharged in an ejaculation (usually somewhat less than a teaspoonful) is composed of sperm cells and secretions from the epididymides, the seminal vesicles, the prostate gland, and the bulbourethral (Cowper's) glands. None of these fluids contains any harmful substances. People who swallow semen, whether by accident or on purpose, have no reason to fear any ill effects. Semen is usually thick and greyish-white in color. However, at times it may also be thin and rather watery. The exact amount, consistency, and composition of semen depends on the frequency of ejaculations.

THE MALE SEXUAL RESPONSE

Every healthy person is able to respond to sexual stimulation. While this response is never exactly the same in any two individuals, its basic physiological pattern is shared by all men and women.

Sexual activity produces many changes in the human body, such as an increase in pulse rate and blood pressure, the swelling of certain organs, muscular contractions, glandular secretions, and many other signs of mounting excitement until, eventually, the tension is released in a pleasurable, seizure-like reaction known as orgasm.

People have, of course, always been aware of these bodily changes. However, until rather recently their true nature and extent remained largely unknown. There simply were no objective scientific studies on the subject. Indeed, the very idea of observing and measuring sexual responses was considered preposterous. In the meantime, the situation has changed drastically. The pioneering work of scientists like Kinsey and his associates of the Institute for Sex Research in Bloomington, Indiana, and Masters and Johnson of the Reproductive Biology Research Foundation in St. Louis, Missouri, has provided us with fresh insights and exposed many traditional beliefs and assumptions as false. Today, there are many researchers all over the world who continue to add to our understanding of the human sexual response.

Human beings can be sexually aroused at nearly all times, in many different ways, and by a great variety of objects. For example, a man's excitement may be triggered at any hour of the day or night, by the sight or touch of certain persons or things, by certain smells or sounds, or simply by some thoughts, recollections, or fantasies. Since the possible sources of sexual stimulation are so numerous and varied, they are not easily listed or classified, and no such attempt is made in the present book. Nevertheless, it may be useful to cast at least a cursory glance at some of the more obvious stimuli that can produce sexual responses.

Of all the human senses, the sense of touch seems to be the one most often responsible for erotic arousal. A person becomes aware of being touched through nerve endings in the skin and some deeper tissues. Since some areas of the body surface contain many more of these nerve endings than others, they are also more sensitive to the touch and, as a result, they may be especially receptive to sexual stimulation. These particular regions have, therefore, also often been called erogenous zones (literally, love-producing zones, from the Greek *eros*: love and *genesthai*: to produce).

The best known erogenous zones are the glans of the penis in men and the clitoris and the minor lips in women, the area between the sex organs and the anus, the anus itself, the buttocks, the inner surfaces of the thighs, the breasts (especially the nipples), the neck, the mouth, and the ears. Touching, stroking, tickling, rubbing, slapping, kissing, or licking these areas can often create or increase sexual excitement. However, this response is by no means automatic. A great deal depends on a person's previous conditioning and on the circumstances under which the stimulation occurs. For instance, when a doctor touches a patient's erogenous zones in the course of a physical examination, there may be no sexual response at all. Neither is such a response likely in cases of rape. In short, psychological factors usually play a decisive role in tactile stimulation. (There are some exceptions to this rule, as in certain cases the body may produce a reflexive reaction to touch. For example, a man who suffers from a certain type of spinal cord injury can have an erection when his penis is fondled, although the stimulation may not register in his brain.)

Because of their different experiences, different individuals are likely to develop different degrees of sensitivity. Negative mental associations can prevent any sexual response to touch. In fact, there are people who want to be touched as little as possible even during sexual intercourse. On the other hand, pleasurable sexual encounters can develop a welcome sensitivity almost anywhere in the body and thus lead to the discovery of new erogenous zones. In the final analysis, people have to find out for themselves which parts of their own (or their partner's) bodies most readily respond to caresses.

Most people are well aware of the fact that they can become sexually aroused not only by persons or things they touch, but also by what they may see, hear, smell, or taste. The sight of a beautiful body, the sound of a musical voice, the smell of a perfume, the taste of certain foods or of a lover's glandular secretions can be powerful stimulants. However, their effect depends entirely on mental associations. A particular individual becomes excited by a particular sight, sound, smell or taste because he associates it in his mind with a previous pleasant sexual experience. (Unpleasant associations, on the other hand, produce a negative reaction. They can reduce or extinguish sexual excitement.)

It follows from these observations that there are no erotic sights, sounds, or smells as such. They only become so through certain erotic experiences. It is not surprising, therefore, that different times and cultures have felt attracted to very different ideals of beauty, or that a certain piece of music may appear stimulating to some but not to others. (Also see "The Development of Sexual Behavior.")

Human beings in general depend very much on psychological factors in their sexual responses, and many people become aroused by mental images alone. Indeed, there are some individuals who are able to reach orgasm simply by fantasizing about sexual matters. It seems, however, that erotic thoughts, fantasies, and anticipations have a more certain effect on males than on females. During sexual intercourse, most women reach orgasm only as a result of continuing physical stimulation. (See "The Female Sexual Response.")

It should perhaps also be mentioned that certain seemingly sexual responses can occur for entirely nonsexual reasons. For example, many men know that they may have erections when lifting heavy weights or when a full urinary bladder causes some physical irritation. There is also a rare pathological condition called priapism in which a man is unable to lose his erection. This disease can be quite painful and may, eventually, do serious damage to the penis.

Once a man has become fully aroused, he tends to seek release through some kind of sexual activity. The type of activity he chooses depends, of course, on the circumstances. However, no matter what his choice, the reactions of his body always follow the same pattern. In other words, from a physiological point of view it makes no difference whether the sexual response is brought about by solitary masturbation or any conceivable form of sexual intercourse. (See "Types of Sexual Activity.") Psychologically, the experience may very well feel quite different, but the basic bodily reactions remain unchanged.

One has to remember, however, that even the physiological reactions are never exactly identical in any two persons or even in the same person on different occasions. People are not machines built on the same assembly line. Any general description of the human sexual response can be only just that—general. The specific responses of a particular individual are bound to show some individual variation. (For example, it is very well possible for some men to experience orgasm and to ejaculate with a limp penis.) The following summary should, therefore, not be considered a norm or an ideal of physical performance toward which everybody must strive. Its only purpose is to shed some light on a previously mysterious subject and to provide men and women with some elementary knowledge of certain bodily functions.

THE FOUR PHASES OF HUMAN SEXUAL RESPONSE

As described in a previous section, the anatomical difference between men and women is not very great. It is not surprising, therefore, that their sexual responses are also quite similar. There are some marked differences, but they are not decisive. In fact, one may very well speak of a basic human sexual response and its male and female variations.

During sexual activity, the human body undergoes a number of physiological changes which form a definite, typical pattern. In the simplest terms, this pattern can be described as a build up and release of tension. However, in an attempt to gain a greater understanding of the processes involved, various scientists have divided the sexual response into not only two but three or four different phases. One has to keep in mind, of course, that every individual human sexual experience is a continuous whole, and that all divisions into stages and phases are always artificial and somewhat arbitrary. Nevertheless, they can help us recognize and understand the many ways in which our bodies respond to sexual stimulation. The following description of the male sexual response is based on the four-phase division proposed by Masters and Johnson. Although there may very well be room for finer distinctions and a more sophisticated terminology in the future, the Masters and Johnson model is quite adequate for our present purposes. (For the application of this model to females, see "The Female Sexual Response.")

1. Excitement

Sexual excitement may mount rather unexpectedly and quickly, particularly in younger men, but it may also build up gradually over a longer period of time. In fact, some individuals deliberately distract themselves repeatedly, in order to prolong and savor their experience of becoming aroused. Especially in its early stages, sexual excitement can easily be reduced by some outside interference or by sudden anxieties or apprehensions. However, with increasing tension such negative influences become less and less effective. The ability for self-control is impaired, and the usual inhibitions are swept away.

The most obvious sign of sexual excitement in the male is the erection of his penis. The three spongy bodies inside of it (the two *corpora cavernosa* and the *corpus spongiosum*) become filled with blood and thus cause the penis to rise and stiffen. At the same time, the smooth muscles of the scrotum contract, its tissue thickens, and the testicles are pulled upward toward the abdomen by the contracting spermatic cords.

As sexual excitement increases, there is a corresponding increase in muscular tension. At the same time, the pulse rate and blood pressure rise. In addition to these symptoms, a number of men also experience what is known as a sex flush, i.e., a red rash that usually begins in the area of the lower abdomen and then spreads to the neck and face or even to the shoulders, arms, and thighs. The sex flush may start only late in the excitement phase and is more likely to appear in the plateau phase. In many cases, however, there is no sex flush at all.

This basic observation also applies to another possible phenomenon: the erection of the nipples. Not all males experience it. In some men, it may be brought about by a direct stimulation of the breasts. When nipple erection occurs, it usually appears toward the end of the excitement phase or during the plateau phase and then lasts through the other phases.

One other fact should be mentioned here: Sometimes a man may fail to achieve or maintain an erection of the penis, although he feels excited and is eager to have sexual intercourse. Obviously, in this case he is also unable to proceed to the other phases of sexual response. Such an occasional lack of erection may have many causes, but can usually be traced to particular circumstances in a specific situation. Both sexual partners should accept the incident with equanimity and perhaps turn to forms of lovemaking that do not require an erect penis. There is no cause for concern. However, if the same problem should occur frequently or even regularly, professional help may be advisable. (See "Sexual Inadequacy.")

2. Plateau

The plateau phase is actually nothing more than the continuation of the excitement phase. The word "plateau" is meant to indicate that a certain even level of excitement has been reached which is then maintained for a while before orgasm occurs. Once sexual excitement has reached this stage, the individual is no longer easily diverted, but becomes gradually oblivious to his surroundings. With increasing sexual stimulation, the entire body experiences an increase in muscular tension, both voluntary and involuntary. At the same time, the pulse rate and blood pressure continue to rise, and breathing becomes faster.

During the plateau phase, the now erect penis does not undergo any new major changes. However, the testicles swell noticeably and are pulled close to the abdomen. The bulbourethral (Cowper's) glands secrete a few drops of a clear liquid which may appear at the tip of the penis. (Such a drop may contain some stray sperm cells. This fact should be remembered by couples who want to avoid pregnancy. Also see "Contraception—Withdrawal.")

The sex flush mentioned earlier may now appear for the first time or, if it had been visible before, grow more obvious. Again, it should be remembered that not all men show a sex flush, and that some show it only occasionally. The same is true for the erection of the nipples. However, if the nipples should become erect during the plateau phase, they will remain so through the other phases.

3. Orgasm

Orgasm (Greek *orgasmos*: lustful excitement) is the sudden release of muscular and nervous tension at the climax of sexual excitement. The experience represents the most intense physical pleasure of which human beings are capable and is basically the same for males and females. An orgasm lasts only a few seconds and is felt very much like a short seizure or rather a quick succession of convulsions which involve the whole body and soon lead to complete relaxation. In sexually mature males, orgasm is accompanied by the ejaculation (Latin: throwing out) of semen. Since women do not produce semen, they do not ejaculate. However, in all other respects the physiological processes are comparable to those in males.

In males, orgasm begins with involuntary rhythmic contractions of the genital ducts and accessory organs (vasa deferentia, seminal vesicles, prostate gland), the urethra, the muscles at the base of the penis and finally the penis itself. The first three or four forceful contractions recur within less than a second, then, as they become weaker, at longer intervals. As a result of these contractions, the accumulated semen is forced through the urethra to the outside where it emerges in several quick spurts. At times, it may be projected a considerable distance; at other times, it may flow out rather gently. The force of a particular ejaculation is not related to a man's strength or virility. The amount of semen ejaculated during one orgasm is usually about a teaspoonful. Repeated ejaculations within a short time produce less and less semen.

The contractions in the sex organs and the subsequent ejaculation of semen produce the most obvious signs of orgasm. However, it is important to remember that the whole body is involved. For example, the anal sphincter muscles contract at the same intervals as the sex organs mentioned above. In fact, there is great muscular tension throughout the body, breathing becomes very fast, and the pulse rate and blood pressure rise even higher than during the plateau phase. It is the sudden, convulsive release from this overall tension that constitutes orgasm. The ejaculation of semen is only incidental to this release.

Orgasm and ejaculation are two different processes. While it is true that, in men, there can be no ejaculation without orgasm, there can very well be orgasm without ejaculation. The most obvious example is the orgasm of boys before puberty. Since their internal sex organs are not yet sufficiently developed to produce semen, there is nothing that could be ejaculated. Nevertheless, these boys can have orgasms.

There are also some adult men in whom ejaculation does not occur until a few seconds after orgasm, and for whom both experiences thus remain completely separated. Certain other men who are capable of several orgasms within a short time may, for a while, exhaust their supply of semen and thus stop ejaculating as they continue to have orgasms. It should be noted, however, that only very few men are capable of multiple orgasms, and usually only while they are young. Multiple orgasms are far more common among women.

Some men claim to experience orgasm without ejaculation while practicing a technique of sexual intercourse known as "karezza" or coitus reservatus. A man who uses karezza tries not to move his erect penis very much once it has entered the vagina. This procedure aims at a spiritual union of the sexual partners who are said to reach thereby a prolonged state of bliss with repeated orgasms. However, it rather seems that at least the men remain in the plateau phase which gives them adequate satisfaction. Their "orgasms," which they may very well experience as special climaxes of intercourse, are not identical with the physiological process discussed here.

A special case is presented by a phenomenon known as retrograde ejaculation. In a few men, certain internal muscles operate in such a way that the semen is not ejaculated to the outside, but instead into the bladder from where it then later is passed off with the urine. From all external evidence these men do not seem to ejaculate at all. There are some men who claim to be able to achieve this particular muscular reaction voluntarily and use it as a means of contraception.

4. Resolution

After orgasm the sex organs (and with them the whole body) need a relatively short time to return to their former, unexcited state. The length of this so-called resolution phase is directly proportionate to that of the excitement phase. The most visible physiological change during this period is the loss of erection which proceeds in two stages. The major loss occurs immediately after ejaculation. However, the penis still retains some firmness which may persist for some time, especially if the excitement and plateau phases were extended. On the other hand, nonsexual activities or distractions can complete the loss of erection rather rapidly.

The sex flush mentioned earlier also disappears quickly. In contrast, the erection of the nipples, if indeed it should have occurred, remains visible for some time. The muscular tension in the body subsides. Breathing, pulse rate, and blood pressure revert to normal. Some men perspire immediately after ejaculation, although even then this reaction usually remains restricted to the palms of their hands and the soles of their feet.

Finally, it should be noted here that immediately following orgasm males experience a so-called refractory period. During this period, which extends well into the resolution phase, the individual cannot respond to any additional or new sexual stimulation, i.e., he is incapable of having another erection and another orgasm. The refractory period may be very short in some individuals, especially while they are young, but it usually becomes longer with advancing age. There may also be such a refractory period in females, although many women can experience several orgasms in rapid succession.

THE SEXUAL RESPONSE IN OLDER MEN

There are many people in our society who consider sexual activity a privilege of the young. Indeed, some of them cannot even conceive of older persons as sexual beings. However, such narrow-minded attitudes are in conflict with the biological facts.

Neither men nor women have to forego satisfying sexual relationships because of advancing age. The sexual reponse described above remains essentially the same. Obviously, older people lose some of their former physical strength, and many of their reactions become slower. For example, a man of sixty cannot run as far and as fast as he could in his twenties. This does not mean, however, that he cannot run at all. Indeed, if he has been practicing regularly he may very well be able to jog along better than certain younger men who lack such practice. The same is true for sexual activity. Men who have been sexually active all their lives can expect to continue sexual intercourse well into old age. Still, they as well as their partners should remember that, within the framework of the basic sexual response, certain minor changes have to be expected.

The most noticeable change concerns the excitement phase. Older men usually need a longer time to achieve an erection. Furthermore, the erection may no longer be as complete as before. However, there is no reason why this should, in any way, diminish the enjoyment of sexual intercourse. In fact, during the ensuing plateau phase an older man has a definite advantage over a younger man because he now can maintain his erection much longer. In later years, the urge to ejaculate becomes less pressing. As a result, older men gain greater control over the timing of their orgasms, and thus have a better chance of truly satisfying their partners.

Further differences in the sexual responses of older and younger men are the natural result of declining physical vigor. They do not have to affect the degree of sexual satisfaction. For example, just as the physiological responses during the other phases are no longer as pronounced as before, orgasm becomes less explosive and forceful. Ejaculations are somewhat weaker, and the subsequent loss of erection is immediate. In addition, the refractory period becomes rather extended, i.e., an older man needs a much longer time before he can again respond to sexual stimulation.

Reference and Recommended Reading

Brecher, Ruth and Edward, eds. *Analysis of Human Sexual Response.* New York: New American Library, 1974.
The Diagram Group. *Man's Body: An Owner's Manual.* New York: Paddington Press —Two Continents Publishing Group, 1976.
Lehrman, Nat. *Masters and Johnson Explained.* Chicago: Playboy Press, 1971 (cloth); 1976 (paper).

THE SEXUAL RESPONSE IN MALES

In modern times, the sexual response cycle was first analyzed and described as the "orgasmic formula" by Wilhelm Reich, who also proposed its division into four major phases: 1. mechanical tension, 2. bio-electric charge, 3. bio-electric discharge, and 4. mechanical relaxation. (W. Reich, *The Function of the Orgasm* [1927] 1942)

More recently, Masters and Johnson have relabeled these phases as 1. excitement, 2. plateau, 3. orgasm, and 4. resolution. In addition, they have introduced the concept of a fifth phase, the refractory period.

Shown here is the sexual response in the male sex organs as described by Masters and Johnson. It must be remembered, however, that the response actually involves the whole body. (For details see preceding text.)

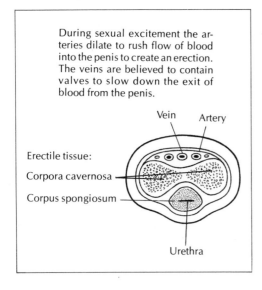

During sexual excitement the arteries dilate to rush flow of blood into the penis to create an erection. The veins are believed to contain valves to slow down the exit of blood from the penis.

Vein   Artery

Erectile tissue:

Corpora cavernosa

Corpus spongiosum

Urethra

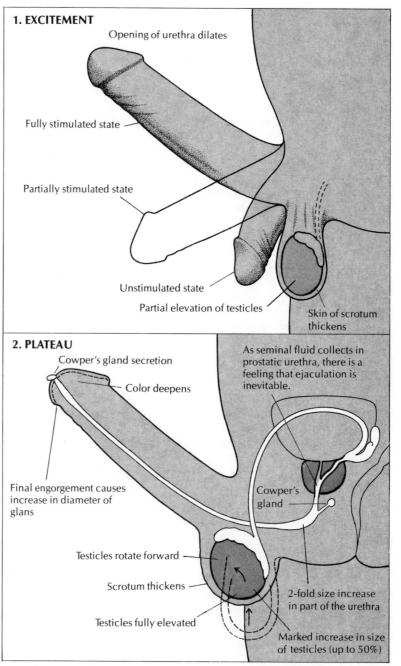

1. EXCITEMENT

Opening of urethra dilates

Fully stimulated state

Partially stimulated state

Unstimulated state

Partial elevation of testicles

Skin of scrotum thickens

2. PLATEAU

Cowper's gland secretion

Color deepens

As seminal fluid collects in prostatic urethra, there is a feeling that ejaculation is inevitable.

Final engorgement causes increase in diameter of glans

Cowper's gland

Testicles rotate forward

Scrotum thickens

Testicles fully elevated

2-fold size increase in part of the urethra

Marked increase in size of testicles (up to 50%)

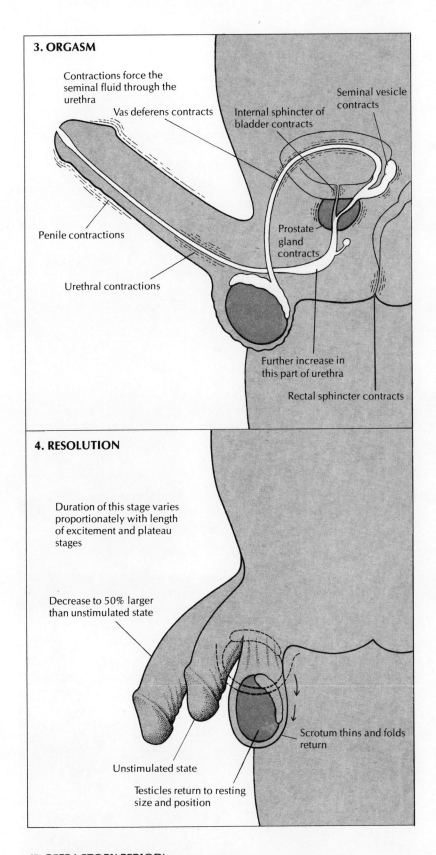

3. ORGASM

Contractions force the seminal fluid through the urethra

Vas deferens contracts

Internal sphincter of bladder contracts

Seminal vesicle contracts

Penile contractions

Prostate gland contracts

Urethral contractions

Further increase in this part of urethra

Rectal sphincter contracts

4. RESOLUTION

Duration of this stage varies proportionately with length of excitement and plateau stages

Decrease to 50% larger than unstimulated state

Unstimulated state

Scrotum thins and folds return

Testicles return to resting size and position

(5. REFRACTORY PERIOD)

After orgasm, there is a period in which males do not respond to new sexual stimulation. This so-called refractory period may be rather short in young males, but usually becomes longer with advancing age.

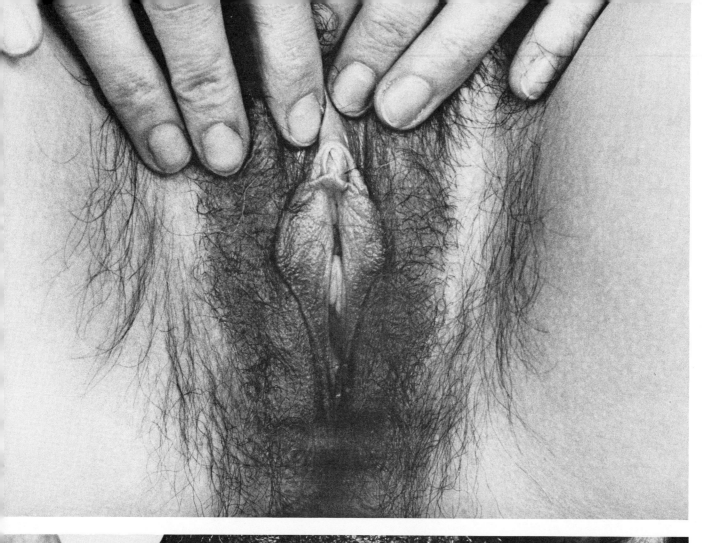
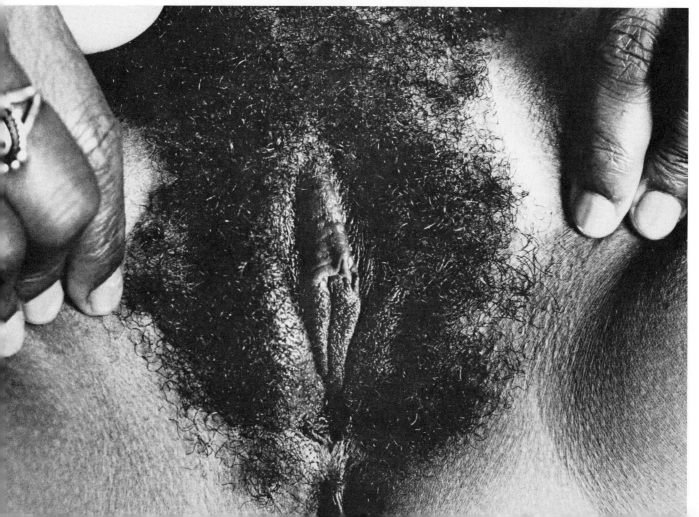

3. THE FEMALE BODY

Females and males are said to have reached sexual maturity when they are able to have children of their own. Since the two sexes play different roles in the creation of new life, the female and male bodies show several obvious differences. An understanding of these differences (as well as the similarities) can help women and men to make each other happy as lovers and to recognize their specific responsibilities as potential parents. It seems useful, therefore, to consider the sexual anatomy and physiology of females and males in two separate sections. The following pages provide a discussion of those aspects of the female body that are relevant to sexual activity and procreation.

THE FEMALE SEX ORGANS

The female and male sex organs have fascinated mankind since time immemorial. However, this fascination expressed itself differently in different historical periods and geographical areas. (For details, see "The Male Sex Organs.") In our culture, most people seem to have mixed feelings about the sexual aspect of their bodies. This is clearly reflected in our language. For example, an expression often used for sex organs is "private parts." This term suggests that certain parts of the anatomy should be considered more personal than others and should therefore not be discussed openly. The same secretive attitude, coupled with a special disdain for women, has produced another word which is normally used only in reference to female sex organs —*pudenda* (Latin: parts of which one should be ashamed). Curiously enough, this priggish term was once very popular with medical authorities.

The language of modern medicine is not entirely adequate either. Terms like "genitals" (Latin *genitalia*: organs of generation) or "reproductive system" do not provide a complete characterization of human sex organs. It is true that some of them (such as the Fallopian tubes in the female) seem to serve only the purpose of reproduction. However, others (like the clitoris) function mainly as organs of sexual pleasure. As a matter of fact, certain societies of the past which took a dim view of such pleasure routinely mutilated their women by clitoridectomies (surgical removal of clitoris). Obviously, such an operation, while nearly destroying a woman's capacity for sexual enjoyment, did not affect her ability to reproduce.

(Top) External sex organs of white woman. (Bottom) external sex organs of black woman

Unfortunately, the expression "sex organs" used in this book is also far from satisfactory. On the one hand, the term simply refers to those organs that differentiate the sexes. On the other hand, however, it also suggests that they are involved in a person's sexual response. Indeed, some people take the term "sex organs" to mean that these are the only organs so involved. However, this interpretation is false. The human sexual response is not restricted to a few particular organs, but is a response of the whole body. This means that the mouth, the skin, and the breasts, for example, are also "sex" organs, since they receive and transmit sexual stimulation. As long as this fact is kept well in mind, the use of the term "sex organs" in the present narrow sense seems defensible.

An objective study of the female sex organs has always been difficult, and thus for a very long time their function was less well understood than that of the male sex organs. One reason for this ignorance was the social emphasis and overemphasis on the reproductive role of women. There simply was not enough interest in learning about their orgasmic potential. Another reason is the anatomical fact that the most important female sex organs are either barely visible or completely hidden from view in the abdominal cavity. A woman's external sex organs, which can be examined easily, offer no clue as to the physiological processes taking place deeper inside. Women thus often find it hard to understand their own bodily functions. Fortunately, modern scientific research has made this task much easier. While many questions are still unanswered, it is now nevertheless possible to provide every woman with enough information for the purposes of everyday life. Such factual information can dispel many lingering fears and old superstitions while helping both sexes to develop a mature and responsible attitude toward the female sex organs.

THE FEMALE SEX ORGANS

1. Mons Veneris
2. Major lip (one of a pair)
3. Minor lip (one of a pair)
4. Clitoris
5. Opening of urethra
6. Urinary bladder
7. Vaginal opening
8. Vagina
9. Cervix
10. Uterus
11. Fallopian tube (one of a pair)
12. Ovary (one of a pair)

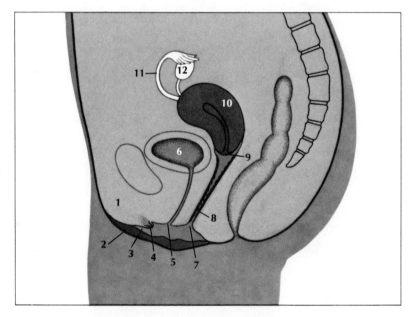

THE EXTERNAL SEX ORGANS

The female external sex organs consist of the mons Veneris, the major and minor lips, the clitoris, and the vaginal opening. All of these parts together are also often referred to collectively as the vulva (Latin: covering).

The Mons Veneris

The mons Veneris (Latin: mountain of Venus) consists of fatty tissue under the skin just over the pubic bone. On the outside, the area is covered with pubic hair, which first develops during puberty, and which makes the mons veneris by far the most conspicuous part of the vulva.

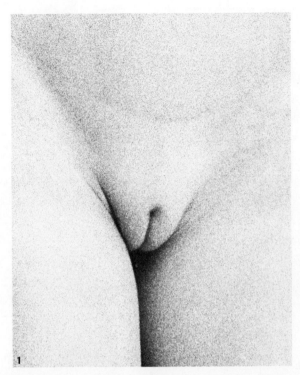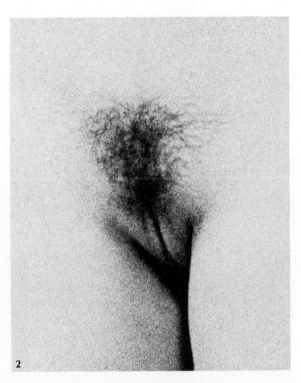

The female external sex organs (1) before and (2) after puberty.

The Major Lips

The major lips (*labia majora*) are two thick and fatty folds of skin which extend from the mons Veneris downward, forming the outer borders of the vulva. On the outside, they are also covered with hair just as the mons Veneris. As the major lips usually lie close together, they seem to keep the other parts of the vulva covered.

The Minor Lips

Just beneath the major lips lie the minor lips (*labia minora*). These are two thin folds of skin richly endowed with blood vessels and nerve endings. As a result, they are quite sensitive to the touch. The minor lips merge at the top forming a single fold of skin covering the clitoris. This fold is also called the foreskin or prepuce of the clitoris, or simply the clitoral hood.

The Clitoris

The clitoris (Greek *kleitoris*: that which is closed in) is located below the mons Veneris at the point where the minor lips meet. The clitoris is a short cylindrical organ composed mainly of erectile tissue, i.e., of two spongy bodies (*corpora cavernosa*) which can quickly fill with blood and thus cause the entire organ to stiffen and increase in size.

The clitoris is partly covered by the clitoral hood or foreskin. It is possible for genital secretions (smegma) to accumulate under this foreskin, thus causing irritation and other problems. (See "Pain During Sexual Intercourse.")

The average length of a clitoris in its unexcited state is less than an inch and most of it is hidden from view. However, in the state of excitement it may swell to twice its usual diameter. In a way, the clitoris can be compared to a very small penis, and its glans, which is normally exposed, is extremely sensitive to the touch as it is studded with innumerable nerve endings. Unlike the penis, however, the excited clitoris does not protrude but retracts under its hood. The clitoris is easily excitable by mechanical stimulation, and it plays an essential role in a woman's sexual excitement. (For details, see "The Female Sexual Response.")

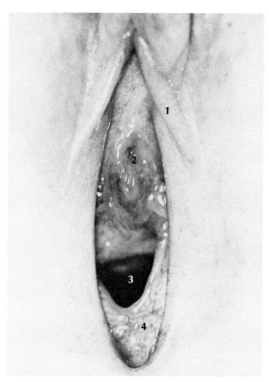

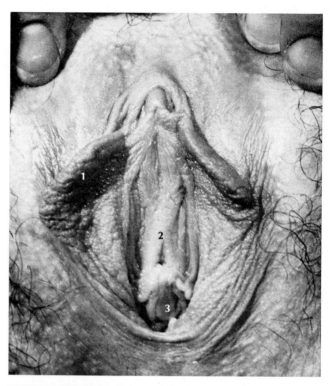

EXTERNAL SEX ORGANS OF A YOUNG GIRL
The clearly visible hymen stretches partly across the vaginal opening. 1. minor lips 2. opening of urethra 3. vaginal opening 4. hymen

EXTERNAL SEX ORGANS OF A WOMAN
The hymen, having been torn, is absent. 1. minor lips 2. opening of urethra 3. vaginal opening

The Vaginal Opening

The vaginal opening lies below that of the urethra which, in females, is independent from the sex organs and is used exclusively for the release of urine. The urethral opening is very small, and it lies roughly halfway between the clitoris and the vaginal opening. By contrast, the vaginal opening is rather large, although it may be partially closed by a thin membrane called the hymen.

The hymen has no known physiological function. Nevertheless, in the past many people ascribed great significance to it. For example, it was believed that an unbroken hymen provided proof of a woman's virginity. However, such a belief is nothing more than a superstition. A hymen usually has one or several holes in it which may be stretchable and thus allow for the insertion of fingers, or even a penis, without tearing. On the other hand, in some women the hymen tears easily, not only as a result of coitus but also because of strenuous physical exercise or sports activities. In some cases, the hymen is even absent altogether. It follows from these observations that the condition of a woman's hymen does not prove anything one way or the other about her sexual innocence or experience. In most cases, the first coitus may very well be the occasion for the breaking of the hymen, but it can, of course, also occur during masturbation and petting, or when the woman first uses menstrual tampons. The tearing of the hymen may cause some initial discomfort and slight bleeding. However, there is no reason for women to fear any great pain.

On both sides of the vaginal opening, between the edge of the hymen and the minor lips, are the greater vestibular glands (Bartholin's glands), which correspond to the bulbourethral (Cowper's) glands in the male. The greater vestibular glands secrete a small amount of lubricating fluid. However, most of the vaginal lubrication needed for coitus is not provided by these glands but by the wall of the vagina itself.

The female internal sex organs consist of the ovaries, the Fallopian tubes, the uterus, and the vagina.

The Ovaries

The ovaries (the female sex glands or gonads) are two walnut-sized bodies which are located inside the abdomen on either side of the uterus.

The ovaries serve a double function:

- They produce eggs which are released into the Fallopian tubes.
- They produce hormones which are secreted directly into the bloodstream.

The Production of Eggs

Before a baby girl is born, all of the cells that will later grow into eggs are already formed in her ovaries. In their primitive beginnings, the cells are called oogonia. These oogonia turn into primary oocytes, some of which eventually give rise to mature eggs (ova).

The process of egg production, called oogenesis, begins in the female fetus, but soon comes to a halt at birth. Thus, every girl is born with nearly 500,000 primary oocytes which remain in their state of suspended development until she reaches puberty. (During this time no new oocytes are produced. On the contrary, most of those that had developed earlier gradually die. By the time a girl reaches puberty, there may be no more than 30,000 primary oocytes left that are capable of further development. At the age of thirty, this number has dwindled even further to about 10,000, and when the woman reaches her menopause, all primary oocytes are gone.) Once the process of oogenesis has resumed during puberty, one or several mature eggs are produced each month by either one of her ovaries until both of them cease functioning following menopause. In the course of her fertile life, a woman may produce some 400 mature eggs. Of course, only a very small fraction of these can ever contribute to conceptions.

All of this provides a striking contrast to the way sperm cells are produced in the male (continuous production of millions of sperm daily, beginning with puberty; for details, see "The Male Sex Organs").

The development of a mature egg proceeds in several steps: Each primary oocyte is contained in a cluster of supporting cells. These clusters lie beneath the outer layer of the ovary. Each month, under the influence of certain hormones, one of the clusters grows to a point where it appears as a rather large blister on the surface of the ovary. This blister is called a Graafian follicle (after the 17th-century anatomist de Graaf). During the period of follicle growth, the primary oocyte, which like any other female body cell contains 46 chromosomes (including two X chromosomes), divides into two new cells of very unequal size: a relatively large secondary oocyte and a minute so-called polar body. In this division, the 46 chromosomes are split apart, and half of them are allotted to each of the new cells. Thus, the secondary oocyte as well as the polar body each contain only 23 chromosomes (including one X chromosome).

The polar body dies and disintegrates. Only the secondary oocyte is destined for further maturation. First, it floats freely inside the growing follicle which contains fluid. Eventually, the follicle bursts, releasing the secondary oocyte into the abdominal cavity. This release is known as ovulation. The secondary oocyte then enters the nearest Fallopian tube. Here it divides again into two new cells of unequal size: a relatively large ootid (mature ovum) and a minute second polar body. However, this time the division reproduces rather than splits the number of chromosomes. Thus, both of the new cells retain 23 chromosomes (including one X chromosome). This last division and the expulsion of the second polar body occur only after fertilization. While the second polar body dies just as the first one, the 23 chromosomes of the ootid unite with the 23 chromosomes of the spermatozoon, thus forming a new cell (the zygote) which again contains 46 chromosomes like all other cells of the body. (For details, see "Conception.")

The Production of Hormones

As described in a previous section, the female and male gonads (ovaries and testicles) also produce certain hormones. These gonadal hormones have been divided into female hormones (estrogens) and male hormones (androgens). However, these terms are somewhat misleading because both "female" and "male" hormones can be found in every female and male body. It is only the quantity of these hormones that differs. Before puberty, the estrogen and androgen levels in girls and boys are nearly equal. Then, during adolescence, the balance begins to shift. In the female body the estrogens rise to a much higher level than the androgens, and in the male body the androgens rise to a slightly higher level than the estrogens. In the female, the increase of estrogens during puberty helps to produce the secondary female sexual characteristics. (In the male, the increase of androgens helps to produce the secondary male sexual characteristics.)

In addition to estrogens (and androgens), the ovaries of a sexually mature female also produce a hormone called progesterone. The production of progesterone takes place mainly in association with the *corpus luteum* (Latin: yellow body) which is formed from the wall of the ruptured follicle after ovulation. During a women's fertile years, the estrogens as well as progesterone play an important role in her reproductive cycle. (For details, see "The Menstrual Cycle.")

There is still much to be learned about the nature and function of hormones in the human body. Nevertheless, a few basic facts have already been established: While the gonadal hormones are necessary for a young person's physical maturation, they are not essential for the continued sexual activity of adults. In other words, females and males need their gonadal hormones during adolescence to develop their full sexual potential. However, once the potential has been attained, they can function sexually without these hormones. Therefore, a woman who approaches menopause does not have to fear that she will lose her sexual responsiveness. Even when her ovaries have ceased their hormone production, she can continue her sexual activities as before. The same is also true, of course, for a woman who has to have her ovaries surgically removed for reasons of illness. (For details, see "The Role of Hormones.")

The Fallopian Tubes

The Fallopian tubes (named after the 16th-century anatomist Fallopius) lead from the ovaries to the uterus. They are also sometimes called oviducts (Latin: paths of eggs), a term that accurately describes their function. They provide a passageway for the egg down to the area where it could implant in case of a fertilization. (They also provide a passageway for sperm cells swimming upward from the uterus trying to reach the egg.) The wide ovarian end of a Fallopian tube has finger-like extensions called *fimbriae* (singular: *fimbria*) which move across the surface of the ovary; the uterine end leads directly into the inside of the uterus.

The fertilization of an egg normally occurs in the upper part of a Fallopian tube. Inside the tube, there are innumerable hair-like growths called *cilia* (singular: *cilium*) whose movements, together with muscular contractions of the tubal wall, sweep the egg toward the uterus. (Inside the male vas deferens, the sperm cells are transported the same way since they are still unable to move by themselves at that point.)

The Uterus

The uterus (Latin: womb) is a muscular organ which is situated between and slightly below the ovaries, approximately in the center of the lower abdomen. The shape of the uterus, which is about 3 inches long, resembles that of a small pear turned upside down. The Fallopian tubes enter the uterus on either side near the top. The wide upper part, known as the body of the uterus, is usually tilted forward over the dome of the urinary bladder, and it is separated from the narrow lower part by a slight constriction. This lower part is called the cervix or neck of the uterus, and it ends in the deep portion of the vagina. The cervix contains a small opening through which sperm cells can travel from the vagina into the uterus. However, except for a certain period during ovulation, the cervical opening is plugged by an impenetrable mucus.

The thick walls of the uterus are made up of three layers: the external cover called the perimetrium, the middle or muscular layer called the myometrium, and the inner layer called the endometrium. This endometrium consists of special tissue which thickens every month as the uterus prepares for the possible implantation of a fertilized egg. (Also see "Conception.") If no implantation occurs, the endometrium deteriorates and is discharged through the cervix and the vagina during menstruation. (See "The Menstrual Cycle.")

In case of a pregnancy, the uterus expands with the growing fetus. The extraordinary muscular structure of the myometrium not only allows for such vast expansion, but also provides the necessary pressure during labor when the fetus is finally expelled. (See "Birth.")

The uterine muscles also contract during orgasm. (For details, see "The Female Sexual Response.")

The Vagina

The vagina (Latin: sheath) is a muscular tube about 3½ inches long extending from the cervix to an external opening which is part of the vulva.

The vagina serves three main functions:

- It provides a passageway for the menstrual flow from the uterus to the outside. (See "The Menstrual Cycle.")
- It serves as a receptacle for a man's penis and his ejaculated sperm which then may move on through the cervix (see "Conception").
- It provides a passageway for the baby during birth from the uterus to the outside. (See "Birth.")

Under ordinary circumstances, the vagina is a collapsed tube, i.e., more a potential than actual space. Its inner surface, like that of the mouth, hosts different kinds of organisms which live in a healthy ecological balance. This balance can be upset, however, as a result of chemical interference. For this reason, vaginal sprays and douches should be avoided. The vagina cleanses itself with its own secretions. It also possesses a special protection against infection. (For vaginal infections and infestations, see "Venereal Diseases.")

The vaginal walls, which lie close together, contain mucous crypts and many blood vessels, but no glands and few nerve endings. (See also "The Female Sexual Response.") During sexual excitement, these walls secrete a watery substance which serves as a lubricant during coitus. Without such lubrication, the insertion of a penis could be painful to both the woman and the man. (See "Pain During Sexual Intercourse.")

The vagina adjusts to the size of any inserted penis, large or small. However, that portion of the vagina which lies closest to the external opening may, in some cases, become too relaxed for the preference of either sexual partner. This can happen after childbirth, for instance, or simply as a result of the aging process. Conversely, it is also possible for the vaginal entry to become so tense and tight that it cannot be penetrated. Such a vaginal spasm is called vaginismus. In either case, it should be remembered that a woman can attain a great deal of control over the function of her vaginal muscles, and that they can be developed by appropriate exercises. Some of these exercises, the so-called Kegel exercises, can easily be performed at all times, anywhere. They are described in another section of this book. (See "Sexual Inadequacy in Women—Lack of Orgasm.")

THE MENSTRUAL CYCLE

A woman becomes capable of reproduction during puberty and then loses this capacity in her early fifties. However, even in her fertile years she can conceive only during a certain time once a month when one of her ovaries releases an egg. The monthly recurrence of this event, together with other regular bodily changes, constitute the female reproductive cycle. Its most obvious external sign is menstruation (monthly bleeding). For this reason, the reproductive cycle may also be called menstrual cycle. Indeed, this latter term has the advantage of referring to a concrete experience which is familiar to practically all women, including those who do not reproduce.

A girl's first menstruation (also called menarche) usually occurs between the ages of 11 and 13. However, the second menstruation may very well be much farther away than just another month. During adolescence, menstrual cycles are rather irregular. It is only later that some definite pattern is established. In a mature woman, menstrual cycles usually last between 28 and 35 days. Still, some irregularity is always possible and quite normal. The irregularity increases again as the woman grows older. Finally, after menopause, her menstruations cease altogether.

In scientific textbooks, the menstrual cycle is usually divided into two, three, four, or more different phases. Such divisions, while always somewhat arbitrary, can nevertheless aid in understanding the biological processes involved. For the purposes of the present volume, a division into three phases seems adequate.

The Three Phases of the Menstrual Cycle

The basic function of the menstrual cycle is easily summarized—it prepares the lining of the uterus for the possible implantation of a fertilized egg. If no implantation occurs, the lining breaks down and is discharged through the vagina. This discharge is known as menstrual bleeding or simply menstruation. When the bleeding has stopped, the preparation of the uterine lining and thus the entire cycle starts again.

Theoretically, a description of the mentrual cycle could begin with any of its phases. For the purposes of medical calculation, for example, the menstrual cycle is assumed to start with the first day of menstruation and to end with the last day before the next menstruation. However, in the present context it seems most useful to begin with the growth of the egg (ovum) and the gradual thickening of the uterine lining (endometrium).

1. Preparing for Ovulation

When the menstrual flow comes to a halt, the uterine lining is very thin. However, it slowly begins to thicken under the influence of estrogen, a hormone that is produced by the ovaries and released into the bloodstream. The rising estrogen level also stimulates the growth of some of the Graafian follicles that encase the immature ova. Eventually, only one of these follicles completes its growth, while the others recede. After approximately two weeks, one follicle ruptures and releases the ovum. This release is known as ovulation. At the time of ovulation, the uterine lining has thickened considerably and is close to becoming ready for a possible implantation.

An ovulation occurs about 14 days before the beginning of the next menstruation. That is to say, if the ovum is not fertilized and implanted, the uterine lining will break down and will be discharged two weeks later. Thus, counting backward, in a menstrual cycle of 28 days, ovulation occurs on the 14th day; in a cycle of 35 days, it occurs on the 21st day. In other words, while the time period between ovulation and next menstruation is relatively constant, that between menstruation and next ovulation can vary considerably. Couples who practice the rhythm method of contraception have to keep this fact well in mind. (See also "Contraception.")

2. Preparing for Implantation

Shortly before ovulation, the follicle that encases the ovum begins to produce a new hormone called progesterone. This production increases dramatically

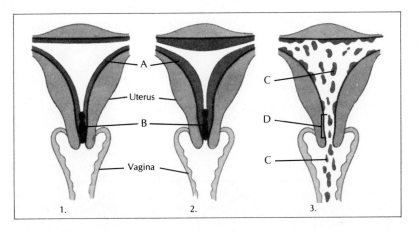

after ovulation when the ruptured follicle is transformed into a "yellow body" (*corpus luteum*). In addition to progesterone, which plays an important part in the final preparation of the uterine lining, the yellow body also continues the production of estrogen. Under the influence of this hormonal stimulation, the lining of the uterus soon achieves its greatest thickness and receptivity for implantation.

After its release from the ovary, the ovum enters the nearest Fallopian tube and begins traveling toward the uterus. Within a few hours, it undergoes its final maturation and becomes ready for fertilization. (For details, see "Conception.") After its fertilization, the ovum develops into a cell cluster which continues its journey through the Fallopian tube to the uterus, where it arrives about three days later. Finally, after another three to four days, it begins to implant in the nourishing uterine lining, thus starting pregnancy.

A pregnancy helps to sustain the yellow body and its production of estrogen and progesterone. As a result, no new ovulation occurs, and the uterine lining does not deteriorate. In other words, in case of a pregnancy, the menstrual cycle is suspended at this point and does not enter the third phase described.

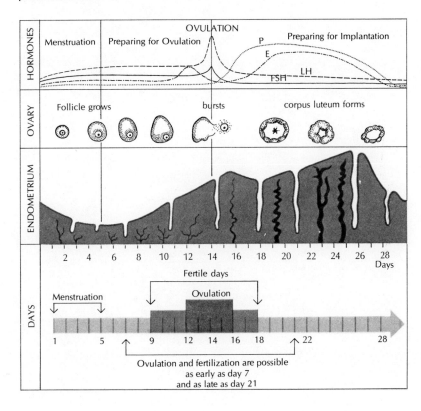

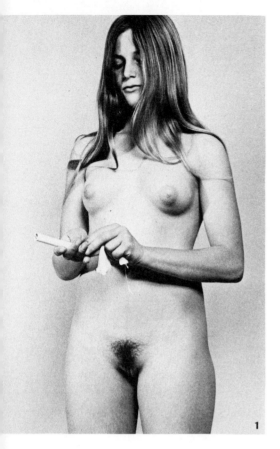
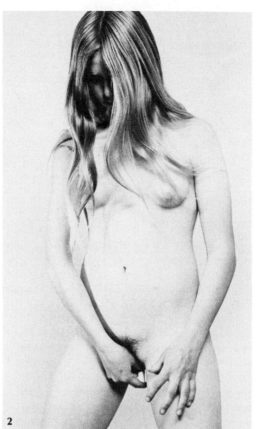
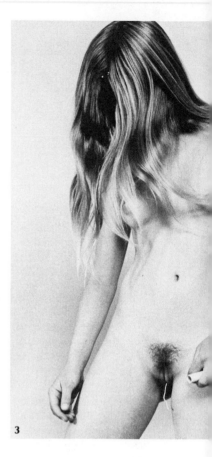

APPLICATION OF MENSTRUAL TAMPON
1. Tampon being revoved from its protective cover. 2. Tampon being inserted into the vagina. 3. Tampon in place where it absorbs the menstrual discharge. (The short string which remains visible allows for the later easy removal of the tampon.)

3. Menstruation

A fertilization is possible only within the first 24 hours after ovulation. If the ovum does not encounter any sperm cells during this time, it simply dies and disintegrates. Obviously, in this case there is no implantation either. As a result, the thick special lining of the uterus is not needed, but soon begins to break down and slough off. The waste material, consisting mainly of mucus, lining tissue, and variable amounts of blood, is discharged through the vagina. This discharge is known as the monthly bleeding or menstruation (from Latin *mensis,* month). It usually lasts between 3 and 5 days. In popular language, these days are also sometimes referred to simply as the "period." The first day of menstruation is usually considered the first day of the entire menstrual cycle.

During her "period," a woman may experience some physical discomfort, such as backaches, headaches, or cramps in the pelvic area. In fact, some women develop some of these symptoms a few days before the menstruation begins. Such premenstrual tension as well as menstrual discomfort can often be alleviated by medication. In any case, there is rarely a need for an interruption of regular daily activities. For example, a menstruating woman can participate in sports without impairing her health in any way.

Most modern women wear tampons during their menstrual periods. These tampons are made of cotton or similar absorbent material, and they are introduced into the vagina where they absorb the menstrual flow. As long as they are replaced often enough, there is no medical objection to their use. In case of heavier menstrual bleeding, the traditional menstrual napkins may be more appropriate.

Sexual Intercourse During Menstruation

In the past, many societies had strong prohibitions against sexual intercourse during menstruation. Generally, women were considered "unclean" during this time, and in some cultures there was a belief that sexual intercourse with a menstruating woman could make a man ill. However, modern medical research has exposed these and similar views as mere prejudices and superstitions. From a purely medical standpoint, there is no reason why sexual intercourse should not take place at any time during the menstrual cycle. In fact, many women are particularly responsive just before or during their periods. Still, some couples may hesitate to engage in coitus because of aesthetic objections to the bleeding. In this case, the use of a diaphragm should be considered. It will not only hold back the blood, but will also act as a means of contraception. After all, sperm cells can stay alive inside a woman's body for several days, and menstrual cycles can be quite irregular. An early ovulation can never be ruled out with complete certainty. (See also "Contraception.")

Menopause

Usually between the ages of 45 and 50 a woman will notice that her menstrual cycles become more and more irregular until, eventually, she ceases to menstruate altogether. This permanent cessation of menstruation is called menopause. A broader term, climacteric (Greek: critical period), refers to the general physiological and psychological changes that occur during this time in a woman's life. As described earlier, the number of a woman's oocytes dwindles to zero over the years. Correspondingly the woman also ceases to produce the hormones necessary for the preparation of the uterine lining. In some women, the resulting hormonal changes may, for a while, produce rather distressing symptoms, such as headaches, dizziness, fatigue, insomnia, and depression. Another symptom that may occur repeatedly is a "hot flash" or brief heat sensation spreading over the body. Such a flash may last from a second to a few minutes, and it may be followed by chills or heavy perspiration. These and other menopausal complaints can often be alleviated or even avoided by hormonal treatment.

In most cases, the entire climacteric does not last longer than about two years. Although menstruations become increasingly rare during this period, ovulations (and therefore conceptions) are still possible. A woman who does not want to become pregnant during her climacteric is therefore well advised to continue the use of contraception. After one year without menstruation, however, she can safely assume that she is no longer fertile.

The loss of fertility does not affect a woman's sexual responsiveness. In fact, many women show a renewed and increased interest in sexual intercourse once they can stop worrying about unwanted pregnancies. (See also "The Role of Hormones.")

THE BREASTS

Although the female breasts cannot be considered sex organs in the narrow sense of the term, they usually play an important part not only in erotic arousal, but also in the nurturing of the newborn. In a sense then, the breasts can be said to have some erotic as well as reproductive function.

The breasts of a mature woman are two cushions of fat and tissue which surround her mammary glands. Whenever she gives birth to a child, these glands begin to secrete milk into special ducts leading to the nipples. The nipples, which are composed of smooth muscle fiber, and which contain many nerve endings, are very sensitive to the touch and can become erect during sexual excitement. (See "The Female Sexual Response.") The area around the nipples is pinkish, but becomes—and then remains—darker as a result of pregnancy.

The female breasts begin to develop fully during puberty as a result of hormonal stimulation. (See "The Role of Hormones.") Their eventual shape and size is determined by heredity.

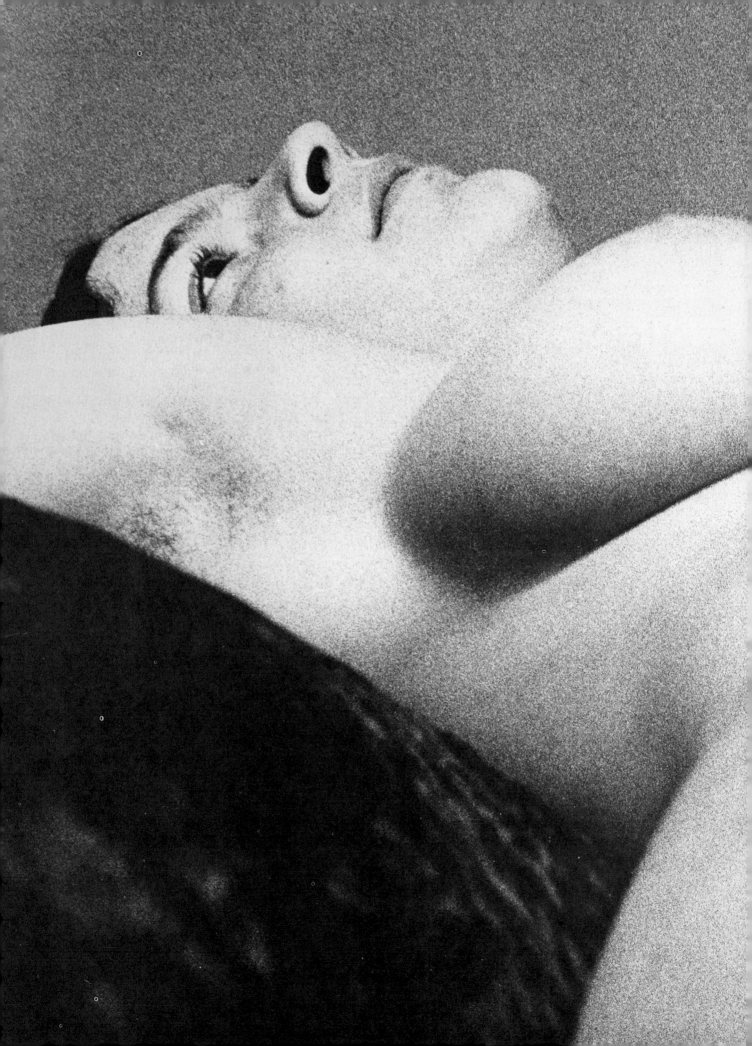

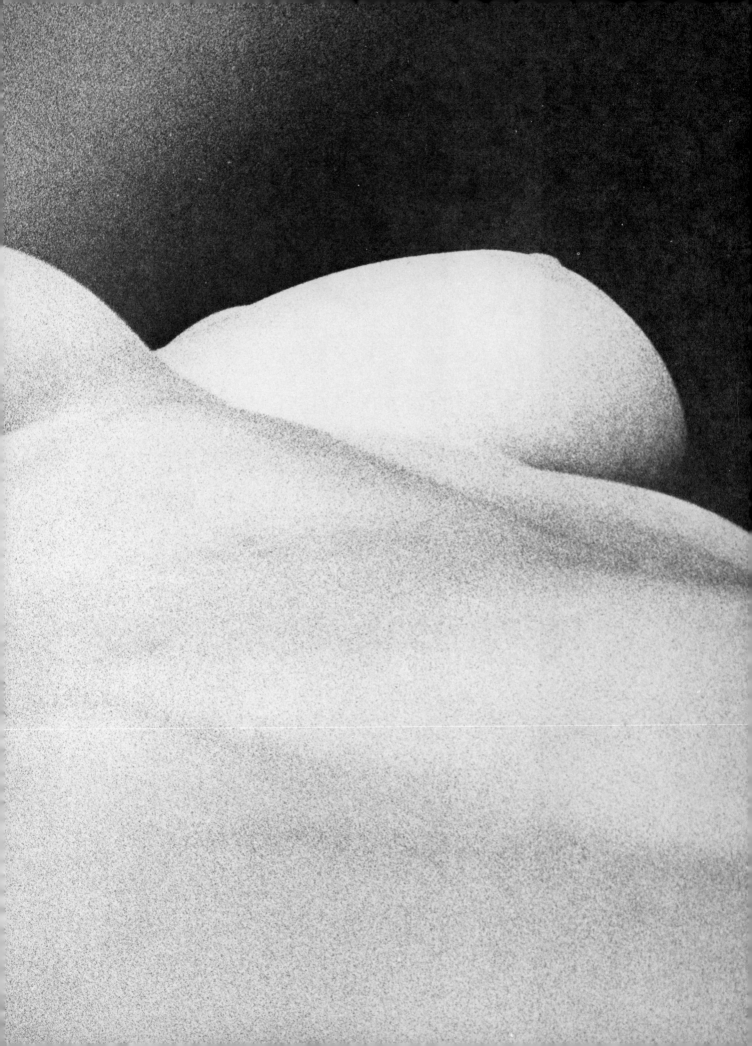

For many men and women, the breasts have a special sexual significance. However, as in all sexual matters, preferences vary widely. In certain societies, long, pendular breasts are considered superior; in others, the taste runs to the round and firm. In some cultures, small breasts are praised as the most beautiful, while in others the ideal is an ample bosom. Even within one and the same culture, the concept of female beauty may change from one generation to the next, indeed from one individual to another.

Men also have breasts, although they are less well developed. Nevertheless, the male nipples may also be very sensitive to the touch. They can also become erect, and they may play an important part in sexual arousal. (See "The Male Sexual Response.") There is one important difference, however—the male breast contains only rudimentary mammary glands. In fact, a male may "give milk" only once in his life—at birth. A newborn baby still shares certain hormones with the mother, including those that stimulate her milk production. For this reason, the baby's breasts also contain colostrum, a pre-milk substance (the so-called witches' milk). This is true for both female and male babies. Naturally, the condition does not last long. (Also see "Male and Female Anatomical Development.")

THE FEMALE SEXUAL RESPONSE

Every healthy woman as well as every healthy man can respond to sexual stimulation. While this response is never exactly the same in any two individuals, its basic physiological pattern is shared by all human beings, regardless of sex.

Sexual activity produces many changes in the human body, such as an increase of muscular tension, the swelling of certain organs, a rise in pulse rate and blood pressure, and many other signs of mounting excitement until, eventually, a pleasurable, seizure-like reaction known as orgasm brings satisfaction and relief. People have, of course, always been aware of these bodily changes, but their true nature and extent remained largely unknown until rather recently when scientists began to observe and measure the human sexual response in the laboratory. The pioneering work of Kinsey and his associates of the Institute for Sex Research in Bloomington, Indiana, and Masters and Johnson of the Reproductive Biology Research Foundation in St. Louis, Missouri, have provided us with many new insights and disproved much of the traditional wisdom in sexual matters.

The importance of this research for women can hardly be exaggerated. In our Western culture, women have, for a very long time, suffered from a social attitude that denied them the full expression of their sexuality. It was generally assumed that men were possessed by a powerful "sex drive" that demanded satisfaction. Women, on the other hand, were considered incapable of strong sexual feelings. Their only recognized biological function was childbearing. As a consequence, men were usually granted considerable sexual license while every effort was made to prevent women from engaging in any nonmarital, nonreproductive sexual activity. Men were encouraged to enjoy their sexual capacities; women were taught to regard sexual desire as base, improper, and degrading. (Also see "The Social Roles of Men and Women.")

This so-called double standard for male and female sexual behavior has had some very unfortunate consequences, not only for the moral health of society but also for the physical well-being of the individual woman. For example, women often find it hard to develop their sexual responsiveness, and a great number of them go through life without ever realizing their erotic potential. While practically all men easily achieve orgasm after a certain amount of stimulation, there are many women who despair of reaching this simple goal. Some women have their first orgasmic experience only after many years of sexual intercourse.

Aside from a few rare cases of physical disability or illness, these strange and unnecessary difficulties are clearly related to the way women are brought up in our society. During their formative years, girls are forced to deny their sexual urges even to themselves in order to maintain an appearance of "decency," "modesty," and "respectability." They are allowed to indulge in romantic and symbolic fantasies, but not to develop their sensory capacities which could turn those vague yearnings into realistic experiences. The resulting inhibitions can become strong enough to prevent any normal sexual functioning. (See also "Sexual Inadequacy.")

For centuries, this deplorable state of affairs was accepted as "natural" and unavoidable. The sexual satisfaction of women was not seen as an attainable or even desirable goal. Those who challenged the double standard found themselves confronted with dogmatic beliefs in a God-given inequality of the sexes and poetic assertions about the "eternal mystery of woman." Nevertheless, in modern times there has been a growing demand for sexual equality, and in recent decades the emancipation of women has made much progress. Part of this progress has been the result of scientific sex research. Undisputable data have now clearly demonstrated that the sexual capacity of females is at least equal to and, in some respects, even greater than that of males. It has further been shown that the sexual response follows essentially the same pattern in both sexes. In an unbiased world, these discoveries would hardly have been startling. Indeed, they only confirm what should have been obvious long ago: Most of the differences between men and women are not inborn but inbred, and sexual behavior in particular is deeply influenced by social conditioning.

Today, we know that both women and men can respond sexually to the same sensory stimuli. Touch, vision, hearing, smell, and taste play an important role in all human sexual arousal. Women as well as men possess a special sensitivity in the same general areas of the body, and they can develop the same erogenous zones. Since these matters have already been discussed in a previous section, there is no need for a repetition here. (For details, see "The Male Sexual Response.") However, it should perhaps be reemphasized that there are a few differences between the female and male responses that may not be due to social influences. For instance, it has been found that the average female is less easily stimulated by mental images alone. Women in general are more easily distracted even when aroused, and many of them reach orgasm only as a result of continuing physical stimulation. (There are exceptions to this rule. Some women can achieve orgasm in response to purely psychological stimuli.) Further biological differences are listed below.

The following summary of the human sexual response is not meant to establish a norm or an ideal of sexual performance. Its only purpose is to provide women and men with some general information about those physiological processes that may accompany sexual activity. Individual variations should always be expected. Still, a particular woman's basic responses are usually the same throughout her life, and it makes no difference whether they are brought about by masturbation or any conceivable form of sexual intercourse. (See "Types of Sexual Activity.") Psychologically, these experiences may very well feel entirely different, but the reactions of the body remain unchanged.

As mentioned earlier, the male and female sexual responses are essentially the same. There are some marked differences, but they are not decisive. In fact, it makes sense to speak of a basic human sexual response and its male and female variations.

During sexual activity, the human body undergoes a number of physiological changes which form a definite, typical pattern. In the simplest terms, this

THE FOUR PHASES OF HUMAN SEXUAL RESPONSE

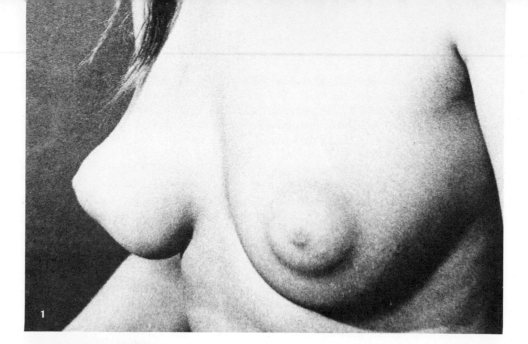

**SWELLING OF BREASTS
UNDER STIMULATION**

1. *Unstimulated breasts.*
2. *Stimulation of breasts.*
3. *Breasts after stimulation.*

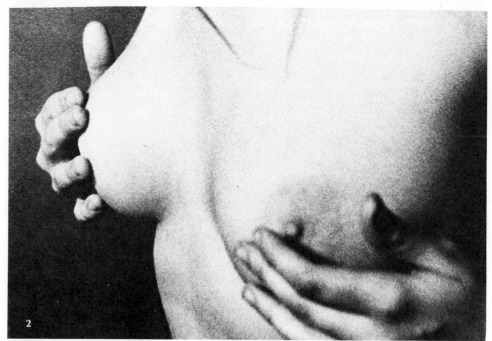

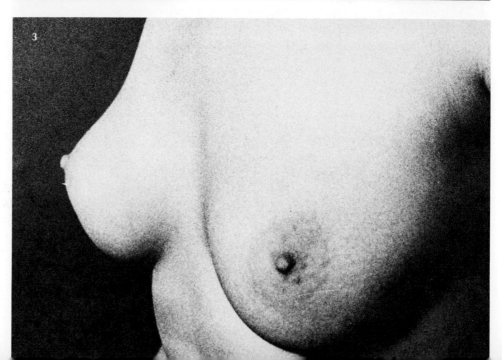

56

pattern can be described as a build-up and release of tension. However, in order to gain greater insight into the processes involved, various scientists have divided the human sexual response not only into two, but three and four different phases. The following description of the female sexual response follows the division into four phases proposed by Masters and Johnson. (For the application of this model to males, see "The Male Sexual Response.")

1. Excitement

It used to be believed that females were slower to respond to sexual stimulation than males. However, this belief is mistaken. Not only men but also women can become sexually aroused very suddenly, and some of them may experience one or more orgasms within a few minutes. As a matter of fact, there are women who reach orgasm fifteen to thirty seconds after they begin sexual intercourse. It seems, however, that during the first stages of arousal women are more easily distracted than men and depend more on continued direct physical stimulation. For this reason, many females seem to need a longer time to reach orgasm during coitus than their male partners, whose excitement is often sustained and increased by psychological factors. In general, females are less easily stimulated by mere sights and sounds, or by erotic fantasies and anticipations. On the other hand, when the average woman is able to concentrate on her preferred method of stimulation (during masturbation, for instance), she achieves orgasm just as quickly as the average man.

In females, the first and most obvious sign of sexual excitement is the lubrication of the vagina. In response to effective stimulation, the vaginal walls begin to secrete a clear fluid which soon provides a moist coating for the entire vagina in preparation for coitus. Without such lubrication, the insertion of a man's penis into a woman's vagina could be painful for both. (The corresponding first sign of sexual excitement in males is the erection of the penis. In short, as the penis becomes ready to enter the vagina, the vagina becomes ready to receive it.) With continued arousal, the inner two-thirds of the vagina increase in both length and width, creating a tenting or ballooning effect. (In its unexcited state, the vagina is a collapsed tube, i.e., its walls are touching.) At the same time, there is a vaginal color change from the usual purple-red to a deep purple that becomes even darker during the following phases.

A woman's major lips (the outer lips of the vulva) respond differently, depending on whether she has given birth to children or not. If she has not given birth, sexual excitement will cause her major lips to flatten out and expose the vaginal opening. The major lips of a woman who has given birth, on the other hand, are rather large and now grow even larger as a result of engorgement. Nevertheless, they also expose the vaginal opening. The minor lips (the inner lips of the vulva) swell considerably in all women and also change their color to a progressively deeper red. The clitoris (just as the penis) increases in size as its erectile tissue becomes filled with blood. This increase is usually most noticeable in the diameter of the clitoral shaft. The uterus also begins to swell and is pulled upward into the abdomen, thus contributing to the lengthening of the vagina mentioned above.

During sexual excitement, the nipples of the breasts become erect and maintain this erection throughout the other phases. However, since the dark area around each nipple, and, indeed the whole breast, soon also becomes engorged and swollen, the nipple erection itself gradually appears less conspicuous. Mounting sexual tension further produces voluntary and involuntary muscular contractions in various parts of the body as well as a rise in pulse rate and blood pressure.

In addition to all the above signs of growing sexual excitement, most women also show a so-called sex flush, i.e., a red rash which begins in the stomach area and then spreads to the breasts and neck. This rash lasts through the orgasmic phase.

2. Plateau

The plateau phase is nothing more than the continuation of the excitement phase. The word "plateau" is meant to indicate that a certain even level of excitement has been reached which is then maintained for a while before orgasm occurs.

During this phase, there is only a slight increase in length and width of the inner two-thirds of the vagina. However, its outer one-third becomes congested with blood. As a result, this part of the vagina, which might have widened somewhat during the excitement phase, now narrows by about 33 percent. This congested and tightening outer third of the vagina has been named the "orgasmic platform" by Masters and Johnson.

While the major lips show no further changes during the plateau phase, the minor lips continue to darken in color, especially in women who have given birth. This marked color change is a sign that orgasm is approaching. Once a certain level of excitement has been reached, the clitoris retracts under the clitoral hood or foreskin, and thus becomes inaccessible to direct stimulation by the woman or her sexual partner. (In the past, it was not always understood that this retraction of the clitoris indicates an increase, not decrease, of sexual excitement.) The greater vestibular (Bartholin's) glands (which correspond to the bulbourethral [Cowper's] glands in the male) may secrete a small amount of fluid during the plateau phase or late in the excitement phase. Also, the uterus is pulled further upward into the abdomen and further increases in size.

The breasts also reach their greatest expansion during the plateau phase, and the sex flush, if indeed it should have occurred, may now become more intense and cover a wider area. Voluntary and involuntary muscular tension greatly increases throughout the body. The pulse rate and blood pressure rise, and breathing becomes faster.

3. Orgasm

Orgasm (Greek *orgasmos:* lustful excitement) is the sudden release of muscular and nervous tension at the climax of sexual excitement. The experience represents the most intense physical pleasure of which human beings are capable and is basically the same for females and males. An orgasm lasts only a few moments and is felt very much like a seizure or rather a series of convulsions which involve the whole body and soon lead to complete relaxation. In sexually mature males, orgasm is accompanied by the ejaculation of semen. Since women do not produce semen, they do not ejaculate. However, in all other respects the physiological processes are comparable in both sexes. (See also "The Male Sexual Response.")

While the experience of orgasm itself is essentially the same in men and women, the latter seem to be better equipped to have more than one orgasm within a short time. There are some rare cases of males who, particularly in their younger years, are capable of several orgasms in quick succession. However, this capacity is quite common in females.

There is one further difference: While the orgasmic pattern of males practically never varies, females may experience orgasm in a number of ways. In some women, orgasm is rather short and mild; in others, it is extended and violent. Even one and the same woman may find herself responding quite differently on different occasions. However, the basic physiological processes underlying these possible variations remain unchanged.

In females, orgasm begins with strong, rhythmic contractions of the outer one-third of the vagina, which Masters and Johnson call the orgasmic platform. These contractions, which may number from three to fifteen, first recur within less than a second, then, as they become weaker, at longer intervals. Almost at the same time, the uterus begins to contract. However, the uterine contractions are irregular. They start at the top, working their way down, not unlike the contractions during the first stage of labor. The sphincter muscles of the rectum may also contract a few times at the same intervals as the orgasmic platform. In general, there is great muscular tension, not only in the entire pelvic area, but also in other parts of the body, such as the neck, arms, hands, legs, and feet. The pulse rate and blood pressure rise slightly even beyond the level reached during the plateau phase, and breathing is very fast. The intensity of all of these physical reactions depends, of course, on the degree and duration of sexual tension.

4. Resolution

After orgasm, the sex organs (and with them the whole body) need some time to return to their unexcited state. During this so-called resolution phase, the congestion in the outer one-third of the vagina (the orgasmic platform) disappears quickly. The major and minor lips again assume their former shape and size. The clitoris reemerges from under the clitoral hood. The uterus also shrinks back to its usual size, and, as it descends from its elevated position in the abdomen, the "tenting" or "ballooning" effect in the inner two-thirds of the vagina is eliminated. The sex flush mentioned earlier vanishes. The nipples of the breasts and the breasts themselves slowly return to their normal state. With the release of muscular tension, the pulse rate and blood pressure decrease, and breathing becomes normal again.

It should be noted at this point that, unlike men, many women do not seem to have a "refractory period," or at least it is not as obvious. In many cases continued or repeated stimulation can bring a woman to a second and third orgasm immediately following the first one. Indeed, many women are capable of having many orgasms in quick succession. Obviously, in this case, the resolution phase as described here does not begin until after the last of these orgasms.

THE SEXUAL RESPONSE IN OLDER WOMEN

There are still many people who believe that women lose their sexual responsiveness after menopause. Still others feel that older women should refrain from sexual intercourse for the sake of dignity or propriety. Fortunately, today such prejudices are fast disappearing as the sexual myths of former ages are replaced with modern scientific knowledge. Neither women nor men have to forego satisfying sexual relationships because of advancing age. The sexual response described above remains essentially the same. Naturally, older people lose some of their former strength, and many of their reactions become slower.

In a woman, there are also certain changes in the sex organs that affect her response. The most noticeable of these changes concerns the functioning of the vagina. Vaginal lubrication, which may appear within fifteen to thirty seconds in younger women, may now take several minutes to develop and be much less profuse. In addition, the vaginal walls become thinner and lose their former elasticity as a result of hormone deprivation. However, hormone replacement can usually improve the condition. Insufficient lubrication can be overcome through the use of an artificial lubricant.

Since the uterus begins to shrink after menopause, uterine elevation during sexual arousal gradually becomes less pronounced. As a result, there is now less of a "tenting" or "ballooning" effect in the inner two-thirds of the vagina. The contractions of orgasm are milder and fewer in number. The resolution phase is much shorter.

None of these possible physical changes have to prevent the enjoyment of sexual intercourse. Indeed, women who have been sexually active throughout their lives can expect to remain responsive well into their old age.

Reference and Recommended Reading

The Boston Women's Health Book Collective. *Our Bodies, Ourselves.* 2d ed. New York: Simon & Schuster, 1976 (cloth); 1976 (paper).
Brecher, Ruth and Edward, eds. *Analysis of Human Sexual Response.* New York: New American Library, 1974.
Lehrman, Nat. *Masters and Johnson Explained.* Chicago: Playboy Press, 1971 (cloth); 1976 (paper).

THE SEXUAL RESPONSE IN FEMALES

In modern times, the sexual response cycle was first analyzed and described as the "orgasmic formula" by Wilhelm Reich, who also proposed its division into four major phases: 1. mechanical tension, 2. bio-electric charge, 3. bio-electric discharge, and 4. mechanical relaxation. (W. Reich, *The Function of the Orgasm* [1927] 1942).

More recently, Masters and Johnson have relabeled these phases as 1. excitement, 2. plateau, 3. orgasm, and 4. resolution. In addition, they have introduced the concept of a fifth phase, the refractory period.

Shown here is the sexual response in the female sex organs as described by Masters and Johnson. It must be remembered, however, that the response actually involves the whole body. (For details see preceding text.)

CHANGES IN EXTERNAL SEX ORGANS

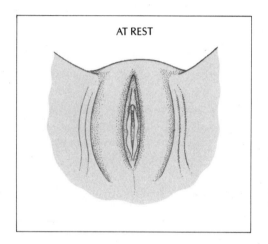

AT REST

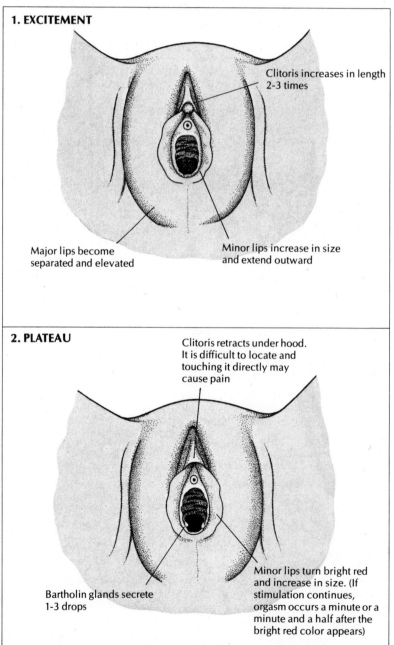

1. EXCITEMENT

Clitoris increases in length 2-3 times

Major lips become separated and elevated

Minor lips increase in size and extend outward

2. PLATEAU

Clitoris retracts under hood. It is difficult to locate and touching it directly may cause pain

Minor lips turn bright red and increase in size. (If stimulation continues, orgasm occurs a minute or a minute and a half after the bright red color appears)

Bartholin glands secrete 1-3 drops

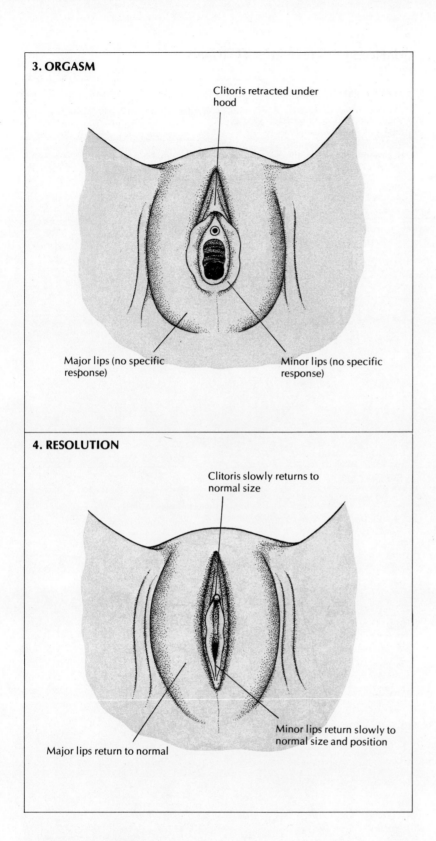

3. ORGASM

Clitoris retracted under hood

Major lips (no specific response)

Minor lips (no specific response)

4. RESOLUTION

Clitoris slowly returns to normal size

Minor lips return slowly to normal size and position

Major lips return to normal

(5. REFRACTORY PERIOD)
There is some evidence that females may also experience a so-called refractory period, i.e. a time after orgasm in which they do not respond to renewed sexual stimulation. However, this phenomenon is not always easily noticed, since many females are capable of several orgasms in quick succession.

CHANGES IN INTERNAL SEX ORGANS

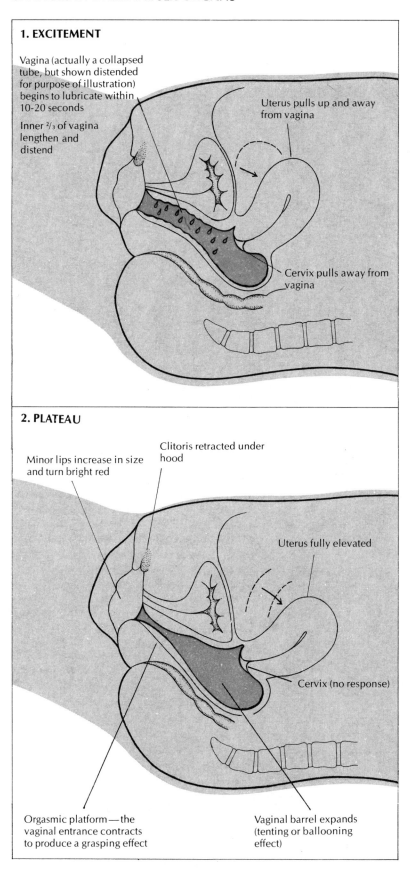

1. EXCITEMENT

Vagina (actually a collapsed tube, but shown distended for purpose of illustration) begins to lubricate within 10-20 seconds

Inner ⅔ of vagina lengthen and distend

Uterus pulls up and away from vagina

Cervix pulls away from vagina

2. PLATEAU

Minor lips increase in size and turn bright red

Clitoris retracted under hood

Uterus fully elevated

Cervix (no response)

Orgasmic platform—the vaginal entrance contracts to produce a grasping effect

Vaginal barrel expands (tenting or ballooning effect)

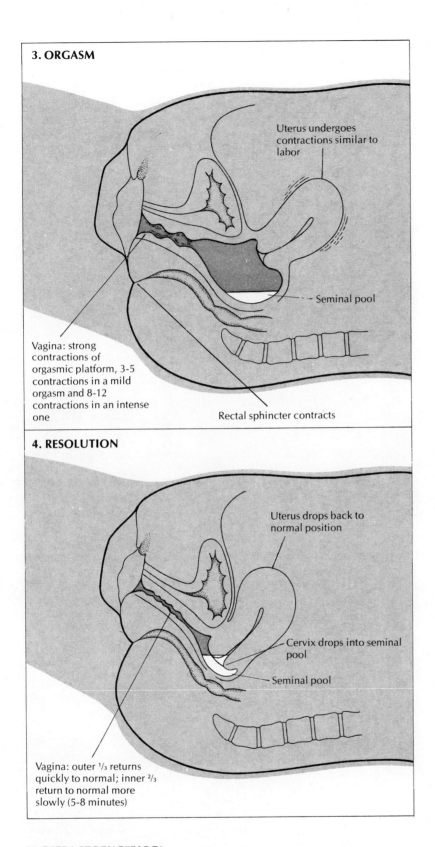

3. ORGASM

Uterus undergoes contractions similar to labor

Seminal pool

Vagina: strong contractions of orgasmic platform, 3-5 contractions in a mild orgasm and 8-12 contractions in an intense one

Rectal sphincter contracts

4. RESOLUTION

Uterus drops back to normal position

Cervix drops into seminal pool

Seminal pool

Vagina: outer ⅓ returns quickly to normal; inner ⅔ return to normal more slowly (5-8 minutes)

(5. REFRACTORY PERIOD)

There is some evidence that females may also experience a so-called refractory period, i.e. a time after orgasm in which they do not respond to renewed sexual stimulation. However, this phenomenon is not always easily noticed, since many females are capable of several orgasms in quick succession.

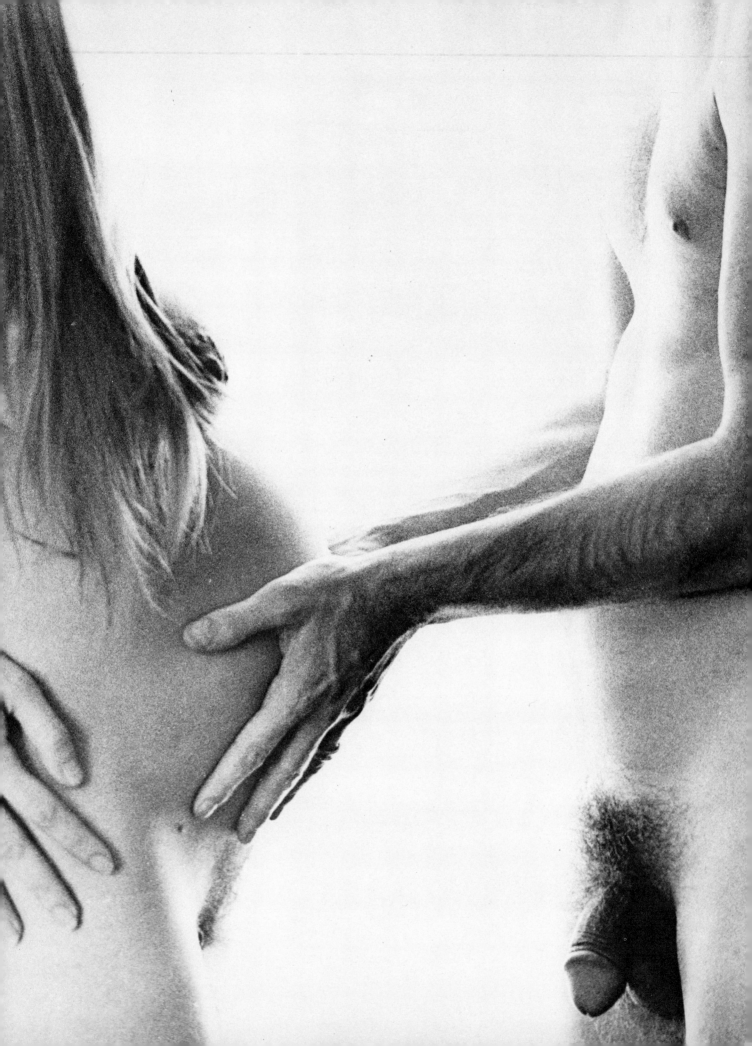

4. HUMAN REPRODUCTION

Human life is reproduced through a special form of sexual intercourse between men and women. The sex organs of males and females can easily be joined together, and such a joining (called copulation or coitus) provides an opportunity for the male and female sex cells (sperm and egg) to unite. This union results in a new cell which may grow into a new human being.

However, while there can be no reproduction without sexual activity, there can very well be sexual activity without reproduction. Men and women can respond sexually at any moment, and they can engage in many non-coital forms of sexual intercourse, but they can reproduce only through coitus and only during certain recurring short periods when an egg is available for fertilization by a sperm.

In spite of these biological facts our culture has long held the belief that the only purpose and justification of sex is reproduction. This belief is reflected in our religious dogmas, criminal laws, and, indeed, in some traditional medical theories. In short, we are conditioned to regard all sexual behavior that cannot lead to conceptions as sinful, illegal, or sick.

Still, there have been peoples on this planet who were quite unaware of the fact that pregnancies are caused by sexual activity. They assumed that a spirit entered the female body where it then grew into a child. Obviously, such an assumption had to lead to a sexual morality very different from our own.

A man who has never heard of the connection between sex and reproduction is, of course, free to enjoy sexual intercourse for its own sake. His attitude may change only when the connection is pointed out to him. Thus, the end of his ignorance could also mean a reappraisal of his moral values. Indeed, he could possibly end up adopting the sexual standards of our society. On the other hand, if, after some time, he should also discover that he is infertile, he might find the newly adopted morality irrelevant and return to his former value system. He would just realize that, in his particular case, there was no connection between sex and reproduction after all.

This theoretical example is not as far-fetched as it may seem. As a matter of fact, it can perhaps serve to illustrate a rather common problem. We know that in every society there are men and women whose sexual intercourse cannot possibly lead to conceptions. They may be too young or too old to reproduce, they may suffer from sterility, or they may prefer members of their own sex as sexual partners. In any case, they all face the same task—developing a sexual morality without reference to reproduction. In the past, the number of people confronted with this situation was always relatively small. For the majority of the population, sex and reproduction remained firmly linked, whether they liked it or not. However, in recent decades the invention of effective contraceptives has made nonreproductive sex a practical possibility for everyone. On the other hand, couples are now also able to reproduce by means of artificial insemination, i.e., without any direct sexual involvement at all. As a result of these developments, sex and reproduction have, once and for all, become separate issues, raising different moral questions.

Our public policies are beginning to take this fact into account. A good example is the official handling of sexual knowledge. Most traditional sex education was never more than reproduction information. When teachers talked to their students about the so-called facts of life, they rarely went beyond a discussion of how babies are conceived, and they almost never explained how conceptions can be avoided. Most people simply assumed that the spread of such knowledge would lead to general immorality. Today, however, there is a growing recognition that it may be immoral to deny young people this knowledge. Indeed, the threat of overpopulation has forced many governments in various parts of the world to reverse their moral positions and to propagate the separation of sex and reproduction for all of their citizens. In most countries, there are now public and private agencies which distribute contraception information in books, films, pamphlets, advertisements, and through personal counseling. At the same time, an increasing number of men and women demand full control over their own reproductive lives without any interference from society.

There is no doubt that the separation of sex and reproduction will eventually revolutionize all our lives. Once sexual intercourse no longer leads to unwanted pregnancies, and the conception of each child is a matter of conscious choice, the attitude of sexual partners toward each other is bound to change. Most probably there will be more mutual understanding and cooperation between the sexes. Many couples already plan their families together and share the experience of the woman's pregnancy all the way through the delivery of the baby. Modern hospitals encourage expectant fathers to remain present during the process of birth and also offer instruction in child care to both parents. These shared interests and responsibilities may soon make the traditional social roles of males and females obsolete and, for the first time in human history, lead to full sexual equality.

In the meantime, there is a clear need for both sexes to become familiar with the basic biological facts. Science has made great progress in exploring the mysteries of procreation and, although the ultimate questions are still unanswered, many time-honored myths and misconceptions have already been laid to rest. Today, men and women who understand the reproductive functions of their bodies have a better chance than ever before to become happy parents of healthy children. The following pages offer a summary of our present biological and medical knowledge in the area of human reproduction. Two special sections deal with contraception and abortion. The various social aspects of these issues are discussed in the third part of this book under "Sex and Society."

CONCEPTION

It used to be said of a pregnant woman that she had "conceived," or that a "conception" had taken place inside her body. Today, these terms are rarely heard in everyday speech, and many people may now find them pretentious and melodramatic. Nevertheless, scientists still fall back on the word "conception" as a matter of course when they want to refer to the beginning of a new life or the beginning of the existence of a new individual. However, these seemingly simple definitions cover a very complex phenomenon that even now is far from being fully understood. Consequently, not all scientists use the word "conception" in the same way.

We know that a woman's pregnancy results from a combination of several biological processes. Among these are:

- The union of a male and female sex cell which produces a new single cell called zygote. This process is called **fertilization.**
- The growth of the zygote by cell division, resulting in a hollow ball of cells called blastocyst. This process is called **segmentation**.
- The attachment of the blastocyst to the lining of the uterus. This process is called **implantation**.

If anything goes wrong with even one of these processes, no pregnancy can occur.

Still, for certain scientific reasons many developmental biologists prefer to speak of a conception as soon as the process of fertilization is completed. On the other hand, some reproductive physiologists believe for their own scientific reasons that a new life begins with the process of implantation. For them, no conception occurs unless the fertilization leads to pregnancy.

These different scientific approaches to the same problem may sometimes confuse the layman who tries to learn at what particular moment a human life begins. However, he may well remember that the advances of modern science have also shattered many traditional assumptions about the exact moment of death. With our increasing scientific knowledge, the beginning as well as the end of life have become more difficult to define. Indeed, it is now very hard to pinpoint any specific moment for either. It seems that we need to know still more (and develop a more precise terminology) before we can really answer these difficult questions.

The following paragraphs offer a summary of what is known today about the main biological processes that contribute to the reproduction of human life.

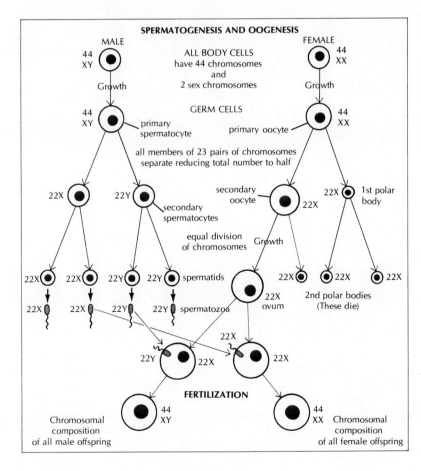

THE DETERMINATION OF SEX

The chart first compares the production of male and female sex cells and then shows the possible results of fertilizations.

1. Spermatogenesis and Oogenesis
While one primary spermatocyte eventually gives rise to four mature spermatozoa, a primary oocyte gives rise to only one ovum. The minute polar bodies which are formed in the process of oogenesis simply die and disintegrate. (See also pp. 29-30 and 45).

2. Fertilization
All mature ova carry an x-chromosome, but the spermatozoa carry either an x- or a y-chromosome. Thus, the union of a spermatozoon and an ovum (fertilization) can result in either one of two possible new cells: one growing into a boy (the xy-combination) or one growing into a girl (the xx-combination).

THE MALE SEX CELL: SPERM

Human life is reproduced sexually, i.e., by the combined effort of two individuals of different sex: a male and a female. In order to reproduce, both the male and the female must be sexually mature, i.e., their bodies must have developed to the point where they produce sex cells (gametes).

The male sex cell is called sperm (spermatozoon, plural: spermatozoa). Sperm cells are produced in the male sex glands (testicles). They are the smallest cells in the human body. While they are invisible to the naked eye, they can be seen and studied under the microscope. An individual sperm cell has a certain vague resemblance to a very skinny tadpole, and it is composed of three main units: head, body, and tail. Its total length is about 1/600th of an inch. The head, which is only 1/10th of the length of the sperm, contains twenty-three special bodies (chromosomes) carrying the man's inheritable characteristics. One of these chromosomes determines the sex of the child that might be produced if this particular sperm should unite with a woman's egg. In other words, sperm cells come in two varieties: those (containing an X-chromosome) that will help produce girls, and those (containing a Y-chromosome) that will help produce boys. Behind the head is the body, which plays an important part in obtaining the energy that enables the sperm to move. The movement itself is caused by the vigorous, whip-like lashings of the tail. The sperm can thus move ahead at the rate of 1/8th of an inch per minute under favorable conditions. This movement is essential since the sperm has to reach the egg deep inside the woman's body (i.e., in one of the Fallopian tubes).

Once the male sex glands have matured during puberty, they produce millions of sperm cells every day. Obviously, only the tiniest fraction of that number can ever contribute to actual conceptions. In the course of a man's life, most of his sperm cells are ejaculated under conditions that offer no chance for a fertilization. Those that are not ejaculated are simply reabsorbed into the body.

THE FEMALE SEX CELL: EGG

The female sex cell is called egg (ovum, plural: ova). Eggs are produced in the female sex glands (ovaries), and they are the largest cells in the human body. They are visible to the naked eye, being about the size of the dot at the end of this sentence. The contrast in volume between egg and sperm is immense. It would take only the combined total length of three sperm cells to span the diameter of one egg, but the egg's volume is 85,000 times greater than that of the sperm. The egg is round in shape and it contains twenty-three special bodies (chromosomes) which carry the woman's inheritable characteristics. However, unlike sperm cells eggs come in one variety only—they all contain X chromosomes. If an egg unites with a sperm that also carries an X chromosome, the child resulting from that union will be a girl. However, if the same egg should unite with a sperm carrying a Y chromosome, the child would be a boy. In other words, the sex of a child is determined not by the content of the egg, but by that of the sperm. The egg does not leave the woman's body in order to unite with the sperm. Instead, the sperm has to be brought to the egg if a fertilization is to be possible.

Once the female sex glands have matured during puberty, they normally release not more than one egg per month. Even so, in the course of a woman's life their total number may very well reach more than 400. Obviously, most of them will never be fertilized and thus never contribute to actual conceptions. Instead, they simply die and dissolve.

COITUS

As mentioned earlier, a conception can occur only inside a woman's body. Here then is the place where sperm and egg have to meet. Their meeting is usually brought about as a result of coitus. This Latin term (literally, going together) refers to the kind of sexual intercourse in which the penis is inserted into the vagina. Other words for coitus are copulation or genital intercourse.

The intimate contact of the male and female sex organs during coitus can give both partners great pleasure. The pleasure mounts as their bodies move

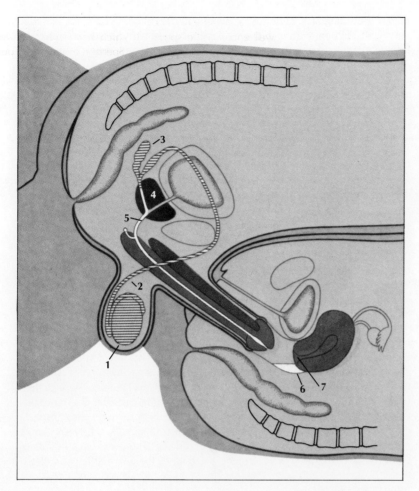

COITUS

The illustration shows the path of the sperm cells from the testicle through the vas deferens. At the end of this journey they are ready to be released through sexual activity. During coitus, the available sperm cells enter the prostate gland where they become part of the semen which is ejaculated into the vagina close to the cervix.

1. *Testicle*
2. *Vas deferens*
3. *Seminal vesicle*
4. *Prostate*
5. *Urethra*
6. *Seminal pool*
7. *Cervix*

to increase the mutual stimulation. Eventually, pleasure and excitement reach a climax. This climax, which provides relief and deep satisfaction, is called orgasm, and for the man it means the sudden release of his semen from his sex organs into those of the woman. This semen contains the sperm cells. Obviously, the man's orgasm is very important for human reproduction. Only during orgasm can he experience the muscular contractions inside his sex organs that are needed to discharge the semen. This sudden discharge is called ejaculation. Without ejaculation the sperm cells remain inside the man's body. However, there are some exceptions to this rule. It is not impossible for a man to release some sperm in advance of his orgasm and even if the orgasm should eventually fail to occur. (For details, see "Contraception—Withdrawal.")

A woman can, of course, very well become pregnant without having an orgasm. (For details on male and female orgasm, see "The Male Sexual Response" and "The Female Sexual Response.")

It should also be mentioned that modern medical techniques have made it possible to bring sperm and egg together by artificial insemination, i.e., without coitus. (For details, see "Infertility.")

When an egg is released from one of the ovaries, it almost immediately enters the open end of the adjacent Fallopian tube. As it travels down this tube toward the uterus, it matures to become ready for the union with a sperm cell. Within a few hours, the egg reaches maturity while it is still in the upper third of the Fallopian tube. This is the time when the sperm should arrive if a fertilization is to occur. The entire period in which egg and sperm can unite is less than twenty-four hours. If no such union takes place, the egg

FERTILIZATION

dies and disintegrates. However, moving into the Fallopian tube, the egg may very well encounter live sperm cells which have arrived and stayed there following coitus several days before. (Sperm cells have been found alive inside Fallopian tubes up to five days after coitus.)

When sperm cells are ejaculated, they are swimming in a thick, greyish-white fluid called semen. Following coitus, the semen is deposited close to the entrance of the uterus. The total volume of semen thus discharged at one time is less than a teaspoonful, but it contains between 200 and 500 million sperm cells, which now try to move into the uterus and onward up into the Fallopian tubes. However, unless an egg has been released by one of the ovaries around that time, the opening of the uterus will be plugged by an impenetrable, thick mucus. Only during ovulation does this mucus become thin enough to be penetrated by sperm cells. Even then, only about 1 percent of them succeed. The others die within a few hours in the slightly acidic, and therefore hostile, environment of the vagina. Those sperm cells that enter the uterus find themselves in a slightly alkaline, and therefore friendly, environment. Furthermore, muscular movements of the uterus and Fallopian tubes help them along on their way. Nevertheless, only a few hundred or a few thousand ever reach that upper part of the tubes where a union of egg and sperm can occur. (Naturally, the sperm cells enter both tubes whether an egg is present or not.)

Usually, several sperm cells reach the egg at the same time. However, only one of them penetrates it, because immediately upon first penetration a chemical change in the outer layer of the egg prevents any additional sperm cells from breaking through. As soon as it enters the egg, the sperm cell loses its tail. The compact sperm swells and forms a small nucleus which then unites with a similar small nucleus developed by the egg. The entire process is called fertilization. It is complete when the twenty-three chromosomes derived from the nucleus of the sperm have joined with the twenty-three chromosomes derived from the nucleus of the egg. Thus, a new cell containing forty-six chromosomes is formed. It combines the inheritable characteristics of both man and woman. This new cell, which is the direct result of fertilization, is called a zygote.

FROM OVULATION TO IMPLANTATION

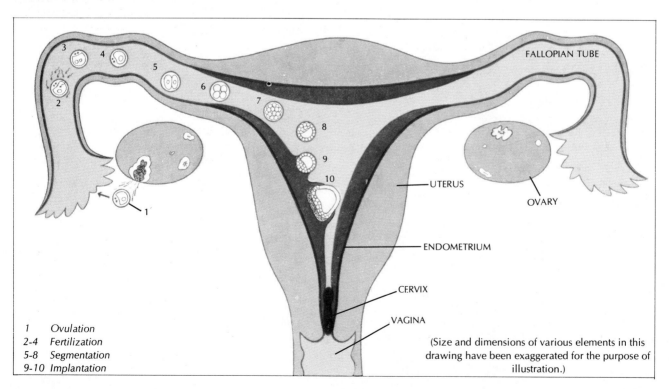

FALLOPIAN TUBE
UTERUS
OVARY
ENDOMETRIUM
CERVIX
VAGINA

1   Ovulation
2-4   Fertilization
5-8   Segmentation
9-10   Implantation

(Size and dimensions of various elements in this drawing have been exaggerated for the purpose of illustration.)

Within a few hours after the nucleus of the sperm has united with the nucleus of the egg, the result of their union, the zygote, begins a process of internal division. First, it divides into two cells, then four, eight, sixteen, and so on, doubling the number with each new division. This process of cell division or cleavage in the zygote is called segmentation. It transforms the zygote into a cluster of cells called a morula which, seen through a microscope, resembles a mulberry. The morula slowly moves down the Fallopian tubes toward the uterus, where it arrives after about three days. By this time, it has developed into a hollow ball of cells called a blastocyst.

SEGMENTATION

After its arrival in the uterus, the blastocyst continues to develop until, after another three to four days, it is ready to attach itself to the uterine lining. About one week after fertilization this attachment begins, and after about another week the blastocyst has completely buried itself in the nourishing tissues that cover the inner surface of the uterus (the endometrium). The entire process is called implantation, and it accomplishes pregnancy.

An implantation can occur only under certain proper conditions. For example, if the zygote should reach the uterus before it has developed into a blastocyst, no implantation is possible and pregnancy cannot be established. The same is true if the uterine lining is not prepared to receive the blastocyst. In both cases, the cell cluster will simply die and disintegrate.

In some very rare instances, the blastocyst will attach itself not to the uterine wall but to the inside of the Fallopian tube or some other place outside the uterus, i.e., in the abdominal cavity. The result is called ectopic pregnancy, which cannot produce a live child and is dangerous to the woman. Therefore, ectopic (Greek *ek*: out + *topos*: place = out of place) pregnancies have to be terminated by surgery.

IMPLANTATION

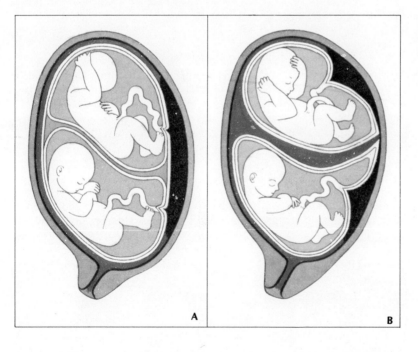

A B

TWO EXAMPLES OF TWINNING

A. Identical Twins *Fetuses are of the same sex and share one placenta. One outer membrane envelops both amniotic sacs.*

B. Fraternal Twins *Fetuses may be of different sex. There are two placentas and two separate amniotic sacs, each with its own membrane.*

In some cases, the zygote may proceed to an external division and split up into two separate cells. These two new cells then continue their development independently as they undergo their own segmentation. Eventually, they both arrive in the uterus where they also implant separately. The result is a twin pregnancy. Since both came from the same egg and the same sperm, the twins will be identical, i.e., they will be of the same sex and, of course, also look alike in every other respect.

MULTIPLE PREGNANCIES

Actually, identical twinning does not necessarily have to begin in the Fallopian tube, but can occur at any time between the second and fourteenth day after fertilization. Thus, even during implantation the blastocyst may still divide and grow into two separate embryos.

There are also some very rare cases of multiple ovulation, i.e., the release of several eggs at the same time. If these eggs are then fertilized, they may, of course, produce multiple pregnancies. Twins born as a result of such a pregnancy are known as fraternal twins. If three of these children are born, they are called triplets, four are quadruplets, five are quintuplets, and so on. Since each of them comes from a different egg fertilized by a different sperm cell, they may be of different sex and will not resemble each other any more than other brothers and sisters.

PREGNANCY

A woman's pregnancy begins with the implantation of the fertilized egg in her uterus and, under normal conditions, ends about nine months later with the birth of a baby. However, for certain purposes of medical calculation the beginning of pregnancy is not dated from the time of implantation, but from the first day of the last menstruation. (The reason for this is that a woman is not aware of an implantation, but usually can recall the date of her last menstruation.) According to this timetable, the woman will give birth 280 days (40 weeks) later. Using the same basis for calculation, the date of delivery can also be predicted by this rule of thumb: "Months minus 3, days plus 7." For example: First day of last menstruation: December 10, or, in numerals, 12/10.

"Months minus 3": 12 − 3 = 9
"Days plus 7": 10 + 7 = 17
Date of delivery: 9/17 or September 17.

Before a woman can deliver a healthy baby, a fascinating and extremely complex process of growth has to take place within her body. Even today, the exact mechanisms of this process are not completely understood. Nevertheless, its main phases can be described. The following paragraphs summarize how the fertilized egg develops through various stages into a viable and independent human being and how this development is experienced by the pregnant woman.

DEVELOPMENT OF EMBRYO AND FETUS

As the fertilized egg develops into the baby we see at birth, it goes through three main stages of growth: 1. the stage of the zygote (before implantation), 2. the stage of the embryo (early in the pregnancy), and 3. the stage of the fetus (later in the pregnancy). Since the first of these stages has already been discussed (see "Conception"), we now turn to a description of how the new organism grows inside the uterus.

The Embryo

The word embryo (Greek: swelling within) refers to the growing organism from the second to the eighth week of its life. During this time, it develops from a tiny cell cluster into a little growth of about 1 inch in length. As this development proceeds, the placenta, a special organ of interchange, begins to grow between the embryo and the uterus. The embryo is connected to the placenta by the umbilical cord. (Soon after the birth of the baby, its umbilical cord is still connected to the placenta which is then expelled from the uterus. For this reason, the placenta is also called the afterbirth.) The placenta acts as a filter and as a barrier. It allows the embryo (and later the fetus) to absorb food and oxygen from the woman's blood and to eliminate carbon dioxide and other waste from its own blood in return. At the same time, however, the two blood systems remain completely separate.

During the first month of its life, the human embryo looks like that of any other higher animal, such as a cat, dog, or pig, for example. Then, during the second month, it slowly assumes human features. It starts to develop a recognizable face, as well as arms, legs, fingers, and toes. Between its legs, the primitive beginnings of sexual organs become discernible, although they are still undifferentiated at this point (i.e., they are the same for both male and female). When the entire growing organism finally becomes clearly identifiable as human, it leaves the stage of the embryo and enters that of the fetus.

The Fetus

The word fetus (Latin: offspring) is used to describe the growing organism from the beginning of the third month of its life to the moment of birth. During this time, it develops from a small growth of slightly over an inch weighing only a fraction of an ounce into a baby of about twenty inches in length weighing approximately seven pounds. In the first weeks of this development, the male-female sex differentiation becomes apparent in the internal sex organs. A little later, the external sex organs develop their characteristic structure. Sometime around the fifth month, the fetal movements become strong enough to be felt by the expectant mother. This so-called quickening was formerly believed to be the moment when life entered the new body.

Throughout its growth, the fetus is well protected from injuries as it floats almost weightlessly inside a fluid-filled sac called the amniotic sac. At the end of the sixth month, the fetus measures about six inches in length and weighs about one and a half pounds. At this time, the centers of the brain which control breathing begin to develop. It is not entirely impossible (although very unlikely) that such a fetus could actually survive a premature birth. However, the probability of brain damage because of still ineffective breathing is great. The last months of fetal development bring further refinements, such as the temperature control mechanism in the brain and a protective layer of fat under the skin. In the case of a male fetus, the testicles descend into the scrotum. If this descent should fail to occur, corrective measures have to be taken sometime after birth. Otherwise, sterility will result. (For details, see "Sexual Malformations.")

During the final weeks before birth, the fetus not only grows rapidly in size, but also gains much of its weight. The birth of a fetus weighing less than five pounds is premature.

Having summarized the development and growth of a new life before its birth, we now turn to the experience of the expectant mother.

The Signs of Pregnancy

The placenta, which develops in response to the implantation of an embryo, produces a certain hormone called chorionic gonadotropin. This hormone acts upon the ovaries, stimulating them to continue the production of the hormones estrogen and progesterone. As a result, no new eggs are released and no menstruation occurs since the uterine lining does not deteriorate but remains in its place for the duration of the pregnancy. (For details on the menstrual cycle, see "The Female Sex Organs.") For this reason, a woman who has had sexual intercourse usually suspects that she has become pregnant as soon as she misses her regular menstrual period. However, this sign alone is not conclusive because the menstruation may just be delayed for one reason or another (sometimes for quite a while). The likelihood of a pregnancy increases if she also experiences an enlargement of her breasts, a darkening of the area around the nipples, nausea (morning sickness), and a more frequent need to urinate. Still, all of these so-called presumptive signs of pregnancy do not mean definite proof.

A greater degree of certainty is provided by the so-called probable signs of

THE WOMAN DURING PREGNANCY

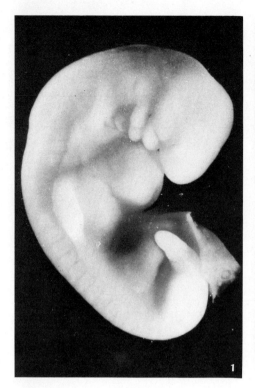
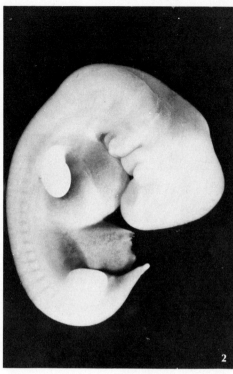
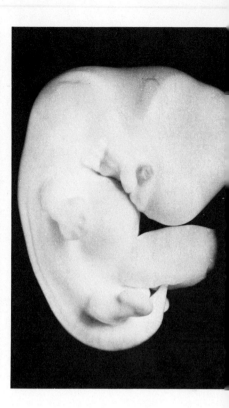

pregnancy, such as an enlargement of the uterus, a softening of the cervix, and an enlargement of the abdomen sometime during the third month. Three weeks after implantation (or about six weeks after the last menstruation) the placental hormone chorionic gonadotropin can be detected in the woman's urine. Such a simple pregnancy test can be made within a few minutes in a laboratory or in a doctor's office. However, although a positive test (detecting the hormone) is almost always correct, a negative result (failing to detect the hormone) is not necessarily reliable.

There are three truly reliable signs of pregnancy: 1. the heartbeat of the fetus, which the doctor can hear through his stethoscope at about the beginning of the fifth month, 2. the active movement of the fetus, which can be felt at about the same time, and 3, the skeleton of the fetus, which will appear on an X-ray picture. (The exposure of fetuses to X rays is usually avoided for medical reasons.)

The First Trimester

Doctors divide the nine months of a pregnancy into three trimesters, i.e., three equal time periods each lasting three months. During the first trimester (dated from the first day of the last menstruation), the woman experiences the early signs of pregnancy. Thus, a lack of menstruation and morning sickness are usually sufficient reason to see the family doctor or an obstetrician. The doctor will try to determine whether a pregnancy has, in fact, occurred. As mentioned above, simple hormonal pregnancy tests are possible about six weeks after the last menstruation. If the pregnancy is confirmed, medical supervision and care should continue up to the time of delivery. The woman's medical history has to be taken, and a thorough physical examination has to determine whether any problems or complications should be expected. In addition, several tests have to be performed. For example, one blood test will find out whether the woman is Rh-positive or Rh-negative; another can detect syphilis. (For details, see "Possible Problems and Complications" and "Venereal Diseases.") All of these measures can contribute to a normal pregnancy and the birth of a healthy baby.

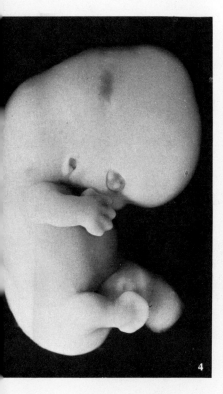
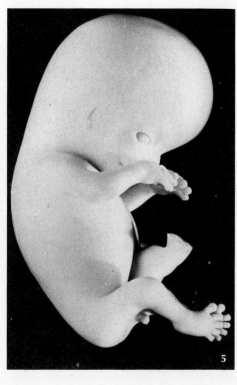

DEVELOPMENT OF EMBRYO
1. 4 weeks
2. 5 weeks
3. 6 weeks
4. 7 weeks
5. 8 weeks

The Second Trimester

The time between the beginning of the fourth and the end of the sixth month is usually the most comfortable for the pregnant woman. The previous morning sickness disappears, and the fetus, being still rather small, does not cause any discomfort. However, sometime around the fifth month the fetal movements can be felt, and the fetal heartbeat can be heard without any elaborate equipment. As the fetus continues to grow, the abdomen begins to enlarge visibly until, toward the end of the second trimester, the pregnancy becomes quite apparent.

The Third Trimester

During the last three months of pregnancy, the woman has to visit her doctor more often because potential complications are most likely to occur during this period. The growth of the fetus becomes even more obvious as the swelling in the woman's abdomen reaches higher above the navel. By the thirty-eighth week of pregnancy, the fetus has attained its maximum growth and is then called term fetus. It is ready to be born.

The exact time from the beginning to the end of pregnancy varies, even with the same woman. Women who engage in vigorous physical exercise usually deliver sooner than others, girls are often born a little earlier than boys, and, in some very rare cases, pregnancies last over 280 days.

Possible Problems and Complications

In the course of a pregnancy, a woman's body changes in many ways. Some of these changes may be experienced as unsettling or unpleasant. For example, nausea, indigestion, constipation, backaches, cramps, and varicose veins are not uncommon in expectant mothers and may cause some concern. However, these complaints do not indicate serious problems in themselves, but are a normal part of childbearing. Nevertheless, there are some complications that require medical attention. A woman can forestall, alleviate, or at least prepare herself for most of these difficulties by regular visits to her doctor during her pregnancy.

Spontaneous Abortion

Almost 25 percent of all pregnancies end with the death of the fetus during the first two trimesters, i.e., in spontaneous abortions or miscarriages. The reason is usually some abnormal development of the fetus caused by a defective egg or sperm, or by some difficulty in implantation. Other reasons are anatomical or functional abnormalities in the woman. The cause may also be found in a poor diet, an illness, or some psychological problem. Strenuous physical exercise as such has no harmful effect. Contrary to popular belief, jumping, falling, or being struck or kicked in the abdomen do not cause a woman to have a miscarriage.

Premature Birth

A miscarriage during the last trimester is called stillbirth. However, the closer the normal date of delivery is at hand, the greater is the chance for survival of the fetus. It is possible (although quite rare) that a fetus born toward the end of the sixth month might survive. After seven months, the chance of survival is fairly good and increases even further during the eighth month. Naturally, in all of these cases expert care is important.

The causes of premature births are not always clear. It has been suggested that certain illnesses or other maternal problems might be responsible. Indeed, there is some evidence that heavy smoking on the part of the expectant mother may be a contributing factor.

The Rh Factor

The Rh factor (short for Rhesus factor) is an antigen present in the blood of most people. These people are therefore called Rh-positive. A problem arises when a woman with Rh-negative blood becomes pregnant by an Rh-positive man. In this case, the fetus may also be Rh-positive. The woman's body may react to this situation by producing antibodies which could harm the fetus. In the case of a first pregnancy, this is usually not much of a problem, although later pregnancies can be adversely affected. Still, such conditions can be controlled by modern medical measures.

Toxemia

Toxemia is a disease of pregnancy which produces symptoms such as high blood pressure, a sudden weight gain, swollen ankles, and protein in the urine. If it goes unchecked, toxemia can lead to dangerous convulsions (eclampsia), or to premature separation of the placenta. There is no complete agreement as to the cause of this disease. It seems, however, that a properly balanced diet can do much to prevent it.

False Pregnancy

There are some very rare cases where a woman who is not pregnant develops symptoms quite similar to those of pregnancy. She may stop menstruating for months and experience morning sickness, a weight gain, an enlargement of the abdomen, indeed even labor, and all this in spite of the fact that there is no fetus that could be delivered. Quite obviously, this condition can be recognized by the absence of reliable signs of pregnancy (fetal movements, fetal heartbeat, and fetal skeleton on an X-ray picture).

SEXUAL INTERCOURSE DURING PREGNANCY

During pregnancy, some women like to have more sexual intercourse while some others would prefer less. Generally speaking, it seems that many women experience an increase in sexual desire during the second trimester of their pregnancy. This desire may then very well diminish during the last trimester.

Whether a woman should have sexual intercourse at any stage of the pregnancy depends, of course, very much on her personal feelings. From a purely medical point of view, there is no reason why sexual intercourse should not take place at any time except when explicitly discouraged by a

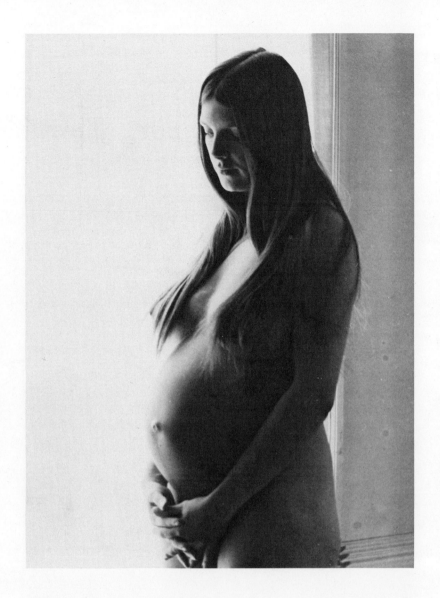

doctor. Usually, he will advise against it only under the following circumstances: 1. if it causes vaginal or abdominal pain, 2. if there is any uterine bleeding, 3. when the membranes have ruptured (for details, see "Birth"), and 4. if there is a danger of miscarriage or premature birth due to uterine contractions during orgasm. (In this latter case, it does not make any difference how the orgasm is reached. In other words, masturbation must also be avoided.) It has also been suggested that air blown into the vagina during pregnancy may cause serious damage to both the fetus and the woman. For this reason, a certain kind of oral intercourse (cunnilingus) may also be inadvisable during this time. In each of the above cases, the doctor's advice should be based on the individual situation, and it should be explained to both sexual partners.

As the pregnancy progresses, the woman's protruding abdomen makes sexual intercourse in certain positions uncomfortable and even impossible. Coitus with the man lying on top of the woman may thus have to be ruled out. A side position for both partners, and positions with the man behind the woman, or the woman sitting on top of the man may be more appropriate and enjoyable. It may also be useful to remember that coitus is only one among many possible forms of sexual intercourse, and that, at least for a while, other kinds of lovemaking can be adequate substitutes. (For details, see "Heterosexual Intercourse.")

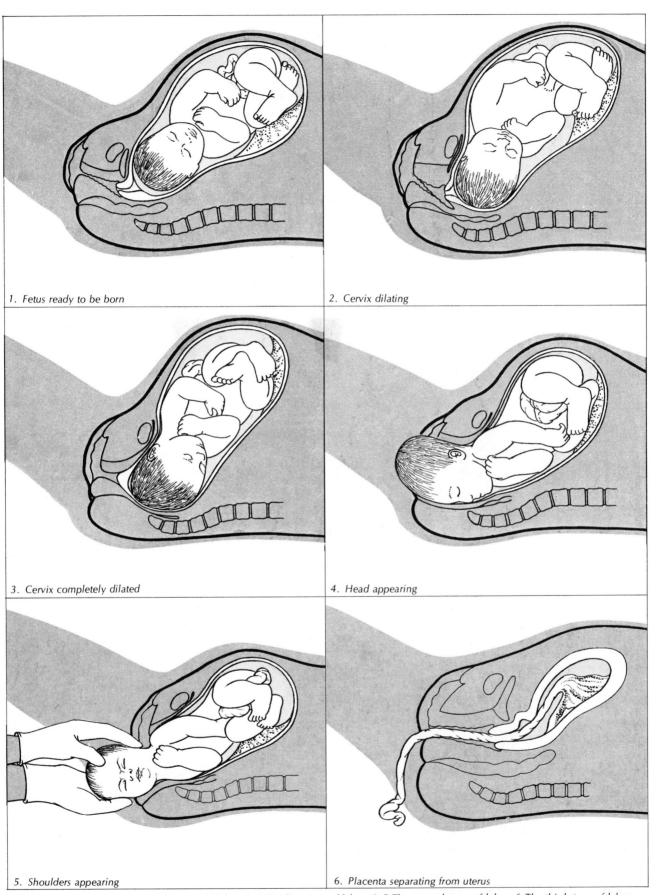

1. Fetus ready to be born

2. Cervix dilating

3. Cervix completely dilated

4. Head appearing

5. Shoulders appearing

6. Placenta separating from uterus

BIRTH OF A BABY *1 Before the beginning of labor; 2–3 The first stage of labor; 4–5 The second stage of labor; 6 The third stage of labor*

BIRTH

The birth of a baby means great physical, emotional, and social changes in a woman's life. If she has consciously chosen her motherhood, she will look forward to most of these changes. In any case, she will have more control over her fate than did most of her female ancestors.

In Victorian times, women were deliberately kept ignorant about their own bodily functions. The entire subject of human reproduction was taboo. Sex organs were considered dirty. Indeed, people were not even supposed to look at themselves in the nude. Conception, pregnancy, and birth were dark and threatening mysteries. As a result, many women were afraid of becoming mothers—they were literally out of touch with their bodies.

In those days, childbirth could be a very depressing, degrading, and dangerous experience. For example, it was widely believed that a woman was destined to bear her children in pain and that such suffering was good for her since it would increase her motherly feelings. She was expected to play a completely passive role. As she had no understanding of the process of birth, she hardly knew what was happening to her. Furthermore, unsanitary conditions in homes and hospitals exposed mothers and their babies to serious infections. Thus, many women died in childbed, and many infants never survived the first few weeks of their lives.

In the meantime, medical advances have brought a drastic reduction in infant mortality, and today the expectant mother is safer on the delivery table than on the highway driving to the hospital. Similar progress has been made in the area of education. The modern woman can actively prepare herself for childbirth and turn it into one of the most rewarding experiences of her life.

The advantages of prepared childbirth were first popularized by Dr. G. Dick-Read, a British obstetrician, who believed that most of the pain during delivery was the result of unnecessary muscular tension. His method of "natural childbirth" was designed to produce relaxation through training in the proper physical and mental attitude.

More recently, the method of "educated childbirth" developed by Dr. F. Lamaze, a French obstetrician, has gained a wide following in this country. This method rests on the assumption that labor is a situation of stress, and that the woman's active participation is the best way of coping with it.

Still another method is the "husband-coached childbirth" developed by the American obstetrician Dr. Robert Bradley. This method uses an extensive training course in which the future mother learns to relax under the guidance of the father. The course takes much longer than the one used in the Lamaze method, but many parents are enthusiastic about it. The aim is a new physical and psychological closeness between mother and father and a birth without the use of drugs of any kind. (It would undoubtedly be more objective to call this method "father-coached childbirth" since not all fathers are husbands and not all mothers are wives.)

Finally, there is a new method called "birth without violence" which was introduced by the French obstetrician Dr. F. Leboyer. This method, which focuses on the child, is aimed at maintaining the natural processes with which the fetus has lived inside the mother's womb: darkness, silence, contact with the mother. Therefore, the delivery room is only dimly lit, a bath of warm water is prepared, and the medical staff is trained to perform quietly. In these surroundings, the babies are born quiet, wide-eyed, and gurgling happily. They are then immediately placed on their mother's stomach. The umbilical cord is left intact and is cut only when breathing has been well established. For a while, the mother gently massages her child who is subsequently bathed in warm water. The entire procedure is aimed at lessening the "birth trauma" and takes into account that the newborn child is a highly sensitive person.

There are still other new methods of childbirth, but the goal is always the same: transforming the birth of a baby from a numbing, passive experience into a conscious achievement. More and more often men also demand to contribute to this achievement by giving support to their women, and hospitals often encourage expectant fathers to remain present throughout the entire process. Childbirth preparation classes for both men and women are offered by many doctors, hospitals, and educational groups. This kind of joint parental instruction often brings the partners much closer together and, in fact, can be seen as a very desirable part of responsible parenthood.

In the meantime, there has also been an increase in home births because many women today do not want to be separated from their newborn children and also like to share their experience with their whole family. In addition, there are now experimental childbirth centers which are not hospitals and which try to avoid a hospital atmosphere.

All of these developments are to be welcomed, as long as they are professionally supervised and as long as emergency medical help remains readily available. The following paragraphs summarize the main biological processes that are part of childbirth.

LABOR AND DELIVERY

Doctors divide the process of childbirth into three stages: 1. the gradual dilation of the cervix, 2. the actual delivery of the baby into the world, and 3. the delivery of the placenta or afterbirth. Using this medical classification, we now discuss each of the stages separately.

The First Stage of Labor

The first stage of labor takes the longest time. (In general, about 16 hours for women delivering their first baby and about 8 hours for the others.) During this period, labor pains begin to be felt and slowly become more frequent and more intense. These recurring pains are caused by rhythmic muscular contractions of the uterus followed by complete relaxation.

At first, the contractions last about 30 seconds and occur about every 15 to 20 minutes. As labor progresses, the periods of relaxation shrink to about 3 to 4 minutes while the contractions last 60 seconds or more. A woman who has prepared herself for childbirth by appropriate exercises can ease much of the physical strain by relaxing and breathing in certain ways which support rather than fight the process taking place inside her body. This process is aimed at dilating the cervix to the point where the baby's head can pass through it into the vagina. Once this is accomplished, the first stage of labor has come to an end and the actual birth is near.

Labor contractions lasting close to a minute and which recur about every five minutes are reason enough to proceed to the hospital. Another sign that birth is at hand is the expulsion of the cervical mucous plug which acts as a barrier between vagina and uterus. (It will be flecked with some light red blood.) Still another sign is the rupture of the membranes of the amniotic sac (commonly called bag of waters). This rupture will produce a flow of clear, water-like fluid from the vagina.

The Second Stage of Labor

The second stage of labor is considerably shorter than the first. (About two hours for women delivering their first baby and about one hour for the others.) During this time, the baby passes head first from the uterus through the vagina into the outside world. The mother can do much to help this process by contracting her abdominal muscles and bearing down with all her strength. Once the head has emerged, the rest of the baby's body follows easily.

The newborn child is still connected to the placenta inside the uterus by the umbilical cord. However, from now on this source of nourishment and oxygen is no longer needed. The sudden change in temperature and atmospheric pressure (sometimes also a slap on the buttocks) causes the baby to draw the first breath. As soon as breathing has become regular, the umbilical cord is cut a few inches from the abdomen. (There is no pain since the cord does not contain any nerves.) After a while, the remaining stub dries up and then falls off by itself.

The Third Stage of Labor

The third and final stage of labor brings the expulsion of the placenta and the umbilical cord from the uterus about fifteen minutes after the baby's birth. The delivery of this so-called afterbirth takes only a few minutes, after which the uterus begins to shrink back to its former shape and size.

Possible Complications

Giving birth is a normal function of the female body. Most dangers and complications popularly associated with childbirth belong to the past. Usually they were caused not by the delivery itself, but by the primitive and unsanitary circumstances under which it took place. A modern woman who has been consulting her doctor throughout the pregnancy and who gives birth with expert assistance has no reason to fear serious problems. Possible difficulties can now be handled quickly and effectively. For example, very often the pressure of the appearing fetus threatens to tear the vaginal opening. In these cases, the doctor makes a small incision (an episiotomy) to prevent such a tear. The incision is easily repaired with some stitches and heals within a short time. Another problem may arise when the baby's feet or buttocks appear first (instead of the head as in most cases). This so-called breech presentation may prolong the process of delivery and can be somewhat risky to the baby. A possible risk for all babies is an eye infection with gonorrhea. In order to prevent such infections, the eyes of each newborn infant are treated with a solution of silver nitrate.

In some rare cases, a normal delivery may be impossible for one reason or another, and a Caesarean section may become necessary. This means that the doctor cuts through the abdomen into the uterus to remove the baby before it passes through the vagina. The term "Caesarean section" refers to the legend that Julius Caesar was born in this fashion.

THE PERIOD AFTER DELIVERY

After delivery, both mother and child are exhausted and need rest. Although most women get up and leave the hospital within a few days, they usually take some time to regain their full strength and to adjust to their new role. Some aspects of this post-delivery period are discussed below.

Recovery

In the weeks following childbirth, the uterus slowly shrinks back to its former size. In the process, the uterine lining breaks down and is discharged through the vagina. First, this discharge is thick and bloody, then it becomes thin and yellowish or whitish in color until, after about three weeks, all waste material has been removed. After six weeks, the shrinkage of the uterus is completed. The process can be helped considerably by appropriate physical exercises. Such exercises can also alleviate certain complaints and discomforts that some women feel during this time, such as loss of appetite or constipation.

In addition to these minor annoyances, many women experience a mild depression. They become overly sensitive, irritable, and may cry without any apparent reason. This kind of unexpected despair has not always been taken as seriously as it should. Many people speak jokingly of "the baby blues." However, there is nothing funny about it. The physical strain of giving birth together with the demands of the new role as mother may, for a while, seem to overwhelm a woman who suddenly feels that she is unprepared for the task. After all, whether recognized or not, becoming a parent is a genuine crisis in everyone's life. Still, like any other crisis, it carries great possibilities for growth. In this situation, a woman can be helped a great deal by her family, and particularly by the baby's father. It is another of those occasions when mutual understanding between man and woman is invaluable.

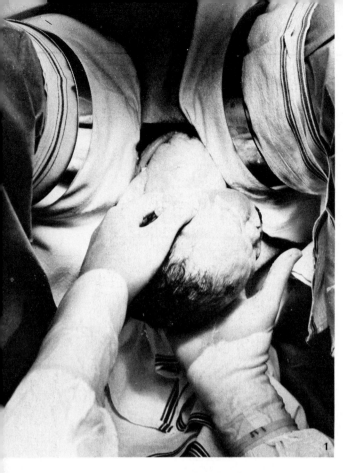

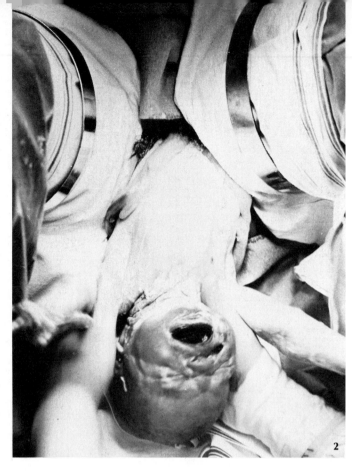

CHILDBIRTH IN THE HOSPITAL

In the United States today most children are born in the hospital. Expert medical attention and emergency help in case of complications have drastically reduced the possible dangers of childbirth for both mother and child.

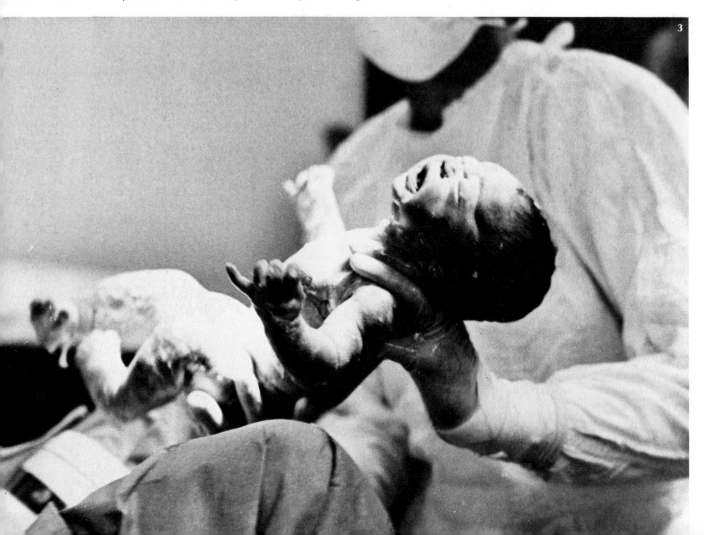

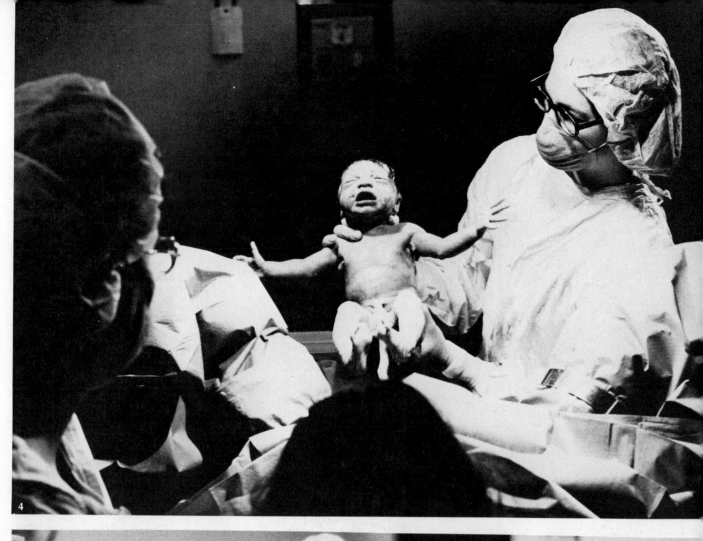

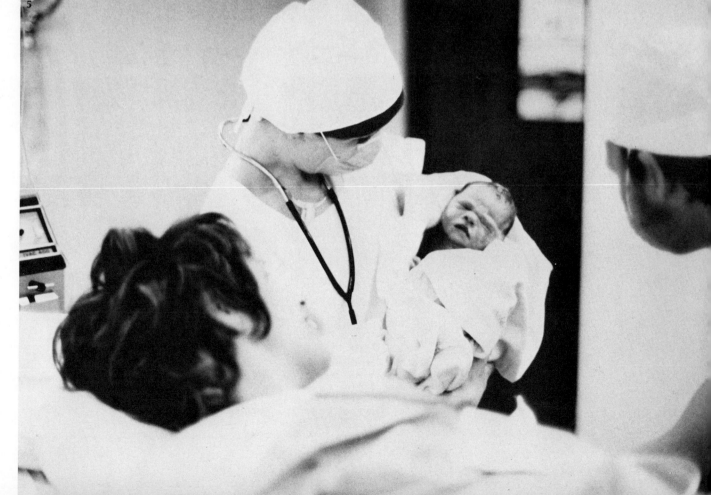

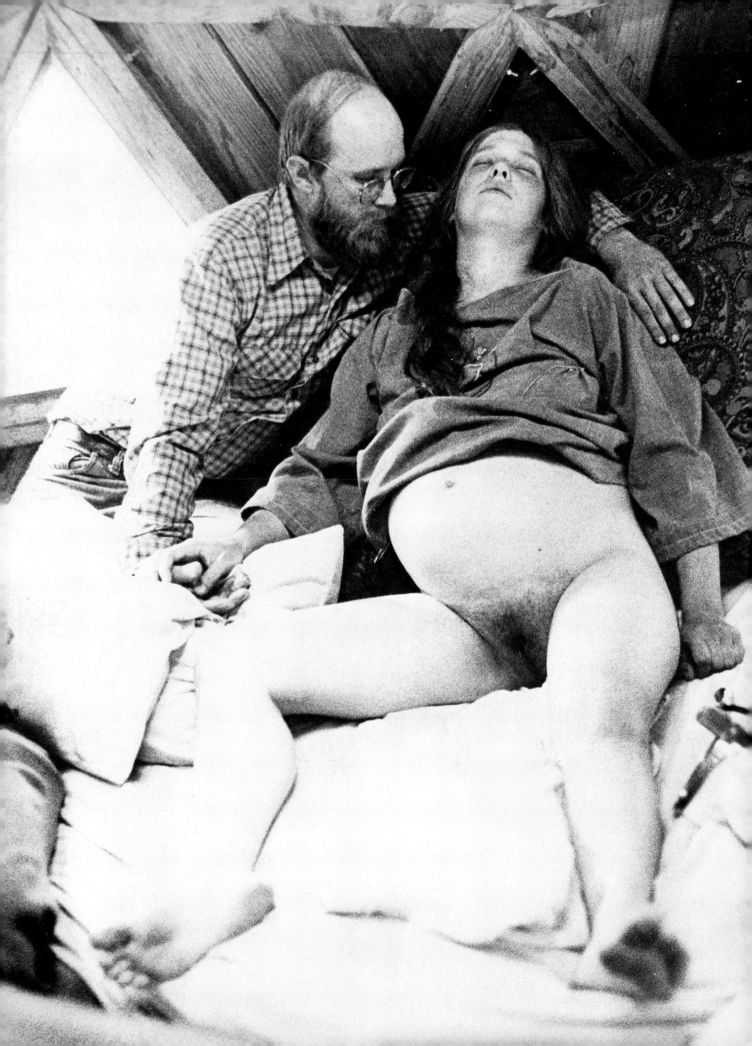

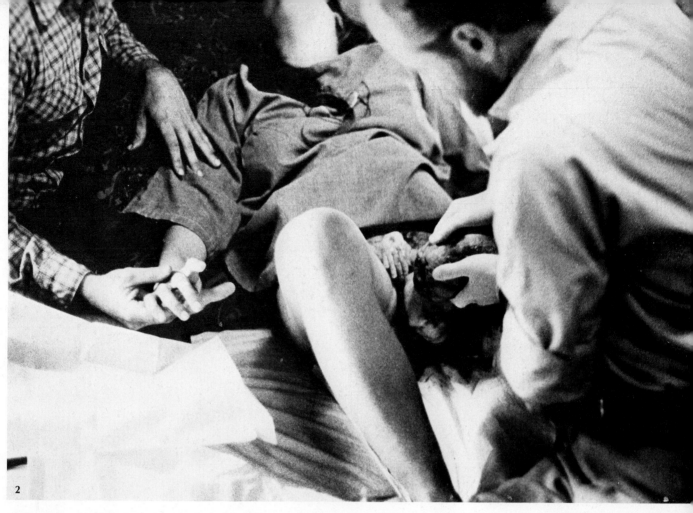

2

CHILDBIRTH AT HOME

In recent years many women have again begun to give birth at home where the event can be shared by the whole family. As long as professional help remains readily available, this practice need not be risky. In the pictures shown here the delivery is assisted by a licenced obstetrician.

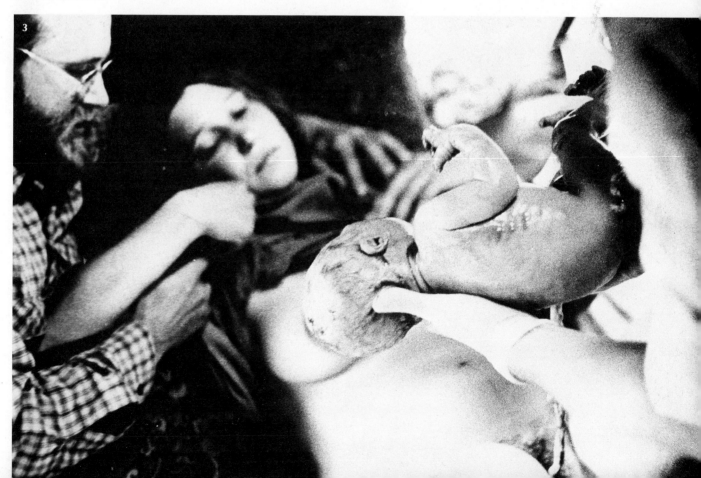

3

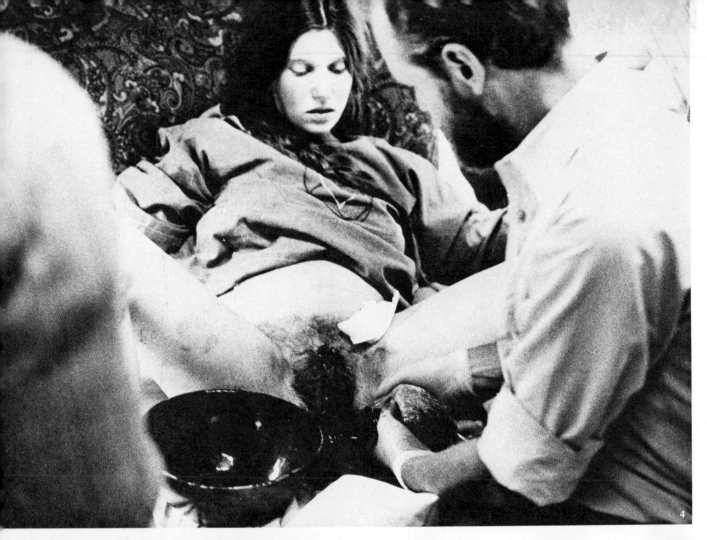

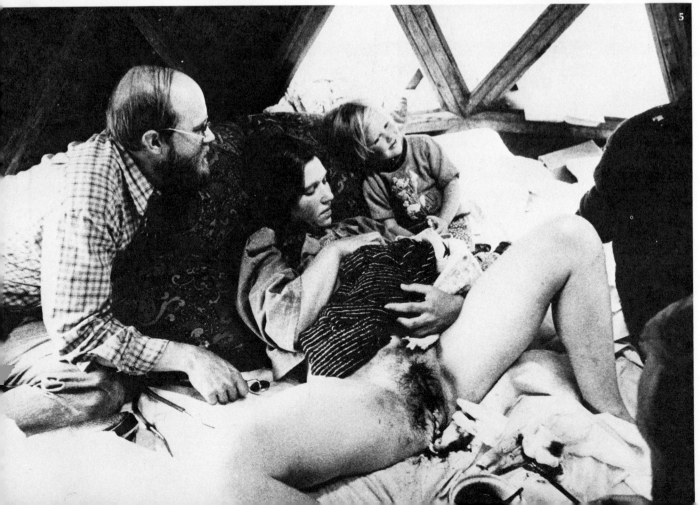

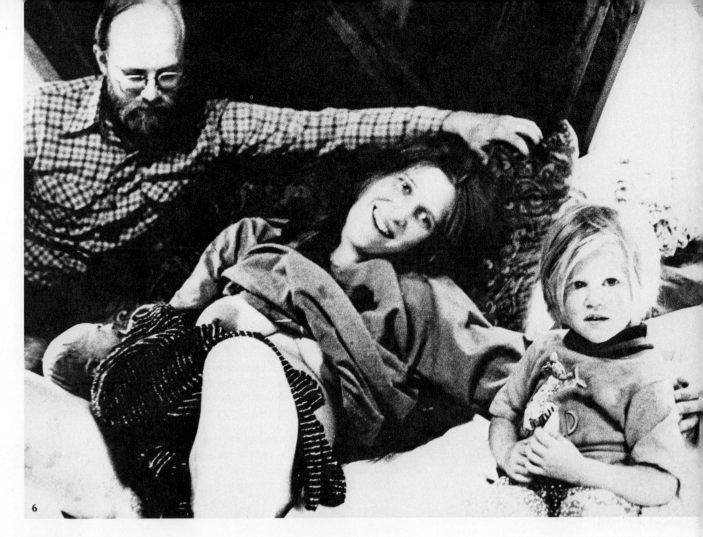

6

Lactation

Immediately after birth, the mother's breasts produce a watery fluid called colostrum which seems to have some immunizing effect on the baby. About three days later, this fluid is replaced by milk. The production of milk is called lactation (from Latin *lac:* milk), and if the mother decides to nurse her child, she will be able to do so for many months.

Most women stop ovulating (and therefore menstruating) during the first few months because of certain hormonal changes in the body. Obviously, this also means that, in the same period, no new conception can take place. However, couples should not count on this "natural protection." Nursing a baby is no substitute for contraception.

It is quite normal for a woman to become sexually aroused while she has her child suckling on her breast. There is no reason whatsoever to become upset or alarmed about this. On the contrary, the experience should be enjoyed as it serves important physiological and psychological functions.

Sexual Intercourse After Delivery

Once the baby is born, some women need time to regain interest in sexual relations, and traditionally couples have been advised not to engage in coitus for at least six weeks after delivery. However, recent research indicates that such general rules are not really helpful and that each case should be judged individually. Very often sexual intercourse can take place much sooner without any harm to the mother. Indeed, from a purely medical standpoint coitus can be resumed as soon as vaginal bleeding has stopped and any tears or incisions in the vaginal area have healed. A slight brownish discharge from the vagina can be disregarded.

Full communication (including sexual communication) between parents, is of course, also in the interest of the newborn child. Still, during this period the woman's personal feelings and desires should be considered first.

CONTRACEPTION

The most obvious and most reliable way of avoiding pregnancy is complete abstinence from coitus. However, throughout history men and women have searched for means of contraception, i.e., for methods or devices that would allow them to engage in coitus without the risk of becoming parents. For thousands of years, such methods as were found remained crude and largely ineffective. Eventually, modern scientists discovered new and better methods (and improved the old ones), until they arrived at the present wide range of reasonable choices. Today, unwanted pregnancies can be prevented with almost complete certainty. Nevertheless, the search for even safer, simpler, and cheaper contraceptives goes on.

The development of reliable methods of contraception has had a profound effect on human sexual behavior. In the past, sex and procreation were inseparable. Sexual intercourse between men and women was restricted to coitus, and potentially it could always lead to the birth of children. Obviously, the interests of these children could best be protected by making sure that the parents stayed together to take care of them. The sexual morals of most societies therefore tried to prohibit sexual activity for everyone but married couples. Sex before and outside of marriage was considered immoral (and was sometimes severely punished). Within the institution of marriage itself, men and women were encouraged to produce as many children as possible. In fact, procreation was declared the true "nature" and only purpose of sex, and all forms of sexual expression that, by their very character, could not lead to pregnancy were called unnatural.

In the meantime, the factual basis of this morality has been all but destroyed by the modern, effective methods of contraception. They have broken the traditional link between sex, parenthood, and marriage. Now a married couple may very well decide to remain childless, or to have children only many years after the wedding. By the same token, fewer young couples are rushed into ill-considered marriages by unwanted pregnancies. As a result, the meaning of marriage itself is beginning to change. Parenthood may no longer be its primary goal. Indeed, love, companionship, professional cooperation, mutual support, or security may now be sufficient reasons to bring and to keep husband and wife together. At the same time, sexual intercourse inside and outside of marriage can be completely divorced from the purpose of procreation. Instead, it is acquiring a new importance as a means of communication.

All of this amounts to a fundamental change in human affairs. There is a new freedom of action and a new need for personal decisions and responsibilities. The challenges of this unprecedented situation cannot be met by prohibitive ethics, restrictive laws, or repressive policies aimed at protecting the people against themselves. On the contrary, they must now be given a chance to develop the capacity for self-determination and to make the right use of their new possibilities.

Nevertheless, the old beliefs and habits die hard. There are still many men and women who either remain blind to the consequences of this contraceptive revolution, or who are honestly afraid of them. For example, there is a widespread concern that the universal acceptance of contraception might lead to universal promiscuity and moral decay. On the other hand, more and more people are becoming alarmed about the dangers of overpopulation. Indeed, there can be no doubt that a further unchecked growth of the population would produce mounting misery in many parts of the world and, paradoxically, could even lead to the extinction of the human race by famine, disease, war, and environmental pollution.

In many countries, these conflicting concerns have produced ambiguous public policies. Certain governments favor the use of contraceptives by married couples, but not by single adults or minors. Some governments support

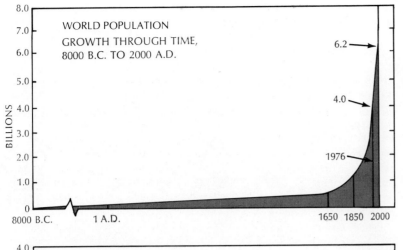

WORLD POPULATION
GROWTH THROUGH TIME,
8000 B.C. TO 2000 A.D.

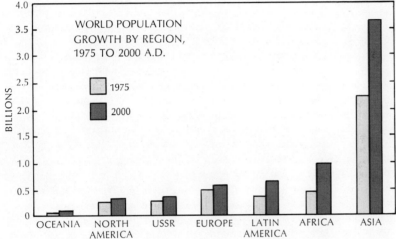

WORLD POPULATION
GROWTH BY REGION,
1975 TO 2000 A.D.

1975
2000

THE "POPULATION EXPLOSION"

Over the last few hundred years the world's population has grown dramatically, and in the future an even more dramatic increase is to be expected. Furthermore, as our graph illustrates, the greatest such increase is likely to take place in the poorest areas of the globe. In view of these developments, many governments have now begun to encourage contraception.

Tables courtesy of Population Reference Bureau, Inc. 1754 N Street, N.W./Washington D.C. 20036

the idea of contraception in order to eliminate the need for abortions which remain prohibited. Others see abortion simply as a welcome additional means of limiting the population. (Where contraception is made difficult, the number of abortions is bound to rise; where abortion is made easy, contraception may be neglected.) In some countries, both contraception and abortion are illegal. Still other countries hesitate to promote voluntary contraception among the general public, but have no scruples about forcing certain people to be sterilized. These sterilizations are usually carried out in order to prevent the transmission of severe genetic defects. (See "Genetic Defects.") However, sometimes forced sterilization has also been used for the purpose of social rather than medical control. (Healthy men and women are made infertile against their will because they are poor or otherwise "undesirable."

The very language in which different authorities speak about contraception often reveals their ideological standpoint. For example, many people today prefer to talk about "birth control." This is a term which includes abortion. (After all, an abortion also prevents a birth.) However, in most cases the issue is not the prevention of births, but of pregnancies, and therefore terms like "pregnancy control" or "conception control" ("contraception" for short) are more precise. Some people insist on using the phrase "family planning." This term implies that contraception is really nothing more than a method of determining the size of a family or, in other words, that it has its place only within marriage. A term like "pregnancy planning" would undoubtedly be more objective. Another term, "responsible parenthood," appeals to certain moral qualities in men and women who might be passive and fatalistic about possible pregnancies. A more neutral term, "planned parenthood," is used by a worldwide organization which offers contraception to all who seek it, whether they are married or not.

This policy springs from the realization that, in the long run, the use of contraception cannot remain restricted to selected groups or individuals. In fact, a growing number of men and women are now demanding full control over their own reproductive lives as a basic human right. The recognition of this right will mean one further step toward a more dignified and humane life. All couples will be able to have children by choice, not by chance, i.e., they will have them when they want them and as many as they want. Many people who know that they are sick, weak, or incompetent as parents will gladly decide not to have any children at all. Many others may postpone parenthood until they have matured emotionally or have achieved some success or financial security. Young people will no longer "get into trouble" or be "forced to marry." Every child will be a wanted child and thus have a better chance to grow up in a healthy environment.

While most people today look forward to this increase in human freedom, many have mixed feelings about the other side of the coin—there may be more sexual intercourse between unmarried couples (including the very young). For this reason, official sex education classes in schools, churches, and youth organizations often shy away from the subject of contraception. Furthermore, while most educators have little difficulty explaining the facts of human reproduction, they are usually ill at ease describing the various contraceptive methods because they then have to discuss the details of sexual activity. Parents of teenagers also find themselves in a dilemma. If they provide their children with contraceptives, they seem to encourage sexual intercourse; if they ignore the problem, they may invite unwanted pregnancies.

The law in regard to contraception for minors is unclear. Actually, in the United States today there is a maze of many different, overlapping, and sometimes contradictory laws and court decisions which make it difficult to determine whether teenagers are legally entitled to contraception at all or, if that is the case, they still need the permission of their parents.

Still, there are now many public and private groups and organizations, such as Planned Parenthood or students' health services, which offer contraception to unmarried minors. Indeed, it seems that teenagers and young adults need such help more than anybody else. Although they are sexually mature, they often have to wait many years before they can get married and support a family. Many of them are still confused about their own feelings, needs, and objectives in life. Very often they do not know enough or do not care enough about contraception. Some young people actually like to gamble in the hope that nature will decide for them, and that a pregnancy, if it should occur, would somehow bring some purpose and order to their lives. They may secretly hope that a baby of their own may prove their independence from their parents, or that it may help them to "get even" with somebody else. Some girls deliberately deceive their boy friends and try to get pregnant in order to force them into marriage or at least a steady relationship.

Most organizations that counsel teenagers about contraception are well aware of these problems. They are, therefore, not content with simply dispensing contraceptive devices, but try to spell out the alternatives and encourage responsible behavior. For this reason, they often invite boys and girls together for a personal discussion. This approach also makes it clear that contraception is always the responsibility of both sexual partners.

Remember:

- Every child should be a wanted child.
- Unwanted pregnancies can be prevented by the careful use of contraception.
- Contraception is the responsibility of both sexual partners.
- Not every contraceptive method is equally effective or suitable for everyone.
- No contraceptive method can work unless used properly.

Although the various contraceptive methods differ in effectiveness and sophistication, the principle of contraception itself is quite simple. As described in a previous section, the process of conception involves the fertilization of an egg by a sperm inside one of the Fallopian tubes leading to the eventual implantation of a growing cell cluster in the uterus, thus starting pregnancy. Obviously then, contraception, or the avoidance of pregnancy, involves an interference with this process by preventing either ovulation, fertilization, or implantation. This interference can take several different forms:

1. Preventing the release of an egg from the ovaries ("the pill").
2. Preventing the passage of the egg through the Fallopian tube (tubal ligation).
3. Preventing the sperm from becoming part of the ejaculated fluid (vasectomy).
4. Avoiding coitus at the time when an egg is available for fertilization (rhythm).
5. Preventing sperm from being deposited inside the vagina (withdrawal, condom).
6. Preventing the sperm inside the vagina from moving through and beyond the cervix (spermicides, diaphragm).
7. Hindering the process of implantation (IUD?, "morning-after pill").

All contraceptive methods listed here have been developed through long and careful observation of the procreative process. They all involve the application of scientific knowledge or rational calculation, and most of them require the use of chemicals, special tools, gadgets, and devices or a calendar and a thermometer. In each case, human cunning prevents nature from simply taking its course. In short, contraception is always the result of a conscious decision which uses certain laws of nature to defy certain others.

This elementary fact has sometimes been obscured by writers who have tried to create a distinction between "natural" and "artificial" means of contraception. Such a distinction is arbitrary and unscientific. However, for the practical purposes of everyday life it is useful to distinguish between those contraceptive methods that require medical consultation and those that do not.

Surgery is needed in the case of sterilization (vasectomy, tubal ligation). A doctor's prescription is needed for contraceptive pills, "morning-after pills," diaphragms, and intra-uterine devices (IUDs). A doctor's advice and supervision are important for the rhythm method. There are three methods of contraception which can be used without any professional help: withdrawal, condom, and spermicides.

Some contraceptives require a doctor's prescription because they could be ineffective or dangerous if used indiscriminately. As a matter of fact, it makes sense to seek professional advice before choosing any method of contraception. Such advice is offered by all Planned Parenthood offices and other family planning clinics as well as by many private physicians. Not every method is suitable for everybody at all times. Making the right individual choice is the first step toward success. In some cases, religious reasons or personal habits rule out certain methods, and what works well with one person today may fail with another tomorrow. It is, therefore, essential to understand how each method works in order to ensure its proper application. Many unwanted pregnancies occur because of careless use of otherwise effective methods.

Some experts have said in the past that any method of contraception is better than none at all. However, some methods are so ineffective as to be practically useless. Among these is karezza, or *coitus reservatus,* a form of coitus in which the man tries to avoid ejaculation. Although such an attempt may have certain emotional and even spiritual values, it does not necessarily prevent pregnancies. Another questionable method consists of inserting a small sponge together with some spermicidal powder or liquid into the vagina. This is not only ineffective, but may also interfere with coitus and cause discomfort. Still another method is vaginal douching after coitus or, in other words, the washing out of the vagina with some sort of solution in the hope of removing the sperm. This procedure is useless because it can never come soon enough to make any difference. There are further certain "feminine hygiene" products which are advertised with hints at contraceptive powers. Nevertheless, they are quite ineffective in that respect and may actually be harmful to the vaginal tissue. In general, vaginal douching and spraying should be avoided because it is unnecessary. The vagina cleanses itself with its own secretions. Too much interference can only upset the vaginal ecology and cause infection or irritation. (See also "Venereal Diseases.") The following pages describe only those methods of contraception that work reasonably well.

CONDOMS

The condom is an excellent contraceptive which also offers some protection against venereal disease. In the United States today various brands of condoms are available to everyone in drugstores or in public vending machines. Many of the newer condoms are prelubricated and some are sold in a variety of colors or with ornamented tips ("French ticklers").

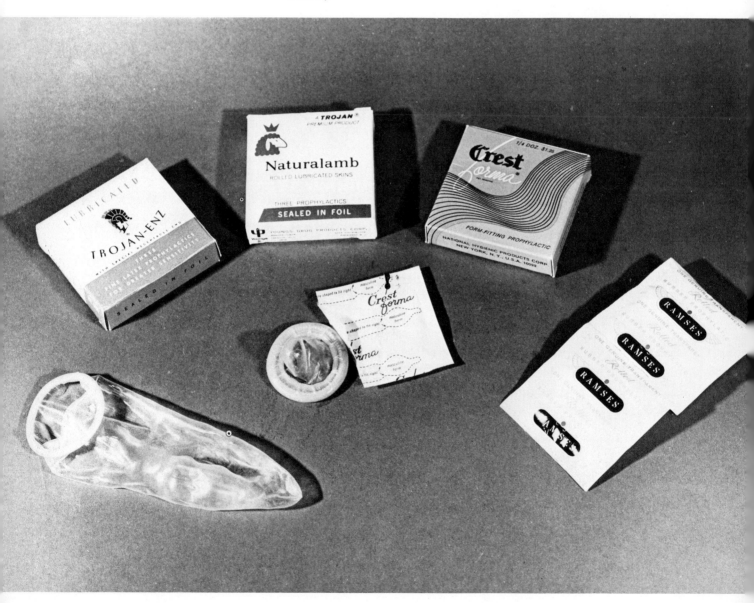

CONTRACEPTIVE METHODS FOR MEN

Withdrawal

The withdrawal method, also known by its Latin name *coitus interruptus*, is probably the oldest method of contraception. It simply means that during coitus the man withdraws his penis from the woman's vagina just before he ejaculates. As a result, his sperm is not deposited inside the woman's body and therefore cannot fertilize the egg.

While this sounds convincing in theory, it does not always work in practice. Many men have difficulty finding the right moment for withdrawal. The resulting worry and the need to control sexual reactions at all times can create considerable tension between sexual partners. It is also possible that some sperm is released from the penis well in advance of the actual ejaculation. Furthermore, even sperm cells that have been ejaculated outside the vagina can move inside by themselves as long as they are in contact with a moist surface. For these reasons, withdrawal is not reliable as a method of contraception. Its only advantage is the fact that it needs no preparation and can be used anytime. However, its disadvantages are so serious that most people will find it appropriate only in unusual circumstances, when no other methods are available.

Effectiveness: not very effective, but better than nothing.

Condom

The condom, also popularly known as prophylactic or rubber, is a sheath made of thin rubber, gut, or plastic. It is shaped like the finger of a glove and it is worn over the penis during sexual intercourse. Because it catches and retains the man's sperm after ejaculation, the woman cannot become pregnant.

The condom is a very effective contraceptive if used properly. It must be put on the erect penis before coitus (not just before ejaculation). At the tip of the penis, some space has to be left to accommodate the expected semen, otherwise the condom may burst. Immediately after ejaculation, the man must withdraw his penis before losing his erection, holding on to the condom at its base so that it cannot slip off. The effectiveness can be increased still further by putting some spermicidal cream or jelly on the outside of the condom after it is in place on the penis, or by having the woman use spermicidal foam at the same time.

Despite its obvious advantages, some people object to the condom either because they do not like the procedure of putting it on during their love play or because they claim that the feeling of rubber dulls their sensation. Nevertheless, all things considered, the condom is still one of the simplest, safest, and therefore best contraceptives available. Moreover, it also provides some protection against venereal diseases. Condoms are not expensive and can be bought in drugstores without a prescription.

Effectiveness: about 95 percent, more if the woman uses foam.

CONTRACEPTIVE METHODS FOR WOMEN

Rhythm

The rhythm method of contraception consists simply of abstinence from coitus during a woman's fertile days. Although this method seems easy and effective in principle, it is quite complicated and unreliable in application.

The first problem is to determine the exact number of fertile or "unsafe" days that require coital abstinence. A woman can become pregnant only as long as an egg is in one of her Fallopian tubes. This means that her fertile or "unsafe" days are those shortly before, during, and shortly after ovulation. Abstinence before ovulation is necessary because sperm cells can stay alive inside a woman's body for some time, and abstinence afterwards is necessary because an egg can be fertilized for some time after ovulation. Since men-

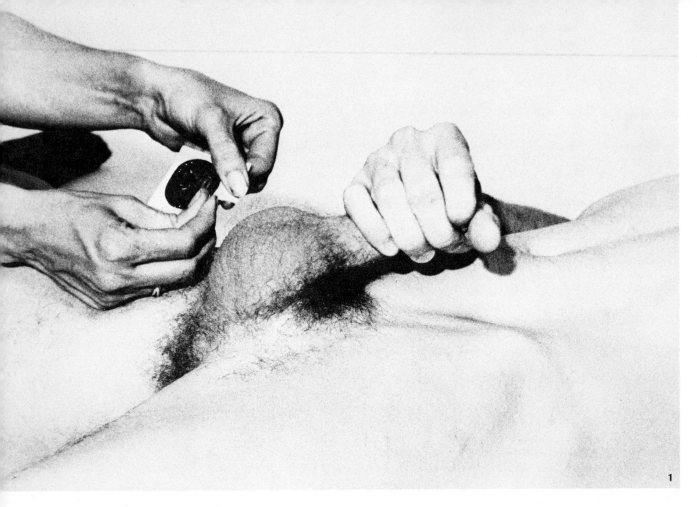

1

APPLICATION OF CONDOM
The application of a condom need not be an awkward interruption of intimacy, but can be a pleasurable shared experience. Indeed, many couples today make it part of their love play. This approach also helps both partners to remember that contraception is their common responsibility. Our pictures show a woman carefully putting a fashionable black condom on her partner's penis.

2

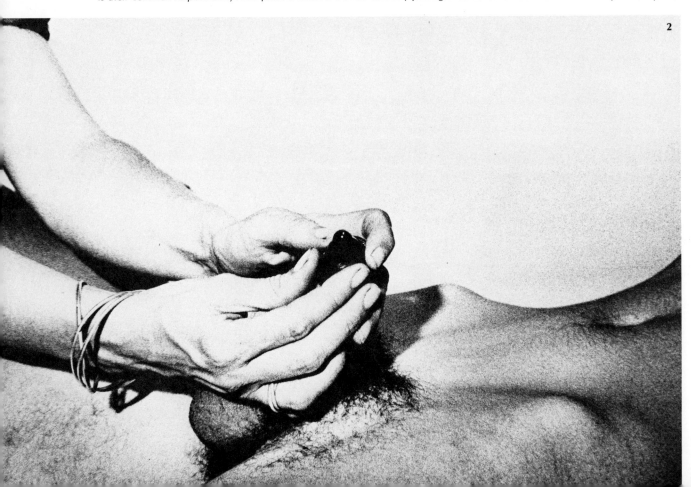

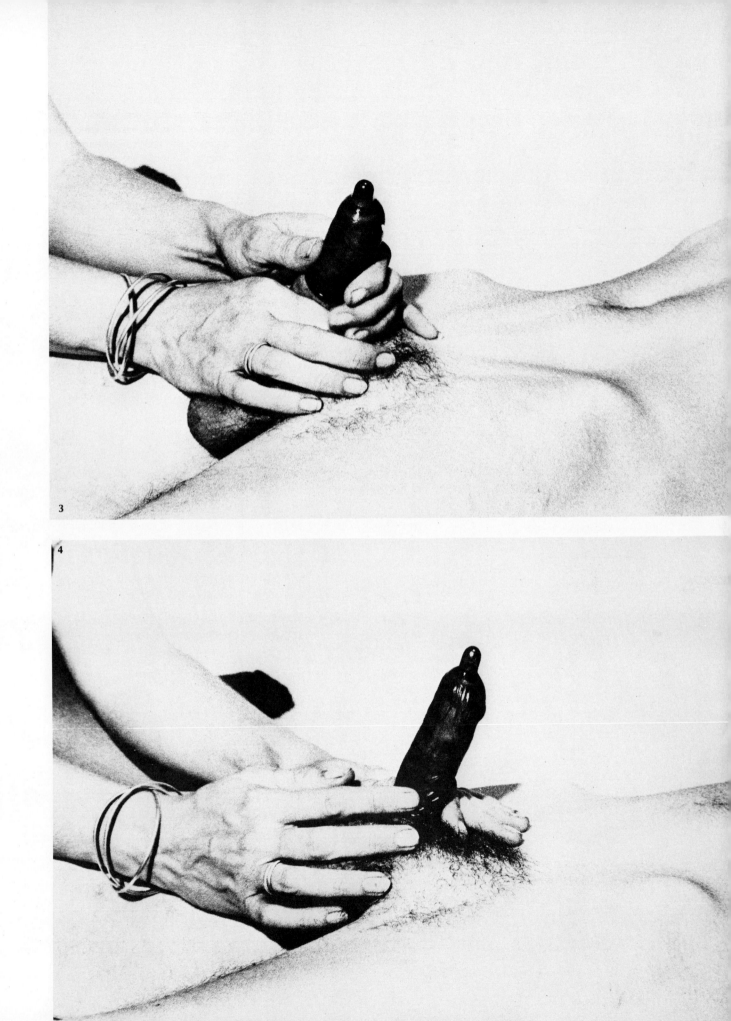

3

4

strual cycles are often irregular and the day of ovulation can therefore not be predicted accurately, one has to allow for a period of at least a week in which an egg could be available for fertilization. To this must be added the possible survival time of sperm cells (up to five days inside the Fallopian tubes), plus another day or two as a margin of safety. Therefore, on the average, the fertile or "unsafe" days add up to about two weeks of each menstrual cycle.

THE RHYTHM METHOD (CALENDAR) HOW TO DETERMINE THE "UNSAFE" DAYS					
SHORTEST CYCLE		FIRST "UNSAFE" DAY AFTER START OF ANY CYCLE	LONGEST CYCLE		LAST "UNSAFE" DAY AFTER START OF ANY CYCLE
21 DAYS	− 18 =	3rd DAY	21 DAYS	− 11 =	10th DAY
22 DAYS	− 18 =	4th DAY	22 DAYS	− 11 =	11th DAY
23 DAYS	− 18 =	5th DAY	23 DAYS	− 11 =	12th DAY
24 DAYS	− 18 =	6th DAY	24 DAYS	− 11 =	13th DAY
25 DAYS	− 18 =	7th DAY	25 DAYS	− 11 =	14th DAY
26 DAYS	− 18 =	8th DAY	26 DAYS	− 11 =	15th DAY
27 DAYS	− 18 =	9th DAY	27 DAYS	− 11 =	16th DAY
28 DAYS	− 18 =	10th DAY	28 DAYS	− 11 =	17th DAY
29 DAYS	− 18 =	11th DAY	29 DAYS	− 11 =	18th DAY
30 DAYS	− 18 =	12th DAY	30 DAYS	− 11 =	19th DAY
31 DAYS	− 18 =	13th DAY	31 DAYS	− 11 =	20th DAY
32 DAYS	− 18 =	14th DAY	32 DAYS	− 11 =	21st DAY
33 DAYS	− 18 =	15th DAY	33 DAYS	− 11 =	22nd DAY
34 DAYS	− 18 =	16th DAY	34 DAYS	− 11 =	23rd DAY
35 DAYS	− 18 =	17th DAY	35 DAYS	− 11 =	24th DAY
36 DAYS etc.	− 18 =	18th DAY	36 DAYS etc.	− 11 =	25th DAY

THE RHYTHM METHOD
(BASAL TEMPERATURE)

BASAL BODY TEMPERATURE DURING THE MENSTRUAL CYCLE

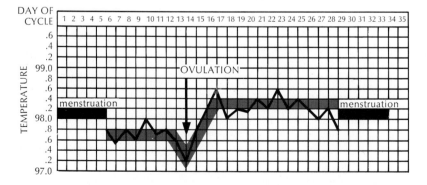

The next question is: When exactly do these two weeks begin? As mentioned above, everything depends on the moment of ovulation. (If it were possible to calculate this moment accurately, the "unsafe" days would be much less than two weeks.) An ovulation usually occurs in the middle of the menstrual cycle or, to be more precise, about two weeks before the beginning of the next cycle. Unfortunately, it is very difficult to predict the beginning of the next cycle. Many women, especially when they are young, or when they are approaching menopause, have irregular cycles, and even for women with regular cycles a variation of two to five days is quite normal. (See also "The Female Sex Organs.")

In order to gain at least some certainty, a woman can use two different strategies (and many women who practice the "rhythm method" actually use both at the same time): First, she can take her body temperature with a special thermometer every morning before getting out of bed (basal temperature). Before each ovulation, there is a slight drop in body temperature followed by a slight rise for the rest of the menstrual cycle. By comparing her temperature records of at least six previous months, the woman can calculate the time of her next ovulation. A second way of finding the "unsafe" days consists of keeping a calendar record of menstrual cycles for at least eight months. Using this calendar record, a woman selects her longest and her shortest cycle. She then subtracts 18 days from her shortest cycle to find the first "unsafe" day of her present cycle. She further subtracts 11 days from her longest cycle to find the last "unsafe" day of her present cycle. For example, if the shortest cycle is 25 days, then $25 - 18 = 7$ (the seventh day is the first "unsafe" day of her present cycle). If the longest cycle is 31 days, then $31 - 11 = 20$ (the twentieth day is the last "unsafe" day of her present cycle).

Each of these two versions of the rhythm method (basal temperature or calendar) requires expert professional guidance. No woman should try them on her own. However, even in combination and with the help of a doctor they are not very reliable. The rhythm method does not work at all for women whose longest cycle differs more than 10 days from the shortest. Physical and emotional problems can change the length of cycles, and there is also the possibility that some women may ovulate in response to coitus itself. Apart from its lack of reliability, the method also has the disadvantage of subjecting coitus to the rule of calendar and thermometer. Nevertheless, many people use the rhythm method for religious reasons, since at present it is the only method of contraception approved by the Catholic church.

Effectiveness: not very effective.

Spermicides
Spermicides are chemical substances that kill sperm cells and thus prevent any possible fertilizations. Spermicidal preparations are available in drugstores without prescription as vaginal foams, creams, jellies, foaming tablets, or suppositories. Some brands of spermicides may cause allergic reactions in some women. In these cases, a doctor should be consulted. Should a spermicidal preparation fail and pregnancy occur, the baby will in no way be affected.

Vaginal Foam
Vaginal foam comes in a small aerosol can with a special applicator. (The best known brand names are Emko, Conceptrol, and Delfen). After shaking the can, the woman fills the applicator with foam and then, lying down, inserts it deep into her vagina. This must be done not more than half an hour before each coitus. Two applications are better than one. The foam kills the sperm and also blocks the cervix mechanically, thus preventing any sperm cells that might have survived from entering the uterus. The protection can be increased further if the man uses a condom at the same time.

Effectiveness: about 90 percent; if the man also wears a condom, close to 100 percent.

Spermicidal Creams and Jellies

Spermicidal creams or jellies are less effective than foam because they sometimes disperse unevenly. Some can be used by themselves, just as vaginal foam. However, they provide much greater protection when used together with a diaphragm. If no diaphragm is available, the man should wear a condom.

Effectiveness: not very effective without a diaphragm.

Vaginal Foaming Tablets and Suppositories

Vaginal foaming tablets and suppositories can only work when they have time enough to dissolve inside the vagina. They must, therefore, be inserted 10 to 15 minutes before each coitus. However, if used alone they do not offer much protection against pregnancy.

Effectiveness: not very effective.

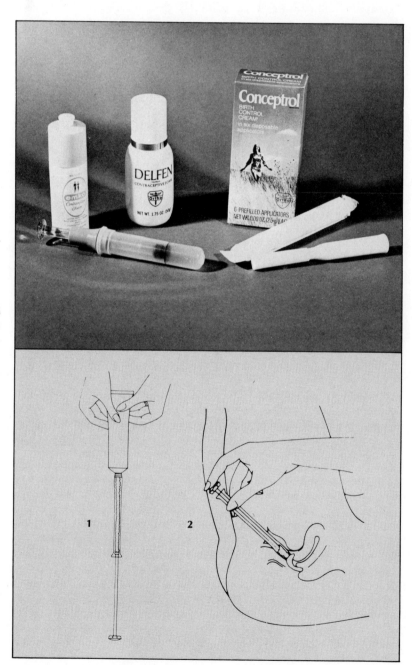

VARIOUS BRANDS OF SPERMICIDAL FOAM
On the left: containers and applicator. On the right: prefitted disposable applicators for one-time use.

APPLICATION OF SPERMICIDAL FOAM
1. Filling the applicator
2. Inserting the applicator into the vagina and releasing the foam
(Courtesy Ortho Pharmaceutical Corporation)

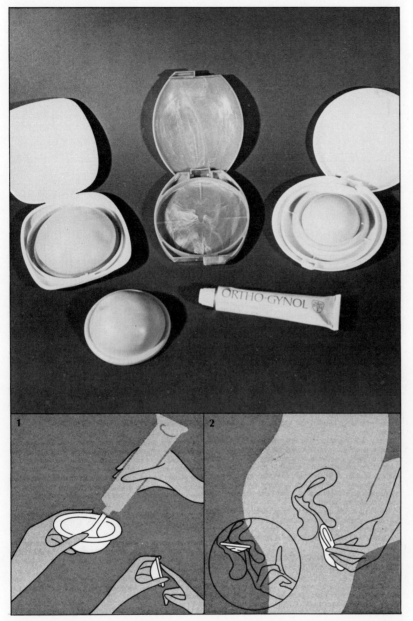

DIAPHRAGMS IN VARIOUS SIZES
In the foreground: spermicidal jelly

APPLICATION OF SPERMICIDAL JELLY AND INSERTION OF DIAPHRAGM
1. Applying the jelly to the diaphragm
2. Inserting the diaphragm into the vagina
(Courtesy Ortho Pharmaceutical Corporation)

Diaphragm and Jelly

The diaphragm is a small, flexible, bowl-shaped device made of rubber that fits closely over the cervix, where it mechanically blocks the sperm cells from entering the uterus. In order to increase its effectiveness, the diaphragm is used together with a spermicidal jelly or cream, which is put inside it and spread around its rim. Since different women are built differently, diaphragms come in different sizes and have to be fitted by a doctor. (A woman should be rechecked for size every two years and after each pregnancy.) The doctor will also teach the woman how to insert the diaphragm properly.

The diaphragm is inserted up to six hours before sexual intercourse and must be left in place for at least eight hours afterwards. If the couple wants to engage in coïtus again before that time, more cream or jelly must be inserted into the vagina (without removing the diaphragm, of course). After the diaphragm has been removed, it is washed with soap and water and can be used again.

Effectiveness: very effective when used with spermicidal jelly or cream.

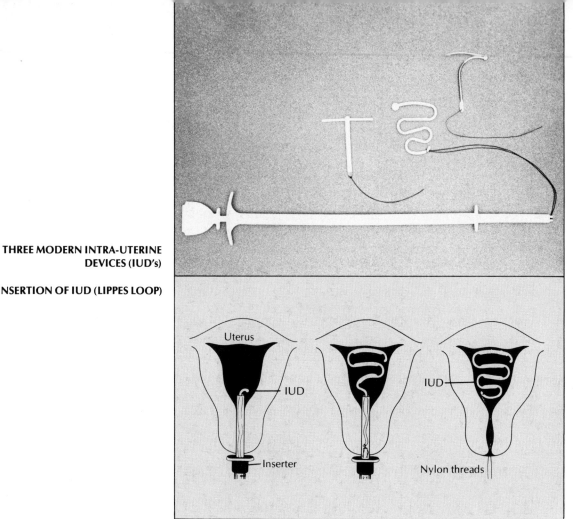

THREE MODERN INTRA-UTERINE DEVICES (IUD's)

INSERTION OF IUD (LIPPES LOOP)

Uterus

IUD

Inserter

IUD

Nylon threads

Intra-uterine Devices (IUDs)

Intra-uterine (contraceptive) devices, or IUDs for short, have been known since ancient times. However, in recent years new types of these devices have been developed. A modern intra-uterine device is a small piece of flexible metal or plastic with nylon threads attached to the bottom. As the name indicates, it is inserted by a doctor into a woman's uterus where it prevents pregnancy. Intra-uterine devices come in various shapes and sizes (the "loop," the "seven," the "coil," and so on).

At present, there is still no satisfactory explanation of how the IUD works. Perhaps it somehow keeps the sperm cells and the egg from meeting under the right conditions, or it prevents the fertilized egg from being implanted in the uterine wall. Several other theories have been suggested. Only one thing is certain: The IUD is very effective as a contraceptive device as long as it is in place. It can be worn for years without interruption and, of course, it can be removed at any time if the woman wants to become pregnant. Recently a new type of IUD has been developed which contains hormones similar to those used in the "pill." The device, known as "Progestasert," thus actually combines the features of two contraceptive methods. However, unlike other IUDs, it must be replaced about once a year.

Unfortunately, in some cases the IUD slips out without the woman's knowledge. It is important, therefore, to check its presence after each menstrual period by feeling for the nylon strings which reach a little way into the vagina. In certain other cases, particularly if the woman has not yet had any children, the IUD may cause severe cramps and bleeding. This may force the doctor to remove it. Many women, however, adapt easily to the IUD after some initial discomfort.

Effectiveness: very effective.

"The Pill"

Contraceptive pills are made of synthetic hormones (estrogen and progestagens) which are similar to those produced by a woman's ovaries. Contraceptive pills prevent any egg from being released from the ovaries. The pills may also have other properties, such as changing the quality of the cervical mucus. This, in turn, may make it more difficult for the sperm to enter the uterus. As a result, the woman cannot become pregnant.

The pills come in packages made to last one month. One pill is taken every day for 20 or 21 days beginning with the fifth day of the menstrual cycle. When the package is empty, the woman stops taking any more pills until the fifth day of her new menstrual cycle. (Some packages contain 28 pills, the last seven without medication.)

The pills can work only if taken regularly. It is advisable, therefore, to take the pill every day at the same time (e.g., when waking up, brushing one's teeth in the morning, at breakfast, at supper, or going to bed). Such a daily routine will prevent a woman from forgetting a pill. If she does forget one pill, she can take two pills the next day at the regular time and continue as usual. However, if she forgot two pills in a row, she should also use another contraceptive method for the rest of the cycle.

Contraceptive pills are available only on prescription, since there are some women who should not take them. Recently several negative side effects have been reported, especially for women over forty. A medical examination will determine whether the pills are appropriate in any individual case.

Some women who take contraceptive pills at first experience some symptoms similar to those of pregnancy: a weight gain, slight nausea, and a tenderness and an enlargement of the breasts. These side effects usually disappear within a few months. However, if they persist, a switch to another brand of pills may be indicated. Occasionally one can read reports that the use of contraceptive pills carries the risk of blood clotting. However, this relative risk is much greater with pregnancy.

Effectiveness: almost 100 percent.

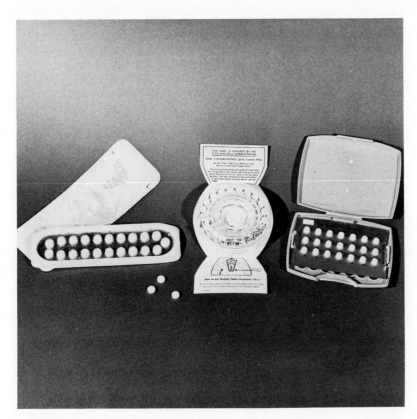

**VARIOUS BRANDS
OF CONTRACEPTIVE PILLS**

The "Morning-after Pill"

A woman who has engaged in coitus without using any contraceptive method, or who knows that the method she used has failed and who has reason to believe that she might become pregnant, can still prevent this from happening by taking a so-called morning-after pill. This pill (a high dosage of estrogen) will prevent any fertilized egg from being implanted in the uterine wall. It must be taken within three to five days after coitus and is available only by prescription. A doctor has to evaluate several health factors before prescribing it. Even where there are no medical objections, the pill may cause very unpleasant temporary side effects, such as nausea and vomiting. In some cases, serious long-term aftereffects have been reported. However, many women would rather endure those than the worry about an unwanted pregnancy. Still, it is obvious that the morning-after pill cannot be used as a regular means of contraception.

Effectiveness: almost 100 percent.

A CONTRACEPTIVE METHOD FOR EITHER MEN OR WOMEN

Sterilization

Men and women who have definitely decided that they do not want any (or any more) children may choose the safest contraceptive method of all, sterilization, i.e., an operation that makes them infertile. The result of this operation should be considered final. Doctors are working on new surgical techniques that would allow for a reversal and thus restore fertility, but at present the chances are still slim at best.

For Men: Vasectomy

The sterilization of a man, called vasectomy, is a relatively simple and safe operation which does not take more than a few minutes in the doctor's office. It involves the cutting and tying of the thin tubes on both sides of the scrotum through which the sperm travels. As a result of the operation, the sperm cells can no longer become part of the ejaculated fluid but are absorbed by the body. This means that the man is now unable to make a woman pregnant. In every other respect, there is no change; erection, orgasm, and ejaculation occur just as before. In other words, a vasectomy does not affect a man's sexual desire or performance, although some sterilized men enjoy sexual intercourse more because they no longer have to worry about causing an unwanted pregnancy.

Effectiveness: virtually 100 percent.

1. Vas deferens
2. Testicle
3. Fallopian tube
4. Ovary
5. Uterus

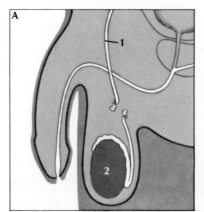 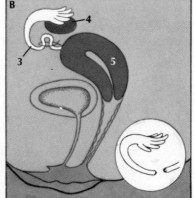

VASECTOMY AND TUBAL LIGATION
A. Vasectomy: *A portion of each vas deferens is removed and the cut ends are tied.*
B. Tubal Ligation: *A portion of each Fallopian tube is tied and cut out. In a few weeks, the cut ends of the tubes are scarred shut and separated from each other (insert).*

For Women: Tubal Ligation

The sterilization of a woman, called tubal ligation, consists of cutting and tying or cauterizing the Fallopian tubes through which her eggs travel to the uterus. Since these tubes are inside the woman's body, the operation is more complicated than for a man. Often hospitalization, at least for a day, is necessary. However, some doctors now use a new surgical technique (laparoscopy) which simplifies and shortens the operation. As a result of a tubal ligation, egg and sperm cells can no longer meet, and thus the woman can no longer become pregnant. In every other respect there is no change; her feelings and her capacity for orgasm are the same as before. In other words, a tubal ligation does not affect a woman's sexual desire or performance, except perhaps in a positive way since she no longer has to worry about an unwanted pregnancy.

Effectiveness: virtually 100 percent.

FUTURE METHODS OF CONTRACEPTION

Medical research has been trying for years to find a contraceptive pill for men. These efforts are beginning to produce some practical results, although at the moment longer-range testing is still necessary. In the meantime, several new contraceptive methods for women are being studied. Among these is a pill that would not have to be taken every day but only before sexual intercourse. Another method consists of the implantation of a small contraceptive capsule under the skin where it could possibly keep releasing its active substances into the bloodstream for years. Still another method involves prostaglandins (substances that can cause uterine contractions) which would prevent pregnancy in spite of fertilization (or could terminate a pregnancy at any time). There is further the possibility of a hormone injection every three or six months which could replace the daily pill known today.

As is obvious from this brief summary, most experimental contraceptive methods still leave the initiative and responsibility for their use mainly to women. It is to be hoped that future research will put renewed emphasis on contraceptives for men. What we really need is a range of contraceptive methods that fulfills the demand for complete sexual equality.

ABORTION

The term "abortion" can be used for both the unintentional and the intentional premature termination of a pregnancy. The unintentional termination of a pregnancy is called abortion if it occurs within the first 4 months; after that time, it is usually called miscarriage. In the nonmedical language of everyday life, however, the word "abortion" most often means the intentional termination of an unwanted pregnancy.

Unwanted pregnancies happen for many reasons. Sometimes people who engage in coitus do not know about contraception, or they are unable to get contraceptives, or the contraceptives they use do not work. Whatever the cause, an unwanted pregnancy often creates very serious problems.

In the case of parents who already have difficulty supporting several children, one more birth can mean misery and despair for the whole family. An expectant mother who is physically weak or who suffers from certain diseases or drug addiction may, by her pregnancy, further endanger her own health or give birth to a sick or deformed baby. A young, unmarried woman may be totally unprepared, unfit, or unwilling to assume the responsibilities of motherhood. Thus, an unwanted birth could be a disaster not only for her but also for the child.

In these and similar cases, a woman may well decide that a voluntary abortion is the only way out. Unfortunately, some women resort to ill-considered, desperate actions and risk their health, indeed their very lives, by trying to abort themselves or by seeking the help of an unskilled criminal abortionist. They do this because our society often makes it difficult to obtain safe abortions. In fact, there is still a passionate debate among many political, religious, and legal authorities as to whether women should have the right to abort at all.

Some of those who argue against abortions do so because they consider themselves friends of the fetus and want to uphold the "sanctity of human life." There can hardly be a motive that deserves to be taken more seriously. Still, the very same motive has led some other people to take the side of the woman who wants to abort and to fight for her right to do so. A reconciliation between these opposing views seems unlikely. It is also obvious that the dilemma cannot be solved by science. There is no scientific way of deciding when a human life begins and under what conditions it may be taken. These are basically moral questions which have to be answered by the individual conscience.

Moral guidance in such matters has traditionally been offered by the various established religions and philosophies. However, their views are not always identical. Some contemporary religious groups favor abortions under certain circumstances and early in the pregnancy, while others are unconditionally opposed to them, considering every abortion to be murder (except to save the life of the mother, in which case it would be self-defense). The Catholic church, for example, maintains today (in contrast to its own teachings during the Middle Ages) that an embryo is a human life "from the moment of conception." However, scientists do not agree as to whether and when such a particular moment should be presumed to occur. In a way, it is a matter of definition. Scientifically speaking, the conception of a human being is best described not as a sudden occurrence but as a gradual, complicated process which begins with the union of an egg and a sperm cell (fertilization) and leads through various stages to the eventual attachment of a growing cell cluster to the uterine wall (implantation). This process is by no means automatic. It depends on a number of interrelated special conditions which are not always present. In some cases, the development takes an entirely different turn, no implantation occurs, and the fertilized egg simply degenerates. Consequently, according to general medical usage, we do not speak of the beginning of pregnancy until the implantation in the uterus has taken place. (For details, see "Conception.")

Until recently, voluntary abortions were prohibited by law in most states of the United States. However, even the most restrictive criminal laws usually recognized the broader scientific view of conception by providing no penalties for the use of "morning-after pills" or intra-uterine devices, which prevent the beginning of pregnancy in spite of possible fertilizations. Indeed, the very fact that such substances and devices are generally considered contraceptives and not abortifacients suggests that the Catholic interpretation is not shared by the public at large. Neither did our laws ever reflect the opinion that abortion is murder. If they had, the penalties for abortionists would have been the same as for murderers: death or life imprisonment. In actual fact, however, the penalties were always much less severe. Moreover, the most important person involved in the crime, the woman who had the abortion performed, was practically never prosecuted at all.

Such curious hesitancy, indeed ambiguity, on the part of the law indicates that the modern secular state cannot support any particular moral or religious viewpoint, but tends instead to seek some position of compromise. In fact, the state, which has to accommodate and protect the adherents of many different and often conflicting beliefs, can meet this obligation only by basing its laws on purely rational considerations. In the case of abortion, such considerations point clearly in one direction: leaving the matter entirely to professional medical judgment and the conscience of the individual.

This is also the direction followed by the U.S. Supreme Court in 1973 when it declared most then-existing state laws banning abortion to be unconstitutional. The court recognized every woman's right to obtain an abortion in the first three months of pregnancy while reaffirming the right of the state to safeguard health, maintain medical standards, and protect potential life. Consequently, the Supreme Court decision allows the individual states to regulate abortions after the third month of pregnancy to the extent that the regulation reasonably relates to the preservation and protection of maternal health. Only after the fetus has reached viability (i.e., the ability to survive outside the mother's womb) may a state continue to prohibit abortions altogether except for the purpose of preserving the life or health of the mother.

It is perhaps useful to remember that the former restrictive abortion laws had been enacted late in the 19th century mainly for medical reasons. At that time, an abortion was a dangerous operation which could easily lead to the death of the woman. In the meantime, however, medical procedures have been perfected to a point where early abortions can be considered quite safe. As a result, the state can now treat such abortions as a private matter and greatly reduce its protective interference. This legal stance does, of course, by no means imply that abortions are desirable. The highest court of the land merely recognizes that it is unwise to make them crimes. Those who are convinced that abortion is murder are still free to reject it for themselves. This is entirely as it should be because forced abortion as well as forced motherhood are incompatible with the ideals of equality, freedom, and self-determination. In the past, these ideals had to remain largely unrealized. Indeed, when it came to abortion the most blatant inequality was a fact of everyday life. Women who could pay for a trip to another state or another country with more liberal laws were not prevented from having a safe and legal abortion any time they wished. It was mainly the poor and uneducated who suffered the consequences of unwanted births or dangerous criminal abortions.

In the meantime it has become apparent, however, that for many Americans the landmark decision of the U.S. Supreme Court has not settled the issue. In fact, there are many individuals and organizations demanding a "right to life" for the unborn and working for a constitutional amendment to criminalize abortions once again. One can assume that much of this campaign is inspired by the highest possible ideals, and there can hardly be any question that, as a matter of principle, abortions are not to be welcomed or taken lightly. Any decision to abort is an unfortunate, hard choice at best. Furthermore, even if one disregards the embryo or fetus, an abortion is always a medical operation for the potential mother which may result in complications. Few sensitive people, therefore, would like to see the practice encouraged as a neutral routine procedure. It would seem much more preferable to arrive at a situation where abortions become unnecessary. Yet the only policy that could reach this goal would be the methodical and nearly universal use of contraception. Consequently, those who want criminal laws against abortion remain unconvincing (and even seem hypocritical) as long as they fail to encourage contraception. (And, let it be noted, such encouragement would have to go well beyond the now "acceptable" standards.) It would seem that, in the meantime, the Supreme Court decision provides a reasonable and practical, and therefore defensible, solution to an unresolved moral dilemma.

It remains to be seen how the various state legislatures will respond to this decision. Fortunately, one fact is already clear: Every woman in the United States who wants a legal abortion can get one if she really tries. Under no circumstances should she put herself in the hands of an unskilled, criminal abortionist, or try to abort herself. The only sensible course of action is to seek a legal, medically competent abortion in a hospital or in a doctor's office. In many cities, the Planned Parenthood offices, the Clergy Consultation Service, women's liberation groups, or free clinics offer the necessary advice and assistance. If no local help is available, information and referral will be provided by Planned Parenthood–World Population, 810 Seventh

Avenue, New York, N.Y. 10019, telephone (212) 541-7800, and by the National Clergy Consultation Service, 55 Washington Square South, New York, N.Y. 10012, telephone (212) 254-6230.

Remember:

- If you are considering an abortion, get expert counseling.
- The earlier an abortion is done, the better.
- You can have a legal and safe abortion in a hospital or in a doctor's office.
- Do not seek the help of an unskilled, criminal abortionist.
- Do not try to abort yourself.

ABORTION METHODS

It makes a great difference whether an abortion is performed early or late in the pregnancy. The earlier it is done, the better. During the first 12 weeks of pregnancy, an abortion is a relatively safe and simple procedure which usually does not require an overnight stay in the hospital. After the 12th week, there is a greater risk of complications, more difficult techniques have to be used, and hospitalization for at least a few days is often necessary. Naturally, a late abortion is also more expensive. After the 20th week, a voluntary abortion, even where it is legal, is usually considered medically indefensible except in the most extraordinary cases. By this time, the fetus has developed to a point where it could actually survive a premature birth. For this and other reasons, most doctors will refuse to perform an abortion at this late stage.

It is important to remember that every abortion, even if done early, is a medical operation which can, under certain circumstances, result in complications. Still, the search for newer and safer abortion methods continues. Some experimental methods involve prostaglandins (substances that contribute to the contraction of uterine muscles). These substances can cause delivery at any stage of the pregnancy. However, since this method still needs to be perfected it is not yet generally available. Any pills, injections, or other abortifacients that can now be obtained either over or under the counter involve grave risks and do not work.

A woman who considers having an abortion should be familiar with the various medically recognized and well-established abortion methods. Thus, she will know what to expect at her doctor's office or at the hospital. Perhaps even more important, she will also be able to judge the techniques of a criminal abortionist and recognize medical incompetence before it threatens her life. Methods other than those described here are either ineffective or dangerous or both.

METHODS USED IN EARLY ABORTIONS

Menstrual Regulation

The usual pregnancy tests do not become reliable until about 40 days or more after the last menstrual period. Women who suspect that they are pregnant but do not want to wait that long to find their suspicion confirmed can ask a gynecologist for a simple procedure called variously menstrual regulation, menstrual aspiration, menstrual extraction, or preemptive abortion. This procedure is similar to the one used for inserting intra-uterine devices (IUDs). Just as in the case of an IUD insertion, the doctor inserts a small tube through the cervix into the uterus. However, instead of depositing the IUD through the tube, he applies a vacuum at one of its ends, thus pulling out (i.e., "aspirating" or "extracting") the lining of the uterus which would normally be shed in menstruation. The procedure takes only a few minutes and can easily be performed in a doctor's office. Obviously, the term "abortion" for this procedure is applicable only if the woman is indeed in the first stages of pregnancy. If she is not pregnant and her menstrual period is simply delayed for another reason, a term like "menstrual regulation" is

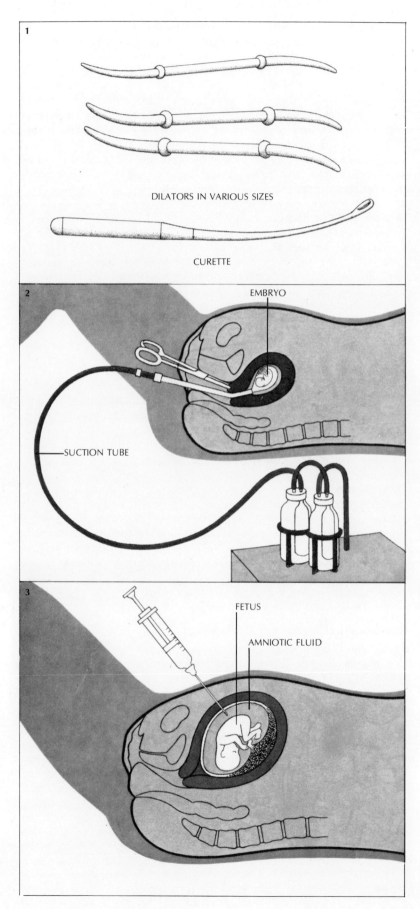

1

DILATORS IN VARIOUS SIZES

CURETTE

2

EMBRYO

SUCTION TUBE

3

FETUS

AMNIOTIC FLUID

THREE ABORTION METHODS

1. Dilation and Curettage
The picture shows some cervical dilators and a curette. The dilators are used to open the cervix for both the older D & C and the modern suction method (see below). The curette is used only for the D & C method to scrape the embryo and placenta from the uterine wall.

2. Suction
An instrument is clamped to the cervix in order to hold it in position, and a suction tube is then inserted through the dilated cervix into the uterus, sucking the embryo into a bottle.

3. Saline Injection
A needle is inserted into the uterus through the abdominal wall. Some of the amniotic fluid is removed and replaced with concentrated salt water which then kills the fetus.

more appropriate. The procedure is mostly designed to fill the gap between "foresight contraception" and "hindsight abortion." It is a fairly new method and may not yet be available everywhere in the United States.

Suction

The suction method, also known as "vacuum curettage" or "uterine aspiration," is today the safest and most commonly used medical technique for an early abortion. After a dilation of the cervix, a tube attached to a suction pump is inserted into the uterus. The pump, which operates on the same principle as a vacuum cleaner, sucks the embryo and the placenta out of the uterus through transparent tubes into a collection bottle. The entire operation takes only a few minutes.

Dilation and Curettage

This older technique, also known simply as "D & C," is in principle not too different from the suction method. Again, the cervix is dilated. However, there is no tube and no vacuum pump. Instead, the entire operation is performed by hand. A surgical instrument with a hollowed out, spoon-like tip is inserted into the uterus. This instrument is called a curette. The doctor uses it to scrape the embryo and placenta from the uterine wall. The operation usually takes about 15 minutes.

METHODS USED IN LATE ABORTIONS

Saline Injection

This method, also known as "salting out," consists of replacing some of the fluid surrounding the fetus with salt water. This is done by inserting a long, hollow needle through the abdomen into the amniotic sac inside the uterus. The salt water kills the fetus. The uterus starts contracting usually within the next two days, resulting in the delivery of the dead fetus.

Hysterotomy

Hysterotomy can be described as a miniature Caesarean section. Fetus and placenta are removed through an incision in the abdomen. This is major surgery requiring hospitalization for several days. A woman who has had a hysterotomy (not to be confused with a hysterectomy, or removal of the uterus) can become pregnant again, but usually needs a Caesarean section every time she wants to give birth.

Reference and Recommended Reading

The Boston Women's Health Book Collective. *Our Bodies, Ourselves.* 2d ed. New York: Simon & Schuster, 1976 (cloth); 1976 (paper).
Bradley, Robert A. *Husband-Coached Childbirth.* rev. ed. New York: Harper & Row, 1974.
Colman, Arthur D. and Libby. *Pregnancy: The Psychological Experience.* New York: Seabury Press, 1972.
Demarest, Robert, and Sciarra, John. *Conception, Birth, and Contraception: A Visual Presentation.* 2d ed. New York: McGraw-Hill, 1976.
Dick-Read, Grantley. *Natural Childbirth Primer.* New York: Harper & Row, 1956.
Group for the Advancement of Psychiatry. *Humane Reproduction.* New York: Scribner's, 1974 (cloth); 1974 (paper).
Hall, Robert E. *A Doctor's Guide to Having an Abortion.* New York: New American Library, 1971.
Lamaze, Fernand. *Painless Childbirth: The Lamaze Method.* Chicago: Henry Regnery Company, 1970 (cloth); New York: Pocket Books, 1976 (paper).
Leboyer, Frederick. *Birth Without Violence.* New York: Knopf, 1975.
Noonan, John T., ed. *Morality of Abortion: Legal & Historical Perspectives.* Cambridge, Mass. and London: Harvard University Press, 1970 (cloth); 1970 (paper).

5. SOME PHYSICAL PROBLEMS

Very few people enjoy perfect health throughout their lives. Most of us sooner or later find ourselves in need of medical attention, if only temporarily. Many of the serious diseases that plague and cripple mankind also have, of course, a damaging effect on the sexual abilities. Wounds and injuries can destroy the sex organs themselves or lead to the loss of control over parts or all of the body. Certain illnesses can affect a person's responses or weaken the body to a point where sexual intercourse becomes difficult or impossible. Usually in such cases, the sexual difficulties are only the by-product of a general infirmity and therefore receive only minor attention. With a full recovery, the sexual capacities are also restored. Even without a recovery the case is not necessarily hopeless. Many permanently disabled and chronically ill patients can now be helped to achieve satisfying sex lives in spite of their problems. (See "The Sexually Oppressed.")

There are, however, certain physical disorders and diseases that affect human sexual activity and procreation directly, and some of them, such as infertility and the venereal diseases, are quite common. Fortunately, many of these formerly hopeless conditions have become responsive to treatment. In some instances, a complete cure is achieved quickly and easily. Nevertheless, since at any given time millions of people all over the world are suffering from one or several of these conditions, every sexually mature person should know about them. The following pages provide some basic information about the main physical illnesses and impairments which can interfere with human sexual functioning. For the sexual difficulties of persons who are physically healthy, see "Sexual Maladjustment."

INFERTILITY

It is estimated that nearly one in every five couples is unable to produce children. In some cases, this infertility creates very little concern and may even be welcome. Most often, however, it becomes a source of frustration and great unhappiness to men and women whose sense of self-esteem is somehow tied to their ability to become parents. Fortunately, the advances of modern medicine have made it possible to help many of them.

A couple's infertility may have one or more of many different causes affecting either the man, or the woman, or both. They range from simple sexual inexperience to poor diet, psychological difficulties, and problems of the male or female reproductive systems. Thus, an apparently healthy young couple (both under 35) who have had no success starting pregnancy after more than a year of conscious effort may be well advised to seek professional help. (If either the man or the woman is over 35, such help should be sought after 6 months.) A careful medical examination of both partners by a specialist can often discover the reason for their failure. Sometimes the diagnosis as well as the therapy are very simple indeed. For example, there have been couples who remained childless just because they never had sexual intercourse on the woman's fertile days. At other times, the problem may prove to be extremely complicated and require extensive treatment involving psychological counseling, hormone replacement, or surgery. One of the more recent and increasingly popular methods of treating infertility is artificial insemination. In some cases (approximately one in every ten couples), fertility cannot be established in spite of all available medical measures. However, these couples may still find fulfillment as parents through adoption.

INFERTILITY IN MEN

A physician who tries to discover the reason for a couple's infertility will usually first examine the man. Not only is the male reproductive system simpler, but quite often the root of the problem can indeed be found in the male. A man's infertility may, of course, result from certain congenital defects (see "Genetic Defects" and "Sexual Malformations"). However, it may also be acquired. Certain diseases, for example, such as mumps in adulthood or gonorrhea, can produce sterility (see "Venereal Diseases"). Another cause of infertility or subfertility (insufficient or low fertility) may be a low sperm count. In this case, the man does produce live sperm, but in quantities insufficient for a successful impregnation. While it is true that only one sperm cell is needed to fertilize the female egg, usually at least 200 million of them have to be ejaculated at one time in order to give this one cell a statistical chance to reach its destination. In some cases, the sheer number of sperm cells is sufficient, but their proper development or their ability to move is impaired. Most often, however, a low sperm count, sperm deformities, and lack of movement are found to occur together. Obviously, this condition does not have to affect a man's sexual desire or performance at all. He is just unable to cause pregnancy in a fertile woman. In other words, such a man is not "impotent," but infertile.

However, there are also some men who are infertile because they are "impotent." They cannot cause pregnancy in spite of their normal sperm production because their inability to have or hold an erection prevents them from even performing coitus. These cases particularly recommend themselves to treatment by artificial insemination.

INFERTILITY IN WOMEN

As mentioned above, the cause of a couple's infertility may lie with the man, or the woman, or both. If medical tests prove the man to be fertile, the examining physician will start a new series of tests on the woman. She may be sterile because of certain congenital defects (see "Genetic Defects" and "Sexual Malformations"), or as a result of certain internal infections, especially gonorrhea (see "Venereal Diseases"). Such infections may have led to a permanent blocking of the Fallopian tubes, thus making fertilization impossible. In some cases of infertility, there simply is no egg to be fertilized because there is no ovulation. In other cases, fertilization does take place, but the fertilized egg invariably fails to attach itself to the uterine wall. In still other instances, both fertilization and implantation occur, only to be followed by early spontaneous abortions (miscarriages). The reason for this may be some abnormality of the uterus or the cervix. In certain women, the cervical mucus is too thick to be penetrated by sperm; in others, the cervical or vaginal fluids are hostile to the sperm and kill it. Sometimes women develop antibodies which appear in the vagina and produce an immunity to all sperm or to the sperm of a particular man.

Since the possible causes of female infertility are so varied and numerous, treatment may sometimes be difficult, and it may involve any number of measures from hormone replacement to surgery. However, in recent decades an increasing number of formerly hopeless fertility problems have been overcome with the help of artificial insemination.

Artificial insemination is a simple procedure in which a doctor uses a fine tube to inject semen into a woman's vagina close to the cervix. This has to be done during a woman's fertile days. A married couple may choose this method of achieving pregnancy in order to overcome certain fertility problems. The semen, which is obtained by masturbation, is usually that of the husband. However, if he should prove to be sterile the semen of an anonymous donor can be used. Such a donor is selected by the doctor and known only to him. In selecting the donor, the doctor normally tries to find a man whose physical characteristics resemble those of the husband, and whose medical history indicates good general health.

ARTIFICIAL INSEMINATION

GENETIC DEFECTS

It has often been said that "nobody's perfect," and this is certainly true in regard to the form and function of our bodies. We all carry through life at least some inherited weaknesses and deficiencies which prevent us from enjoying complete physical and mental vigor from birth to old age. Most often these deficiencies are relatively inconsequential, such as premature baldness or flat feet. However, in certain cases they may be very serious, such as hemophilia, sickle-cell anemia, or some forms of muscular dystrophy. There is no doubt that much human suffering could be prevented if these and similar genetic defects would cease to be transmitted from one generation to the next.

Unfortunately, some genetic defects can be transmitted by hidden carriers, i.e., men and women who themselves remain unaffected and therefore often unaware of the possible danger to their offspring. The reason for this can be found in the laws of heredity.

Generally speaking, genetic defects come in two varieties: dominant and recessive. A dominant genetic defect can be transmitted through one parent alone. In other words, even if only one of the parents has a dominant genetic defect they will transmit it to half of their children. A recessive genetic defect can be transmitted only by both parents. In other words, if only one of the parents has a recessive genetic defect they will not transmit it to any of their children. However, if both parents have the same recessive genetic defect they will transmit it in the following way: On the average, for every four children, one child will be completely unaffected, two children will be hidden carriers, and one child will show the defect.

In view of these facts, some people may find it useful to seek genetic counseling before they decide to have children. A careful examination of a couple and their family medical histories can provide valuable clues as to their chance of transmitting serious genetic defects. Most couples will find that they have little to worry about. However, a few may learn just in time that they cannot have a healthy baby of their own, and that they can find greater happiness through adoption. There are also some rare cases where severe genetic defects or other serious abnormalities of an unborn baby are discovered in the course of a woman's pregnancy. Even in the more restrictive past, such a discovery has usually been considered sufficient reason for a legal abortion.

In the United States there are now several hundred laboratories offering various genetic services. More than 200 of these offer genetic counseling. Further information is available from: The National Genetics Foundation, 250 West 57th St., New York, N.Y. 10019; The National Foundation–March of Dimes, P.O. Box 2000, White Plains, N.Y. 10602; and the Information Office, National Institute of General Medical Services, National Institute of Health, Bethesda, Md. 20014.

SEXUAL MALFORMATIONS

Most people take the healthy development and functioning of their bodies for granted. They usually do not see a doctor until they experience some illness or breakdown in familiar bodily functions. This is, of course, also true in the area of sex. However, there are some persons who are born with certain sexual deformities and handicaps which require medical treatment before any satisfactory sexual activity can even begin. Such a handicap may be due to chromosomal or hormonal anomalies, and it may involve the internal or external sex organs, or both. These anomalies can result in a number of problematic conditions, which sometimes have been conveniently grouped together as "sex errors of the body," and most of them do not have to be considered here. Fortunately, today many of them can be corrected by proper treatment, just like other physical handicaps. Two of the most obvious sexual malformations are discussed in the following paragraphs.

UNDESCENDED TESTICLES

The testicles (male sex glands)—like the ovaries (female sex glands)—are formed within the abdomen during the development of the embryo. However, before a baby boy is born they descend from his abdomen into his scrotum (the bag of skin which hangs between his legs just behind the penis). In some rare cases, the testicles fail to descend. This can be due to some hormonal deficiency or some other reason. If a boy approaches the age of puberty in this condition, treatment becomes necessary because the testicles cannot produce sperm at body temperature, and thus infertility would result. Hormone replacement or surgery can usually bring about the proper development.

There are also (even rarer) cases where the testicles prove to be imperfect or absent altogether. Boys with this problem can also be given hormonal treatment so that they develop physically just as other boys. However, for obvious reasons they will remain sterile. A normal physical appearance can be achieved by a surgical insertion of artificial testicles into the scrotum.

HERMAPHRODITISM

As a baby grows inside the mother's womb, its internal and external organs (including the sex organs) form and develop gradually to the point of completion we see at birth. However, in some very rare instances something interferes with this development, and the baby is born with the sex organs still uncompleted. In such a case, the baby's sex may be difficult to determine because the unfinished sex organs of both sexes look very much alike. The child may be a male (pseudo-) hermaphrodite (if two testicles are present), a female (pseudo-) hermaphrodite (if two ovaries are present), or a so-called true hermaphrodite (if both testicular and ovarian tissue is present). In some cases, there may be no problem of external appearance, but some internal ambiguity of sex. (See also "The Process of Sexual Differentiation.")

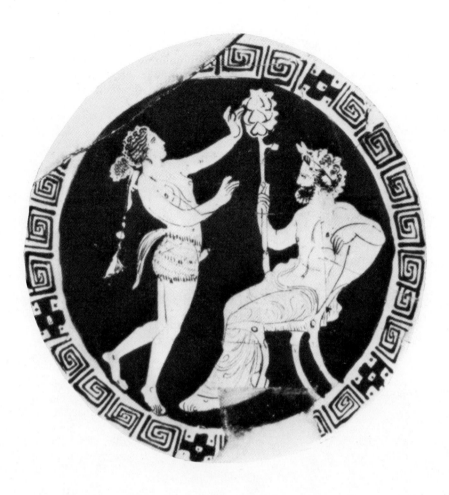

HERMAPHRODITE

A hermaphrodite is a person whose body shows both male and female sexual characteristics. In ancient times such persons were often believed to have special magical powers. In some societies they were also sought after as sexual partners. This ancient Greek pottery painting shows a young hermaphrodite dancing in front of an admirer.

The word "hermaphrodite" has been used since ancient times for a person whose body shows both male and female sexual characteristics. (In Greek mythology, Hermaphroditos, the son of Hermes and Aphrodite, was a handsome, but prudish young man. When he rejected the love of a nymph, she embraced him so passionately, that her body merged with his and he literally became "two in one flesh.") Fortunately, modern hormonal and surgical treatment can go a long way toward completing the development of a baby born "sexually unfinished." At the same time, psychological counseling can help the parents to raise their child in the appropriate sexual role, regardless of an initially misleading appearance. If all factors are given their due consideration, the assignment of sex will prove workable and, in time, a definite sexual identity will be established. In other words, although there may be permanent sterility in some cases, persons born as hermaphrodites can today benefit from many advances of medicine and may grow up to be otherwise ordinary men and women.

There are also some cases where men or women whose biological sex is clearly not in doubt express the wish for a "sex change." This phenomenon, known as transsexualism, is more of a psychological than a physiological problem and is therefore not discussed here, but in the section on "Sexual Maladjustment."

PAIN DURING SEXUAL INTERCOURSE

For a healthy human being, the purely physical aspect of sex is usually not much of a problem. After some initial uncertainty and experimentation, the sexual response simply becomes another bodily function which requires no further worry or analysis. However, there are exceptions. Some men and women, for example, experience pain during sexual intercourse. Obviously, such an experience can be very frustrating and even force some people into complete sexual abstinence. Fortunately, a careful examination by a doctor can very often discover the cause and thus lead the way to successful treatment. The following paragraphs deal with the main physiological causes of pain during sexual intercourse. (Possible psychological causes are discussed in the section on "Sexual Inadequacy.")

PAINFUL SEXUAL INTERCOURSE IN MEN

Apart from obvious genital injuries and diseases, the most common cause of pain during sexual intercourse in men is a tightness of the foreskin called phimosis. This condition occurs in some uncircumcised men who have such a small opening in their foreskin that it cannot be pulled back over the glans of the penis. This can result in irritation and pain during every erection. Some simple surgical treatment, possibly including circumcision, can eliminate the problem.

Circumcision, or the complete surgical removal of the foreskin, also prevents another condition that can develop in uncircumcised men. If the foreskin is not periodically pulled back over the glans to allow for a thorough washing with soap and water, there may be a buildup of certain secretions which can cause infection and inflammation.

Infections of the penis may also be contracted during sexual intercourse (see "Venereal Diseases").

Finally, some men develop an abnormal sensitivity of the glans or allergic reactions to the vaginal environment or certain spermicidal or douching preparations. Naturally, the treatment consists of a change in douching habits or method of contraception. The use of a condom may also provide at least a temporary solution of the problem.

PAINFUL SEXUAL INTERCOURSE IN WOMEN

Apart from genital injuries and diseases, the most common cause of pain during coitus in women is a lack of sufficient vaginal lubrication. This may be due to the aging process and can then be treated with hormone replacement. In other cases, insufficient lubrication simply indicates that the woman is not sufficiently aroused and is not ready for coitus. (The male parallel would be lacking erection.)

Some women may experience pain because of an unusually thick hymen which prevents the penis from even entering the vagina. In such a rare case, local minor surgery can help. (Some slight discomfort may be felt by many women during their first attempts at coitus. However, the penetration of the hymen is usually accomplished easily, and any discomfort disappears quickly.)

Another cause of pain, burning, and itching in the vagina is infection by a venereal disease. Trichomonal organisms or an overgrowth of yeast (monilia) may cause similar symptoms. (For details, see "Venereal Diseases.") Such symptoms may also occur when a couple engages first in anal and then in vaginal intercourse without a thorough washing of the penis in between. In such cases, the penis carries rectal bacteria into the vagina where they cause infection. The obvious solution is washing the penis with soap and water immediately after withdrawal from the rectum and before resuming any other form of sexual intercourse. Coitus can also become painful for women who suffer from cystitis (an inflammation of the bladder). Clearly, in such cases, medical treatment is indicated.

Vaginal sensitivity can develop as a reaction to chemicals used in contraceptive or douching preparations. In such cases, the use of the offending substances has to be discontinued. (As a rule, vaginal douching is unnecessary and may be harmful.)

Still another cause of pain during coitus is a thinning of the vaginal walls in older women. The condition can be improved by hormonal treatment.

Finally, some women may develop an unpleasant sensitivity of the clitoris, either because some secretions have accumulated under the foreskin of the clitoris causing irritation or because the head of the clitoris has been overstimulated by the male partner. (This misguided practice may be the result of bad advice given in some marriage manuals.)

VENEREAL DISEASES

Sexual intercourse can be among the healthiest and most enjoyable experiences in life. Unfortunately, it is sometimes also allowed to become the source of needless misery, suffering, and even death. For example, our society today is still perpetuating and indeed aggravating a serious health problem that could have been eliminated a long time ago: the venereal diseases.

The vague and poetic term "venereal diseases" (literally, diseases attributed to Venus) is a euphemism for those contagious diseases that are transmitted through intimate physical contact, especially sexual intercourse. There are, of course, many other diseases that can be transmitted by intimate contact with another person, such as the common cold, smallpox, tuberculosis, and other infectious diseases. Nevertheless, the so-called venereal diseases have been singled out as a distinct group because they are almost always contracted by close contact with a diseased sexual partner, and they usually first affect the sex organs by which this contact has been made.

The various venereal diseases produce very different symptoms but are transmitted the same way: They are caused either by viruses or by germs which thrive in the warm, moist inner surfaces of the body (particularly in the mucous membranes of the sex organs, mouth, and rectum). Outside of this favorable environment, they quickly die. For this simple reason, they cannot be picked up from toilet seats, doorknobs, or similar objects (although in some very rare cases some venereal diseases have been picked up from used towels, underwear, and other clothing). On the other hand, sexual intercourse provides ideal conditions for all of these microorganisms to be transmitted from one person to another. It is very well possible to become infected with several venereal diseases at the same time. While all of them can be cured, there is never an immunity against them. One can catch all venereal diseases again and again.

In the United States today, the most common and most dangerous venereal diseases are gonorrhea and syphilis. Both have a long history dating back to ancient times, and for thousands of years nothing could be done about them. They not only remained incurable, but ever-increasing sexual taboos eventually made them unmentionable. Finally, in 1910, the first at least partially effective cure for syphilis was discovered (with Salvarsan, an arsenical compound also known as "606"). Still, it was not until the arrival of penicillin in the 1940s that successful treatment of both syphilis and gonorrhea could be assured. Nevertheless, it is now apparent that this scientific breakthrough was not enough. There also has to be a drastic change in society's attitudes.

In the past, when venereal diseases were poorly understood, they were often seen as a moral rather than a medical problem. Intolerant minds called them "the wages of sin" and believed them to be the just punishment of debauchery. According to this philosophy, "nice" people did not get venereal diseases. It was also believed that a young person should not learn too much about them. Fear and ignorance were supposed to keep him chaste. There was even the opinion that a successful cure could only encourage sexual license and would thereby undermine the moral health of society. Compared to this danger the threat to people's physical health seemed somehow less important. These and similar misguided views often led to irresponsible public policies for which we are paying a heavy price today. Moreover, in recent years the invention of new contraceptive methods has reduced the use of condoms which had always helped somewhat in the prevention of venereal diseases. Finally, inefficient self-treatment by ignorant patients in some parts of the world has contributed to the development of new and stronger strains of gonorrhea which, in our age of increasing travel, are quickly spread to other countries. These and other factors have now produced what can only be called a venereal disease epidemic.

This epidemic is hurting young people most of all. The greatest increase in reported infections is among teenagers. Because of inadequate education, they are often totally ignorant about the causes and symptoms of venereal disease. Consequently, many of them do not realize that they have become infected and thus may infect others. Some young people are also too afraid or embarrassed to seek treatment because they do not want their parents to find out that they had sexual intercourse. (In a number of states, a physician is not allowed to treat a minor for venereal disease without informing the parents.) However, the consequences of an untreated venereal disease are much worse than any momentary family crisis.

Fortunately, free tests and treatment for venereal disease are offered by departments of health in most cities. Such treatment always remains completely confidential. Nevertheless, every doctor is required by law to report any case of venereal disease to the appropriate public health agency. This is necessary in order to trace contacts who might also need treatment. Naturally, their privacy is protected as well.

The fight against venereal disease can still be won if everybody cooperates with those measures. Obviously, people who have become infected must immediately stop having sexual intercourse until they are cured. They should also ask their partners to get tests and, if necessary, treatment. Beyond such individual contributions, however, the most important task is this: Our society as a whole must make sure that every sexually mature person, including teenagers, learns the facts about venereal disease.

Fortunately, in recent years much progress has been made toward that goal. For example, the National Community Service Corps has established a national hotline that can be called toll-free from anywhere in the United States. It is operated mostly by teenagers who are well informed about the venereal diseases and who can give advice as to where to go for free examination and treatment in each community. This telephone service is available during regular business hours. The number is (800) 523-1885.

Remember:

- Venereal diseases are dangerous.
- You can have a venereal disease without having any symptoms.
- You can have several venereal diseases at the same time.
- Venereal diseases can easily be cured if treated early.
- Free tests and treatment are offered by your local department of health.
- All treatment for venereal diseases remains completely confidential.
- Self-treatment is ineffective.
- You can catch venereal diseases again and again.

The following paragraphs provide some basic information about the different venereal diseases.

Gonorrhea, also popularly known as "the clap" or "the drip," is by far the most common venereal disease today. It is caused by a bacterium, the gonococcus, which is transmitted from one person to another through the mucous membranes of the sex organs, the mouth, or the rectum. Outside of these warm and moist areas, the gonococcus quickly dies. It is therefore nearly impossible to contract the disease from toilet seats, doorknobs, towels, and other such objects.

Symptoms

An infection of the sex organs with gonorrhea (in the case of genital intercourse) will usually be noticed by a male within 2–10 days because of a sudden burning sensation when urinating. At the same time, a thick, green-yellowish discharge ("the drip") will appear at the opening of the penis. In females, on the other hand, the infection can often go unnoticed for quite some time. The early symptoms may be the same as in the male: a burning sensation and a discharge. However, it is also possible that no symptoms appear at all. In this case, the female may not realize that she is infected. Thus, she may not only risk later complications for herself, but also unknowingly transmit the disease to others.

An infection of the throat with gonorrhea (in the case of oral intercourse) may produce symptoms similar to those of an ordinary sore throat ranging from scratchiness to severe pain upon swallowing. However, very often there are no symptoms at all.

An infection of the rectum with gonorrhea (in the case of anal intercourse) may cause itching, burning, or bleeding, a yellowish discharge and pain when defecating. These symptoms are often mistaken for a simple case of diarrhea or hemorrhoids, and the necessary treatment may be delayed for this reason. Unfortunately, sometimes there are no symptoms at all.

If gonorrhea remains untreated, its early symptoms may disappear by themselves, but it will then spread inside the body and cause internal abscesses, arthritis, and sterility (the latter especially in women). The baby of a mother who has gonorrhea may be infected during its birth. In order to prevent possible eye infections with gonococci, the eyes of newborn children are routinely treated with a special solution.

Diagnosis

Gonorrhea can be properly diagnosed only by a physician, primarily by means of a bacterial culture which is taken from the infected area, i.e., the sex organs, the throat, or the rectum.

Treatment

Gonorrhea is a serious disease requiring the earliest possible treatment. Fortunately, modern medicine has made such treatment simple, fast, and effective. If treated early, gonorrhea can usually be cured within a few days with penicillin. Occasionally, some other medication is indicated. A successful cure does not mean immunity, however. A person can catch gonorrhea again and again.

Prevention

The only certain way to prevent an infection with gonorrhea is to avoid sexual intercourse with an infected partner. However, since the disease is so widespread today and symptoms may sometimes be unnoticeable or absent, this advice almost amounts to a demand for complete sexual abstinence. Those who do engage in genital or anal intercourse can at least partially protect themselves by wearing a condom, and by urinating and washing with soap and water immediately afterwards. In the case of coitus, some protection is also provided by spermicidal foams and jellies which are introduced into the vagina. Perhaps gargling with some antibacterial mouthwash after oral intercourse is not entirely useless either. Still, all of these measures are, at best, only marginally effective. Sexually active females are therefore well advised to have vaginal cultures taken at regular intervals. Males as well as females who engage in oral intercourse should also ask for a throat culture. A rectal culture is necessary in cases of anal intercourse. In any case, it may be useful to remember at least this: Someone who has an exclusive sexual relationship with only one partner is in less danger of catching gonorrhea than a person who changes partners frequently.

SYPHILIS

Syphilis (or lues), also popularly known as "the siff" or "bad blood," is the most dangerous venereal disease. Although it is not nearly as common as gonorrhea, it is by no means rare. Syphilis is caused by a bacterial organism, the spirochete, which is transmitted from one person to another through intimate physical contact, particularly the touching together of the moist inner body surfaces during sexual intercourse. Outside the human body, the spirochete cannot survive more than a few seconds. It is therefore practically impossible to contract syphilis from toilet seats, bath tubs, towels, bed linens, or other such objects. Neither can the disease be transmitted through the intact skin. However, the spirochete, which may be present in the mucous membranes, the saliva, semen, or blood of an infected person, can enter any cut or even slight skin abrasion of his sexual partner.

Symptoms

The first symptom of a syphilitic infection is a painless ulcer or sore (chancre) which appears within ten to ninety days at the point where the spirochete entered the body. Depending on the kind of sexual intercourse, this can be anywhere: on or near the sex organs, the mouth, the rectum, or some other area. The ulcer may be large and obvious or small and hardly noticeable. If it should appear inside the vagina or rectum, it might easily go undetected. Unfortunately, sometimes there is no outward symptom at all. In any case, the ulcer heals itself after a while. An infected person may thus gain the false impression that he is cured. In reality, however, the disease has now entered its second stage.

At the second stage of syphilis, the spirochetes have entered the bloodstream and thus spread through the whole body. The result is a rash, which usually appears 3–6 weeks after infection. This rash may take almost any form and may cover a small or large surface of the skin. In some cases, no rash may appear at all. Both the rash and the primary ulcer are infectious. There may also be a loss of patches of hair.

After the rash has disappeared, the disease enters its third stage which may last from a few months to several years. There may be no symptoms at all for quite a long time. However, this stage is the most dangerous of all because the disease may now suddenly attack various areas inside the body, destroying normal tissue and causing serious heart disease, blindness, paralysis, brain damage, and even death.

Syphilis can be transmitted to a baby before its birth through the mother's bloodstream. Because of this danger, expectant mothers need to have a blood test for syphilis early in the pregnancy.

Diagnosis

A diagnosis of syphilis can be made only by a doctor, usually by means of a blood test.

Treatment

Syphilis is a very dangerous disease which requires the earliest possible treatment. Fortunately, it is easily curable today, although any damage that has occurred before treatment is started cannot be repaired. The usual treatment consists of a series of penicillin shots. Occasionally, some other medication may be indicated. In order to insure success, follow-up blood tests are necessary. Successful treatment does not result in immunity. A person may catch syphilis again and again.

SYPHILIS AT A U.S. HIGH SCHOOL
Each figure represents at least one sexual contact. Some 40 per cent of those exposed escaped infection altogether. How many of those treated preventively may have been infected is unknown.

INFECTED

TREATED PREVENTIVELY

NOT INFECTED

Note that the disease is spread by both heterosexual and homosexual contact. In the case cited here, the total number of individuals is 63. Of these, 44 had only heterosexual contact; 16 had only homosexual contact; 3 had both heterosexual and homosexual contact. (Source: Newsweek, Jan. 24, 1972)

Prevention

The only certain way to protect oneself against syphilis is to avoid sexual intercourse with an infected partner. However, since there may be no noticeable symptoms and people may therefore have the disease without knowing it, the best advice for any sexually active person is to have regular blood tests (one every 3–6 weeks). Such tests, together with proper treatment (where necessary), are offered free by public health clinics in most cities.

Wearing a condom during genital or anal intercourse and urinating and washing with soap and water immediately afterwards also offer at least partial protection, as will the use of vaginal contraceptive foams or jellies.

SOME TROPICAL VENEREAL DISEASES

There are some other, less common, venereal diseases which deserve to be mentioned. Although they are found mainly in tropical countries, it may be useful to know about them in our age of increasing travel.

Chancroid

The chancroid, also known as "soft chancre," is a bacterial infection which results in one or several large, painful, and destructive ulcers within a few days. The disease can be effectively treated with antibiotics.

Granuloma Inguinale

This is another bacterial infection which causes ulcers. It can also be treated effectively with antibiotics.

Lymphogranuloma Venereum

An infection caused by a virus. The disease produces an ulcer and a swelling of the lymph nodes in the groin. Effective treatment is possible.

OTHER DISEASES THAT CAN BE SPREAD BY SEXUAL INTERCOURSE

In addition to the "classic" venereal diseases, there are numerous other diseases that can be spread by sexual contact. Some of them are very serious, such as salmonellosis, typhoid fever, amoebic dysentery, and hepatitis. Infectious hepatitis, for example, can be transmitted through fecal contamination during oral-anal intercourse (anilingus). Some viruses causing hepatitis appear in semen and saliva and thus can also be transmitted sexually. Needless to say, in all of these cases immediate medical attention is essential. Fortunately, these serious infections are relatively rare. The following paragraphs deal only with more common, less serious diseases.

Monilial Vaginitis

Women may sometimes experience an upset in the ecological balance of the many organisms living in the vagina. Such an upset can result from vaginal douching, taking antibiotics or birth control pills, or from a variety of other causes. As a consequence, there may be an overgrowth of a yeast called monilia. The symptoms are itching, burning, a whitish discharge with a characteristic odor, and often a dryness of the vagina. It is also possible to transmit the condition to a man through sexual intercourse, causing an inflammation at the tip of the penis. The man, in turn, can reinfect the woman. Monilial vaginitis is quite common and does not have the same serious consequences as gonorrhea and syphilis. It is treated with locally applied medication.

Trichomonal Vaginitis

The trichomonas vaginalis, a single-cell organism, is present in the urethra and bladder of many men and women. While it usually does not produce any symptoms in males, it may, under certain conditions, cause problems in women who may develop a burning sensation when urinating and a vaginal discharge which is whitish, foamy, and has a characteristic odor. There may also be some reddening and swelling of the vaginal opening. The condition

VD

A CHECKLIST OF SYMPTOMS

It is very well possible to suffer from gonorrhea and syphilis without having any symptoms. Every sexually active person should therefore have periodic medical tests. However, if there are symptoms they may appear in the following parts of the body:

The Whole Body:
A slight fever accompanied by an overall feeling of sickness may be a symptom of either *syphilis* (second stage) or *gonorrhea* of the throat.

The Skin:
Itchy raised areas or red bumps which look like mosquito bites but do not cure themselves may be caused by *scabies*. Also, *syphilis* chancres can appear anywhere on the body where contact has been made. A body rash may be a symptom of *syphilis* (second stage). A syphilitic rash is likely to extend to the palms of the hands and the soles of the feet.

The Scalp:
A sudden loss of patches of hair may be a symptom of *syphilis* (second stage).

The Mouth:
A harmless looking "cold sore" may actually be a *syphilis* chancre.

The Throat:
A sore throat may be caused by *gonorrhea* after oral intercourse. However, in most cases gonorrhea of the throat does not show any symptoms.

The Penis:
A painless open sore may be a *syphilis* chancre. Burning sensations and a white or yellowish discharge may be symptoms of *gonorrhea* or *nonspecific urethritis*. Small, painful blisters which appear and then heal themselves only to recur again may be *herpes*. As long as the blisters are present, the virus is very contagious. Small, cauliflower-shaped warts may be *venereal warts*.

The Vulva and Vagina:
Chancres appearing on the major or minor lips may indicate *syphilis*. although this disease rarely shows symptoms in the female sex organs. A whitish discharge and abdominal cramps may indicate *gonorrhea*. Vaginal discharges are more likely to be caused by *monilia* or a *trichomonas* infestation. The vulva may also be affected by *herpes*, *venereal warts*, and *crabs*.

The Anus:
Small cauliflower-shaped warts may be *venereal warts*. A discharge of blood or mucus on feces, especially if accompanied by rectal itching, may be a symptom of anal *gonorrhea*. However, at this site the disease most often does not show any symptoms. The anal area and rectum may also develop a *syphilis* chancre after anal intercourse.

is treated with oral medication and has to involve both sexual partners. This is necessary because a man who harbors the trichomonas organisms, while usually developing no symptoms of his own, may very well retransmit the condition to a woman. Trichomonas infestations are common. They do not result in the same complications as gonorrhea and syphilis.

Venereal Warts
Venereal warts are the result of a viral infection. Since this infection usually occurs during sexual intercourse, the warts appear on or near the sex organs or anus of both men and women. Treatment is relatively easy and effective.

Herpes Progenitalis
Cold sores or herpes are due to a viral infection which appears at the various openings of the body, particularly around the mouth and nose. An infection of these areas can, of course, occur without sexual contact. However, herpes of the sex organs are caused by a different virus and are transmitted from one person to another by sexual intercourse. The symptoms are painful ulcers on or around the male or female sex organs or the anus. The ulcers may hurt for several weeks, then gradually heal themselves and disappear. Unfortunately, there may also be recurrent attacks. There is no simple and effective treatment. Nevertheless, men and women who discover these ulcers on their sex organs or anus should see a doctor in order to rule out other more serious diseases.

Nonspecific Urethritis
Nonspecific urethritis is the name given to some infections which may result in an inflammation sometimes producing symptoms similar to those of gonorrhea: a discharge and discomfort when urinating. However, the condition is less serious than gonorrhea and can often also be successfully treated within a few days.

CRAB LICE
Crab lice, also known as "crabs," live and breed mostly in pubic hair and thus can be transmitted from one person to another by close sexual contact. In rare instances, the transfer may also be through infested clothing or bed linen. In any case, their presence will soon be noticed since they cause a persistent itching in the pubic area. The condition is treated with a prescription item, Kwell (ointment, lotion, or shampoo), or with A-200 Pyrinate, which is available without prescription. Before using any medication, a hot bath and extensive washing with soap are important. Wearing clean clothing afterwards will prevent reinfestation. Clothing and linen which may be infested should be dry cleaned or laundered and dried in a hot dryer.

SCABIES
The itching of scabies is caused by a tiny mite which burrows through the skin. The mite can be transferred from one person to another by sexual and other physical contact as well as through infested clothing or bed linen. As in the case of crab lice, the infestation is treated with locally applied lotions (Kwell).

Reference and Recommended Reading

Grover, John W., and Grace, Dick. *VD: The ABC's.* Englewood Cliffs, N.J.: Prentice-Hall, 1971.
Money, John, ed. *Sex Errors of the Body: Dilemmas, Education, Counseling.* Baltimore and London: Johns Hopkins University Press, 1968.
Morton, R.S. *Venereal Diseases.* Baltimore: Penguin Books, 1970.
Nicholas, Leslie. *How to Avoid Social Diseases: A Practical Handbook.* New York: Stein & Day, 1973 (cloth); 1973 (paper).
Rosebury, Theodore. *Microbes and Morals: The Strange Story of Venereal Disease.* New York: Ballantine Books, 1973.

HUMAN
SEXUAL BEHAVIOR

oday, the term "human sexual behavior" sounds so familiar and is so widely used that it may be hard to imagine a time when it was unknown. After all, the human race has always consisted of two sexes and these have always felt drawn to each other. Indeed, men and women have always engaged in intimate physical intercourse and thereby produced new life. Moreover, we can assume that most of them knew what they were doing, and thus, when we talk about human sexual behavior, we seem to be talking about a simple and universal concept as old as mankind itself.

However, the realization that people have always done certain things does not necessarily allow us to conclude that they have always thought of them the same way. Actually, as any historian and anthropologist knows, human perceptions of even the most elementary "facts of life" vary greatly from one time and place to another. Linguists also know that seemingly simple words often have no exact equivalents in other languages and that, as the years go by, they may very well change their meaning.

This is particularly true of the word "sex" and all its derivations. We know, of course, that in ancient and medieval times people had dozens or even hundreds of words for the male and female organs and for the act of copulation. We also know that they talked about being fruitful and reproducing their "own flesh and blood." They knew what was meant by kissing, embracing, or fondling another person. They were familiar with sensual pleasure, physical stimulation, and excitement. They spoke proudly of love, desire, affection, tenderness, passion, minne, amour, Eros, Cupid, and Venus. Some men and women enjoyed displaying their nude bodies or observing nudity in others. Some tried to suppress their "concupiscence" and spoke with disgust of wantonness, lechery, lewdness, lust, or temptation by the devil. They warned against being "unclean," having "pollutions," or "wasting one's seed." Some also praised chastity, modesty, continence, innocence, and virginity while condemning carnal impurities, abominations, sins against God, and crimes against nature. Still, as a closer look reveals, our distant forebears had not yet summarized all of this in the single, unifying concept of "sexual behavior." They did not see these varied human experiences, actions, and attitudes as having the same source or even as being related to each other.

At the same time, people were not yet used to isolating a specific "sexual drive" in the wide spectrum of human motivations. In the prescientific mind, human life was not yet neatly compartmentalized. The bodily functions were not divided into separate categories, nor were there sharp distinctions between different kinds of physical needs. Erotic impulses were like other passing moods which arose suddenly and then died down by themselves. The occasional urge to touch, caress, or make love to someone was not seen as an autonomous instinct in its own right, but rather as a minor aspect of the general human condition. Men and women shared a common basic experience. Together they belonged to the world; they were all links in the "great chain of being," humble elements in some eternal plan. The same divine law governed the stars, the seasons, dead matter, and living organisms. Everything was connected with everything else. All normal inclinations were part of the same continuum, and thus there was little reason to grant them a character and a significance of their own.

This may explain why the expression "sexual behavior" does not appear in any European language until modern times. It is not used anywhere in the Bible and was unknown to the classical Western writers from Homer to Dante, Shakespeare, Racine, and Goethe. As a matter of fact, even the word "sexual" alone, which by now dates back several hundred years, only gradually acquired its great variety of present meanings. At first, it was nothing but a narrow, purely technical term and simply referred to the attribute of being either male or female.

Of course, before the adjective "sexual" could even come into existence, the noun "sex" had to be introduced. For the English language, this was accomplished by a translation from the Latin Bible in 1382. In this famous translation, which was inspired by the religious reformer John Wycliffe, God commands Noah to select two specimens of every animal for his ark: "the maal sex and femaal" (Genesis 6:19). Here the word "sex" simply meant something like gender, sort, set, class, type, race, or breed. In fact, until well into the 18th century the word was often used in the same sense as the word "sect," i.e., as referring to a group of followers, a denomination, faction, caste, or school. Thus, one could speak of various "large and small sexes," a "new sex," or a "sex of hermits." Until the 19th century, "sex" was also used as a synonym for "women" (the [female] sex), and there was even a verb "to sex," which meant to characterize somebody or something as being of male or female sex. (For the origin of the Latin word *sexus*, see "The Process of Sexual Differentiation.")

By the same token, the adjective "sexual" originally had only a very limited use and never implied anything more than a category of some kind. It was not until the 18th century that the word broadened its meaning and began to refer also to the process of reproduction. This was, in part, a consequence of scientific progress. For example, in 1735, the Swedish botanist Linné devised what he called a *methodus sexualis*, i.e., a sexual classification method or system in which plants were listed according to the character and number of their reproductive structures. This method (which is now obsolete) greatly impressed most scholars and even many laymen at the time. However, there was also some rather peculiar opposition. Linné's system was violently attacked by certain religious leaders who noted that it allowed for the cohabitation of a male stamen with several female pistils in one and the same flower. This was clearly indecent and a defamation of God who could not possibly have created such depravity. Biology teachers were therefore implored not to mention it to their young students.

From our present point of view, it is, of course, easy to ridicule these concerned moralists, but, to a certain degree, their objections were understandable. It seemed to them that Linné and other scientists were trying to "sexualize" nature or, in other words, that they were imputing a lascivious purpose to the growth of every last leaf of grass. This charge was unfair, but it articulated a valid general impression. With the rapid advance of biological and medical research, more and more areas of life were fearlessly investigated, anatomies and behaviors were compared, and connections were demonstrated where none had ever been noticed before. Once people started to think of roses and daffodils as sexual beings, the concept of sex gained entirely new dimensions. Sex suddenly became all-pervasive, and this realization, in turn, was bound to have a bad influence on the excitable minds of the young. (Ironically, however, after a while the moralists themselves took advantage of the enlarged new perspective and explained human reproduction to their children by talking about "the flowers, the birds, and the bees.")

At any rate, the controversy surrounding Linné's "sexual system" indicates that the formerly neutral and very narrow concept of sex had begun to expand. It now embraced not only gender, but also the process of generation and the various physical and psychological responses connected with it. Thus, within the next 150 years a number of new and evermore specific expressions were coined which quickly entered most European languages. The English language reflects the general trend as well as any of these. For example, the *Oxford English Dictionary* lists the following terms together with the dates of their first use in print: "sexual intercourse" (1799), "sexual function" (1803), "sexual organs" (1828), "sexual desire" (1836), "sexual instinct" (1861), "sexual impulse" (1863), "sexual act" (1888), and "sexual immorality" (1911).

It is also interesting to note that, in turn, many of these new expressions themselves began to expand their meaning soon after they had been introduced. For example, the term "sexual organs" at first merely meant male and female organs (i.e., organs that have to do with sex as an anatomical distinction). Then, after some time, it was also understood to mean organs of erotic gratification (i.e., organs that have to do with sex as a pleasurable activity). As a result, very soon any behavior involving the stimulation of these organs could be described as "sexual." Therefore it even became possible to speak of "sexual" contact between members of the same sex who shared the same basic anatomy.

Furthermore, at the beginning of the 19th century the new noun "sexuality" appeared in the scientific discussion. Again, at first this word referred only to the quality of being male or female. Within a few decades, however, it was also used to denote a preoccupation with sexual matters, and finally it came to mean the possession of sexual powers or the capability of erotic feelings. In short, it gradually turned from a relative into an absolute term. Thus, by the 1880s, one could discuss a person's sexuality as a special phenomenon all by itself. This phenomenon represented more than mere maleness or femaleness, and it was not necessarily always related to male-female encounters. Neither gender attraction nor any reproductive process had to be implied. Even solitary masturbation could now be perceived as "sexual" behavior, i.e., as an expression of someone's "sexuality."

With the beginning of our own century, and under the growing influence of psychoanalytic thinking, the concept of sexuality became even more inclusive. It now referred not only to procreation and the pursuit of erotic pleasure, but also to the need for love and personal fulfillment, i.e., to the "lust for life" itself. The sexuality of men and women was now regarded as an important aspect of their personality, a fundamental and all-pervasive characteristic, the sum total of their feelings and actions as human beings capable of sexual responses. Indeed, Freud and his followers learned to see a sexual element in nearly all human activity and then described it as the expression of a primary instinct, the manifestation of a basic and powerful inner "drive."

There is no question that these semantic shifts and the discovery of human "sexuality" as a natural force in its own right reflected a very significant change in the image people had of themselves. After all, since the end of the Middle Ages the style of living in Europe had undergone a thorough and ever-accelerating transformation. The transition from a feudalistic to a capitalistic economy, the growth of trade, and the advance of technology gave rise to new attitudes, habits, and moral values. The emerging urban middle class or *bourgeoisie* trained itself for a greater degree of discipline, self-control, and self-denial than had ever been known before. Efficiency, punctuality, productivity, and profit were proclaimed as the new ideals. The human body came to be seen as a machine which had to perform in the most regular and rational manner possible. Spontaneous physical responses and desires which interfered with such smooth functioning were rigorously suppressed. Waste and idleness could not be tolerated. Even love had to be justified as a means to an end—the procreation of children, i.e., new workers, soldiers, and other "useful" members of society. In the 18th century, masturbation was declared to be a serious threat to health. A growing prudery alienated men and women from themselves and each other, and by the middle of the 19th century virtually all natural bodily functions had become taboo.

Curiously enough, it was this very suppression, subjugation, exploitation, and fear of the body which increasingly focused attention on its "sexual" qualities. No matter how much people tried to steel themselves, their bodies remained capable of experiencing sensual pleasure and "useless" ecstasy. In fact, the more such pleasure was condemned, the greater grew the temptation to indulge in it. The danger was ever-present, and everyone had to be on his guard. Finally, when the general prudery reached its height, the forbidden flesh became a powerful, secret obsession. The Victorians saw "sex" everywhere.

At the same time, however, they also found themselves with a greatly reduced vocabulary for the sensual or erotic. The fantastic variety of medieval English, French, and German words for sex organs, bodily functions, and lovemaking had gradually been replaced by some embarrassed euphemisms and a small number of incomprehensible Greek and Latin terms. The rich vernacular was suppressed as "vulgar" and "dirty." As a result, a few "acceptable" terms now had to be stretched considerably in order to cover the same semantic field. Thus, the word "sexual," for example, continued to acquire certain new meanings simply by filling the newly created terminological vacuum. Modern Europeans and Americans often had no choice but to use the single word "sexual" when talking about many formerly distinct and unrelated phenomena. Such usage, in turn, could not remain without influence on the general public consciousness. People became accustomed to finding sexual implications in all sorts of behavior which before had been seen as "pure" or sexually indifferent. In other words, men and women began to develop a highly sensitive, hypersexual attitude toward each other. Perhaps one can best illustrate this change in perception by citing a simple example: It is a common experience of modern psychotherapists that in sexually mixed encounter groups many interpersonal problems are defined as being sexual in nature. However, these same problems are often defined quite differently in all-male or all-female groups. Here the sexual aspect does not seem very important, and thus the participants are prepared to look for another explanation.

It is also well known that many so-called primitive peoples fail to see the "sexual" element in certain situations which seem to suggest nothing but sex to the modern Western observer. This is true even for peoples who put great emphasis on sexual satisfaction. They are simply much less concerned with the ramifications, connotations, or symbolic meanings of their behavior. Thus, while sex is important to them, it remains a rather limited issue.

The same can be said of young children in our own culture who engage in "sexual" activity. Much of this activity is not regarded by them as being sexual at all. Indeed, the seemingly obvious adult interpretation is adopted only gradually and often reluctantly.

These and similar observations indicate that it takes a special frame of mind to detect "sexual" signals everywhere and to conceive of "sex" as a fundamental and all-pervasive force. Moreover, this frame of mind does not necessarily reflect a greater capacity for sensual pleasure or a more vigorous love life. In fact, it may very well be the sign of a crippled or impoverished sensuality. A preoccupation with sex is not the same thing as erotic fulfillment. In any case, it seems only prudent to approach the entire subject with caution. We must always remember that when we talk about human "sexual" behavior, we are not simply describing some objective factual occurrences. We are also choosing a very special point of view from which to focus on these occurrences. In short, we are expressing a certain subjective (and perhaps shortsighted) philosophy.

When we examine the professional language of our own time, we discover that the term "sexual behavior" can have three different basic meanings, depending on the background and scientific interest of the writer:

1. The term "sexual behavior" can refer to all actions and responses that make fertilization possible.
This is the oldest, simplest, and narrowest definition. It reflects the observation that each species of the higher animals is divided into two groups or sexes, male and female, and that they reproduce sexually. That is to say, males and females produce different but complementary sex cells (gametes). New life may begin to develop when a male sex cell (spermatozoon) unites with and thus fertilizes a female sex cell (ovum). In order to effect this fertilization, a male and a female individual have to go through a certain characteristic and very specific sequence of physical motions and responses. This sequence (or any part of it) is properly called sexual behavior.

In the lower mammals, sexual behavior is firmly regulated by certain specific physiologic controls. At certain times when fertilization is possible, males and females respond to certain behavioral "cues" in each other and thus begin to interact in such a way that the male and female sex cells are brought together. For example, the male may mount the female, their sex organs may be joined together, and he may ejaculate into her body where fertilization can then take place. However, the entire sequence of actions and responses can be completed only if all necessary cues are received by both partners. Male and female sexual behaviors have to reinforce each other at every step and in very specific ways. The animals are "programmed" to effect fertilization, but the program breaks down or even fails to develop without such mutual reinforcement. This means, among other things, that the sexual behavior of these animals is not "instinctive," i.e., entirely directed from within. Instead, it is "built up" or "put together" in response to certain stimuli at the time of its occurrence.

In the higher mammals, the inborn physiologic controls of sexual behavior are not sufficient to guarantee "successful" mating, but have to be augmented by learning. For example, monkeys and apes raised in isolation who had no opportunity to observe or practice copulation still possess the capacity to respond to the cues of suddenly appearing partners, but may not know how to interact with them. Their bodily movements remain clumsy and inappropriate. As a result, fertilization cannot take place. Thus, it is obvious that the "normal" sexual behavior of these animals depends, to a great extent, on training and experience. Furthermore, it is clear that the sexual behavior of many higher animals is quite varied and elaborate and serves more than a mere reproductive function. It also helps to maintain social coherence and coordination.

The behavioral pattern becomes even more flexible and complex in the highest mammal—man. Human beings are born with the capacity for certain basic sexual responses, but are not in any specific way programmed for mating. Thus, they depend almost entirely on observation and experience. Their sexual behavior is exceedingly variable, and fertilization may no longer be its primary function. Instead, individual satisfaction and various social goals may turn out to be much more important. In short, when we talk about humans we cannot simply equate sex with reproduction. Human sexual behavior is more than reproductive behavior, and it therefore requires another, much broader definition than the one provided above.

2. The term "sexual behavior" can refer to any behavior that involves a "sexual response" of the body.
This is a more recent and rather pragmatic definition. It reflects the observation that, when they mate, most higher animals experience certain bodily changes which show a characteristic pattern and which may be summarized in the term "sexual response." It has further been noticed that this response can occur even in situations where fertilization is impossible. Thus, some animals have been seen stimulating their own sex organs when alone, or mounting partners of their own sex, or trying to copulate with members of other species (including man). In all of these cases, an obvious sexual response is involved.

It follows that sexual behavior in the above sense cannot be explained only in terms of reproduction and male-female relations. Indeed, in some instances this so-called sexual behavior could very well be described quite differently and much better as "warning behavior," "greeting behavior," "appeasing behavior," "rank-demonstrating behavior," or the like. For example, certain monkeys display an erect penis as a warning to intruders into their territory; they greet or appease higher ranking animals in their group by presenting themselves for copulation; or they demonstrate their own rank by mounting their inferiors. Therefore, when we call such behavior sexual we are purely (and selectively) descriptive and do not imply anything about its significance. We are saying only that the behavior involves some sexual response (however rudimentary). We are not saying what this response *means*. As a matter of fact, in some animals it may take very extensive observations to determine the meaning.

In human beings, the meaning of sexual behavior in this sense is sometimes even less clear. The sexual response as such may be obvious enough, but its motivation and purpose may remain entirely obscure. Using a popular expression, we may then say that someone uses "sex for nonsexual ends." However, the debate over what these ends are often remains unresolved. (Actually, the curious notion of "sex used for nonsexual ends" neatly pinpoints the whole problem of defining sexual behavior. After all, on the face of it the phrase is meaningless. It is very much like speaking of "politics for nonpolitical ends." Obviously, it all depends on what you mean by "political.")

Needless to say, there is an advantage in speaking about sexual behavior without reference to its possible meaning. A neutral usage can protect us from prejudging the issue. Therefore, this usage is now very popular with sex researchers who try to get an objective and detailed description of what someone does before they declare why he does it. Clearly, the definition covers all types of human sexual activity (sexual self-stimulation, heterosexual and homosexual intercourse, and sexual contact with animals), but it does not imply any hierarchical order among them. Moreover, it leaves each of these activities open to interpretation. In short, the above definition does not equate sex with reproduction or any other particular purpose. It merely calls attention to a certain physical response common to a variety of activities. Still, we know that, at least in human beings, this response is often accompanied by strong sensual pleasure.

3. The term "sexual behavior" can refer to all actions and responses related to pleasure seeking.

This is a modern, very wide definition which can be traced to Sigmund Freud and his psychoanalytic theory. It was Freud who advanced the concept of "libido" (Latin: lust) which for him at first summarized the physiological energy associated with sexual urges, and later all constructive human endeavor. Eventually, he saw human life as a whole dominated by two opposing basic instincts: Eros (the life instinct) and Thanatos (the death instinct). This view was not shared by all of his followers, but the notion of a powerful innate erotic instinct or drive was widely adopted and even became part of modern popular wisdom. Thus, in many minds "the sex drive" came to stand for man's pursuit of pleasure in all its forms. "Sex" was the underlying motive of every life-enhancing activity.

As we can see, when used in this fashion, the term "sexual behavior" becomes quite inclusive. It then may refer not only to all forms of lovemaking between men and women, but also to all sorts of other human activities. Indeed, it may be applied to infantile breast- and thumbsucking as well as to adult eating, drinking, and smoking, to dancing, singing, bicycle riding, collecting art, or applauding an artist. It may even refer to hunting, wrestling, fencing, or firing a gun. The only question in all of these cases is one of motivation. If the behavior is somehow motivated by the wish for pleasure, if it is prompted by an individual's inner need for self-fulfillment, if it satisfies him or gives him comfort, if it heightens his sense of being alive—then it is clearly sexual.

As a matter of fact, one could go further and speak of sexual behavior in individuals who daydream about love or who act out their erotic fantasies in an unrecognizable, symbolic fashion. One could also say that the "sex drive" is blocked, warped, or disturbed in some men and women, and that they therefore offend, attack, hurt, maim, or even kill other people in a "perverted" attempt to obtain sexual satisfaction. In some of these cases, obvious sexual clues might even be entirely absent. Nevertheless, a psychoanalyst could perhaps track them down and thus reveal the "true" motivation. (On the other hand, in the end the "true" motivation may also turn out to be entirely negative, i.e., a manifestation of the death instinct. Then the suspected sexual behavior would stand revealed as not having been sexual at all.)

These few examples may suffice to show that the above definition of sexual behavior is problematical. Certainly, it is not descriptive and neutral as were the two earlier definitions. Instead, it is evaluative and contains a strong element of speculation. One may also question whether it would make any sense when applied to animals. In any case, it has not proved to be very useful to scientists. By the same token, however, it has often had great appeal for moralists and philosophers.

By now it should have become sufficiently clear that, even on a theoretical level, "sex isn't that simple." Furthermore, it is obvious that the way in which people commonly talk about "sex," "sexual behavior," or the "sex drive" is quite imprecise. It certainly is not adequate for an objective analysis. For example, if there is such a thing as a sex drive, what exactly is it? Is it a drive to reproduce? Or is it a drive to release a specific tension in a specific way? Or is it a drive to experience pleasure? Indeed, what exactly is a drive to begin with?

The English term "sex drive" or "sexual drive" was coined early in our century in analogy to the German *Sexualtrieb* which was sometimes also translated as "sexual instinct." Instincts or drives were said to be innate forces or energies which "drove" animals to behave in certain predictable ways. Specifically, drives prompted an animal to avoid discomfort, like hunger or thirst, and to release physical tension through sexual activity. Thus, for example, the animal's hunt for food indicated the workings of a hunger drive, the search for liquid those of a thirst drive, and the attempt at sexual activity those of a sex drive.

Originally, therefore, the word "drive" was simply a narrow biological term. However, as we have seen earlier, for Sigmund Freud the concept of a sex instinct or sex drive soon acquired much larger dimensions. Under the name of libido, and later that of Eros, it became part of his increasingly ambitious psychoanalytical theory which tried to explain the (largely unconscious) motivations of all human behavior. Indeed, to this day Freudians continue to use the term "sex drive" in a special way of their own which is not very widely shared, but which is justified in the context of other psychoanalytic assumptions. Still, also to this day, psychoanalysis has remained more a matter of faith than of scientific proof.

In contemporary scientific discussions, the word "drive" is no longer used as often as before. Many scientists have, in fact, rejected the concept altogether. They do not see any real advantage in describing hunger as a hunger drive, and instead of talking about an animal's thirst drive, they prefer to say simply that the animal is thirsty. Furthermore, the idea that animals are basically inert and have to be "driven" into activity is increasingly being questioned. Nevertheless, the concept of "drive" has retained some appeal for psychologists who want to describe motivations that have some physiological basis. Thus, in textbooks on psychology one can still find the term "drive" defined as "an urgent basic need which is rooted in some physiological tension, deficiency, or imbalance, and which impells an organism to action." Sometimes "drive" is also defined as an "aroused condition in which an organism's behavior is directed toward avoiding discomfort or a state of physiological imbalance." Drives in this sense are, for example, hunger, thirst, the need for sleep, and the need for moderate temperatures. A lack of food, liquid, and sleep, or a temperature that is either too hot or too cold activates the drive. The greater the imbalance, the stronger the drive. By the same token, when sufficient food, liquid, and sleep, and a moderate temperature have been obtained, the drive is satisfied until a new imbalance activates it again. Finally, it is clear that these drives perform a vital function for the organism. Without food, liquid, or sleep, and in boiling or freezing temperatures, the organism would eventually die.

As we have already mentioned, scientists argue whether, even in these "simple" cases, the concept of drive really explains very much. However, be that as it may, we can easily see that, at least in the case of sex, this concept makes little sense. First of all, sexual activity is not necessary for the survival of any organism. A lack of food or liquid will lead to death, but a lack of sex has never killed anyone. Secondly, the strength of sexual desire does not depend on the degree of sexual deprivation. Sexual abstinence does not always increase sexual desire, and frequent sexual activity does not always diminish it. On the contrary, some people who have been abstinent for a long time eventually lose all interest in sex, while others who are extremely active continue to be easily aroused. Furthermore, people usually do not make themselves deliberately hungry or thirsty, but they often actively seek sexual arousal. Also, unlike hunger or thirst, this arousal may be caused and increased by psychological factors alone. Finally, hunger and thirst are experienced as unpleasant, while sexual arousal feels good and is thus rewarding in itself even if it remains "unsatisfied."

In view of these facts, modern sex researchers have practically abandoned the general concept of a sex drive. Instead, there has been a tendency toward breaking it into components. As early as 1940, R. L. Dickinson differentiated between "sex endowment, capacity, and drive." In 1948, Alfred C. Kinsey spoke of sexual "capacity" as opposed to "actual performance"; and in 1958, Lester A. Kirkendall proposed a distinction between "sexual capacity, sexual performance, and sexual drive." ("Toward a Clarification of the Concept of Male Sex Drive," *Marriage and Family Living*, 20, November 1958). So far this latter approach seems to be the most promising, and therefore we should perhaps adopt Kirkendall's argument here (while slightly modifying his language). When talking about human sexual behavior, it seems useful to distinguish between three basic factors:

1. Sexual **capacity**, i.e., what the individual *can* do.
2. Sexual **motivation**, i.e., what the individual *wants* to do.
3. Sexual **performance**, i.e., what the individual *does* do.

Sexual *capacity* (i.e., the ability to become sexually aroused and reach orgasm) depends on a person's general physical condition and especially on the functioning of the nervous and muscular systems. This capacity varies from one individual to another and even from time to time in the same individual. (For example, the same person usually has quite different sexual capacities in infancy, childhood, adolescence, adulthood, and old age.)

Sexual *motivation* (i.e., the desire to engage in sexual activity) may be influenced by the level of certain hormones in the body, but seems mostly dependent on psychological factors. Very important are social conditioning and the special circumstances in any particular situation. Thus, sexual motivation also varies greatly from one individual to the next and from one time to another in the same individual.

Sexual *performance* (i.e., the objective amount of sexual activity) depends not only on physiological and psychological factors, but also on opportunity. Needless to say, at its upper extreme performance is limited by capacity.

Simple common sense tells us that sexual capacity, motivation, and performance do not always coincide. After all, when it comes to sex, very few people have the opportunity to do everything they can do and want to do. At any rate, sex researchers have demonstrated that in males, for instance, the greatest sexual capacity is usually reached many years before the peak of actual sexual performance. Or, to take another example, it has been shown that in females the sexual capacity is often much greater than the sexual motivation. In some people, one may also find a high level of sexual performance combined with a low level of sexual motivation. Instead, the motivation may be mostly financial (as in the case of a prostitute) or social (as in the case of a tired wife who wants to hold on to a husband).

Under these circumstances, it no longer appears justified to speak simply of a human "sex drive." Such a summary approach is not likely to lead very far. It seems much more promising to investigate clearly defined special aspects of human sexual activity. Actually, in the meantime many such investigations have been carried out which have produced useful, and sometimes surprising, results. After Kinsey's statistical count of "total outlets" (i.e., units that measure sexual performance), William H. Masters and Virginia E. Johnson measured human sexual capacities in the laboratory. These and many other new studies have done a great deal to clarify the issue. At the present time, scientists are also conducting more detailed research in the area of sexual motivation. For example, a promising start was made several years ago by R. E. Whalen, who divided sexual motivation into two components: *arousal* and *arousability*. According to this distinction, people's arousal depends on specific stimuli in specific situations, while their arousability depends on their physiological condition (i.e., in part on the presence of certain hormones as well as on their particular learning experiences. The latter are very important, because sexual arousability can vary a great deal even in individuals with the same hormone level. (Whalen, "Sexual Motivation," *Psychology Review*, 73, pp. 151-63, 1966.) Of course, in a sense Whalen's two-component model can also be understood as a simplified alternative to Kirkendall's. After all, while "arousal" is obviously an aspect of motivation, "arousability" also implies some capacity. In any case, these and similar distinctions offer new insights into a formerly obscure subject, and thus we can hope that the future will bring us much closer to understanding the puzzling complexity of human sexual behavior.

In the present book, the term "human sexual behavior" is used both in a wider and a narrower sense. In the wider sense, it simply means everything people do as sexual beings. Among other things, this covers the way in which they perform their masculine and feminine gender roles and how they choose and approach their sexual partners. This usage may be vague, but it is widely accepted and generally understood. Therefore it does not present any serious problem.

However, as we have seen, in the narrower sense the term is more difficult to define. Undoubtedly, sexual behavior is somehow related to reproduction, or at least originally it evolved in connection with reproductive behavior. Still, we also know that in the higher animals and especially humans this is not the whole story. Finally, we know that Freud and his followers assume the existence of a powerful basic sexual instinct or drive in every human being.

Fortunately, for our limited purposes it is not necessary to decide whether this assumption is justified or not. Instead, we can restrict ourselves here to a more practical view. In the following pages, therefore, sexual behavior in the narrow sense simply refers to behavior which involves the stimulation and excitation of the sex organs. We make no prior judgment as to the causes, motives, or purposes of such behavior.

6. THE DEVELOPMENT OF SEXUAL BEHAVIOR

In the first part of this book, we have seen that the anatomical differences between men and women, their sexual responsiveness, and their ability to reproduce do not appear suddenly and all at once, but result from a slow and gradual development. We have also seen that this development can be thwarted in various ways. For example, certain chromosomal or hormonal anomalies may prevent the normal growth of a fetus and lead to the birth of a baby who is "sexually unfinished." Even boys and girls born without sexual malformations may later fail to develop the typical appearance of mature males or females if they are deprived of their gonadal hormones by injury, illness, or castration. In this case, their sexual capacities also remain rather limited and, of course, they never become able to produce children of their own. Finally, there are many adults who are infertile in spite of an otherwise healthy development.

What is true of human physical growth also applies to the development of human sexual behavior. Masculine and feminine attitudes and the preference for certain sexual partners or certain forms of sexual activity are not established once and for all at one particular moment, but are acquired gradually over a period of time. The outcome of this process depends not only on a child's inherited abilities, but also on social influences, such as the reactions of parents, teachers, playmates, and friends. In some cases, these influences can be quite negative. For example, an infant boy may consistently be treated like a girl by his family and thus learn to consider himself female. This early role assignment may then become irreversible and lead to lifelong difficulties. Even boys and girls who develop the appropriate sexual self-identification may later have traumatic experiences that prevent them from attaining their full sexual potential and lock them into narrow patterns of compulsive or destructive behavior. Finally, there are many adults who, after an otherwise healthy development, find themselves strangely inhibited, poorly coordinated, and thus sexually inadequate.

The realization that adult human sexual behavior results from a long, complex, and often hazardous development is relatively new. Until about the beginning of our century, sex was believed to be largely instinctive, i.e., the result of biological heredity. Most people simply assumed that, at some time after puberty, sexual desire and sexual activity "came naturally" to every male and female, and that no social conditioning was involved. Sexuality was a "force of nature" which appeared suddenly and then, all by itself, found its full "natural" expression. Society could suppress this force, but had no part in shaping it.

The first serious challenge of this traditional view came from Sigmund Freud (1856–1939) and his followers. In his practice as a physician, Freud encountered many patients suffering from what was then called hysteria, i.e., a severe disability, such as paralysis or blindness, for which no physical cause could be found. Indeed, according to all standard medical tests, the patients should have been able to function normally. After interviewing these men and women over long periods of time, Freud noticed that their disabilities seemed somehow related to painful or disturbing childhood experiences. He further discovered that these early experiences, of which the patients were no longer consciously aware, were of a sexual nature. Finally, he found that once the experiences were again clearly remembered and understood by the suffering adults, their mysterious disabilities disappeared.

On the basis of these and other findings, Freud gradually developed his psychoanalytic theory which since then has had a profound influence on European and American thought. However, when it was first proposed the theory was greeted with outcries of public indignation. It was plainly inconceivable to most people that a long forgotten childhood experience should continue to have any decisive influence on a person's adult life, and they were positively outraged at the suggestion that such experiences were sexual. In their view, children were "innocent" and "by nature" utterly incapable of sexual feelings or responses. For Freud, on the other hand, the sexuality of children and, indeed, infants was an indisputable fact of the utmost importance.

According to psychoanalytic thinking, there is a basic sexual instinct or drive present universally in all human beings from the moment of birth. This instinct, which strives for sensual pleasure, is at first diffuse and attains its eventual proper direction and focus only through a process of "psychosexual maturation." Human infants first seek their gratification in a direct, unhampered, and undiscriminating way, until they learn to modify and control their instinctual urges through social conditioning. Human sexuality thus unfolds under the influence of two opposing forces: the "pleasure principle" and the "reality principle." In other words, a child's personality development can be described as a contest between biological drive and cultural constraint. This contest proceeds in three major steps, which are coordinated with the child's physiological maturation: the oral, anal, and phallic phases.

In the oral phase (from Latin os: mouth), the chief source of pleasure is the mouth. As it sucks the mother's breast, the infant finds not only nourishment, but deep physical and psychological satisfaction. In this phase, the mouth also serves as an organ of exploration. The infant puts everything in its mouth in order to get to know it. "Taking in" the world is the first attempt at mastering it.

In the following anal phase (from Latin anus: the rectal opening), the main source of sensual gratification shifts from the mouth to the anal area. The child now begins to gain control over the bowel movements and thereby, indirectly, over the attending adults, whom it can now please or displease by eliminating or withholding feces. At the same time, the child learns to grant or withhold affection, say yes or no, in short, to master the world by "holding back" and "letting go."

While the oral and anal phases, which extend roughly through the first three years of life, are the same for both sexes, the now following phallic phase (from Greek phallos: penis) brings an increasing awareness of sexual differences and of the male and female sex organs. The most pleasurable zones of the body are no longer the mouth or the anus, but the penis (for boys) and the clitoris (for girls). This is the phase in which children become actively curious about their surroundings, poke their fingers into things, look inside their toys by taking them apart, and also investigate their own and each other's bodies. The most important aspect of this phase, however, is the development of the so-called Oedipus complex, i.e., the child's erotic attachment to the parent of the opposite sex and a feeling of rivalry toward the parent of the same sex. (The term "Oedipus complex" alludes to the legendary Greek king Oedipus who unknowingly killed his father and married his mother.) For example, it is the rule for a four-year-old boy to be deeply in love with his mother. She is, for him, the only woman he knows and cares to know. However, this woman already has a husband—the father. The boy is jealous of him and would like to push him aside in order to assume his position. This desire is usually expressed openly and spontaneously, as for instance when the boy climbs into his mother's bed announcing: "When I grow up, I'll marry you." Obviously, this situation can be compared to that of King Oedipus, although there is one important difference: Oedipus actually did remove his father forever from his mother's side, and he did marry her. The normal development of a child takes another course. The boy replaces his desire to marry his mother with the wish to marry a woman like his mother, and his urge to take the place of his father turns into the determination to become a man like his father. The boy can make this transition easily, if the father provides an attractive model to follow, and if he actively encourages his son to become a man. At the same time, it is the mother's task to help her son realize that she has already chosen and is no longer available as a sexual object. These parental attitudes will lead the boy to seek his sexual gratification elsewhere. (In the case of a girl, the development takes the opposite course: she loves her father and is jealous of her mother. The respective psychoanalytic term is "Electra complex," after Electra, a legendary Greek princess who, after the death of her beloved father, helped kill her mother who had murdered him. [It must be pointed out, however, that the notion of an Electra complex was advanced by some of Freud's followers, not by Freud himself, who did not subscribe to it.])

Freud believed that every child normally progressed from the oral to the anal and finally to the phallic phase, unless some negative influence interfered with this development. However, if the particular needs of any one of these phases were either unfulfilled or gratified to excess, the child could become "fixated" and thus hampered in its psychosexual growth. For example, a child's too rigid or overindulgent toilet training could lead to a fixation at the anal level of satisfaction. As an adult, such a child would then turn into an "anal character," i.e., a person who is obsessed with discipline, order, and cleanliness, who hoards money (the unconscious equivalent of feces, which can be "withheld" from others) or who prefers anal stimulation to all other forms of sexual intercourse. An "oral character," on the other hand, would continue to depend mainly on his mouth even for sexual satisfaction, or he might become a compulsive eater, smoker, or drinker.

Children who do not become fixated in this manner eventually reach "genital maturity." That is to say, after a so-called latency period, during which obvious sexual interests seem largely suspended, the sexual instinct reawakens with puberty and seeks satisfaction through genital intercourse. Oral and anal stimulation may still be enjoyed to a limited extent, but they now take second place to coitus which, for adults, is the one truly "mature" form of sexual expression.

As can be gathered from this brief and superficial sketch, Freud's concept of human sexuality is extraordinarily broad. Indeed, he stretches this concept to cover responses and activities that, before him, were considered to be completely nonsexual. Even today, the average layman may find it difficult to see any sexual implications in a baby's suckling on the mother's breast, or in an adult's compulsive eating habits. As a matter of fact, many scientists also continue to challenge the psychoanalytic view. For example, anthropologists who have studied various primitive cultures suggest that the Oedipal conflict may not be a universal human experience. Social psychologists have raised serious doubts as to whether an innate sexual drive or instinct even exists at all. Finally, many behaviorists and learning theorists maintain that Freud's whole theory is unnecessarily complex and that there are simpler (and therefore more convincing) explanations of human behavior. Moreover, the fact remains that this theory has never been scientifically tested on a sufficient scale to be proven or disproven.

It is therefore obvious that Freud's teachings cannot simply be accepted as dogma, but have to be studied and evaluated within the cultural context of his particular time. Eventually, such a critical evaluation may even lead to a better understanding of our own post-Freudian culture. Freud was one of history's most brilliant and uncompromising thinkers as well as a great writer, and his works (which comprise 24 volumes in their English language edition) contain deep insights not only into human sexuality, but also into the history and character of Western civilization.

Some of Freud's disciples and followers, however, have shown little allegiance to his critical spirit, but instead have converted elements of his theory into convenient tools of social control. As a consequence, the liberating impulse of psychoanalytic thinking has often been obscured and perverted. This tendency has been particularly noticeable in America where, contrary to Freud's own intentions, some of his hypotheses have been used to justify the persecution and oppression of sexual minorities. (See "Conformity and Deviance" and "The Sexually Oppressed.")

The scope of the present book does not permit a detailed discussion of the various psychoanalytic schools or even of Freud's original theory. On the other hand, experience has shown that this theory does not lend itself to simplification and popularization. Where such simplifications have been attempted, they have all too often led to serious misunderstandings. It is true that Freudian terms have long since entered our everyday language, and that today we can read about the "Oedipus complex" and "the subconscious" in newspapers and popular magazines. We hear of "Freudian slips," "ego," "superego," "libido," and "sublimation" in movies, on radio, and on television. Nevertheless, when taken out of their theoretical context, these words can create considerable confusion, and, among laymen, they are usually misapplied.

Fortunately, in the meantime, it has become very well possible to describe the development of sexual behavior without any reference to psychoanalytic concepts. Recent empirical sex research has provided us with a great deal of new information as to how people learn to act the way they do. We have also gained some understanding of the statistical frequency of certain behaviors. This, in turn, has forced us to reexamine many traditional assumptions about the "nature" of human sexuality. As a result, we are now able to take another entirely fresh look at the subject.

Around the middle of our century, Alfred C. Kinsey and his associates of the Institute for Sex Research in Bloomington, Indiana, published two monumental studies of human sexual behavior which were based on personal interviews with thousands of individuals from all age groups and all walks of life. Previously, such studies had always been forced to rely on small samples of medical patients or sex offenders, and the full range of "normal" sexuality was therefore largely unknown. Kinsey's work provided the first reliable statistical data on the behavior of healthy, average men and women. (*Sexual Behavior in the Human Male*, 1948, and *Sexual Behavior in the Human Female*, 1953.)

At about the same time, Clellan S. Ford and Frank A. Beach, an anthropologist and a psychologist, wrote a cross-cultural study in which they compared the patterns of sexual behavior in 191 different societies. (*Patterns of Sexual Behavior*, 1951.) More recently, John Money of Johns Hopkins University and some fellow researchers have conducted extensive research into sexual malformations and the problems of gender identity. (*Sex Errors of the Body*, 1968; *Man and Woman, Boy and Girl*, 1973; and *Sexual Signatures*, 1975.) In addition, William H. Masters and Virginia E. Johnson of the Reproductive Biology Research Foundation in St. Louis, Missouri, have carried out a thorough scientific investigation of human sexual functioning and malfunctioning. (*Human Sexual Response*, 1966; *Human Sexual Inadequacy*, 1970; and *The Pleasure Bond*, 1975.)

These and many other new studies of human sexuality owe little or nothing to psychoanalytic theory, and on certain issues they sharply disagree with Freud. Nevertheless, they confirm at least some of his basic contentions. For example, it is today generally accepted that sexual behavior does not "come naturally" to human beings, but is, in fact, shaped by social conditioning. It is further quite obvious that this conditioning has different goals and produces different results in different societies. There is also no longer any doubt that children are capable of sexual responses, and that certain early childhood experiences can have a crucial influence on a person's later sexual development.

Unfortunately, it is less clear than ever what all this social conditioning really means. The physician Freud had been mainly concerned with helping his patients, and for him and his followers sexual childhood experiences could easily be defined as either beneficial or harmful according to a single criterion: they were beneficial if they furthered the individual's "genital maturity," and they were harmful if they hindered or prevented it. Sexual behavior was thus described in terms of maturity and immaturity, health and sickness, norm and deviation.

In the meantime, however, sex researchers have become much more cautious. They now realize that sexual norms change a great deal from one time and place to another and that, in regard to human behavior, terms like "maturity" and "health" are value judgments rather than judgments of fact. In Freud's time, sexual health and maturity were believed to manifest themselves in a monogamous marriage devoted to the procreation of children. Sex, love, marriage, and procreation were therefore seen as inseparable. Indeed, sexual activity without any of its "socially redeeming" features was considered evil: sex without love (masturbation and prostitution), sex without marriage (premarital and extramarital intercourse), sex without procreation (childhood sex play, sex after the menopause, homosexuality). Today, we know that this particular value system is far from universal, and that it was typical only of the Western middle classes during a certain historical period. Medieval farmers or feudal lords, for example, lived by an entirely different value system, and the same must be said for people in the traditional African and Asian cultures. Finally, we see that in our own society more and more men and women are breaking away from their inherited middle class morality and are searching for new values. Under these circumstances, we have to be very careful about establishing any specific goals, norms, or standards for sexual behavior. Our first obligation is simply to understand it, and we therefore need an objective description in morally neutral terms.

Objectivity is not the only requirement, however. The description also has to be clear and precise, and this is a difficult task in itself. Nowhere is the terminological confusion greater than in the area of human sexuality. In fact, this confusion already begins with the very concept of sex.

We know that the term "sex" somehow refers to the difference and the attraction between males and females, but the extent of this difference and the character of this attraction are still largely disputed. Nevertheless, modern research has done a great deal to clarify the issues, and particularly the study of childhood development has provided us with some very valuable clues. It has been observed, for instance, that hermaphroditic children (i.e., children who are "sexually unfinished") may be raised as either boys or girls and develop all the "appropriate" attitudes, including their choice of sexual partner. To put it another way, children whose sex is misdiagnosed at birth learn to identify with the sex that is assigned to them. Furthermore, once a certain critical period has passed, this identification is permanent. Even if the mistake is later discovered, it cannot be corrected. After a certain age, a boy raised as a girl will continue to consider himself female and, in most cases, feel sexually attracted to males, while a girl raised as a boy will continue to consider herself male and, in most cases, feel sexually attracted to females. In other words, if "sex" has to do with the contrast between male and female, then a person's "sexual" development has at least three aspects:

1. The male or female characteristics of the body (biological sex),
2. the social role as male or female (gender role), and
3. the preference for male or female sexual partners (sexual orientation).

A great deal of confusion can be avoided if these three aspects of human sexuality are considered separately, and it seems useful, therefore, to keep the following definitions firmly in mind:

Biological Sex

Biological sex is defined as a person's maleness or femaleness. It is determined on the basis of five physical criteria: chromosomal sex, gonadal sex, hormonal sex, internal accessory reproductive structures, and external sex organs.

People are male or female to the degree in which they meet the physical criteria for maleness or femaleness.

Most individuals are clearly male or female by all five physical criteria.

However, a minority fall somewhat short of this test, and their biological sex is therefore ambiguous (hermaphroditism).

Gender Role

Gender role is defined as a person's masculinity or femininity. It is determined on the basis of certain psychological qualities that are nurtured in one sex and discouraged in the other.

People are masculine or feminine to the degree in which they conform to their gender roles.

Most individuals clearly conform to the gender role appropriate to their biological sex.

However, a minority partially assume a gender role that contradicts their biological sex (transvestism), and for an even smaller minority such a role inversion is complete (transsexualism).

Sexual Orientation

Sexual orientation is defined as a person's heterosexuality or homosexuality. It is determined on the basis of preference for sexual partners.

People are heterosexual or homosexual to the degree in which they are erotically attracted to partners of the other or same sex.

Most individuals develop a clear erotic preference for partners of the other sex (heterosexuality).

However, a minority are erotically attracted to both men and women (ambisexuality), and an even smaller minority are attracted mainly to partners of their own sex (homosexuality).

It is important to realize that not only biological sex but also gender role and sexual orientation are matters of degree, and that they may be independent of each other. Thus, they may appear in different combinations in different individuals. A few examples of biological males may illustrate the point:

- *Male—Masculine—Heterosexual*
  A person of male sex usually adopts the masculine gender role and develops a heterosexual orientation. Such an individual then conforms to our image of the "typical" male.
- *Male—Masculine—Homosexual*
  A person of male sex who has adopted the masculine gender role may very well develop a homosexual orientation. Such an individual may then look and behave like any other "typical" male in all respects but one—his choice of sexual partner.
- *Male—Feminine—Heterosexual*
  A person of male sex may adopt the feminine gender role. Such an individual may then try everything possible (including a "sex change operation") to make the body conform to the feminine self-image. In this case, an erotic preference for males, would, of course, have to be considered heterosexual.

- *Male—Feminine—Homosexual*

  A person of male sex may adopt the feminine gender role and try everything possible to make the body conform to the feminine self-image. If such an individual then also developed an erotic preference for females this sexual orientation could only be called homosexual.

Obviously, the last two examples represent rather extreme cases, and it should be remembered that even where a man identifies with the feminine gender role, this identification does not have to be complete. He may adopt that role only partially or occasionally, and he may not consider himself female at all. He may only cultivate feminine mannerisms and prefer feminine clothes or feminine occupations. It should further be noted that, in any or all of these cases, he may be heterosexual, ambisexual, or homosexual. In short, the four examples given here are not meant to establish new norms, classifications, or human stereotypes. They should simply be taken as a hint at the wide range and astonishing variety of human life. We must never forget that each individual person is unique, that few people ever fall into tidy sexual categories, and that there are countless shades and gradations.

Indeed, the very distinction between biological sex, gender role, and sexual orientation can help us to avoid hasty judgments and unwarranted generalizations. It can remind us, for instance, that not every effeminate man is a homosexual, and that not all homosexuals are effeminate. It also makes clear why somebody can think of himself as less than a "real man" when he knows very well that he is male. Finally, it shows us the possible extent and the limitations of a "sex change."

Once we realize how social conditioning influences our development as males and females, we have taken the first step toward understanding the development of our "sexual" behavior. Moreover, we can now make another useful distinction. In the preceding text, we have used the term "sexual orientation" very broadly to indicate an erotic preference for male or female partners. However, most people know that erotic preferences are usually much more specific. For example, a "typical" male is by no means attracted to all females, but only to those of a certain age, height, weight, hair color, etc. In fact, he may prefer not only a special type of female, but a special type of sexual intercourse under special conditions. These particular preferences and tastes within the general framework of a person's sexual orientation are best described as personal sexual interests. They too are the result of conditioning.

It is, of course, true that all human beings are born with the capacity to respond to many kinds of sensual stimulation. We also know that erections of the penis, the lubrication of the vagina, muscular contractions, and rhythmic pelvic movements can be observed in very young infants. In short, nobody has to learn the physiological responses that lead to orgasm. Still, everybody does learn under which specific circumstances these responses may be triggered. From their first years of life, children learn to react positively to certain stimuli and negatively to certain others. As a result of their personal experiences, they then acquire their individual behavior patterns. Thus, as already mentioned, human beings learn to be masculine or feminine, heterosexual or homosexual. They also learn to masturbate, to engage in coitus, and to feel happy or guilty about sex. They learn to prefer younger or older partners, blondes or brunettes, Europeans, Africans, or Asians. Some persons develop a strong attachment to one particular partner and are unable to respond to anyone else; others change their partners frequently. Some like variety in their erotic techniques; others stick to a single approach throughout their lives. Some men and women depend on complete privacy for their sexual responsiveness; others find additional stimulation in the knowledge that they are being watched. There are people whose sexual advances are passionate, inconsiderate, and even brutal, and there are others who enjoy making love slowly, gently, and deliberately. Certain individuals may even prefer solitary masturbation to any sexual intercourse, and certain others may seek sexual contact with animals.

Since these and many other personal sexual interests, choices, and preferences are developed through learning, they may appear natural, reasonable and, indeed, inevitable to the person involved. Even behavior which seems outrageous, fantastic, meaningless, or absurd to most people may be meaningful and rewarding to a certain individual because of the way in which he has been conditioned. A man who becomes sexually excited at the sight of a wooden horse may merely reflect some early experience in which sexual pleasure was associated with a merry-go-round, and his behavior may be no more difficult to explain than that of another man who becomes aroused while watching a striptease show. The latter response may have a certain advantage over the former, but neither of them should be of any social concern. A great number of people, however, seem to find comfort in the assumption that there is only one right way of doing anything. They take no joy in the infinite variety of human sexual behavior, but instead see it as an affront to their sense of stability and order. Such people are always tempted to set up their own preferences as universal norms, and to condemn everybody who disagrees with them.

On the other hand, it is clear that every society has a right to protect itself against sexual acts that involve force or violence, or which take place in front of unwilling witnesses. Such acts may be satisfying to the person who commits them, but since they obviously violate fundamental rights of others, they are socially unacceptable. Traditionally, they have always been treated as serious crimes which deserved severe punishment. However, in modern times there has been a growing tendency to view such acts as symptoms of mental illness rather than crimes. By the 19th century, psychiatrists began to argue in court that certain sexual offenders should not be sent to prison but to a mental hospital, and that they should not be punished but cured. In support of this argument, numerous attempts were made to classify sexual acts as normal or abnormal, healthy or sick. The best known of these attempts is perhaps that of Richard von Krafft-Ebing, a Viennese psychiatrist. In his book *Psychopathia Sexualis* (1886), he presented a long list of supposedly pathological sexual interests, for which he invented a number of rather fanciful special terms. Since then many other psychiatrists have followed his example, the lists have grown longer, and the special terms have become even more outlandish and exotic. Unfortunately, these lists usually do not restrict themselves to socially harmful acts, but include many types of behavior that are merely uncommon, unconventional, or disliked by the writer. Indeed, to this very day studies on "sexual psychopathology" have rarely been more than moralistic tracts in scientific disguise. They are important mainly as historical documents which reflect the sexual standards and moral obsessions of a particular time. (For further details, see "Conformity and Deviance.")

Nevertheless, it cannot be denied that some people develop behavior patterns which are unacceptable even to themselves. For example, a man may realize that his sexual acts are harmful to others, but he may have great difficulty controlling himself. In another case, such compulsive behavior may not be antisocial, but since it creates a sense of helplessness in the individual, he may still find it highly disturbing. There are also some men and women who feel guilty and apprehensive about any kind of sexual activity, and some others are so self-conscious and inhibited that their sexual responses are inadequate.

It is fair to say that all of these people are sexually maladjusted. In other words, their particular learning experiences have rendered them incapable of full sexual communication. They either have become insensitive to the needs of others, or are unable to fulfill them. They cannot relate to their sexual partners as complete persons, or adapt their own desires to different circumstances and situations. Instead, they seem condemned to repeat the same frustrating and self-defeating acts. In short, they fail to achieve the full amount of physical and emotional satisfaction of which most human beings are capable. (A detailed discussion of these problems can be found in the section on "Sexual Maladjustment.") The following pages simply summarize our present knowledge about the "normal" development of human sexual behavior from infancy to old age. Obviously, such a summary cannot give a complete account of the innumerable ways in which this development is influenced. A few broad hints have to suffice. However, some additional information on this subject is provided in the third part of this book, "Sex and Society."

INFANCY AND CHILDHOOD

When, at the beginning of our century, Sigmund Freud first wrote about the sexuality of children, he was vehemently attacked as an evil-minded man bent on destroying purity and innocence. Most of his contemporaries were convinced that children had no sexual feelings or capacities whatsoever. Indeed, there are still some people today who are deeply troubled by the suggestion that children start having a "sex life" the moment they are born.

However, even in our Western civilization, people have not always felt that way. Indeed, the very notion of childhood as a "pure," protected period of life is only a few hundred years old. In ancient and medieval Europe, children were not treated very differently from adults and shared in most of their activities. They did the same work, played the same games, sang the same songs, and wore the same kind of clothes. Medieval painters portrayed boys and girls as miniature adults with sinewy bodies and serious faces. Medieval poets and writers took no special notice of children and mentioned them only in connection with adult experiences and concerns. There was no special children's literature. If they could read at all, children read the classical Greek and Latin authors in the original language. As a matter of fact, there were no special schools for children. Most children had no formal schooling of any kind, but simply worked for their parents, became apprentices to some artisan, or lived as pages with a noble family. Some exceptional children had private tutors, and others attended classes for students of all ages. It was not until the 16th century that certain religious orders founded exclusive schools for the young.

The sexuality of children was not considered a problem. In general, sex was equated with reproduction, and thus people paid little attention to sexual behavior before puberty. As long as boys and girls were unable to reproduce, they remained free of sexual restrictions. It also has to be remembered that nobody made any effort to determine a person's exact age. Children often did not know how old they were, and neither did their parents. In any case, as soon as a girl had her first menstruation, she was believed ready for marriage.

These traditional attitudes began to change toward the end of the Middle Ages. Technological progress, the increasing specialization of labor, the growth of the cities, and the rise of the middle classes produced a new family structure and a new way of life. The churches started to keep accurate birth registers. Age differences became more important, as did the efficient use of time and the strict observation of schedules. Between the 16th and the 18th centuries, childhood began to be perceived as a separate phase of life with special needs of its own. People created schools, fashions, books, games, and toys that were considered suitable for children. Thus, the emotional, intellectual, and social maturity of boys and girls was postponed for quite a while. Beginning with the 18th century, this "protection" of the young was extended into still another special period of life—adolescence. In short, young people began to live in a world very different from that of adults. (For further details, see "Adolescence.")

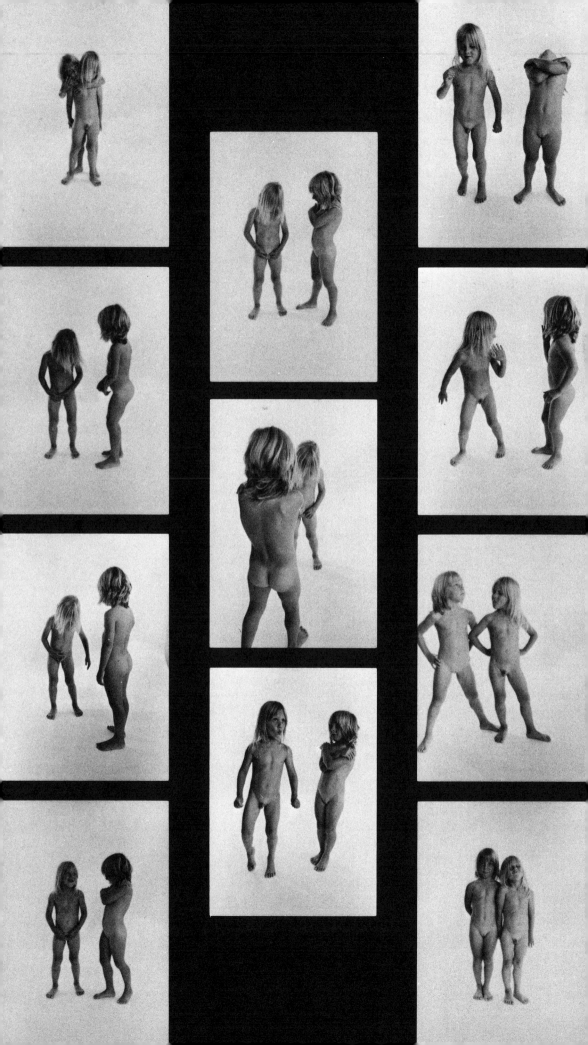

This new world was one of growing sexual repression. As mentioned earlier in this book, the modern age with its emphasis on efficiency and performance demanded a great deal of self-control from each individual. People could no longer afford to follow their impulses, and they became very sensitive about their spontaneous bodily functions. Open coughing, sneezing, yawning, belching, and farting, which had been considered healthy and natural, were now unacceptable in polite society. Nudity was no longer tolerated. The organs of excretion and reproduction began to be seen as disgusting and dirty, and finally they were completely taboo.

In the 18th century, physicians suddenly claimed to have discovered a horrible new danger to physical and mental health—childhood masturbation. According to many popular medical books of the time, masturbation was at the root of nearly all human disabilities and diseases, and it could actually prove fatal. Parents endangered the lives of their children by ignoring the practice. Among the "pampered" children of the rich, there were only a few who did not indulge in this "solitary vice" between the ages of 6 and 12. (These are the same years that were later believed to constitute the "latency period.") Only desperate measures could save these unfortunate boys and girls from death or insanity.

The crusade against masturbation, which lasted more than 200 years, led to many bizarre educational practices. Their goal, however, was always the same: protecting children against their own sexuality by denying its very existence. Children had to be kept ignorant about sexual matters, and they had to be isolated from all "bad" influences. In fact, they had to be watched and controlled at all times, lest their "purity" became contaminated with "filth." (At the same time, adults saw nothing wrong with child labor. Even in Victorian England, poor children were forced to work more than 12 hours every day in coal mines and factories.) Eventually, childhood masturbation was no longer openly mentioned. Parents and teachers began to act on the assumption that it was nothing but an "unnatural" habit of evil or sick children, and that "normal" boys and girls had no taste for it. By the end of the 19th century, most adults had persuaded themselves that childhood was indeed the one period of life in which the individual was totally free from any sexual urges.

It is easy to understand why people who held this belief were shocked and dismayed by Freud's writings. After all, he seemed to be saying the exact opposite. According to his theory, every child was born with a powerful sexual instinct, and the first years of life were decisive for its eventual proper expression. In spite of considerable opposition, this psychoanalytic view gradually gained a wide following. However, it did not change the protective attitude of parents and educators. On the contrary, while they no longer denied the child's sexuality, they were now all the more concerned about the possible influences on its development. Moreover, they became aware of their own responsibility in this respect, and this awareness sometimes created new apprehensions and anxieties.

Today, Freud's influence seems to have passed its peak. Many contemporary sex researchers no longer accept his assumptions, and, in general, they are much less preoccupied with the experiences of childhood. There is now a greater awareness than ever before that men and women are capable of learning, unlearning, and relearning many sexual attitudes and reactions throughout their lives. Nevertheless, the importance of sexual conditioning in infancy and childhood remains well recognized. There is also no doubt that parents and close relatives have a great influence on a child's sexual development. The discipline they demand, the routines they establish, and the examples they set give boys and girls the first concept of sexual differences and teach them how to relate to their own bodies. Adults convey their sexual attitudes to children in a thousand different ways: through their sense of modesty and privacy, the way they answer questions about sex, the words they use for sexual organs and sexual activity, their tone of voice, their gestures and facial expressions.

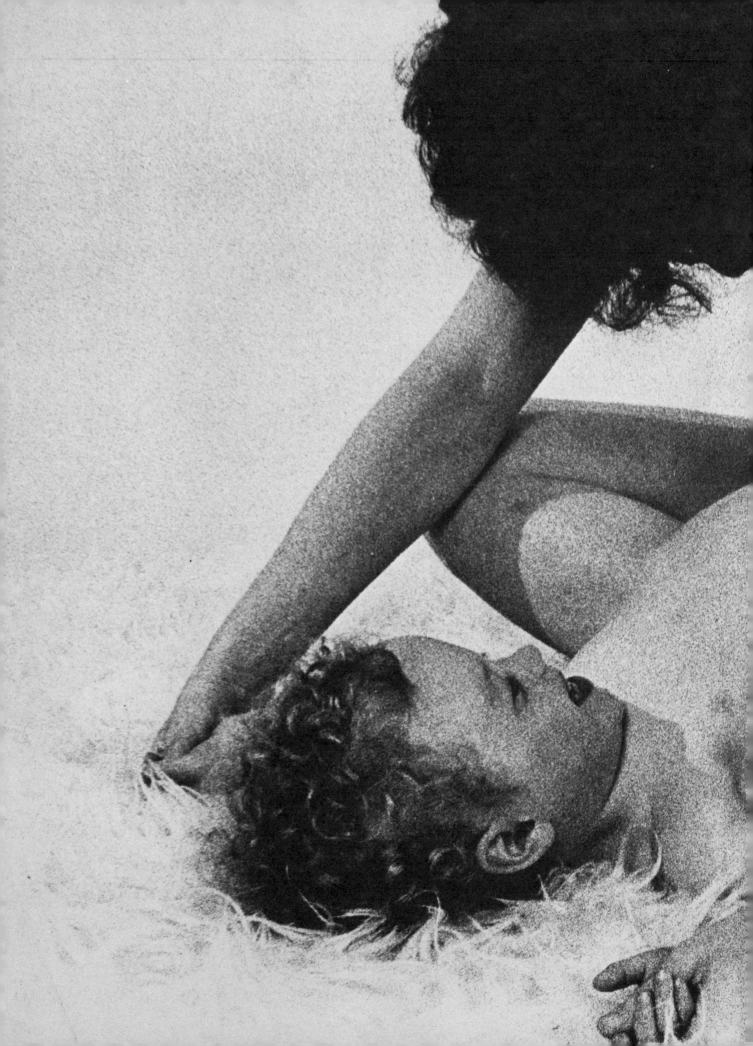

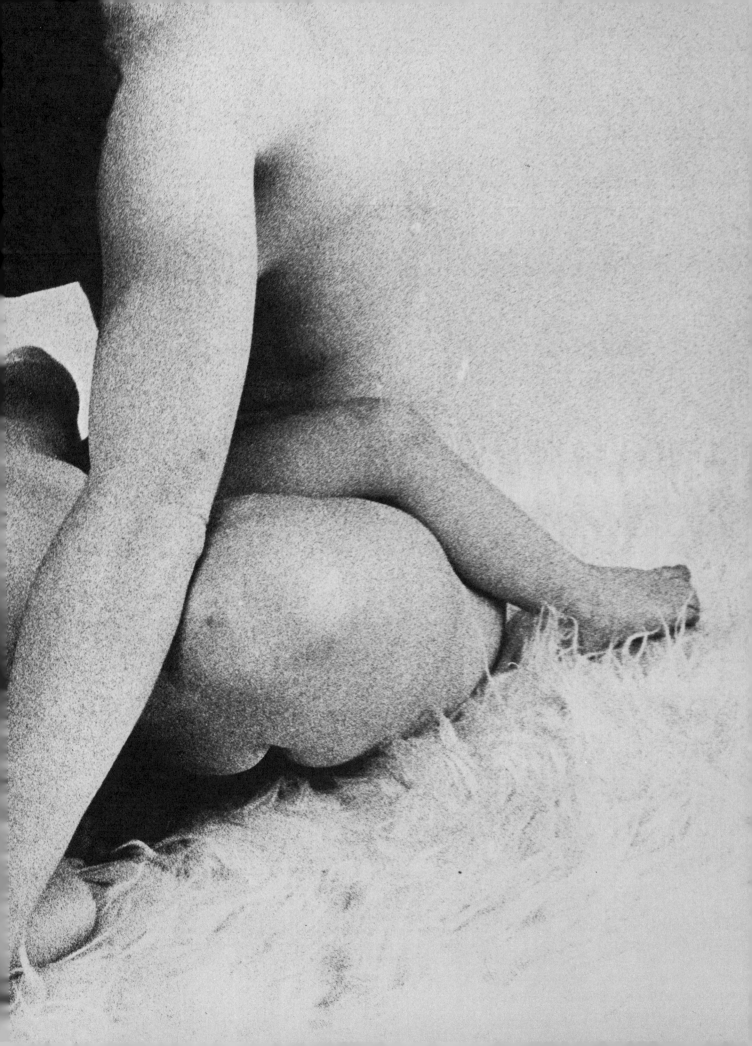

Unfortunately, in our culture many adults are rather uncomfortable with their own sexuality, and thus they are unable to accept their children as happy and healthy sexual beings. As a result, there often develops a serious communication gap between the generations. Children who are made to feel ashamed and guilty about their natural physical responses lose confidence in their parents and soon stop asking them sexual questions. When this happens, some parents may secretly feel relieved, and they may even conclude that their children have lost interest in sexual matters. At any rate, most adults today have become accustomed to viewing the years of late childhood as a period of sexual "latency," i.e., a phase of life when the sexual development comes to a temporary halt.

Indeed, as children approach puberty their social interests and obligations expand considerably, and their sexual activity may therefore seem to decrease for a while. Furthermore, older children are often sexually segregated in their leisure activities. There is less opportunity for physical contact between boys and girls. Especially girls are warned against kissing, embracing, exposing their bodies, or having sexual intercourse. Still, those children who have begun masturbating to orgasm usually continue to do so. In other words, if there is indeed a latency period, it does not seem to have a biological basis. This conclusion is also supported by various anthropological studies. Children in sexually permissive "primitive" societies do not give up their sex play in late childhood. (For further details on social attitudes toward childhood sex play, see "The Sexually Oppressed.")

THE SEXUAL RESPONSE IN INFANTS

Modern sex researchers have often compared the development of sexual behavior to the learning of a language, and this comparison is indeed very illuminating. For example, we know that people in different cultures display different sexual behaviors, just as they speak different languages. Furthermore, there are differences within one and the same culture. Just as an individual may acquire an exceptional mastery over his native language, some persons may show a greater sexual responsiveness than others; and just as certain people suffer from speech impediments, some men and women are sexually inhibited or completely unresponsive. Finally, it is clear that human beings can learn to respond to a great variety of sexual stimuli, just as they can learn to understand several languages. In short, all healthy children are born with the capacity to learn any possible human language and to adopt any possible human sexual behavior. In both cases, their development is greatly influenced by cultural conditioning.

Very young children who are still unable to speak are called infants (from Latin infans: someone who cannot speak). While they have all the necessary physical equipment for speech (mouth, tongue, vocal cords, etc.), they cannot yet form any words that another person can understand. Instead, they produce a random flow of many different vocal sounds, including vowels and consonants that are not even part of the language they are about to learn. These "extra" vowels and consonants are suppressed and forgotten as children learn to repeat the proper sounds of their mother tongue. In fact, when they later study a foreign language, they may spend a great deal of time and energy relearning the very sounds they were once taught to forget.

The early development of sexual behavior proceeds along very similar lines. All babies are born with a certain physical equipment which enables them to respond to sexual stimulation. Infant boys may have frequent erections of the penis, and infant girls may very well experience lubrications of the vagina. They feel pleasure when their sex organs or other erogenous zones are touched, and they may even reach orgasm fairly early in life. Nevertheless, infants are still "sexually inarticulate." They respond rather indiscriminately to all kinds of stimuli, and their responses are not yet fully integrated and coordinated. Only gradually, under the influence of social conditioning, do children begin to structure their sexual behavior in a way that is acceptable to the culture in which they grow up. In other words, they not only learn the "proper" responses, but also suppress and forget the "improper" ones. In fact, when they later try to increase their sexual responsiveness, they may spend a great deal of time and energy relearning the very responses they were once taught to suppress.

For infants, the main source of sensual stimulation is the mother. As they are being touched, caressed, and nursed, they learn to feel loved and accepted and to gain confidence in the world. Physical closeness gives them the sense of security they need for a healthy development. It is therefore very unfortunate that some hospitals still separate newborn children from their mothers, thus depriving both of the first essential communication. Later, this initial mistake may be compounded by the mothers themselves when they avoid any skin contact with their infants and keep them clothed even while playing with them. By the same token, a mother who does not breastfeed her baby misses an important opportunity to build a more intimate relationship. Babies want more than just nourishment. They also hunger for human warmth and reassurance. Some mothers realize their children's needs in this respect, but refuse to meet them after a rather short time. However, just as infants cannot learn to speak unless they are spoken to, they cannot learn to show love and affection unless they are hugged, stroked, tickled, and kissed by their parents or nurses. Parents who deny their children such physical and emotional gratification leave them frustrated and, in fact, teach them to feel uncomfortable with their bodies. There is no doubt that such negative early experiences can deeply affect the child's future attitude toward sex.

SELF-EXPLORATION IN INFANCY
Unless their natural curiosity is suppressed by their parents, children begin to explore their bodies as soon as they are capable of doing so. In this picture a little girl examines her sex organs as she plays with her mother.

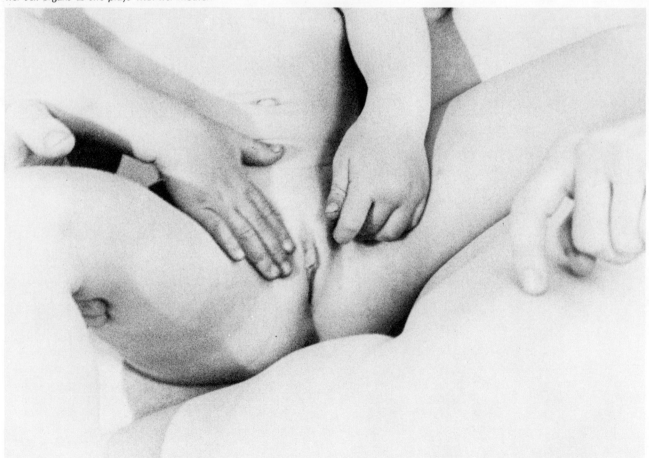

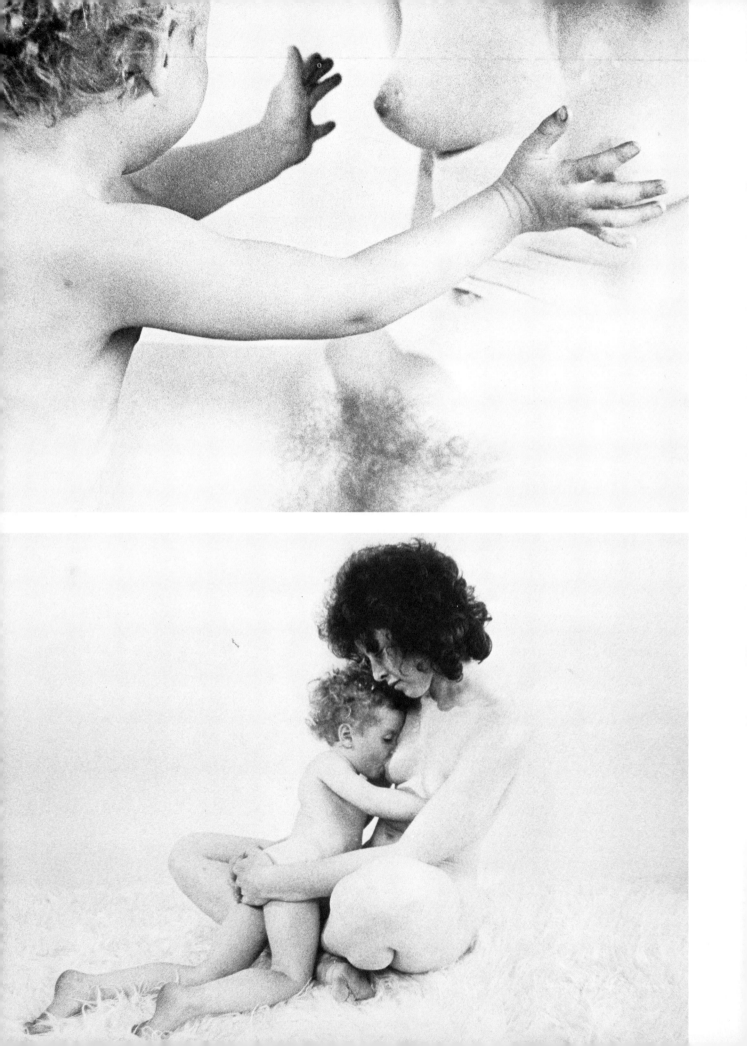

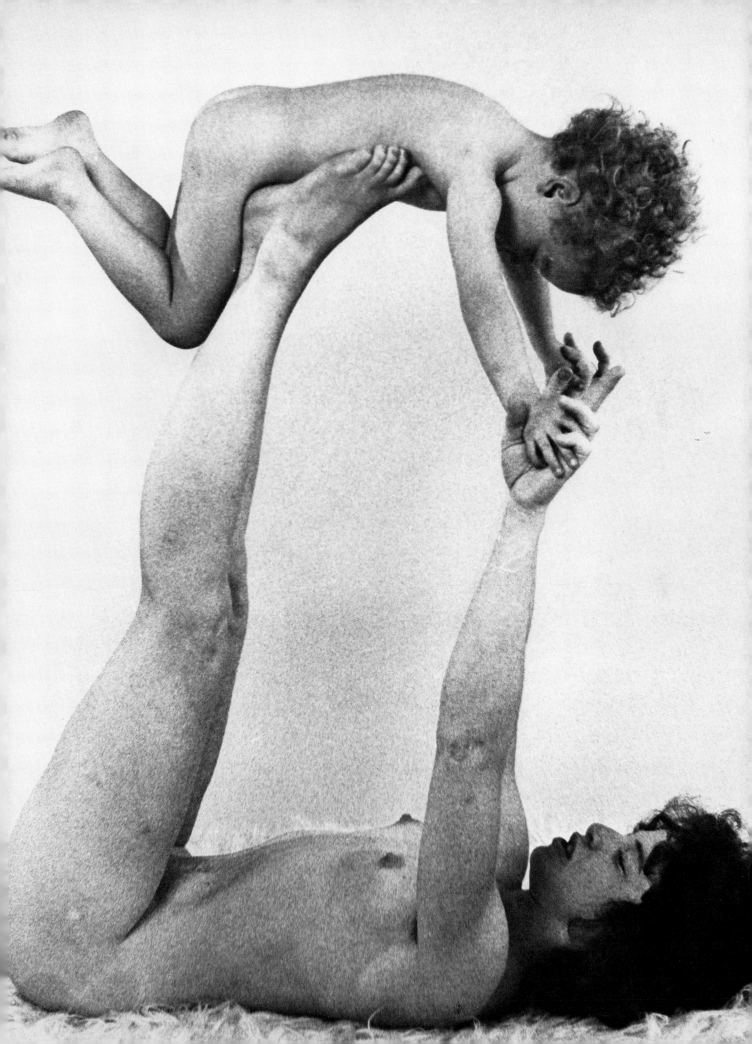

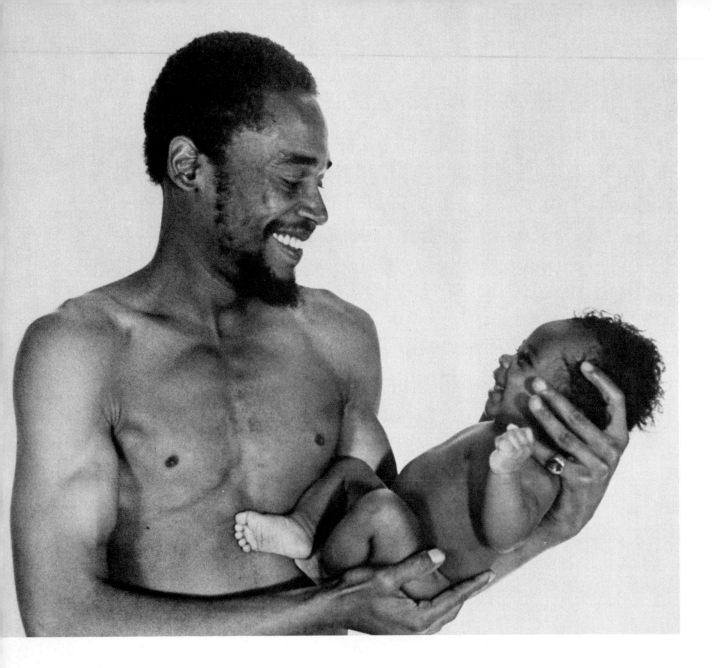

LEARNING A
GENDER ROLE

Human beings are either male or female, and children learn at an early age to identify themselves as one or the other. At the same time, they also learn to behave in a way that is considered typical of males or females. In short, they learn to adopt a masculine or feminine gender role.

The concept of gender role has been explained by John Money, one of the leading researchers in this field, as "all those things that a person says or does to disclose himself or herself as having the status of boy or man, girl or woman, respectively. It includes but is not restricted to sexuality in the sense of eroticism. A gender role is not established at birth, but is built up cumulatively through experiences encountered and transacted, through casual and unplanned learning, through explicit instruction and inculcation."

When a child is born, the parents, relatives, friends, and neighbors first try to find out whether it is a boy or a girl. One look at the baby's external sex organs normally supplies the answer, and this answer has immediate social consequences.

An adult is used to approaching boys and girls very differently. For example, he is more likely to praise a baby boy for his strength and a baby girl for her pretty face than vice versa. In our particular culture, boys are usually dressed in blue, girls in pink. (Most Americans consider pink a feminine color.) Boys are given different names than girls, and their hair is usually cut in a different style. They are presented with different toys and encouraged to play different games. Indeed, even in his first months of life a boy may be touched, picked up, and held in a different manner, and he may receive different and fewer caresses than a girl. As he grows up, he is told that "big boys don't cry" and that he should learn to control his emotions. A girl, on the other hand, is expected to show tenderness and affection. According to a popular nursery rhyme, boys "are made of snips and snails and puppy dog tails," while girls "are made of sugar and spice and everything nice." Thus, boys do not find themselves rewarded for a gentle, quiet demeanor, and girls soon learn to suppress their aggressive impulses. (See also "The Social Roles of Men and Women.")

Under the influence of these adult attitudes, approaches, hints, examples, and expectations, boys and girls gradually develop a concept of themselves as sexual beings. They also learn how the two sexes relate to each other. By the time children begin to have a command of language (between 18 months and 2 years of age), the establishment of their gender roles is well under way. In this period, they strongly identify with the parent of their own sex and, after about another 2 years, their self-identification as male and female is

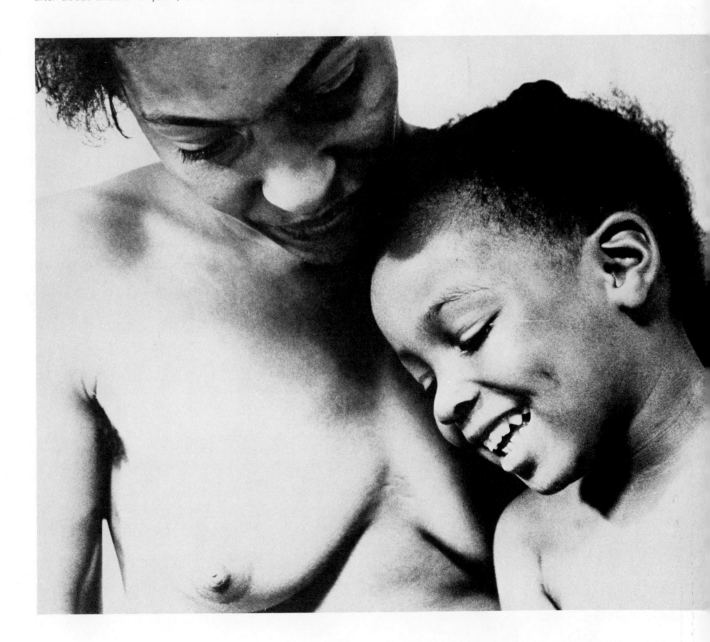

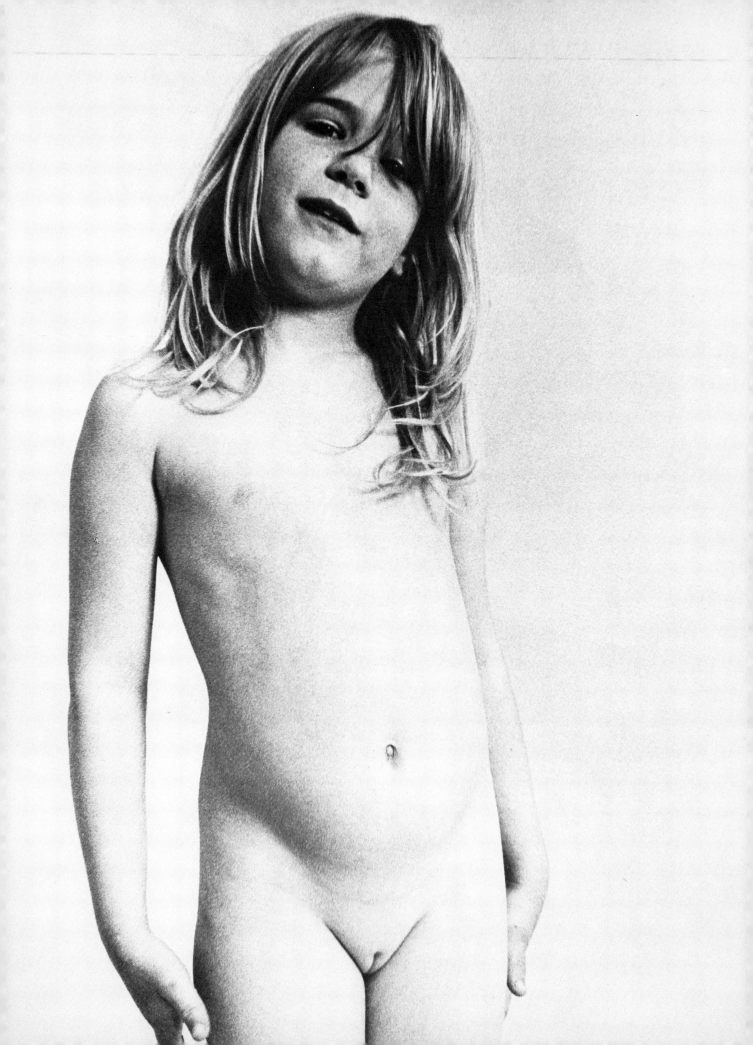

usually irreversible. It should be noted that 4–5-year-old children may still be confused about male and female sex organs, and that they may define males and females according to other criteria, such as height, shape, clothing, hairstyle, etc. This does not mean, however, that they have any doubts about their own masculinity or femininity. It only indicates that, for children of this age, the sex organs are not yet of any decisive importance.

There are some rare cases in which children with sexual malformations are misdiagnosed at birth and thus brought up in a gender role inappropriate to their biological sex. When the mistake is later discovered, it may become necessary to reverse the sex assignment. In the early months of life, such a reassignment of sex is often possible if all adults who come in contact with the child are consistent and completely firm about it. However, after the first 18 months the attempt is less likely to succeed, and after the child's fourth birthday it is virtually guaranteed to fail. (See also "Sexual Malformations.")

There are also certain cases where children who are clearly male or female adopt an ambiguous, defective, or erroneous gender role. The problems of these individuals are discussed in another section of this book. (See "Transsexualism.")

CHILDHOOD SEX PLAY

Children develop their concept of sex only gradually. Thus, as already mentioned, they are taught to identify themselves as male or female and to act accordingly. It is important to realize, however, that the rehearsal of a gender role involves many things that acquire a sexual meaning only after puberty. In other words, children learn some "sexual" behavior patterns long before they realize their true implications. For instance, on many American and European beaches little girls are made to wear two-piece bathing suits while boys are allowed to wear simple trunks. From a strictly logical standpoint, this difference in clothing may at first be hard to understand. After all, before puberty the breasts of males and females look exactly alike. Nevertheless, in anticipation of future differences, girls already learn to be modest about this particular part of their anatomy. As a result, the female breast is "eroticized," and the male breast is not. (In certain non-Western cultures, on the other hand, the female breast remains exposed throughout life and has no special erotic significance.)

As this example shows, children may adopt certain sexual attitudes well in advance of any actual sexual encounters. However, they may also have intimate physical contact with other people without considering it sexual at all. They have to be told by adults or older children that some things or actions have to do with "sex" and are therefore especially important, mysterious, secret, exciting, or naughty. It is quite obvious, therefore, that the parents have a decisive influence on a child's sexual development. If they feel uncomfortable or even guilty about their own sexuality, they are bound to convey these negative feelings to everybody around them and, as a result, the child may become confused and apprehensive. This would be very unfortunate. Children cannot develop properly if they are not encouraged to experiment, to seek new experiences, and to exercise all their faculties. With such encouragement and proper guidance, however, their "sex play" will eventually turn into purposeful, responsible behavior.

Self-Stimulation

As noted above, very young infants are already capable of certain sexual responses. Indeed, many boys are born with an erection of the penis. Infants of both sexes may be observed rubbing their sex organs against the bed, the floor, or some toy in a thrusting motion, and there is no doubt that they derive physical pleasure from it. For some time, they are still unable to coordinate their movements and to use their hands for a more direct stimulation. However, after a while, they may learn to do so and begin to masturbate. Quite often such deliberate masturbation is carried through to the point of orgasm.

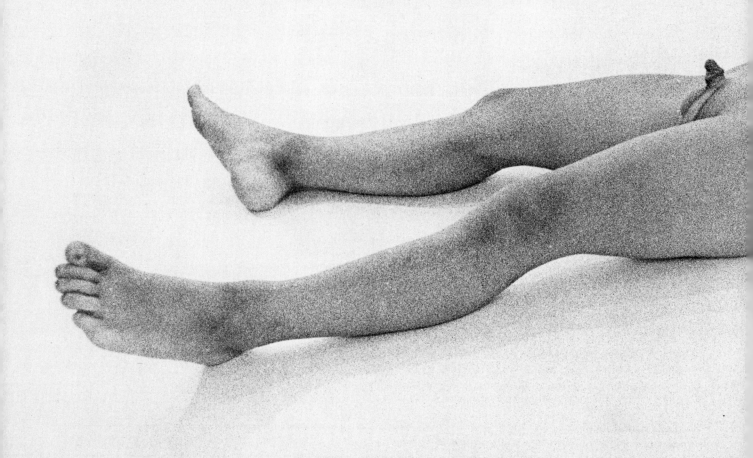

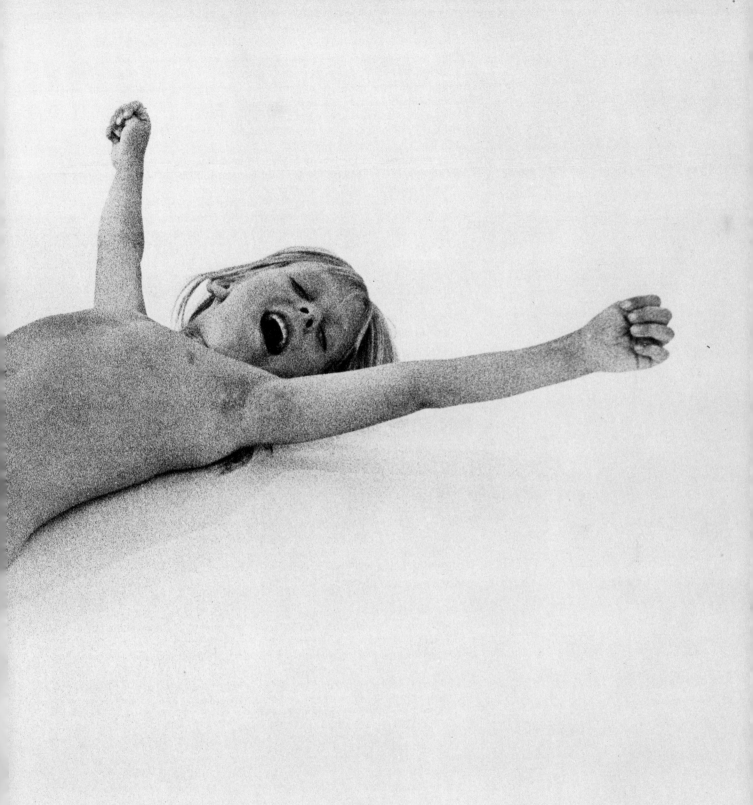

A child's orgasmic capacity increases with advancing age. By their fifth birthday, more than half of all boys have reached orgasm, and for boys between 10 and 13 years of age the figure rises to nearly 80%. Naturally, the orgasms of these boys are not yet accompanied by ejaculations, since no seminal fluid is produced before puberty. (Even then the ejaculated semen may not contain any sperm cells for some time.) On the other hand, some boys are capable of several orgasms in quick succession. They normally lose this capacity as they grow older.

It seems that, on the whole, fewer girls than boys masturbate to orgasm at an early age. One reason for this may be found in the different anatomy of the two sexes. (A penis is comparatively easy to manipulate, and its erection is more difficult to ignore than the lubrication of the vagina.) A second reason may be the passive, nonsexual attitude that girls learn to adopt as a result of social conditioning. In our culture, little girls are usually not encouraged to be sexual beings.

Parents who see their boys or girls masturbate make a serious mistake if they become alarmed about it and force them to stop under the threat of punishment. This will only create needless feelings of guilt in the children as they continue the practice in secret. The sexual response is a normal function of the human body at any age and, as such, cannot possibly do any physical harm. Neither can it stunt a child's growth. On the contrary, for many children masturbation is simply part of growing up, and there is no medical reason why they should not enjoy it. Nevertheless, children can and should learn that, in our particular culture, masturbation is a very personal and private activity which is unacceptable in public. At the same time, they should be made to understand that what is done in private is not necessarily bad, shameful, sinful, or dirty. As long as such negative connotations are avoided, childhood masturbation creates no problems.

Sex Play with Other Children

Children are naturally curious and, as they grow up, they try to learn everything they can about themselves and the world around them. Once they have explored their own bodies, they are eager to find out whether the other children are in any way different. This is especially true for children who have never seen their parents or brothers and sisters in the nude.

Just as boys and girls compare their height and physical agility, they are also likely to compare the various parts of the body, including those that are kept covered by clothing. Usually, they find a practical way of doing this by playing "doctor," or "house," or "mummy and daddy." Such games give them an opportunity to study each other's bodies at leisure, to touch and fondle the sex organs, or even to engage in mutual masturbation. Indeed, they may lie on top of each other and try to imitate coitus or anal intercourse. Boys as well as girls may also take a penis in their mouths and suck on it.

Such behavior is not necessarily sexual in the adult sense of the word. Children learn only gradually to invest certain activities and social situations with erotic meaning. At first, childhood sex play is just another way of becoming familiar with the human anatomy. Thus, boys play not only with girls in this fashion, but also with other boys, and girls often play with each other. As a matter of statistical fact, before their tenth birthday boys have more sex play with other boys than with girls. It would be foolish, however, to view such incidents as early evidence of homosexuality. While the term "homosexual behavior" may be technically correct whenever partners of the same sex are involved, it is quite misleading in this context because same-sex play in childhood in no way precludes an adult heterosexual orientation. The premature application of labels to the behavior of children only creates unnecessary problems. By the same token, it is unwise to speak of a "homosexual phase" in every boy's personal development. It may very well be true that many boys go through a period of "hating girls" in which they prefer to associate with other boys. However, this attitude is much better explained as an attempt to consolidate the masculine gender role. (The theory that children progress from self-love through love of the same sex to that of the opposite sex has never been proven, and recent scientific findings strongly suggest that it is false.)

Almost all children play sexual games at one time or another, and very often it is a wholesome, pleasant experience for them. They may not realize the erotic potential of these games right away, but sooner or later they will become aware of it. If their sex play then continues to be enjoyable, it may help them to accept their own bodies and to grow up without sexual fear and guilt.

Unfortunately, this positive outcome is not always assured. Indeed, under certain circumstances, sexual games can become quite disturbing for children. This is the case, for example, if they are threatened or exploited by older friends or some playground bullies. Children can be cruel and are very well capable of mistreating those who are timid or weak. Obviously, any sex play that involves unwilling participants must be considered harmful.

Another potential source of trouble is the reaction of parents. Many parents are horrified when they discover that their child has been involved in sex play and, in some cases, they feel that such "bad" behavior deserves drastic punishment. This attitude is incomprehensible to children, and thus they may, for the first time in their lives, feel misunderstood, betrayed, and abandoned. They also may become so fearful and suspicious of anything sexual that their further personality development is seriously impaired. Some sensitive children never outgrow such an early traumatic experience. It is therefore very fortunate that, in recent decades, adult sex education has made great progress and that, generally speaking, parents have now become more sophisticated and tolerant in these matters.

Sexual Contact with Adults

As mentioned earlier, our Western civilization has not always believed that children should be protected from all sexual contact. In medieval Europe, children were still freely touched, caressed, and fondled by every member of the household. Particularly in rural areas, parents, nurses, or servants were accustomed to masturbating small children to please them or to keep them quiet. (This practice is also found in many non-European societies. In the United States today, it is still alive among the Hopi Indians.) However, in modern times there has been a growing tendency to view children as asexual beings. Only in this century, under the influence of Freud and his followers, has the sexuality of children regained at least partial acceptance. Nevertheless, most people continue to believe that there cannot possibly be any harmless sexual contact between children and adults.

There are indeed some adults who abuse children sexually, and parents are justly concerned about this danger. Unfortunately, this concern leads some parents to become overcautious and overprotective. Children who are constantly warned against strangers, and who are taught to be suspicious of any friendly gesture of the part of adults, may become nervous, hostile, and withdrawn. Eventually, they may learn to fear all adults and all sexual feelings and thus become emotionally crippled. This may also happen if they have a pleasant sexual encounter with an adult which is then discovered and misinterpreted by other adults. Even if the encounter was unpleasant, it may in itself cause less psychological damage than the overreaction of parents, neighbors, and public officials. A case in point is the public attitude toward exhibitionists. Children who are familiar with the nude human body may be startled, but are unlikely to be seriously shocked when they see a man exposing his penis. Moreover, since such a man is usually nonviolent, no great harm will be done if the parents remain calm and explain the incident properly.

Nevertheless, as a general rule boys and girls in our culture are well advised to keep away from strangers and to avoid any sexual contact with adults, or even with much older children. A child is clearly better off playing sexual games with close friends of the same age.

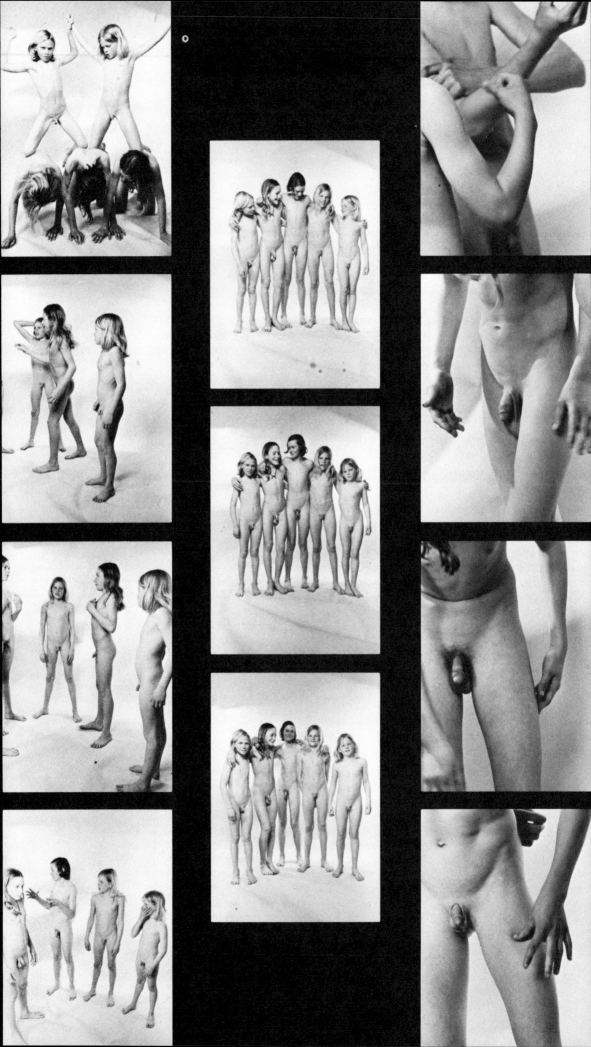

ADOLESCENCE

Adolescence (from Latin *adolescere:* to grow up) is the period of life between puberty and adulthood. In the last several centuries, this period has become rather extended, but throughout most of human history it was relatively short. Indeed, today there are still "primitive" peoples in many parts of the world to whom an adolescence in our modern sense is completely unknown. Instead, they use so-called initiation rites to confer the status of adults on their children as soon as they reach puberty.

Puberty is, in essence, a process of physical maturation which produces the secondary sexual characteristics and leads to fertility. In contrast, adolescence is better described as a process of psychological and social maturation which leads to full citizenship. Puberty is a biological phenomenon, adolescence a cultural one. Puberty normally begins in a person's early teens and ends a few years later. Adolescence begins with puberty and today may very well last a decade or more.

Many people are unaware of the fact that even in our own Western culture things have not always been this way. For example, in medieval Europe boys and girls reached legal adulthood fairly early in life. Most ancient Middle European tribes declared their children adults at the age of 12, the Angles and Saxons even at the age of 11. A 13th-century German legal code *(Schwabenspiegel)* still allowed males of 14 and females of 12 to marry without their father's consent.

In order to understand these laws and customs properly, we have to remember that they were tailored to the needs of a largely agrarian culture, that the average life span was very short, and that young and old shared in practically all daily activities. Under these circumstances, there was no need for an extended special period of transition from childhood to adulthood. Indeed, the social contrast between a child and an adult was much less pronounced than it is today. Children were not sentimentalized as weak, pure, and innocent, but simply worked alongside their parents and older brothers and sisters as best they could. In this manner, they gradually adopted adult attitudes and assumed adult responsibilities.

We have mentioned earlier that the beginning of the Modern Age brought a growing awareness of generational differences. Children became more "child-like," and adults more "serious." To be an adult now meant to be able to control oneself, to submit to a greater degree of discipline than ever before. The specialization and mechanization of labor in the developing cities made it necessary to find new, exact methods of measuring time. Fixed schedules for work and leisure had to be established. Young people were trained in a craft or business according to a certain timetable, or they were sent to a school with a definite curriculum. The number of years spent in such training increased. The opportunities for individual early achievement dwindled. Once special schools for the young had been founded, they provided a temporary escape from the demands of real life, a closed environment with values of its own. Students had many duties but few rights, and, for a long time, they remained dependent on their parents and teachers. Beginning with the 16th century, childhood emerged as a special, protected period of life. In the 18th century, a second such period began to be recognized—adolescence.

Thus, within a few centuries the social attitudes toward young people underwent a dramatic change. This change was particularly obvious in the area of sex, as we can learn from a comparison between two important educational books of the 16th and 18th centuries: *Colloquia Familiaria* by Erasmus of Rotterdam (1522) and *Emile* by Jean-Jacques Rousseau (1762). Erasmus wrote the *Colloquia* for his six-year-old godson "in order to teach him good Latin and to educate him for the world." The text therefore deals with all sorts of everyday experiences and problems, including sexual ones.

There are detailed and very frank discussions of sexual desire, sexual pleasure, and sexual intercourse, conception, pregnancy, birth, marriage, divorce, prostitution, and venereal disease. The language is straightforward and sometimes humorous. Sex appears as a natural and pleasant part of life which must be approached with understanding and common sense.

For Rousseau, on the other hand, who sets out to describe an utopian, ideal education, sex is a highly problematical, potentially dangerous subject. He therefore no longer writes for children, or even for their parents, but for professional educators. Even so, his language is evasive and ambiguous, important points are deliberately left unexplained, and all possible negative connotations of sex are heavily emphasized. In contrast to Erasmus, Rousseau clearly distinguishes between childhood, adolescence, and adulthood. In his "modern" view, children must be kept completely ignorant about sex, and adolescents must learn as little as possible. Only direct and persistent questions are to be answered, and then the utter seriousness of the subject must be stressed. The longer a young person's "innocence" can be preserved, the better. Youth must be protected from sexual knowledge, and his book therefore tells enlightened adults how to provide such protection.

We have to realize, of course, that Rousseau, like Erasmus before him, merely expressed the spirit of his times. The new ideal was the "pure," asexual, idealistic adolescent who "saved his strength" for the somber duties of adult life. It is no coincidence that, early in the century, the first medical pamphlets describing the dangers of masturbation had appeared in England and Germany. Indeed, a few years before the publication of *Emile,* a respected Swiss physician by the name of Tissot had joined the campaign, which then quickly spread all over the Western world, leading to unprecedented excesses of adult hysteria over the "moral and physical corruption of youth." In this climate of growing prudery, young people soon lost their right not only to sexual information, but also to any and all sexual activity. (For further details, see "Types of Sexual Activity—Sexual Self-stimulation.")

It has to be stressed, however, that at first these developments affected only the children of the middle classes. The aristocracy and the lower classes, such as farmers, workers, soldiers, and domestic servants, held on to their traditional sexual practices and attitudes. It was not until after the industrial revolution, when the middle classes became socially dominant, that their way of life became a model for all of society. Even today, there are still social groups within our culture which do not accept this model. In the United States, these groups are often defined by their ethnic origin. For example, the Indians on their reservations, the Blacks in the urban ghetto, the Eskimos in Alaska, and the Polynesians on various American Pacific islands all have their own sexual morality and their own view of adolescence. (To a lesser extent, such cultural differences can also be found among the various white ethnic groups.) Furthermore, in recent years many members of the middle class have "dropped out" and gone back to the historically older "lower-class" values.

Nevertheless, generally speaking, the sexual laws and customs in most industrial societies reflect the needs, hopes, and fears of the middle classes that emerged with the beginning of the Modern Age. Thus, adolescence has become accepted as a rather long special period of adjustment in which young people must be protected not only against the harsh realities of life, but also against their own immaturity. Adult rights, privileges, and responsibilities cannot be bestowed upon the individual all at once in a particular ceremony, but have to be acquired gradually over many years. Indeed, some people may not become fully independent adults until their middle or late thirties.

In the United States, the first small step toward adult status is now usually taken at the age of 12 when children lose the right to special price reductions and are treated as fully grown customers by movie theaters, museums, zoos, bus companies, airlines, and so on. The next change in status occurs four years later. At the age of 16, boys and girls can obtain a driver's license, and they escape many of the restrictions of the child labor laws. In some states, they also gain the legal competence to consent to sexual intercourse. Another significant change occurs at the age of 18. For females, this is the "age of consent" in most states. Males may be drafted into the armed forces. (This rule remains in effect even if the military draft is temporarily suspended during peace time.) In most states, both sexes may marry without the consent of their parents. They also win the right to vote and to run for public office. In fact, in most states they are now considered adults for most legal purposes. However, in a number of states they have to wait until the age of 21 before they are allowed to drink alcohol or enter a bar or night club where alcohol is served. Even then, they may not yet become full adults in the functional sense. For example, as college students they may still be financially dependent on their parents. In fact, if they choose to enter a highly specialized profession, they may remain unable to support themselves for another decade or more.

Thus, we see that, depending on their social background and their aims in life, young people in our culture may not achieve complete legal and economic independence until 5, 10, or even 20 years after puberty. To a great extent, this delay is, of course, unavoidable because of the growing complexity of the modern world. It can even be seen as beneficial because it allows for a gradual adjustment to the many demands of today's adult life. However, it also creates many serious problems, including sexual ones.

Our official morality restricts sexual intercourse to married partners, but physically mature males and females often are not allowed, cannot afford, or do not want to get married before they are well into their twenties. As a result, they are forced to go through a difficult period of sexual frustration. Fortunately, in the meantime, the antimasturbation campaign of the last two centuries has lost most of its impact, but premarital coitus is still largely condemned. Thus, for many adolescents masturbation is the only available outlet. Some experiment with various "petting" techniques, and others turn to homosexual contacts as a temporary substitute.

There can be no doubt that the sexual oppression of the young creates much genuine misery. Contemporary scholars and scientists have clearly demonstrated that, on the average, males reach the height of their sexual responsiveness during their teens, and that it is then virtually impossible for them to go without some sort of regular sexual activity. An adolescent female may find it somewhat easier to remain abstinent, but her chances for sexual satisfaction in marriage are greatly improved if she experiences orgasm earlier in her life.

Thus, modern research has rediscovered what had always been obvious to former, less repressive ages. Indeed, as Alfred C. Kinsey reemphasized decades ago, many of the great romances of world literature celebrate the passionate love affairs of the young. Eros and Psyche, Acis and Galatea, Pyramus and Thisbe, Daphnis and Chloë, Floire and Blancheflor, Aucassin and Nicolette, Romeo and Juliet—all of these famous lovers were underage according to modern standards. Margarethe was a teenager when she fell in love with Faust, and Helen was only twelve years old when she left her husband Menelaos and followed Paris to Troy. Narcissus was sixteen "when many youths and many maidens sought his love." Ganymede was even younger when Zeus made him his favorite. Hyacinth was an adolescent when Apollo and Zephyros quarreled over his possession, and so was Hylas when Hercules abducted him from his parents. In short, as every student of cultural history knows, Western mythology and poetry abound with references to such youthful "objects of love," but if any of them came to life today, they would simply be considered juvenile delinquents, and their lovers would be imprisoned for the "corruption of a minor."

One can only hope that, in the future, our society will abandon these negative and unrealistic attitudes. It is a good sign that a growing number of adults already accept and defend the sexual rights of adolescents. Even some public and private schools, foundations, and health agencies have dropped

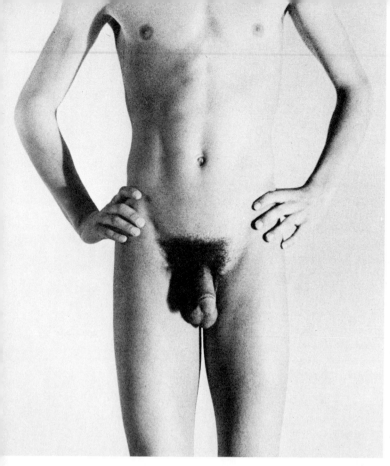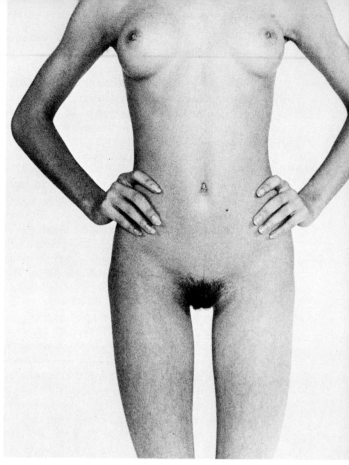

THE PHYSICAL CHANGES OF PUBERTY
During puberty, the male and female bodies develop their secondary sexual characteristics. The so-called pubic hair begins to appear, and males experience an increase in the size of their external sex organs. In females, the breasts start to develop. (For a more detailed comparison see chart on p. 20.)

the traditional pretenses and now take a certain amount of adolescent sexual activity for granted. In many parts of the country, young people also receive an adequate sex education and are given effective help with their personal sexual problems. (See also "Contraception," "Abortion," and "Venereal Diseases.") Nevertheless, in spite of such recent progress, there are still many males and females for whom adolescence is the most trying period in their lives. (For a more detailed discussion of these issues, see "The Sexually Oppressed.")

The following pages first briefly summarize the physical changes of puberty and then describe some of the ways in which adolescents in our society may learn to express themselves as sexual beings.

THE PHYSICAL CHANGES OF PUBERTY

Puberty (from Latin *puber:* adult) is the period of life when boys and girls turn into young men and women. That is to say, their bodies begin to show the secondary male and female sexual characteristics, and they become capable of reproduction. These physical changes occur under the influence of various hormones, especially the gonadal hormones. (For details, see "The Process of Sexual Differentiation.")

Puberty arrives at different ages for different individuals, and it may last between one and several years. Much depends on hereditary factors, diet, climate, cultural influences, and emotional conditions. In recent decades, the age of puberty seems to have been lowering for both sexes. However, now as before, the physical maturation of females begins somewhat earlier than that of males. In girls, the enlargement of the breasts and the growth of pubic hair start at an average age of 10 to 11 years, and the first menstruation occurs at about 11 to 13 years. In boys, the enlargement of the testicles and the growth of pubic hair normally begin during the ages of 12 to 16 years, and the first ejaculation occurs from 13 to 17 years of age.

Since the physical changes of puberty may appear early or late, quickly or slowly, individuals of the same chronological age may find themselves in very different stages of development. For an adolescent, this is often a matter of great concern. Boys may worry about their height, the breadth of their shoulders, the strength of their muscles, the size of their penis. Girls may be afraid of growing too tall, and they may anxiously measure the size of their breasts and the width of their hips. Indeed, during this period, young people tend to become extremely sensitive and self-conscious about their appearance. In many cases, the hormonal changes in the body produce acne, an inflammatory skin disease which, although otherwise harmless, may temporarily disfigure the face, neck, and back. Some adolescents also consider themselves unattractive because they seem to be gaining too much weight. Still another potential source of embarrassment is the heightened sexual responsiveness. For example, boys may resent the fact that they have sudden erections at very awkward moments. To some extent, this may also have happened in childhood. However, with the arrival of puberty these responses occur more often, and they now become more clearly defined as sexual. Paradoxically, the sexual awareness of girls lags well behind that of boys. While the secondary sexual characteristics may appear much earlier in females than in males, the female capacity for sexual arousal and orgasm often develops much later. There may be some biological reason for this, but social conditioning undoubtedly also plays a role.

As already mentioned, children are capable of sexual responses well before puberty. For example, they may become aroused in the course of their games and other physical activities. Indeed, they may have an orgasm while riding a bicycle, climbing a tree, sliding down a bannister, or wrestling with a playmate. However, at first they do not define these experiences as sexual in the adult sense of the word. They learn to do so only gradually as they grow older. Indeed, boys and girls normally do not become fully aware of their sexuality until they have reached puberty.

Adolescence can therefore be seen as a time when many sexual attitudes and reactions that were rehearsed in childhood begin to reveal their true meaning. Most important of all, it is a period in which experimental and exploratory sex play turns into purposeful adult sexual behavior.

Unfortunately, in our culture young people are severely limited in their sexual opportunities. Because of social and religious taboos, most adolescents have difficulty beginning sexual intercourse with a partner of the opposite sex. Even if they find such a partner, they often feel that they have to restrict themselves to "petting," i.e., sexual contact that stops short of coitus. For the vast majority of adolescents, the main sexual outlet is solitary masturbation, although some boys may occasionally masturbate together in small groups. A few boys who live in the countryside may also have sexual contact with animals.

On the whole, adolescent girls engage in much less sexual activity than adolescent boys. One reason for this is undoubtedly the double standard of morality which threatens females with much harsher punishment for sexual infractions than males. (Also see "The Social Roles of Men and Women.") Furthermore, girls are usually not encouraged to develop sexual needs. It is true that they are taught to be sexually attractive, to move gracefully, to dress seductively, to experiment with flattering hairstyles, and to use facial makeup. At the same time, however, their own sexual feelings remain rather weak and unfocused. Instead, they tend to fantasize in a general way about their future roles as brides, wives, and mothers. At other times, they dream vaguely about some ideal lover or some romantic situation. In short, they are less concerned with the physical aspects of sex than with its social implications.

SEXUAL ACTIVITY IN ADOLESCENCE

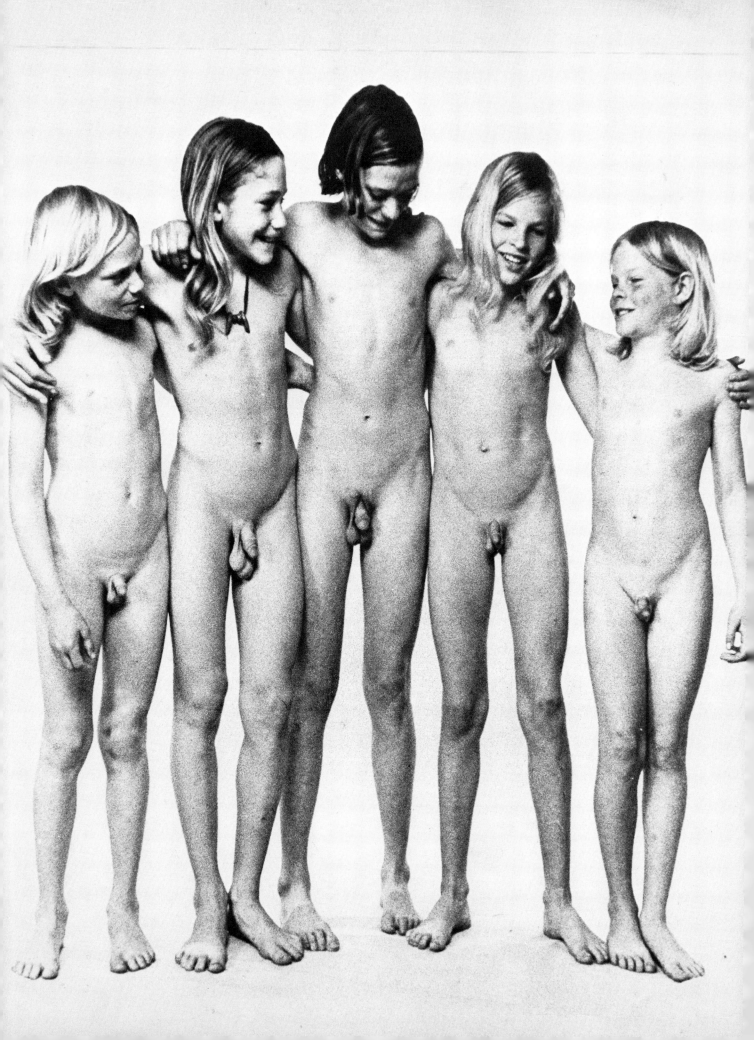

In contrast, the sexual fantasies of boys are much more specific. They are mainly interested in the sexual activity itself. For most of them, sexual desire and satisfaction are immediate physical experiences quite unrelated to any particular social setting. Their sexuality is detached, private, and personal. Thus, for a while, the two sexes are out of step in their personal development. Where adolescent girls may seem coquettish, conformist, and unresponsive, adolescent boys may appear inconsiderate, irresponsible, and selfish. It is only toward the end of adolescence that males begin to see sex as a means of human communication, and that females discover the full sexual potential of their bodies.

Self-stimulation

The hormonal changes of puberty produce a great increase in sexual responsiveness. Especially boys are very easily "turned on," and their bodies become ready to produce and release seminal fluid. In some cases, the ejaculation of semen occurs spontaneously while the boy is asleep. In other words, he has a "wet dream." There are boys who experience their very first ejaculation this way.

Since girls do not produce any semen, they do not ejaculate. Nevertheless, they also may have orgasms in their sleep, although for them this is a much rarer experience than for boys.

The same is true for deliberate masturbation. By the time they reach the age of 15 years, only about 25% of all girls have masturbated to orgasm, while the comparative figure for boys is nearly 100%. It can be said, therefore, that masturbation is a universal experience of male adolescence. However, there is much individual variation in regard to frequency and technique. Some boys masturbate regularly and often, others only occasionally or for a short period of their lives. As for technique, many boys use one or both hands to squeeze and stroke the penis. Some rub it against the mattress of their bed, a blanket, or a pillow. Others try to approach the feeling of coitus by inserting the penis into the wide mouth of a bottle, a toilet paper tube, or a pair of rolled-up socks. Still others try to take their own penis into their mouths, although they normally find this to be anatomically impossible. (Only about 1% of all males can do it.) It is not unusual for a boy to experiment with these and similar masturbation techniques and to switch from one to the other according to the circumstances. However, no matter what method is used, the adolescent male soon learns how to reach orgasm at will. He becomes familiar with the reactions of his body and gradually gains some control over them. Thus, he develops a sense of mastery over his new sexual capacities.

Girls also employ different masturbation techniques. In most cases, they move a finger or the whole hand gently over the clitoris and the surrounding area. Since a prolonged direct stimulation of the clitoris can become painful, many girls prefer to caress the entire vulva. Some of them insert a finger or some round, cylindrical object into the vagina and thereby try to approach the experience of coitus. They may also rub the vulva against the corner of a chair, some firm cushion, or a stuffed animal. There are girls who reach orgasm simply by pressing their thighs closely together while rhythmically moving one leg or contracting the muscles of their buttocks. Hardly any two girls masturbate in quite the same way.

While many boys are taught how to masturbate by other (mostly older) boys, girls usually develop the practice by themselves. Actually, in some instances girls masturbate regularly for years before they find out that this is what they have been doing. They may then be quite shocked and feel guilty

THE BEGINNING OF PUBERTY IN MALES
Not all children reach puberty at exactly the same age. The picture shows five boys aged 10, 12, 14, 12, and 9 (from left to right). The 14-year old in the middle has clearly entered puberty, and even the 12-year old on the left shows some first signs of it. However, the 12-year old on the right, just as the two younger boys on the outside, still has the sex organs and the body of a child.

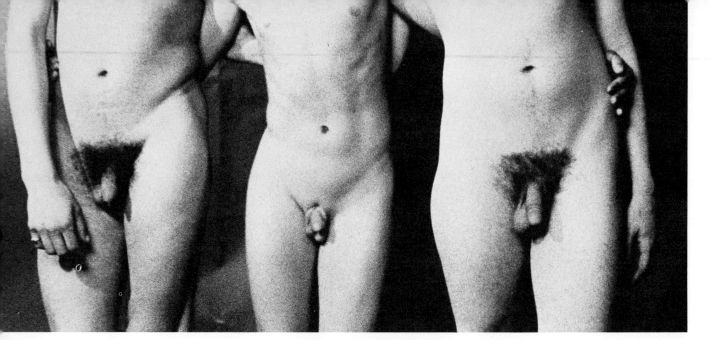

PUBERTY AND THE MALE SEX ORGANS
The remarkable growth of testicles and penis during the relatively short period of puberty is demonstrated in this picture which shows three young males aged 14, 12, and 15 years (from left to right).

about it. After all, most people in our culture consider masturbation wrong, and, in spite of all the propaganda to the contrary, many adolescents still adopt the moral values of their elders.

Since nearly all adolescent boys masturbate, the moral problem is particularly acute for them. Until a few decades ago, they were told not only that masturbation was sinful, but also that it could cause physical and mental illness. Even today they are sometimes warned that "excessive" masturbation can somehow weaken the body. (This "excess" is always left undefined.) As a result, many boys feel a double guilt: They seem to displease God and to ruin their health at the same time.

In view of these common worries, responsible adults have the duty to provide young people with the scientific facts: Masturbation as such cannot possibly cause any harm, and it can never be excessive. Some individuals can have more orgasms within a short time than others, but nobody can masturbate too much, because after a while the body simply no longer responds until it is given some rest.

Some adolescents are also disturbed by the sexual fantasies they have while they masturbate. Such fantasies are especially common among boys. They may imagine having sex with one or several girls, with other boys, with their brothers and sisters, or even with their own parents. They may picture themselves in bizarre and outlandish sexual situations, or fantasize that they rape somebody or are being raped themselves. These fantasies do not have to mean that a boy is sick, or that he will carry them out in real life. Many boys also dream of being a millionaire, a great movie star, a Roman emperor, or the strongest man in the world. Daydreams of this sort do not prove anything particular and do not deserve to be taken seriously. Still, pleasant sexual fantasies can strengthen the powers of imagination and creativity. They can also prepare an adolescent for future encounters with a real partner.

It seems that, on balance, adolescent masturbation has much to recommend it. It feels good, releases tension, and stimulates one's fantasy life. It is legal, always available, and not hazardous to anyone's health. It does not cause pregnancy and cannot lead to venereal disease. Moreover, it may help boys and girls to become better lovers. A boy who masturbates frequently can learn to delay his ejaculation by interrupting or slowing down his movements. This ability may later help him to provide greater satisfaction for his female sexual partners. A girl, on the other hand, can practice to reach orgasm quickly. This can also help her later when she engages in coitus.

The case against masturbation rests mainly on religious grounds. Traditionally, Jews and Christians have always disapproved of the practice, although this disapproval was never as strong as in the last two centuries. In any case, those adolescents whose religion does not allow them to masturbate are unlikely to derive any benefits from it. Masturbation is definitely bad if it causes fear, shame, anxiety, and guilt. Fortunately, some Christian churches have recently changed their attitude and are now much more tolerant in this matter. Finally, it should perhaps be mentioned that, occasionally, some adolescents masturbate almost obsessively because they are frustrated, lonely, or bored. They may be under great pressure at home or at school, or they may be experiencing some other nonsexual problem. Masturbating may then become a false escape or an excuse for not facing up to a difficult situation. Obviously, in such a case the underlying problem should be solved, if necessary, with the help of counseling. (For further details on masturbation, see "Types of Sexual Activity.")

Homosexual Contact
It is not unusual for adolescent boys to masturbate in groups. Occasionally, two or more boys may also masturbate each other. Indeed, they may even experiment with oral or anal intercourse. Such behavior can be called homosexual because it occurs between members of the same sex. However, it does not necessarily follow that these boys are homosexuals and have no sexual interest in girls. Strictly speaking, to be a homosexual and to engage in homosexual behavior are two different matters. There are many homosexuals, i.e., people falling in love mainly with partners of their own sex, who never proceed to any actual sexual contact. On the other hand, there are many heterosexuals who, for one reason or another, participate in homo-

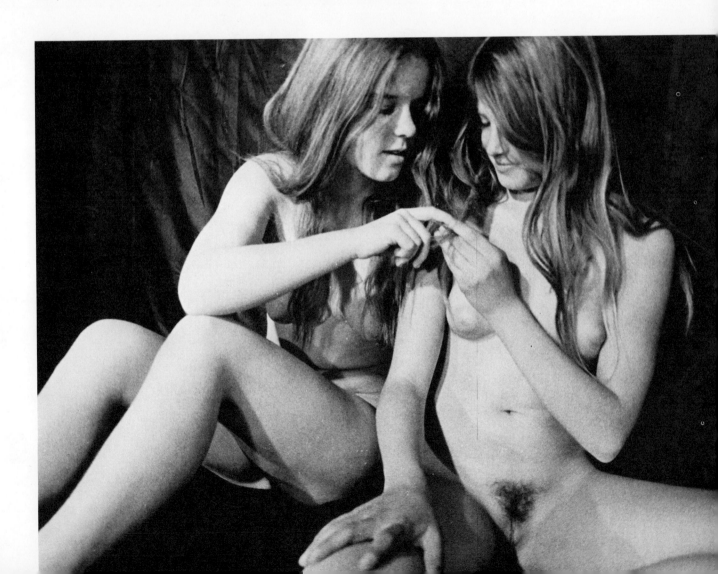

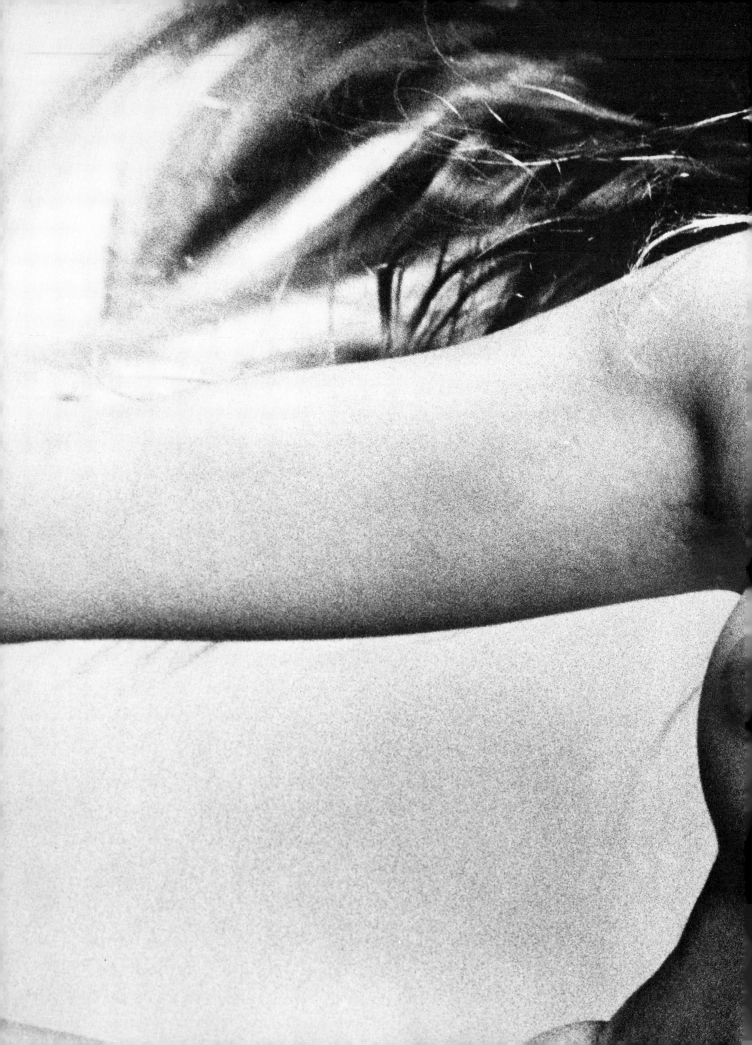

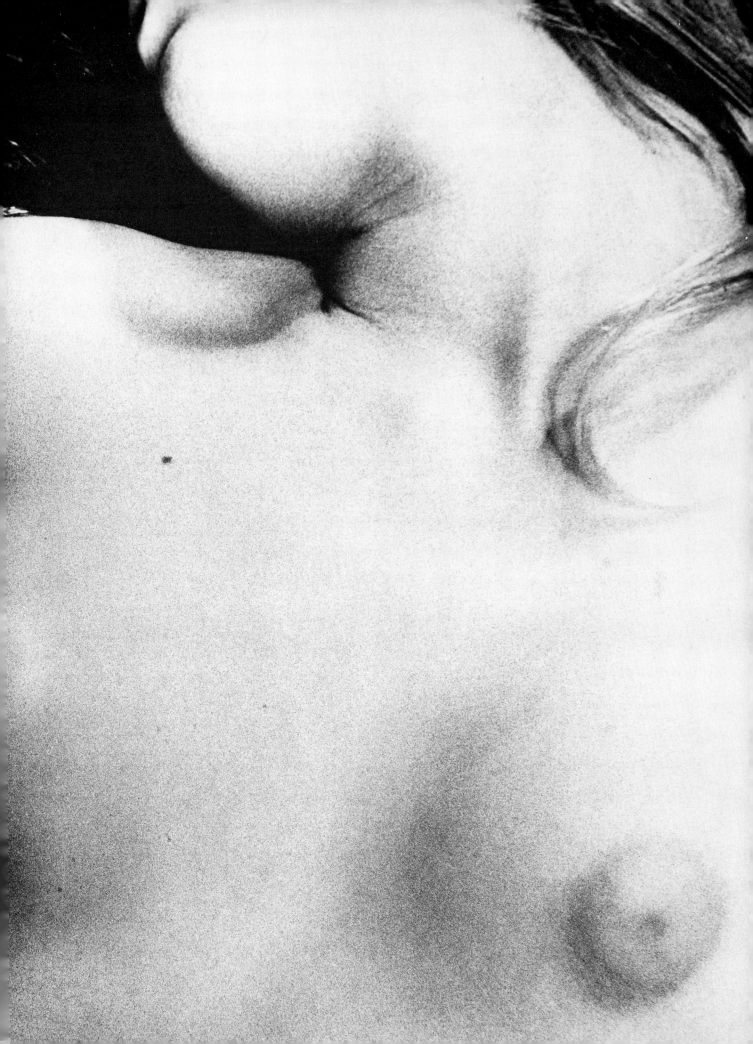

sexual acts. For example, in prison, in a labor camp, or aboard a ship men may temporarily have sex with each other because no women are available.

Adolescent boys sometimes find themselves in a very similar situation. That is to say, when their sexual contact with girls is severely restricted, they may turn to the next best choice—their male friends. Such a relationship may then satisfy them for a while until they are a little older and have more opportunities for heterosexual intercourse. Most often, however, adolescent homosexual contact is even more casual than that. In many cases, boys simply enjoy demonstrating their sexual prowess to their buddies, or they try to defy adult moral standards by sharing some "forbidden" experience. A great number of boys have such experiences, but most of them just go on becoming "typical" heterosexual men.

Under the circumstances, it seems sensible to avoid any labeling of same-sex behavior among adolescents. Indeed, it is downright foolish to call a boy homosexual just because he has sex with another boy. Such a label can have serious social consequences and thus become the main reason for later heterosexual failure. An adolescent who is told that he is "queer" may feel compelled to live up to the image society has of him, even if it is false.

Because of the widespread fear of homosexuality in our culture, males are usually not allowed to show love and tenderness for each other. While men in some other cultures freely hold hands, kiss, and embrace in public as an expression of friendship, Americans are conditioned to see sexual implications in such behavior. Indeed, when they discover it in their own country, they are likely to have the men arrested for "lewdness." In this poisonous atmosphere of general apprehension, many boys sooner or later begin to question their own proper sexual development. For instance, if they feel a special affection for another boy, they may wonder whether they are turning into homosexuals. Such idle worries can torment an American adolescent for years and ruin many friendships.

In this respect, a girl enjoys a definite advantage over a boy. When two girls are seen touching, hugging, and kissing each other, nobody thinks much of it. As a result, girls are free to develop intimate friendships. Even a relationship with clear erotic overtones may attract no special attention, and no social label may be attached to it. A few girls actually have sexual contact with other girls, but since they themselves normally do not dramatize such experiences, they rarely come to light. In any case, the social condemnation of adolescent female homosexuality is relatively mild, and a later heterosexual adjustment is almost never ruled out.

If our society had the same attitude toward male adolescents, their lives would undoubtedly be much easier. Their occasional homosexual contacts would no longer be seen as a threat to their basic sexual orientation, and a great number of them who are now trying to conform to some rigid sexual stereotype would learn to be proud of their individuality. A generally more relaxed approach to the problem would, of course, also benefit the small minority of adolescents who actually do turn out to be homosexuals. (For further details on homosexuality, see "Types of Sexual Activity," "Conformity and Deviance," and "The Sexually Oppressed.")

Heterosexual Contact

Beginning with late childhood, boys and girls in our society become increasingly separated in their daily activities. Even where they attend the same schools and receive the same instruction, they join exclusively male or female athletic teams, are encouraged to take up "masculine" or "feminine" hobbies, and attend sexually segregated summer camps. By the time they reach puberty, they live in different worlds with different values and concerns. As a result, adolescent boys and girls often know little about each other and have to go through a difficult period of reestablishing personal contact.

In many parts of the United States, these efforts follow a rather formalized pattern known as dating. A boy asks a girl for a date, then borrows the family car, picks her up at her home, takes her to a movie or a dance and, by a certain hour, brings her back to her parents. It is understood by all concerned that, while the boy and the girl are alone, they may have some close physical contact, such as holding hands, embracing, and kissing. In some cases, even more intimate caresses are permitted, as long as they do not lead to coitus. This is where both families and the girl herself usually draw the line.

The specific forms of dating vary a great deal according to region, social class, and ethnic background. Furthermore, in recent years America has seen a great general change in young life-styles. An increasing number of teenagers today do not care to repeat the almost ritualistic dating patterns known to their parents, but prefer more spontaneous meetings and associations. Indeed, it cannot be denied that the traditional form of dating had a number of undesirable features, and that in many cases it took on competitive aspects, or even turned into a popularity contest or a fight for social success. Thus, instead of contributing to a better understanding between the sexes, it could lead to a disregard for the dating partner, whose availability became a means to some egoistical end. In the future, young people may very well try to develop new, more meaningful forms of dating. However, in one form or another the custom itself is bound to survive because it also serves some very useful purposes: It gives boys and girls an opportunity to meet each other, it strengthens their self-confidence, it develops their sense of courtesy and good manners, and it can help them to find a suitable partner for marriage.

Some boys and girls feel apprehensive about their first dates because they do not know how to behave. They fear that they will find themselves in some embarrassing situation and lose the respect of their partner. This problem is easily solved by double-dating or group dating. When several boys and girls go out together, they find it much easier to be entertaining and to overcome awkward moments, and once they have gained some experience, they have little difficulty enjoying a single date.

Dating teaches boys and girls a great deal about each other, but it also helps them to understand themselves. For example, they may realize that they can get along with partners of very different character. Furthermore, they may learn to accept the fact that not everybody likes them, and that this is no reason to be upset. Being able to live with an occasional rejection is the mark of adulthood. They may also learn that some people like them for what they really are, not for what they pretend to be. This experience can relieve them of many unrealistic fears and help them to be true to themselves.

Eventually, many young couples decide to "go steady," i.e., to stop dating other partners and to spend most of their leisure time together. Such a decision has its advantages and disadvantages, and both deserve to be considered. The case for a steady relationship of this sort is obvious: It provides emotional security. The boy as well as the girl can stop worrying about dates. They know that their partner is always available, and that they do not have to get used to a new face every time they want to go out. Neither do they run the risk of ending up with unpleasant company. On the other hand, going steady also may deprive them of many interesting and broadening experiences, and they may miss meeting an even more suitable partner. These arguments have to be weighed by the adolescents themselves. However, knowledgeable adults can perhaps point out to them that, as a general rule, it seems best for young people to keep their options open.

Couples who go steady normally wonder how far they should go in their physical relationship. There are very few parents who like their adolescent sons or daughters to engage in coitus. However, they often tolerate or even encourage other forms of sexual contact, such as "necking" and "petting." These terms may mean different things to different teenagers, and today they sound slightly stuffy and obsolete. Originally, they were meant to describe caresses that avoided "real intercourse." (Necking usually just involved the face and the breasts, petting the whole body, including the sex organs, and heavy petting implied reaching an orgasm. In any case, the point was always the same: preserving the girl's "virginity.")

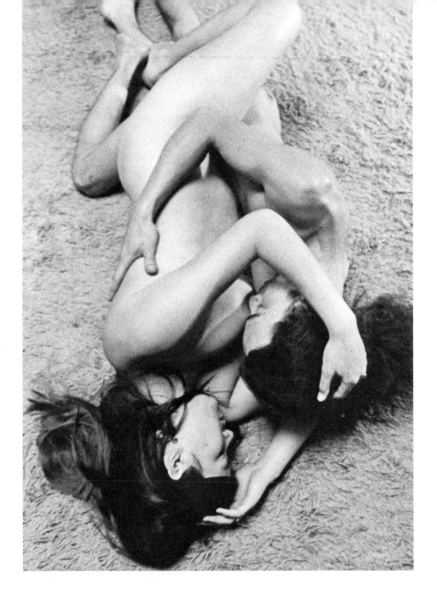

There are still many males today (although their number seems to be declining) who insist that they will only marry a "virgin." Unfortunately, the concept of virginity is not as clear and simple as it may seem at first glance. In the past, the word "virgin" was used to describe a girl or a woman who had had no sexual intercourse, and who was therefore sexually "innocent." Proof of this innocence was her unbroken hymen (i.e., the thin membrane that stretches across the vaginal opening). Today, we know that such proof is inconclusive because the hymen may be torn not only by sexual intercourse, but also by masturbation, or as a consequence of certain athletic activities. In some cases, the hymen may even be absent. Furthermore, the hymen of some girls stretches so easily that they can have coitus without tearing it. There are also some girls who preserve their "technical virginity" by avoiding coitus itself, while freely engaging in oral or anal intercourse. (The French call such girls *demi-vierges* or half-virgins.)

In view of these facts, the traditional obsession with the hymen seems rather misguided. Basically, it is a relic of former times when a man bought his bride like a piece of property and therefore demanded some physical evidence that she was free of "damage." However, as we have seen, this demand rested on false assumptions. On the other hand, a new definition of virginity can hardly serve any useful purpose either. This becomes especially clear when the term is applied to males, as is sometimes done today. At what point does a boy lose his virginity? When he has his first orgasm? When he first ejaculates in his sleep? When he begins to masturbate alone? When he masturbates with other boys? When he has an orgasm caressing a girl? When he has his first coitus? It is obvious that the answer can only be arbitrary.

As these examples show, the discussion of a person's virginity can easily degenerate into a quibble over technicalities. It is therefore more reasonable to approach the issue from an entirely different angle. Instead of worrying about the distinctions between necking, petting, heavy petting, making out, intercourse, and real intercourse, young people would be better advised to examine their motives. After all, a boy can do wrong even by simply kissing a girl, if he knows that she is not ready for it and that it upsets her. In other words, it is not the type of sexual activity that counts, but the intentions behind it.

It is also important to realize that not everyone has the same sexual needs, and that some people can live quite happily without sex. Adolescents are often too self-centered to respect such individual differences. Moreover, they may want to live up to the standards of their peer group, and thus try to "go all the way" simply because they hear that "everybody's doing it." In fact, this kind of pressure can cause some boys and girls to feel inferior or inadequate if they do not follow the crowd. However, conformism is never a good basis for personal growth, and sexual conformism is no exception. Sexual intercourse of any kind is, above all, a means of communication between individuals, and it is therefore their individual needs, wishes, hopes, and fears that must be considered first. For instance, when a boy finds that his girl friend is not so much interested in coitus than in human warmth, understanding, tenderness, and sensitivity, he should try to develop these qualities. Only then can he expect a corresponding effort on her part to understand his expectations too. In short, any intimate personal relationship requires some mutual adjustment and shared responsibility.

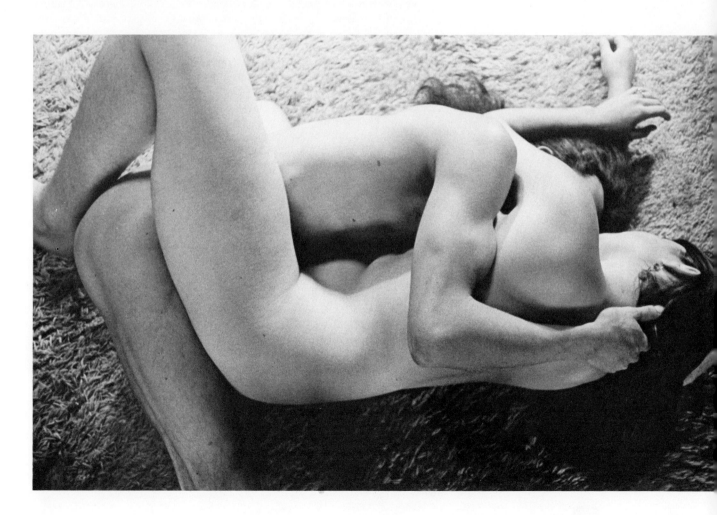

When seen from this standpoint, all forms and degrees of sexual contact can be meaningful and rewarding in their own right. Thus, a young couple may, for a while, very well be content with few and simple caresses. Then, as they become accustomed to each other, they may gradually progress to ever more intimate forms of lovemaking without necessarily comparing themselves to others or worrying about some abstract rules and regulations. This deliberate and individualistic approach to sex gives both boys and girls a freedom of choice and allows them to make intelligent decisions. Once they have learned to appreciate each other as persons, they are much better equipped to decide whether they really want to engage in coitus.

Coitus (i.e., the insertion of the penis into the vagina) is the only form of sexual intercourse that can lead to the conception of a child. This puts a great deal of responsibility on a young couple because an unwanted pregnancy can have very serious consequences, especially for the girl. In our society, unwed mothers and "illegitimate" children still encounter much public and private discrimination. On the other hand, an abortion is never a happy experience, even under the best of circumstances. Putting the baby up for adoption may not be very pleasant either, and the only other possible choice, a premature "forced" marriage, may be the worst solution of all.

As previously noted, boys may remain sterile for a while even after their first ejaculation, and for girls this adolescent sterility can even extend over a period of several years after their first menstruation. However, this is not something to be counted on. It is much safer for adolescents to assume that they become fertile as soon as they reach puberty. By this time, at the latest, they should also have acquired an adequate understanding of contraception. Fortunately, today many parents, schools, and church groups provide young people with all the necessary information. In addition, there are Planned Parenthood centers in almost every city offering their assistance. Under these circumstances, responsible teenagers no longer run the risk of unwanted pregnancies.

However, even the careful use of contraception does not necessarily make coitus "safe," harmless, and desirable for unmarried adolescents. For one thing, they may encounter unexpected legal difficulties. If they are over the age of consent for sexual intercourse (different from state to state, but usually 16 or 18 years), they may be violating the law against fornication. Many states in the United States have such laws, and the punishment can range up to 1 year in prison. If both adolescents are under the age of consent, they may still be treated as delinquents, and the same fate may await them in states where fornication as such is not a crime. (If only the girl is underage, the boy may be convicted of "statutory rape.") The existence of these laws may come as a surprise to many people, and it must be admitted that they are very rarely enforced. Nevertheless, they can be used at any time against "undesirables" who, for one reason or another, displease the authorities. (For further details, see "Conformity and Deviance—Legal-Illegal.")

Another point to be considered is the danger of venereal disease. While it is true that venereal diseases can be transmitted by oral and anal intercourse and, indeed, in some rare cases by kissing, coitus offers by far the greatest opportunity for an infection. There is, unfortunately, a venereal disease epidemic among young people today, and boys and girls therefore have the duty to learn all they can about the symptoms, the treatment, and the prevention of gonorrhea and syphilis. (For details, see "Venereal Diseases.")

Still another potential source of trouble is the repressive, anxiety-laden atmosphere in which adolescent sexual intercourse often takes place. As long as young people live with their parents or in college dormitories, they may find neither the right place nor the right time for true intimacy. Thus, their attempts at coitus may turn into hurried, frustrating, and ultimately disappointing experiences. Furthermore, religious condemnation and strong social disapproval of sex without marriage may create deep feelings of guilt. Finally, it must be recognized that adolescents of both sexes may have intercourse for nonsexual reasons, and that they can use it as a means to manipulate, hurt, or degrade their partners. Such behavior can only lead to misery and distrust and therefore condemns itself.

However, it is a fact of life that many teenagers do engage in all forms of sexual contact, including coitus, and that by no means all of them suffer any negative consequences. On the contrary, those that go about it in a mature, responsible manner can find strength and happiness in their sexual relationships. There is also little doubt that males as well as females find it much easier to train their own sexual capacities and to adjust to each other while they are still young. In this sense, early regular coitus can be seen as an excellent preparation for marriage.

In sum, there are valid arguments not only against, but also for unrestricted sexual intercourse between adolescents and, in the final analysis, the decision is theirs. All any adult can hope for is that they make this decision in full knowledge of all its implications. (For further details on heterosexual intercourse, see "Types of Sexual Activity.")

Sexual Contact with Adults

Throughout human history, there has always been sexual intercourse between partners of widely different ages. For thousands of years, middle-aged men married girls in their early teens, and boys who had just reached puberty were quite often introduced to the "art and science of love" by experienced older women. These practices are still alive today in many "primitive" societies where an adolescence in our modern sense of the word is unknown, and where children are granted the status of adults as soon as they become capable of reproduction. This change in status may be rather abrupt, and usually it is connected with certain magic ceremonies or initiation rites. Indeed, these rites themselves may include some sexual contact with adults. For example, girls may be "deflowered" by some priest or chief, and boys may become "passive" partners in anal intercourse with older members of the tribe. A variation of this latter custom could also be found in ancient Greece where a male adolescent sometimes entered into a sexual relationship with a man who then became his spiritual mentor. Similar arrangements existed in some traditional Asian societies. More recently, young men in Mediterranean and Latin American countries were often expected to "establish their manhood" with prostitutes.

However, in the last 200 years most Western societies have developed the belief that even physically mature teenagers need protection from sexual contact with older persons. Thus, many countries have established age limits for sexual partners. That is to say, outside of marriage a person over a certain age (called adult) may no longer have sexual intercourse with another person under a certain age (called minor). The exact age at which a minor becomes an adult varies from country to country.

In the United States, full legal adulthood is usually not reached before the age of 21. Nevertheless, young people may acquire a number of adult privileges well before that date. For instance, they are granted the privilege to consent to sexual intercourse as soon as they reach the "age of consent." Unfortunately, this age is not the same in every state, but can range anywhere from 12 to 18 years. Furthermore, it is often different for males and females as well as for heterosexual and homosexual intercourse. As a result, some "minors" and "adults" unexpectedly find themselves in frightening and absurd situations.

A good example is the crime of "statutory rape." (This curious term can perhaps best be translated as "rape created by statute" or "rape by nobody's definition but the law's.") Before a girl has reached the age of consent to sexual intercourse, the law believes her to be unable to give such consent. Since sexual intercourse without the girl's consent is known as rape, any lover of hers is automatically considered a rapist. The following case may illustrate the point: An 18-year-old boy is seduced by a 17-year-old prostitute. The state in which the seduction occurs has established 18 as the age of consent for girls. Therefore, the boy is guilty of statutory rape. The fact that she took money from him and that he was a rather reluctant participant makes no difference. She is a minor who needs to be protected, and he is an adult who needs to be punished. On the other hand, if the state's age of consent for girls is 16 or younger, he cannot be accused of rape at all. (However, depending on the state, both he and the girl may have broken several other sex laws.)

Cases like this one make it quite obvious that the "protection of minors" can be carried too far. In fact, when examined closely, the whole problem seems to be more a matter of arbitrary legal definition than anything else. From a logical standpoint, it is hard to understand why a 17-year-old girl in one state should be judged unable to consent to sexual intercourse when a 12-year-old girl in another state is legally entitled to such a decision. What the law seems to be saying here is that emotional maturity is a matter of geographical location, and that a morally incompetent girl can win instant competence simply by crossing a state line. Even more ironic, in some states a girl can consent to marriage several years before she is allowed to consent to sexual intercourse. Fortunately, in the meantime, a number of states have abolished some of these irrational laws and have adopted a more realistic attitude. Thus, the new criminal code of Hawaii, which can perhaps serve as a model for the nation, has lowered the age of consent to 14 years for both sexes. As a result, many unnecessary problems have disappeared in that state, and its youth-oriented counseling and health services have become much more effective.

Boys and girls who understand their own sexuality and who know the various methods of contraception are not very likely to be sexually exploited by adults. Where sex between adolescents and older persons nevertheless seems to create problems, counseling can often be helpful. Unlike the law, such counseling can address itself to the specifics of each case and thus avoid the danger of attaching inappropriate social labels to individuals and their actions. For instance, a teenage girl who develops a "crush" on her teacher, or who actually starts dating a middle-aged man, may very well profit from a personal, open discussion with another, disinterested adult. She may not realize that few responsible older men would consider very young girls adequate partners.

Counseling can also dispel many misconceptions and needless fears. There is, for example, great concern among many parents that their adolescent son or daughter might become a homosexual as a result of seduction by a homosexual adult. However, most scientific opinion today doubts this possibility. Isolated sexual acts in adolescence do not seem likely to establish a permanent sexual preference, unless there is a definite predisposition which would manifest itself sooner or later even without premature encouragement. Moreover, the great majority of reports by homosexuals themselves show that seduction has not been decisive in their own development. In short, a few homosexual acts (whether with adults or other adolescents) do not, in themselves, cause or indicate a homosexual orientation.

ADULTHOOD

As we have emphasized, the sexual development of human beings neither begins nor ends with their physical maturation. People acquire many sexual attitudes and capacities well before puberty, and they may acquire many more in the course of their adult lives. They may also lose certain capacities with advancing age, or they may learn to view them differently. They may develop new sexual tastes and habits and, over the years, they may go through several periods of increased or diminished sexual activity.

These changes, adjustments, and reorientations occur not only for natural biological reasons, but also in response to varying cultural demands. For example, in our culture people are held to very different sexual standards depending on whether they are male or female, heterosexual or homosexual, single or married, young or old. Furthermore, men and women may also be forced to adopt different sexual attitudes when they rise to a higher social class, move from a small rural town to a big city, or emigrate to another country. Individuals who do not live up to the expectations of their community may be made to feel guilty or inadequate, and, in some cases, they may risk criminal prosecution or forced "rehabilitation." Even a person who tries to avoid all such trouble and leads an unoffensive "normal" life may suddenly be affected by larger social movements and events. Thus, the invention of reliable contraceptives and the legal emancipation of women have forced many otherwise "stable" adults to change their behavior and to search for new sexual values.

In short, there is sexual development as long as there is life, and it is therefore impossible to offer a definite description of adulthood. All we can do here is to provide a few broad hints at some of the sexual problems encountered by adults today. More detailed discussions of specific issues can be found in other relevant sections of this book.

THE SINGLE ADULT

Our official morality allows sexual intercourse only within marriage, and young males and females are therefore under tremendous social pressure to get married. Indeed, today more people get married than ever before, and this in spite of the fact that one-third of all marriages now end in divorce. Men and women who are divorced usually do not come to the conclusion that there is something wrong with the institution of marriage or that they as individuals have no talent for it. On the contrary, most of them continue to feel that they will find lasting happiness only with the right marriage partner. Thus, there are people who go through four, five, six, or more marriages and divorces in the course of their lives. In short, there is now a nearly universal and unshakable belief in our society that everybody should marry, and that only marriage offers complete sexual fulfillment.

Former ages have not always shared this belief. In fact, until well into the 19th century it was taken for granted that a certain number of people were unfit for marriage. Those who could not support themselves were often prohibited by law from getting married. Others who faced no such legal obstacles were nevertheless deliberately denied the opportunity to meet suitable partners. Thus, many parents insisted that at least one of their daughters be kept at home to take care of them in their old age. By the time the parents died, the daughter had usually become an "old maid" without any hope of finding a husband.

However, it would be wrong to conclude that the "spinsters" and "perpetual bachelors" of the past always resented their fate. First of all, on the whole, marriage was much less romanticized than it is today. Furthermore, single adults were not necessarily deprived of the joys and the comfort of family life. The traditional extended family consisted of children, parents, grandparents, great-grandparents, various other close and distant relatives, plus domestic servants. In such a household, there was room for several unmarried men and women. (For further details on the extended family, see "Marriage and the Family.")

Today, most single adults live alone. While this can be very dull and even depressing at times, it also has its advantages. Indeed, in many of our big cities the single way of life can be very attractive. There are special apartment houses, retirement homes, and residential hotels which cater to singles and which try to make their lives as comfortable and enjoyable as possible. As a matter of fact, the cities themselves, with their libraries, museums, theaters, clubs, sports facilities, health spas, restaurants, cafés, etc. offer so many pleasures that perhaps only a single person can take full advantage of them. Most important of all, the anonymity of city life results in a great deal of sexual freedom. Unmarried men and women meet in social groups, at parties, in special singles bars, or even through newspaper ads. They can live together for longer or shorter periods of time, then separate and find new partners without too much difficulty. All of this is true for those who have never been married as well as those who are widowed or divorced, for the young as well as the old, heterosexuals as well as homosexuals. In short, it may seem that, at least sexually, the modern single adult lives in the best of all possible worlds.

In many cases, this impression is deceptive, however. For instance, those unmarried adults who have to live in suburbs, small towns, or rural communities still find their sexual opportunities severely restricted, especially once they reach middle age. Even in the big city, older men and women may run into trouble if they openly defy the sexual standards of their neighbors. Nevertheless, sometimes a couple has no choice but to avoid marriage because it would mean the loss of a pension or other financial benefit. Thus, many poor older couples today live together while remaining legally single. Unfortunately, as a result, they may suffer several other disadvantages. Single persons usually pay higher taxes, and they may have a harder time finding a job than married persons. Such job discrimination may even be quite open and blatant if the applicant is a homosexual. Furthermore, because of the antiquated sex laws in most states of the United States, single adults who engage in any sexual intercourse at all are technically criminals and thus live under the constant threat of arrest and conviction. (Again, homosexuals suffer the most from these laws, although heterosexuals may be prosecuted as well.) Finally, it has to be realized that many adults remain single because they are physically unappealing, crippled, deformed, or chronically ill. Still others are sexually inadequate or have unusual sexual interests that make them unsatisfactory as marriage partners. Such adults may lead very unhappy lives. Some of them may find at least some satisfaction with prostitutes, but here again our lawmakers and the police try to interfere.

At least in the United States today, single adults are justified in seeing themselves as members of an underprivileged group. On the whole, they are met with hostility and suspicion because our society regards only the "family man" and the "wife and mother" as fully "responsible" citizens. Thus, the social pressure to get married continues. It may take some time before people realize that this pressure is not necessarily in the general interest. Some individuals simply cannot find happiness in marriage. Others are quite unfit to be parents, and, in a sexually less conformist culture, they might well feel less tempted to reproduce. Indeed, since the world is now threatened with overpopulation, many countries may eventually have to discourage marriage (or at least early marriage) and to reward those of their citizens who remain single.

Fortunately, modern contraceptive techniques have made it possible for men and women to have sexual intercourse without risking unwanted pregnancies. Thus, there is no longer any valid reason why single adults should be forced to remain abstinent. (For more details on the problems faced by single adults, see "The Social Roles of Men and Women.")

SEXUAL ADJUSTMENT IN MARRIAGE

Most men and women today seek their sexual fulfillment in marriage. However, not all of them realize that such fulfillment has to be worked for. A permanent sexual relationship requires a great deal of tolerance, patience, and mutual effort. There is nothing automatic about marital bliss.

It is therefore important that people develop a realistic understanding of their own sexual interests and abilities. At the same time, they should accept the fact that they will have to adjust to their partners. Furthermore, every couple needs at least some basic factual knowledge about the physical aspects of married life, such as sexual intercourse in its various forms, pregnancy, childbirth, contraception, and so on.

Even couples who have thus prepared themselves for marriage may experience much anguish and frustration. To begin with, as a result of various political, economic, and technological developments in our culture, the social roles of men and women are now changing very fast. The traditional concepts of masculinity and femininity are increasingly being questioned, and this may become a source of marital conflict (also see "The Social Roles of Men and Women"). The conflict may even manifest itself in the impairment or complete blockage of normal sexual responses. Thus, men who begin to fear for their dominant status or women who begin to resent male dominance may become sexually inadequate. It may then take a lot of mutual education (sometimes with outside professional help) to reestablish a satisfying sexual relationship.

Another possible cause of disappointment is the modern preoccupation with sexual "efficiency" and "performance." Today, married couples (just like everybody else) are exposed to a constant barrage of commercial propaganda which seems to suggest that everybody can be romantic and beautiful all the time, that sex is the way to total ecstasy, and that only such regular ecstasy makes a marriage worthwhile. However, real life is not like that. For instance, unless the partners have been living together before their marriage, they need some time to get used to each other. They may very well make love passionately and frequently, but they may not achieve full mutual satisfaction until several months or even years after the wedding. Husband and wife may also differ in the intensity of their sexual urges. Early in the marriage, it is often the husbands who have the greatest interest in sexual intercourse. Later, when the wives have lost their inhibitions and begin to feel more secure, the situation may well be reversed. Indeed, with the approach of middle age, many men experience a marked decline in their sexual capacities. Such a decline rarely has a biological cause, but is instead usually related to the man's increasing absorption in his work, vague apprehensions about the loss of his physical strength, lack of imagination, boredom, and routine. A woman, on the other hand, may feel that her menopause finally frees her from all worries about an unwanted conception, and thus she may become sexually more active than ever before.

It is not uncommon for married couples to disagree about the frequency and the techniques of sexual intercourse. Sometimes such disagreements simply spring from a difference in temperament. However, at other times they result from ignorance or prudery, and, in a few instances, they have still other, more complex causes. For example, there are men and women who try to use sex for nonsexual ends. Thus, they may refuse intercourse because they want to punish their spouses, or they may agree to it only in return for some special favor. Needless to say, in the long run, such egoistical behavior is self-defeating.

Some couples also face sexual difficulties because they are afraid to communicate their true wishes and feelings to each other. As a consequence, they settle into a single standard pattern of intercourse, and the sheer monotony of their life together then gradually kills their interest in sex. On the other hand, there are individuals who suddenly seem to acquire highly unusual sexual tastes and preferences which cannot be satisfied within their marriage. Others make repeated and increasingly desperate efforts to bring variety to their lovemaking, only to be rejected or ridiculed by their partners. Still others seek new excitement in extramarital affairs. These and similar developments can put a considerable strain on a marital relationship, and, in some cases, the partners themselves may be unable to find a workable accommodation. Still, if they are seriously concerned for each other, they can often save their marriage by seeking professional help. (Also see "Sexual Maladjustment.")

Marriage partners may also have to make new sexual adjustments when they become parents. For instance, in the later stages of a pregnancy and for some time after the birth of a child, they may have to vary their approach to coitus or even avoid it altogether in favor of other forms of sexual inter-

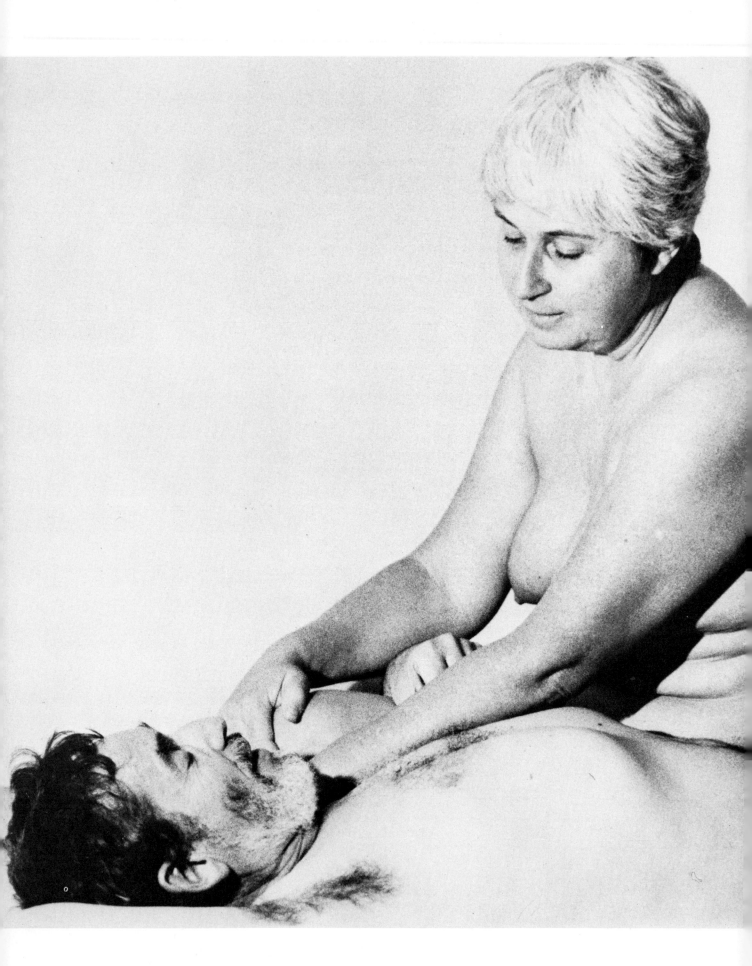

course. (See "Pregnancy," "Birth," and "Heterosexual Intercourse.") The roles of mother and father soon pose new challenges of their own. Children have to be accepted as sexual beings and also need an adequate sex education. Many parents, however, are so uncomfortable with their own sexuality that they cannot discuss sex freely and openly with a child. As the child grows up and the parents begin to age, they may be reminded of old, long-suppressed conflicts and thus experience new sexual anxieties. Many parents therefore have ambiguous feelings about the approaching maturity and growing sexual attractiveness of their offspring. Here again professional counseling can be very useful. (Also see "Sex Education.")

None of the foregoing is meant to suggest that marriage and parenthood are unrewarding. On the contrary, all marital conflicts mentioned here carry the opportunity for personal growth. Indeed, they can become a source of strength and thus contribute to a fuller, more meaningful life. Couples who avoid rigidity and who do not take each other for granted can very well find lasting happiness in marriage. (For a more detailed discussion of marriage, see "Marriage and the Family.")

SEX AND THE AGING

Sexual activity was once considered the exclusive privilege of the young. Women expected to lose their sexual responsiveness after their menopause, and men resigned themselves to the rapid decline of their virility once they reached late middle age. However, modern sex research has shown that these assumptions are false, and that human beings can continue to be sexually active well into their old age. (See "The Male Sexual Response" and "The Female Sexual Response.")

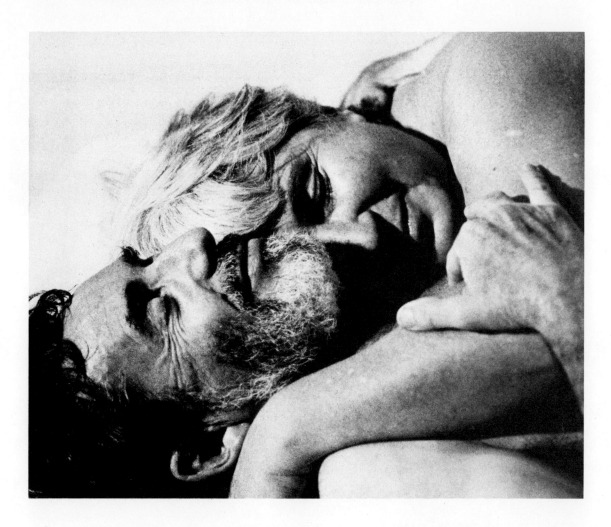

Still, many individuals do experience a gradual weakening of their sexual urges in later years. Sometimes other satisfactions, such as the joys of parenthood and grandparenthood, professional success, or the preoccupation with some hobby can diminish a person's interest in sex. At other times, older people find it undignified or bothersome to look for sexual partners. Some men also feel that the loss of their physical strength signals the end of their sex lives, and thus they simply give up. In short, people often deny themselves sexual pleasures long before it is biologically necessary.

In many respects, this is quite unfortunate. Sexual intercourse can help older people to preserve their self-esteem and confidence. It can give them a sense of well-being, renew their interest in life, and thus prevent them from aging prematurely. A certain lack of strength and the infirmities of age do not have to be an obstacle to sexual satisfaction. Moreover, specific physical problems can often be alleviated by hormone replacement and other therapeutic measures.

The reasons that keep older men and women from remaining sexually active are mostly psychological. However, it is almost certain that the various modern movements toward sexual liberation will sooner or later also affect the aging and allow them to develop new sexual attitudes. (See also "The Sexually Oppressed.")

Reference and Recommended Reading

Freud, Sigmund. *Three Contributions to the Theory of Sex.* New York: Johnson Reprint Corp., 1910 (cloth); New York: Dutton, 1962 (paper).
——— *The Sexual Enlightenment of Children.* New York: Macmillan, 1963.
Group for the Advancement of Psychiatry. *Normal Adolescence: Its Dynamics and Impact.* New York: Scribner's, 1968 (cloth); 1968 (paper).
Kinsey, Alfred C., *et al. Sexual Behavior in the Human Female.* Philadelphia: Saunders, 1953 (cloth); New York: Pocket Books, 1965 (paper).
LeShan, Eda J. *Sex and Your Teenager: A Guide for Parents.* New York, McKay, 1969 (cloth); New York: Warner Books, 1973 (paper).
Pomeroy, Wardell B. *Boys and Sex.* New York: Delacorte Press, 1968.
——— *Girls and Sex.* New York: Delacorte Press, 1969 (cloth); New York: Dell, 1973 (paper).
———*Your Child and Sex: A Guide for Parents.* New York: Delacorte Press, 1974.
Sherfey, Mary Jane. *The Nature and Evolution of Female Sexuality.* New York: Aronson, 1974 (cloth); New York: Random House, 1973 (paper).

7. TYPES OF SEXUAL ACTIVITY

There are many ways of classifying human sexual behavior. For example, one can select one particular type of sexual activity as the standard or norm and then describe all other types as "variations" or "deviations." This is the approach traditionally used by religious, legal, and psychiatric authorities.

However, the sexual norms established by the church, the law, or the psychiatric profession are subject to change and do not always agree with each other. Thus, a certain behavior may be declared normal in one historical period and deviant in another. Furthermore, theologians, legislators, and psychiatrists often have different concepts of what is right and wrong in a person's sexual conduct. In other words, one cannot assume that every moral sexual act is legal and will be considered healthy. By the same token, not every sexual sin is also a sexual crime, and not every sexual crime signals a sexual disorder. (For details, see "Conformity and Deviance.")

In view of these facts, it seems advisable to seek another, more neutral system of classification. Indeed, if we do not want to prejudge the issue, we best avoid all value judgments and keep the distinctions strictly technical. One possibility is to describe sexual behavior simply in terms of the "objects" involved. For instance, we can distinguish between those acts that a person performs alone and those that require contact with others. Such contact, in turn, can take place with a partner of the opposite sex, a partner of the same sex, or an animal. Thus, we arrive at four basic types of sexual activity:

1. Sexual self-stimulation,
2. heterosexual intercourse,
3. homosexual intercourse, and
4. sexual contact with animals.

It has to be emphasized, of course, that these distinctions refer only to different kinds of behavior, not to different kinds of people. In other words, one and the same person may very well engage in all four types of sexual activity. There are individuals who first rely mainly on sexual self-stimulation, then go through a brief period of sexual experimentation with animals, and then turn their interest to human partners of the opposite sex. Others engage in both homosexual and heterosexual behavior throughout their lives. Still others have varied sexual experiences in their youth, but eventually find complete satisfaction in a traditional marriage. On the other hand, the loss of a marriage partner through death or divorce may prompt some men and women to revert to earlier behavior patterns.

Modern sex research has shown that human sexual behavior is not guided by a fixed and unerring biological instinct, but is greatly influenced by social conditioning. Furthermore, historical and anthropological studies reveal that different societies condition their members very differently in this regard. In short, it is now generally understood that people choose their sexual objects according to the circumstances and as a result of their individual learning experiences. (See "The Development of Sexual Behavior.")

However, there is also no doubt that most societies strongly favor one particular object choice over all others: an adult human partner of the opposite sex. Thus, heterosexual intercourse is and has always been by far the most common type of sexual activity. The reason for this is not very hard to find: only sexual contact between males and females can lead to reproduction and thereby ensure the survival of the species and of the social group. Any society that developed a bias in favor of sexual self-stimulation, homosexual intercourse, or sexual contact with animals would simply condemn itself to extinction.

Still, as we all know, human survival can be threatened not only by a lack of reproduction, but also by an excess of it, and, in this latter case, a society may very well have no choice but to change its sexual values. For example, the ancient Greek philosopher Aristotle mentions in his *Politics* (Book II, Chapter 10) that the threat of overpopulation once forced the inhabitants of the island of Crete to institute homosexual behavior as a means of lowering the birth rate. This legend may be true or false, but in any case it reveals that even over 2,000 years ago some people were aware of the fact that sexual object choices may, to a certain extent, be dictated by the shifting needs of society.

These observations should not be taken to mean that human sexual behavior is completely uninfluenced by biological factors. On the contrary, it seems that a certain inclination toward heterosexual intercourse is part of man's mammalian heritage. While it is true that many of the higher mammals can and do engage in sexual self-stimulation, homosexual activity, and sexual contact with animals of other species (including man), their predominant mode of sexual expression is heterosexual copulation within their own species. It is safe to assume that human beings, as the highest mammals, have inherited at least a vestige of this general behavior pattern. At the same time, we have to recognize, however, that human societies usually do everything they can to reinforce the natural tendency toward heterosexual intercourse and to discourage the other equally natural kinds of sexual behavior. In sum, the available evidence clearly suggests two conclusions: First, in a society without any taboos and prohibitions, heterosexual intercourse would still be the most common type of sexual activity. Second, the other types would be a great deal more common than they are in most societies today.

In recent years, our own society has experienced a considerable increase in sexual freedom, and, as a result, more people than ever before have become aware of the wide range of human sexual behavior. However, it is difficult to say whether this behavior itself has changed, since the first reliable statistical data were collected only a few decades ago. We know that, in theory, at least our Victorian ancestors were much more restricted in their sexual activities. Still, in actual practice, their behavior may very well have been quite similar to our own.

Nevertheless, it is obvious that people are now better informed and have more opportunities to explore their sexual potential. The invention of reliable contraceptives has freed many couples from the fear of unwanted pregnancies. The economic and legal emancipation of women has brought a greater degree of honesty to male-female relationships, and the modern mass media have begun to provide a constant flow of sexual information which helps both the young and the old to understand and accept themselves as sexual beings.

It is to be hoped that these and similar positive developments will eventually lead to the general realization that love can flourish only in a climate of tolerance, that there is no need for a rigidly enforced single standard of sexual behavior, and that the interest of society is best served by granting everybody the right to sexual self-determination.

The following pages provide some general information about the four basic types of sexual activity and also offer brief descriptions of the most common sexual techniques. The social significance of these various behaviors is discussed more fully in the third part of this book under "Conformity and Deviance" and "The Sexually Oppressed."

SEXUAL SELF-STIMULATION

Human beings (and many animals) can very well become sexually aroused and reach orgasm without partners. Such self-stimulation is possible at any age. It may be brought about voluntarily by masturbation, or it may occur involuntarily while the person is asleep. In short, our bodies are always capable of sexual responses regardless of whether we are in the company of others or alone with ourselves.

In ancient times, it was often thought that involuntary orgasms occurred when an angel of the night, a spirit, or a demon visited people in their sleep. During the Middle Ages, it was believed that the devil himself could seduce good Christians at night by appearing as an *incubus* (i.e., lying upon a woman) or a *succubus* (i.e., lying under a man). It is interesting to note, however, that Jewish and Christian religious authorities were usually much less concerned with the spontaneous orgasms of women than with those of men. One reason for this was undoubtedly their conviction that male semen was not meant to be "wasted" in nonreproductive activities. Some medieval physicians also declared that semen was an essential, life-sustaining fluid, more precious than blood, and that too many ejaculations therefore weakened the body. A loss of semen was healthy only under special conditions, just as forced bleeding was beneficial only as a treatment of certain diseases. Since women do not ejaculate any semen, none of these considerations applied to them, and, as a result, not much attention was paid to their orgasms.

The Judeo-Christian concern over the possible "waste" of semen also led to a general disapproval of male masturbation. While it is true that masturbation is never mentioned in the Bible, traditional rabbinical teaching always considered it a grave sin, and for at least one Talmudic authority it was a crime to be punished by death (Niddah 13a). The Christians later simply adopted the negative Jewish attitudes.

Still, in medieval Europe masturbation was not seen as much of a problem. While it was condemned in various penitentials, the other theological and pastoral writings of the time hardly mentioned it at all, or referred to it in a rather oblique fashion. Even the popular catechisms that began to appear in the 16th century contained nothing on the subject. This omission may appear strange at first glance, but it becomes understandable when we remember that the medieval concept of sexuality was still relatively narrow. Indeed, the very term was unknown. Instead, people spoke of love, desire, or Venus, and they recognized only one kind of activity as being strictly sexual: coitus among adults. It seems, therefore, that at least women and children had no great feelings of guilt about masturbation, but simply thought of it as a way of relieving physical irritations, comparable to scratching.

All of this began to change in the 18th century. In 1710, an anonymous pamphlet appeared in England under the title, *Onania, or the Heinous Sin of Self-Pollution and All Its Frightful Consequences in Both Sexes, Considered with Spiritual and Physical Advice.* The author Bekker was a former clergyman turned quack who offered his readers an embellished rehash of older theories about the dangers of "wasting" semen. He called this behavior onania in reference to Onan, a biblical character who was punished by God for refusing to impregnate his brother's widow. As required by custom, he engaged in coitus with her, but prevented any possible pregnancy by practicing the withdrawal method of contraception (Genesis,38:8–10). Unfortunately, Bekker's absurd ideas and his misleading term soon found wide acceptance. The pamphlet was quickly translated into several European languages and eventually went through more than eighty editions.

In 1760, a respected Swiss physician by the name of Tissot published an even more influential book entitled, *Onanism, or a Treatise Upon the Disorders Produced by Masturbation*. The author claimed that masturbation was not only a sin and a crime, but that it was also directly responsible for many serious diseases, such as "consumption, deterioration of eyesight, disorders of digestion, impotence, . . . and insanity." Tissot's success was spectacular. He was widely quoted as the greatest authority on the subject of masturbation, and he was universally praised as a benefactor of mankind. Within a few decades, his views became official medical doctrine. Physicians all over the Western world began to find masturbation at the root of almost every physical problem.

By 1812, when Benjamin Rush, known as the father of American psychiatry, published his *Medical Inquiries and Observations Upon the Diseases of the Mind*, the harmful effects of masturbation were taken for granted everywhere, and their number had greatly increased. According to Rush, "onanism" caused not only insanity, but also "seminal weakness, impotence, dysury, tabes dorsalis, pulmonary consumption, dyspepsia, dimness of sight, vertigo, epilepsy, hypochondriasis, loss of memory, manalgia, fatuity, and death."

As these examples indicate, the first modern fighters against the evils of masturbation were physicians, and their arguments were mostly medical. Very soon, however, they found themselves supported by "enlightened" educators who feared for the moral health of their students. The churches, on the other hand, at first showed little interest in joining the crusade. Some clergymen pointed out, for example, that they could not find a single reference to masturbation in the Holy Scriptures, and that they were therefore unable to condemn it. It seemed that the only solution was a new, much broader interpretation of the biblical commandment against adultery. However, in the long run this procedure could easily make matters worse. It would require a great deal of detailed sex education, and particularly the young and innocent would suddenly have to be told about sins of which they had never heard before. Moreover, the exact definition of masturbation appeared far from easy. After all, the term had first been applied only to adult males. The notion that women and children also masturbated was new. Indeed, it is evident from the antimasturbation pamphlets of the time that the authors had great difficulty explaining to the public exactly what they were talking about. Nevertheless, after some initial reluctance even the clergy became "progressive" enough to recognize the dangers of masturbation, and soon everybody was convinced that these dangers demanded the most drastic and extraordinary measures of protection.

Here again, the medical profession pointed the way. First of all, it knew how to discover the masturbators. General apathy and laziness, dim or shifty eyes, a pale complexion, a slouching posture, or trembling hands were symptoms of secret "self-abuse." Whenever these symptoms were found, a thorough investigation was in order. Fortunately, a sudden confrontation with the evidence often prompted the culprits to make a full confession, and once the facts had been established, the "therapy" could begin.

In the 18th century, a confirmed masturbator was usually given a special diet. (Different doctors recommended different diets, not unlike their modern colleagues who fight obesity.) It was also believed that a hard mattress, a thin blanket, frequent washing with cold water, and generally low room temperatures were helpful in breaking the habit. In addition, simple and practical clothing was considered essential. (There was even a campaign to introduce skirts for men and to abolish trousers, "because they are too warm and irritate the sex organs.") Finally, it was obvious that the "patient" needed constant supervision.

This relatively harmless treatment became much more elaborate and cruel in the 19th century. Psychiatrists found that the insanity caused by masturbation was of a particularly disagreeable kind. As explained in 1867 by Henry Maudsley, the greatest British psychiatrist of his time, it was "characterized by . . . extreme perversion of feeling and corresponding derangement of thought, in earlier stages, and later by failure of intelligence, nocturnal hallucinations, and suicidal and homicidal propensities." In other words, masturbators were mad potential killers, and it seemed only prudent to have them locked up in an asylum.

To make matters worse, in its later stages "masturbatory insanity" was considered incurable. All medical science could really do was to concentrate on the prevention and early detection of the disease. Parents were therefore advised to tie the hands of their children to the sides of the bed, or to make them wear mittens spiked with iron thorns. Special bandages and "chastity belts" were to render the sex organs inaccessible. Doctors with a knack for mechanics invented ingenious contraptions that would "protect" people from "abusing themselves." (One of the more bizarre of these inventions was an "erection detector" which rang a little bell in the parents' bedroom as soon as their son had an erection in his sleep.) Finally, if everything else failed, surgery was recommended. The most popular surgical treatments were infibulation for males (i.e., putting a metal ring through the foreskin, thus preventing an erection) and clitoridectomy for females (i.e., cutting out the clitoris). However, cauterization and denervation of the sex organs and even castration were sometimes also deemed necessary.

Needless to say, all of these mechanical devices and surgical procedures constantly focused attention on the sex organs and their functions. Thus, it became nearly impossible for the "patients" to forget their "problem" even for a moment. Small wonder, then, that for many the concern with masturbation turned into a complete obsession.

One cannot help but feel that the authorities who administered these painful, dangerous, and useless "treatments" were not so much interested in preventing masturbation as in punishing it. Their unfortunate victims, on the other hand, often seemed curiously eager to accept this punishment. Indeed, some guilt-ridden individuals punished themselves by mutilating their bodies or committing suicide.

Today, we may wonder how intelligent men and women could ever develop such attitudes. After all, a little common sense and the simple observation of humans and animals could have told them that masturbation is a universal and harmless practice which cannot possibly be more unhealthy than sexual intercourse. Furthermore, even if one believed, contrary to all evidence, that the loss of semen somehow weakened the male body, there could never be any such danger for women and children. In short, the medical arguments against masturbation were illogical and invalid from the start. The fact that they were nevertheless believed obviously demands some explanation.

It seems that the real reason for the antimasturbation campaign was simply a growing sexual prudery. It is hardly a coincidence that the doctors, educators, and clergymen who figured most prominently in this campaign were all members of the middle classes. We have pointed out earlier in this book how the rise of the middle classes in Europe and America affected the treatment of children and adolescents, and how it changed the general attitude toward the human body and its functions. (For details, see the introductions to "The Human Body," "Infancy and Childhood," and "Adolescence.") In the middle-class view, the body was, above all, a machine, an instrument of labor which had to function in the most efficient and economical manner. Inefficiency, idleness, and waste, which had been of little concern to the ancient and medieval mind, now came to be seen as the supreme vices. Sexual activity was permissible as long as it produced children and thereby increased the labor force. Pure sensuality without purpose, however, was subversive and dangerous. Solitary masturbation posed a particular threat because it did not even require the cooperation of a partner. Moreover, it was always available to males and females of all ages and social classes, reminding them that their bodies could also be used as instruments of pleasure. Such a use was frivolous and could not be tolerated. Thus, the pseudoscientific theories about the dangers of masturbation were nothing more than rationalizations and excuses for the increasing repression of nonreproductive sex in general.

This repression was apparently also linked to the beginning industrialization of the West and the resulting demand for disciplined, docile labor. Not surprisingly, therefore, we find that the persecution of masturbators reached its greatest extent and intensity in Victorian times. It was only toward the end of the 19th century, when most Western societies had become fully industrialized and started to enjoy the fruits of their new affluence, that a slow process of sexual liberalization began to set in.

Thus, over the last hundred years we can observe a gradual softening of the original harsh psychiatric attitude toward masturbation. First, some psychiatrists began to wonder whether it might not be the result rather than the cause of a person's insanity. Then it was doubted that any connection existed at all. "Self-abuse" was perhaps only a "bad habit" or a symptom of "arrested development." Still, it remained potentially harmful, at least for males. Some doctors insisted that a young man's proper physical growth depended on the preservation of his semen and that he could therefore weaken his body by wasting it prematurely. Naturally, soon even this theory had to be abandoned for lack of evidence. It therefore became fashionable to warn only against "excessive" masturbation, and, for a while, this proved to be a comfortable fallback position. Since the "excess" was never clearly defined, no scientific proof had to be offered, and any prospective masturbator was nevertheless deterred. However, modern sex research finally succeeded in demonstrating the obvious: Masturbation as such cannot do any physical or mental harm, and "excess" is a relative term. While some people never masturbate at all in their entire lives, others masturbate several times a day for decades, and the one behavior is just as "natural," "normal," or "healthy" as the other.

Unfortunately, it takes more than the simple presentation of facts to overcome centuries of negative propaganda. Even today, many people still have their doubts and fears about masturbation. They may be unable to give any valid reason for these fears, but somehow they just cannot get rid of them. Thus, certain educational writers still denounce masturbation as a "nonproductive," "noncreative," and "parasitic" habit. They admit that it cannot do any physical harm, but continue to warn that any "excess" will turn it into a "false lead," like alcoholism and compulsive gambling. Some writers also hint vaguely that masturbation might lead to egoism, loneliness, or a hatred of the opposite sex.

These and similar superstitions survive only because our society has not yet fully freed itself from the sexual repression of the past. However, it seems that in the future more and more people will learn to see masturbation simply as another form of sexual activity which can help them in developing their erotic potential, and which can greatly enrich their lives.

ORGASM DURING SLEEP

It has always been well known that human beings are capable of experiencing sexual responses while they are asleep. In certain cultures and historical periods, however, people ascribed this capacity only to males. For example, the Bible tells us that, among the ancient Hebrews, a man who had an orgasm in his sleep was required to take a ritual bath for purification. His involuntary ejaculation of semen was called a "pollution" which made him "unclean" (Leviticus 15; Deuteronomy 23). There was no comparable requirement for women. Since women do not ejaculate anything, nobody paid any attention to their spontaneous orgasms. Indeed, until fairly recently the religious and medical authorities in our Judeo-Christian culture were used to discussing the entire matter only under the heading of "nocturnal pollution" or "nocturnal emission." It was not until around the middle of our century that Kinsey and his associates presented some reliable statistics as to the frequency of this type of sexual outlet. The figures showed that not only males, but also many females, have orgasms in their sleep (although the percentage of females is smaller). As a consequence, Kinsey no longer spoke of "nocturnal emissions," but of "nocturnal sex dreams." This was a term that could be applied to both sexes. However, it also covered cases where no orgasm was reached. In order to be more precise, other sex researchers therefore replaced Kinsey's term with "nocturnal orgasm" (i.e., orgasm during the night). Unfortunately, this now popular expression is very misleading, because in our culture most orgasms occur at night, including those reached by coitus. Sexual dreams, on the other hand, may very well occur during an afternoon nap, in which case they would have to be called "diurnal sex dreams" (i.e., sex dreams during the day). It seems then that "orgasm during sleep" is the simplest and most accurate term available.

Involuntary orgasms are almost always accompanied by sexual dreams, especially in males. These dreams may depict unusual and forbidden behavior, such as sexual intercourse with close relatives, children or animals, group sex, exhibitionism, and many other activities that the individual would never contemplate in his waking hours. However, during sleep our normal inhibitions and learned controls are much less effective, and many of our unconscious wishes may thus be acted out in a harmless, symbolic fashion. The lack of conscious restraints also accounts for another phenomenon: Many people (particularly women) reach orgasm much faster in their sleep than while they are awake.

Today, the religious and medical attitudes toward such experiences are generally very lenient. Some Christian churches have stopped being concerned about them at all, and the Catholic church considers them sinful only if they are somehow consciously planned, welcomed, or enjoyed. Certain psychiatrists once used to regard involuntary orgasms in women as symptoms of some neurotic disorder, but, in the meantime, this curious opinion has been completely discarded. Instead, there is now a widespread belief that orgasms during sleep are necessary and healthy, and that they can even provide a "natural" compensation for sexual abstinence. In other words, it is assumed that persons who do not engage in any conscious sexual activity will instead find sexual relief while asleep. This popular assumption seems to be false, however. For instance, according to Kinsey's findings, women who suddenly lost the opportunity for several coital orgasms per week had only a few more orgasms in their sleep per year. As a matter of fact, for some women the number of involuntary orgasms increased only when they also had more voluntary orgasms. In short, an orgasm during sleep is a possible natural function of the human body, but it is no substitute for conscious sexual activity.

MASTURBATION

The word masturbation is derived from the Latin verb masturbare: to defile by hand or to disturb by hand (i.e., manus: hand + either stuprare: to defile, or turbare: to disturb). The term was introduced into the English language only about 200 years ago. Before that time, people apparently used less definite references and descriptions, such as "youthful passions" or "solitary pleasures." Today, however, the word "masturbation" has become part of most European languages, and in professional textbooks it has replaced all other expressions. Under the circumstances, we have no choice but to follow the common usage in the present book.

Still, it is important to realize that the term is actually quite imprecise and misleading because both males and females can masturbate without using any hands. Therefore, when modern sex researchers speak of masturbation, they refer to "any deliberate bodily self-stimulation that produces a sexual response." Such deliberate stimulation can take many different forms. In a great number of cases, of course, the hands are indeed used. Thus, males may fondle, rub, or stroke their penis with their hands until they reach orgasm. At the same time, they may also use one hand to manipulate other erogenous zones of the body. For instance, in order to increase their overall sexual arousal, they may touch and lift their scrotum, or insert a finger into their anus. There are even some very rare cases in which men insert a solid object, such as a wire, into their urethra for stimulation. (It goes without saying that this latter practice is painful and potentially dangerous.) Recently some mechanical and even electric male masturbation aids (Accu-Jac) have appeared on the market. These gadgets, which apply some rhythmic air suction to the penis, may have a certain therapeutic use for physically handicapped men. However, otherwise they do not seem to offer any advantages over more "traditional" forms of masturbation. They are also rather expensive.

Females may also use one or both hands to masturbate. Most often they manipulate the entire vulva, or gently stroke the shaft of the clitoris and the minor lips (labia minora). Some women simultaneously play with the nipples of their breasts, and, in some cases, this breast stimulation alone may lead to orgasm.

Instead of using their hands, both males and females may also simply rub their sex organs against some object, such as a pillow, a towel, the bed cover, or the mattress. Indeed, some females reach orgasm by riding a bicycle. Many females can also masturbate by crossing their legs or pressing them together while moving rhythmically back and forth. In certain instances, rhythmic muscular tension alone is sufficient to produce an orgasm.

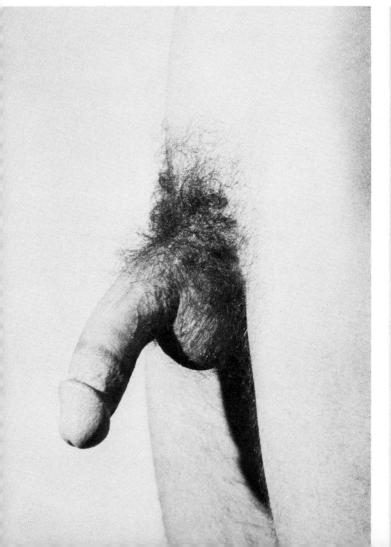
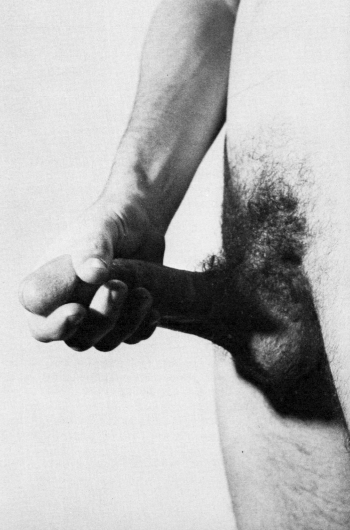

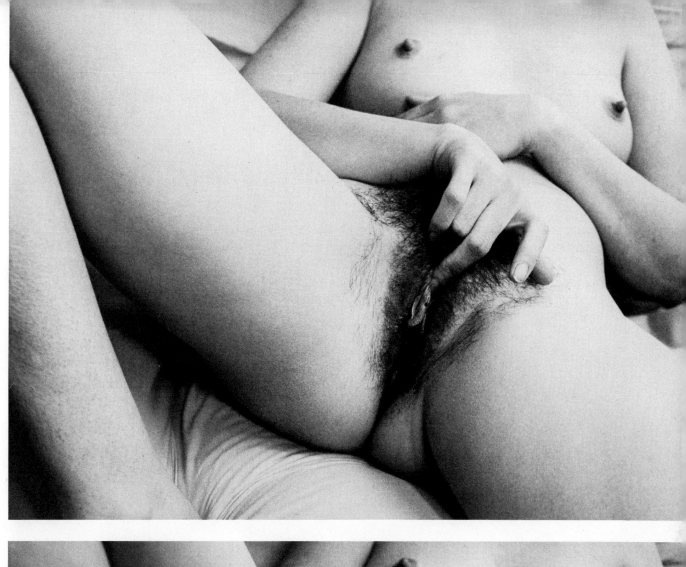
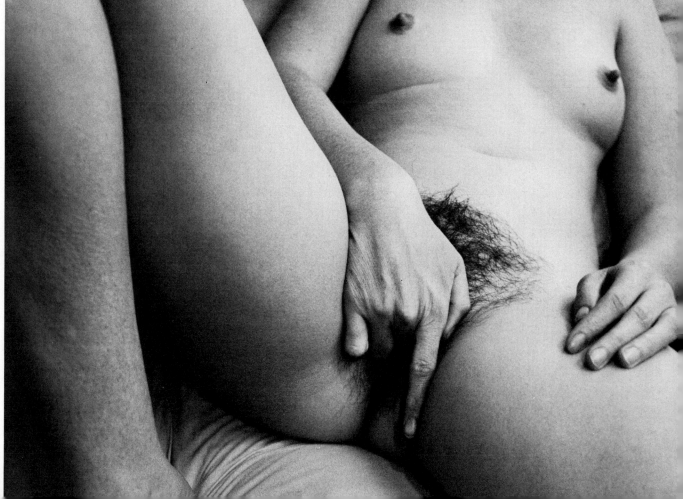

EJACULATION
The picture captures the moment of
ejaculation in a young man, with the
semen (upper left) being propelled
over a considerable distance. Not all
ejaculations are equally vigorous,
however, even in the same individual,
and with advancing age they gradually
become weaker.

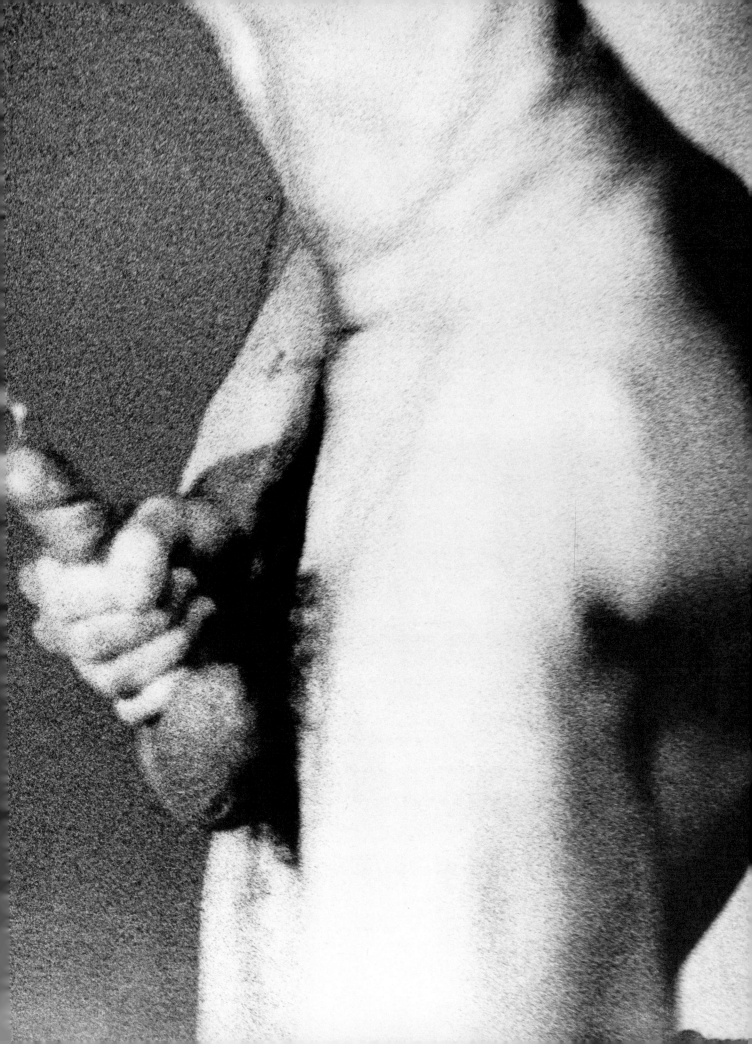

Many men imagine that women insert their fingers or some cylindrical object into the vagina when they masturbate. However, only relatively few women ever do so. There is almost no sensation in the vagina itself because its walls contain hardly any nerve endings. Instead, the most sensitive and excitable female organs are the clitoris and the minor lips. Thus, women may, on occasion, insert a finger into the vaginal opening in order to gain a firm hold for the rest of the hand which then stimulates the external sex organs.

Those women who insert various objects deep into the vagina often do so only to please and entertain men. The objects used for this purpose are usually simple household items, such as candles, cucumbers, or bananas. However, today there are also special masturbation aids on the market. The most common of these is the artificial penis, also known as a dildo (probably from the Italian *diletto*: delight). Dildos are made of wood, rubber, or plastic, and some of them can even be filled with warm liquid which, when suddenly released, simulates an ejaculation. Furthermore, in recent years penis-shaped electric vibrators have appeared in many American drugstores. The Japanese have developed still another device called *ben-wa* or *rin-no-tama*. It consists of two hollow metal balls, one of which contains a smaller ball of lead or mercury. The two balls are introduced into the vagina and held in place by a tampon. The woman's normal bodily movements then cause the balls to click together and to send pleasant vibrations through her entire pelvic region. It is doubtful, however, whether they can cause much sexual arousal or lead to orgasm. They never touch the clitoris at all, and the vagina itself contains virtually no nerve endings. Only its outer third (the so-called orgasmic platform) narrows in response to sexual stimulation.

Finally, there are also some electric vibrators or massagers which are meant to be used on the female external sex organs. Such a vibrator usually consists of a small electric motor which is encased in plastic and which is equipped with a vibrating rubber cup. The cup is placed near the clitoris and the vaginal opening where it provides a much more effective sexual stimulation than could be achieved by vaginal insertions. (For details, see "Sexual Inadequacy in Women—Absence of Orgasm.")

Both males and females may learn to masturbate all by themselves while still in their infancy. As they play with their sex organs, they may discover some plesurable feeling and then simply try to repeat the experience. However, in most cases, conscious and regular masturbation does not begin until adolescence. Boys are often taught how to masturbate by other boys, or they hear about it in their conversations. Since boys seem to discuss sexual matters much more openly than girls, they usually obtain more sex information at an earlier age. In contrast, girls are more likely to discover masturbation alone and by accident. Some of them are introduced to it through "petting" with a boy, and others read about it in books or magazines. There are even cases of girls who masturbate for years before they realize what they are doing.

In many popular sex guides (and even in some medical textbooks), masturbation is seen almost exclusively as an adolescent activity. In actual fact, however, it is also practiced by many adults, including married couples. Particularly older men and women may find themselves regaining great interest in masturbation when they live alone, or when their partners are sick, weak, or unavailable for some other reason. In these and many other cases, masturbation can be a very satisfying substitute for sexual intercourse which relieves tension, exercises the body, stimulates the imagination, and keeps the sexual capacities alive.

Still, generally speaking, in our society only the better-educated adults seem to take full advantage of the possibilities of masturbation. Many people at lower educational levels apparently stop masturbating at some time in late adolescence because they consider all sexual practices other than coitus to be childish, improper, immoral, or even unhealthy. High school and college graduates, on the other hand, usually know that masturbation is no danger to health, and they may, in fact, view it as useful and therapeutic. Moreover, a well-educated person normally also cherishes the sexual fantasies which can make the experience more rewarding.

We know that for many teenagers in our culture masturbation is the most common or even the only sexual outlet. However, this does not mean that it is typical for the earlier phases of human sexual development and that it is "appropriate" only during adolescence. It simply means that adolescents do not have sufficient opportunity for sexual intercourse. Adults who masturbate when they cannot find a sexual partner have no reason to feel that they are "immature."

HETEROSEXUAL INTERCOURSE

According to the dictionary, the word intercourse (from the Latin *intercurrere:* to run between) can refer to any interchange or communication between persons. Thus, one may speak of social intercourse in general or, more specifically, of visual intercourse between people who wink at each other, of oral intercourse between people who talk to each other, and of manual intercourse between people who shake hands. However, today many doctors, lawyers, and other professionals use the term in a much narrower sense. When they speak of intercourse, they mean only one particular kind of communication: sexual intercourse. Indeed, they often mean only one particular kind of sexual intercourse: coitus.

Unfortunately, in the meantime, this narrow professional usage has also been widely accepted by the general public. For example, popular marriage manuals now often distinguish between "intercourse" (coitus) and "petting" (all other forms of sexual intimacy). They also declare that the dramatic event of "intercourse" itself should be preceded by "foreplay" and followed by "afterplay." In short, they imply by their very language that the only sexual contact that really counts is that between penis and vagina.

This is a very shortsighted view. After all, as we have seen in the first part of this book, the human sexual response involves the whole body, and orgasm can be reached in many different ways. (See "The Male Sexual Response" and "The Female Sexual Response.") Statistically speaking, coitus may very well be the most common form of sexual contact, but it is by no means the only one. Indeed, for many men and women it is not even the one they like best. Furthermore, there are countless individuals who are physically unable to engage in coitus because of certain handicaps, injuries, or diseases. Nevertheless, many of them can and do have satisfying sexual relationships.

Coitus is, of course, the only form of sexual intercourse that can lead to the procreation of children, and in our culture it has therefore long been extolled as superior. According to Jewish and Christian religious traditions, sex and procreation were meant to be inseparable. Any sexual activity that, by its very nature, could not lead to pregnancy was considered sinful and had to be discouraged. As a result, in most Western countries the sin also became a crime. Noncoital intercourse was declared a serious offense, and the punishment could be very severe. Finally, modern psychiatrists turned the crime into a disease by claiming that adults who did not prefer coitus to any other sexual activity were mentally ill, or at least "immature." (For further details, see "Conformity and Deviance.")

Today, we are beginning to realize that these negative attitudes toward all sexual intercourse except coitus have needlessly impoverished many lives. Indeed, there is little doubt that the constant preoccupation with penis and vagina and the neglect of other "erogenous zones" of the body can actually

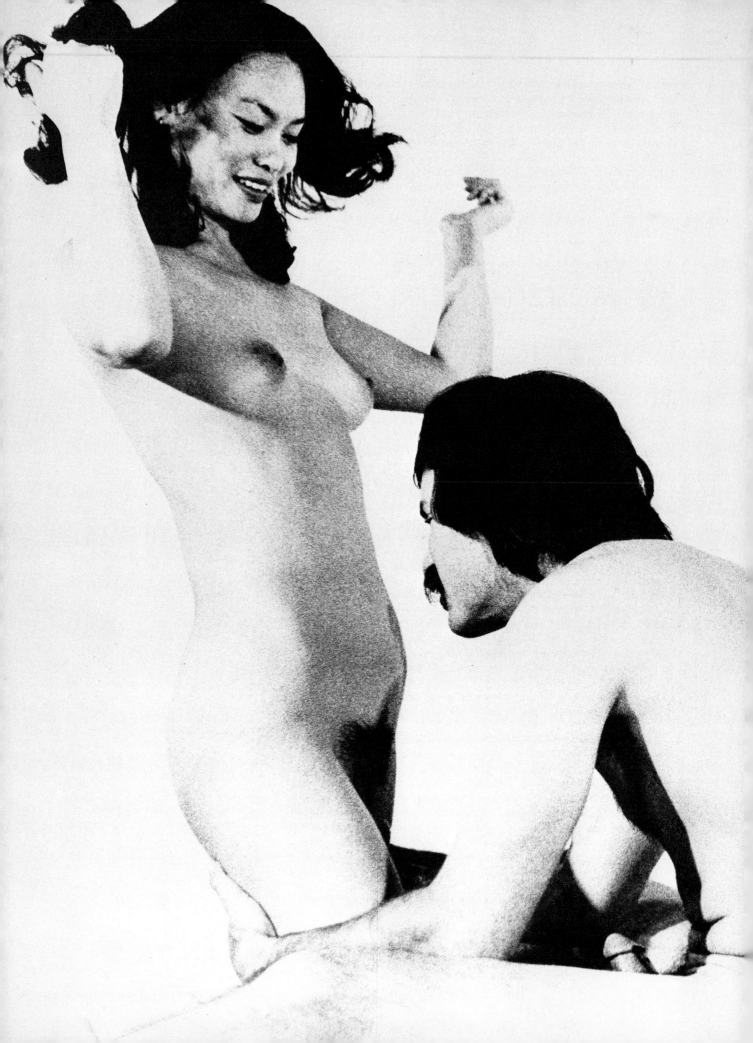

make men and women insensitive and thus prevent their normal sexual functioning. (See "Sexual Inadequacy.") This is exactly why so many modern "sex experts" emphasize the need for "petting" and "foreplay." However, even these well-meaning people still fail to recognize the real issue. As long as coitus is described as the supreme and ultimate form of sexual intercourse, all other forms will obviously have to be considered inferior. At best, they will be treated as "variations" or "substitutions," and their main function will always be to serve as some sort of "prologue" or "epilogue" to the "main event." In other words, couples will still feel obliged to justify their spontaneous sexual experiments by trying to lead up to coitus. They will continue to divide sexual intercourse into acts, chapters, or escalating phases, and they will remain unable to develop their full erotic potential.

It is for this reason that, in this book, we do not follow the standard approach of other sex guides and marriage manuals, but treat the subject in a more general way. Thus, instead of trying to impose a specific sexual preference on the reader, we begin with a very simple definition:

Sexual intercourse is any communication between persons that involves a sexual response.

Such communication can, of course, take many different forms. People may respond sexually to each other when they embrace and kiss, but also when they just look into each other's eyes or talk to each other on the telephone. In other words, they may never touch each other's sex organs and, indeed, may have no direct physical contact at all. Still, as long as there is some interchange and a mutual awareness of sexual feelings, there is sexual intercourse in the true sense of the word.

This is where the entire matter might well rest were it not for the clergymen, lawyers, and doctors who feel that they must somehow specify, classify, and categorize what people do to each other when they make love. Naturally, each professional discipline has its own perceptions and concerns, and anybody who likes professional jargon can easily come up with new special terms of his own. The possibilities are virtually endless. Even sexual intercourse without direct physical contact can be divided into several subcategories. For example, a person who is stimulated by an obscene phone call, and who actually encourages the caller, may be said to engage in "vocal and aural intercourse." In the same vein, the relationship between an exhibitionist and a voyeur may well be called "visual intercourse." Indeed, there is no reason why one should not speak of "postal intercourse" between people who send each other sexually arousing letters or photographs.

However, as the examples illustrate, this kind of terminology can eventually become so specific as to be ludicrous. For practical purposes, some professionals have therefore agreed on just a few basic terms which describe only those forms of sexual intercourse that involve direct physical contact with the sex organs of at least one of the participants. This compromise approach is not perfect, but it simplifies the matter considerably, and, since it has found wide popular acceptance, we might as well use it here to give some shape and structure to our discussion. Thus, following modern general usage, we distinguish between four basic types of sexual intercourse:

- We speak of **manual intercourse** (from Latin *manus:* hand) when the sex organs of one partner are in contact with the hand(s) of the other.
- We speak of **oral intercourse** (from Latin *os:* mouth) when the sex-organs of one partner are in contact with the mouth of the other.
- We speak of **genital intercourse** (from Latin *genitalia:* organs of generation) when the sex organs of one partner are in contact with the sex organs of the other.
- We speak of **anal intercourse** (from Latin *anus:* rectal opening) when the sex organs of one partner are in contact with the anus of the other.

These are, of course, purely technical distinctions, and they are not meant to suggest clear-cut alternatives or separate and exclusive approaches. It is true that there are some men and women who restrict themselves to only one type of sexual intercourse, but most couples today prefer to make love by freely switching from one approach to another. Thus, their intercourse may first be manual, then oral, and finally genital. Indeed, if one wanted to be pedantic about it, one could introduce several more distinctions and speak, for example, of "femoral intercourse" (from Latin *femora*: thighs) and "mammary intercourse" (from Latin *mamma:* breast) when a man places his penis between the thighs or breasts of his partner. After all, a couple may spend hours in each other's arms trying all possible variations of lovemaking before they reach orgasm. At other times, they may simply relish the process of mutual stimulation itself without reaching any orgasm at all. None of this makes any difference for the purposes of our definition. It is always the whole of a couple's sexual interaction that matters, not just its possible last phase.

On the other hand, we have to remember that it is only the sexual character of this interaction that concerns us here. For example, our definition of manual intercourse does not apply to the manipulation of a patient's sex organs by an examining physician. The mere fact that the sex organs of one person come in contact with the hands, mouth, sex organs, or anus of another is, in itself, no reason to speak of sexual intercourse. The term is justified only if at least one of them shows a sexual response which is noticed and encouraged by the other. (This also means, among other things, that children who touch each other's sex organs out of sheer curiosity are not engaging in sexual intercourse.)

While it is relatively easy to agree on a general definition of sexual intercourse, it would be foolish to attempt a standard description of it. Among human beings, sex is essentially a personal matter. Each individual has different sexual interests, and therefore no two couples ever make love in quite the same way. Some follow a single pattern throughout their lives, some try specific approaches on specific occasions, and some just go on seeking variety for its own sake. There are couples who need only a few minutes or even seconds for their lovemaking, and there are others who prolong it for hours. Some men and women never repeat the experience at all, others repeat it regularly, but at rather long intervals, and still others continue to have sexual intercourse several times a day for many years.

There is nothing wrong with any of these choices as long as they are satisfying to those directly involved, and it is preposterous for any religious, legal, or medical expert to tell them otherwise. Unfortunately, this is exactly what, in the past, many such experts tried to do. Instead of encouraging people to find their own way to happiness and to develop their individual capacities for pleasure, they established a rigid ideal of "natural," "normal," and "healthy" sexual intercourse toward which everyone was supposed to strive. All deviations from this ideal were declared to be "unnatural," "abnormal," and "sick."

As already mentioned, in our own particular culture coitus was, for a very long time, the only acceptable sexual activity. In fact, even today many states of the United States still punish noncoital sex as a "crime against nature." Thus, even married couples who engage in oral intercourse are to be regarded as depraved and dangerous criminals, and if their "crime" should come to the attention of a court, they may be sentenced to long prison terms.

These laws are not any less absurd because they are rarely enforced. Indeed, their necessarily selective enforcement renders them all the more scandalous. However, at least as objectionable as the laws themselves is the primitive view of human sexuality that inspired them. In this view, sexual intercourse between human beings is nothing but a means of producing offspring, just like the mating of cattle. There is no room for refinement and cultivation. Indeed, any attempt at such refinement is a perversion of the "natural order." Man may strive to perfect himself in all other spheres of life, but in his sexual activity he must never rise above the level of beasts.

Fortunately, in the meantime, most people in our society have adopted a more civilized attitude. They realize that a sexual relationship involves each partner as a whole person, and that the demand to restrict sexual contact to

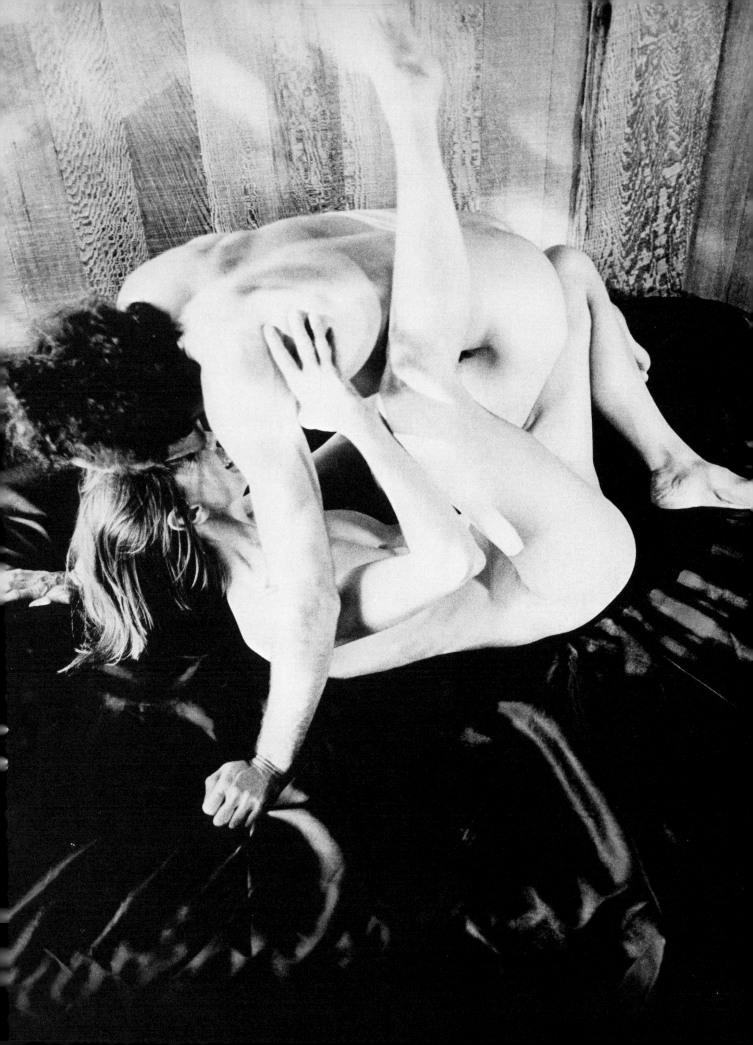

specific areas of the body is, in itself, perverse. Thus, at least in practice, sexual experimentation has now become widely accepted.

Nevertheless, even today there are many couples who fail to develop their full erotic potential, if for a slightly different reason. They may no longer fear to bring variety to their lovemaking, but they may continue to see it merely as a means to an end. That is to say, just like their forebears, they are still concerned with the product rather than the process of sexual intercourse. From a means of producing offspring, they have simply turned it into a means of producing orgasm. In short, they still lack the capacity to relish sexual pleasure as an end in itself. However, it is this very capacity that binds men and women together, provides for their deepest satisfaction, and ensures their sexual functioning well into their old age.

The following pages offer a few broad hints at some forms of sexual intercourse without any special emphasis on either reproduction or orgasm. Here, as elsewhere in this book, the main purpose is simply to clarify some terms, to describe certain techniques, and to point out various possibilities. The choice among these possibilities has to be left to each individual. The text makes no attempt to establish any standard, norm, or goal of sexual intercourse except that of mutual pleasure.

MANUAL INTERCOURSE

Manual intercourse is here defined as involving sexual contact between the sex organs of one person and the hand(s) of another.

In older marital guides, this kind of sexual intercourse was often described as "petting" or as a "foreplay" to coitus. Intensive manual stimulation of a woman's sex organs was considered necessary for her complete arousal, and husbands were therefore admonished to make it a regular habit in order to please their wives. (These books always pretended to be written exclusively for married couples.) Unfortunately, many men came to think of this "foreplay" as just another unpleasant male duty. Furthermore, since they knew little about the female sexual response, some of them overstimulated the female clitoris to the point where they caused more pain than pleasure. Women, on the other hand, were often reluctant to touch the male sex organs at all. In short, manual intercourse was rarely seen as a mutually enjoyable experience in its own right.

Today, however, a general change in sexual attitudes seems to be taking place. Many men and women now frankly tell each other what they like sexually, and they are much more willing to experiment. Thus, they begin to realize that coitus is by no means the only road to sexual satisfaction. Indeed, they may find that they can give and receive great pleasure by simply touching, stroking, and massaging each other's bodies. Moreover, modern sex therapists have discovered that such mutual pleasuring can unblock long inhibited sexual responses and thus help overcome male and female sexual inadequacies. (See "Sexual Inadequacy.")

As the partners gently explore each other's erogenous zones, they are likely to return again and again to those that are the most sensitive—the sex organs. Thus, very naturally, they may find themselves engaging in manual intercourse. They may also discover that either of them can take the initiative, or that they can very well act simultaneously. In this latter case, one may, of course, speak of mutual masturbation. Obviously, a man who wants to masturbate a woman should ask her where and how she likes to be touched. (Hardly any two women masturbate in quite the same way.) Most often he will be told that the glans of the clitoris is too sensitive for any direct stimulation, and that it is far better to stroke the side of the clitoral shaft and the minor lips (labia minora). Furthermore, as the woman becomes sexually excited, her vagina begins to lubricate naturally, and the man should then use his fingers to spread this lubrication to the clitoris in order to avoid possible irritation. He should also remember that, with mounting excitement, the clitoris withdraws under its hood or foreskin and therefore becomes inaccessible. However, as long as he follows the woman's own instructions

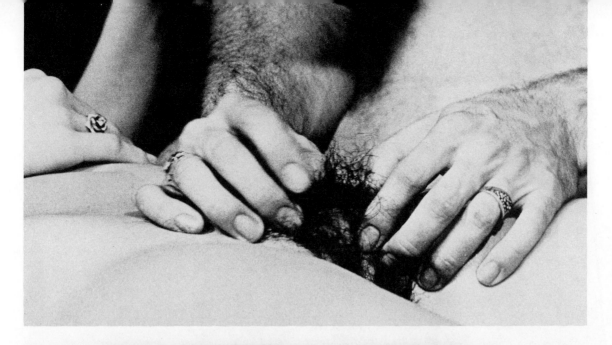

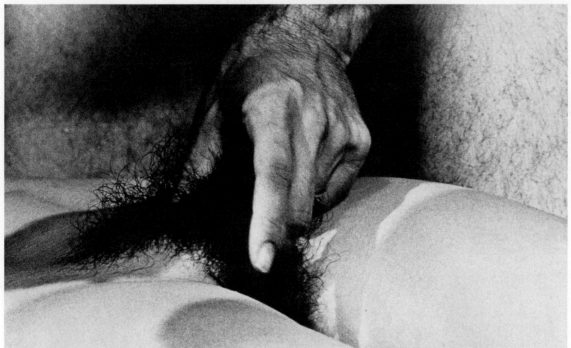

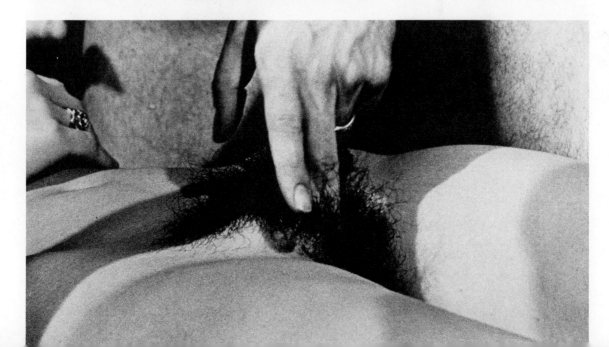

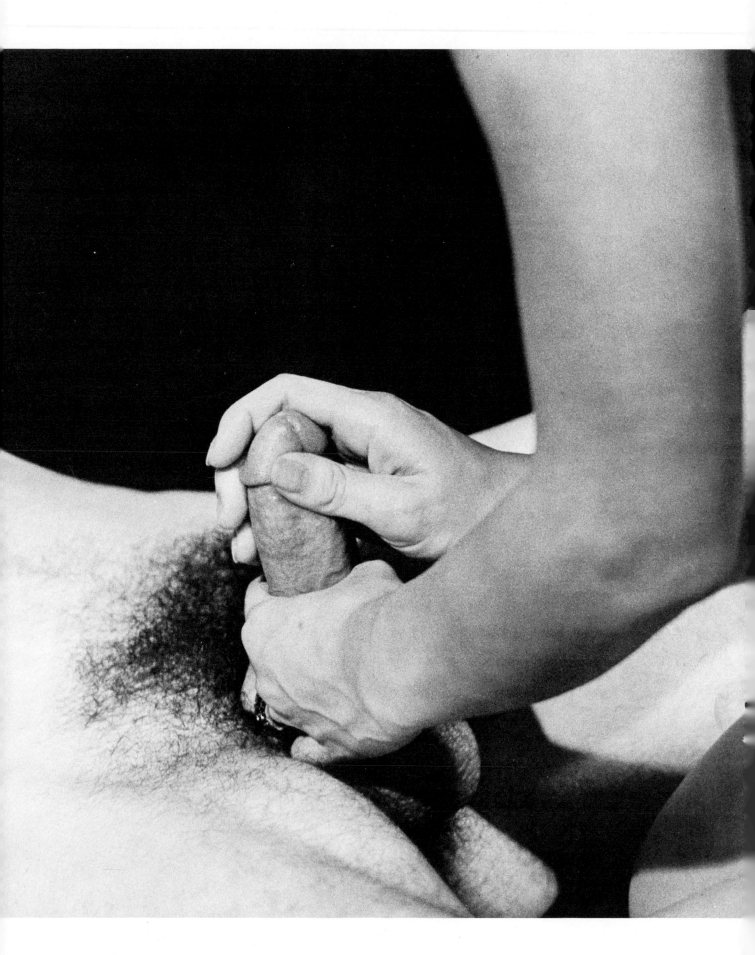

Cunnilingus

The term "cunnilingus" (from Latin *cunnus*: vulva and *linguere*: to lick) is used to describe the licking or sucking of the female sex organs.

A woman's external sex organs and the surrounding areas usually represent the most sensitive erogenous zones of her body. They are easily stimulated by regular, soft strokes of the hand, or by gentle and passionate kisses. Thus, a man may greatly arouse a woman by licking the inside of her thighs, the space between the sex organs and the anus (the perineum), and the anus itself. He can further heighten her pleasure by kissing, licking, and sucking the minor lips of her vulva and the shaft of the clitoris. Indeed, with some practice, he may very well bring her to orgasm this way.

A man who licks a woman's sex organs should, of course, ask her how she likes it best and then follow her instructions. In some situations, where the man cannot get an erection and therefore cannot begin coitus, he may be glad to discover that prolonged oral stimulation alone often leaves a woman completely satisfied. On the other hand, a man may also use cunnilingus simply as a means of arousal before switching to other forms of sexual intercourse. At other times, he may continue it until the woman has had several orgasms and then bring her to orgasm once more through coitus.

With mounting sexual excitement, a woman's vagina secretes some special lubricating fluid. In a healthy woman, this fluid is quite clean and can be swallowed without any ill effects. In fact, many men learn to love its peculiar, slightly acidic taste. However, in recent years the cosmetics industry has begun to produce certain "feminine hygiene" sprays and sweet-smelling vaginal douches. These superfluous products may upset the vaginal ecology and thus cause infection and irritation. Furthermore, they may also prove harmful to the sensitive areas of a man's penis or mouth. It is therefore advisable for a woman to avoid all vaginal douching and to restrict herself simply to washing her vulva with soap and water. The vagina cleanses itself with its own secretions. In short, there is no need for either the woman or the man to fear that cunnilingus might be unpleasant or unhealthy. Unusual vaginal secretions or odors are a sure sign that something is wrong. In such a case, a physician should be consulted.

Just as fellatio, cunnilingus can be practiced in many different positions. Individual sexual partners have to find out for themselves which position gives them the greatest pleasure. Some couples may avoid cunnilingus during the woman's menstrual period for aesthetic reasons. This is a matter of personal preference. However, it has been suggested that no man should lick or suck a woman's sex organs in the last stages of pregnancy because air blown into the vagina may then cause serious damage to the woman and the fetus. This danger may be somewhat exaggerated, although in the late stages of pregnancy some caution and circumspection is advisable for all forms of sexual intercourse. (See "Pregnancy.")

"69"

The slang term "sixty-nine" (or French *soixante-neuf*) is used to describe a form of oral intercourse in which the partners simultaneously lick each other's sex organs. In doing so, the position of their bodies in relation to each other is similar to that of the inverted numerals in the number 69.

Simultaneous mutual oral intercourse can be very enjoyable for both partners, and it can, of course, lead to orgasm. However, most men and women will probably use it only as a means of stimulation and then proceed to other forms of lovemaking because they may find it difficult to keep adjusted to each other in this unusual position. Such adjustment is a little easier if they take their time and lie on their sides rather than on top of each other. However, even then only one of the partners may be able to reach orgasm. In this case, it may be better to continue sexual intercourse in some other way.

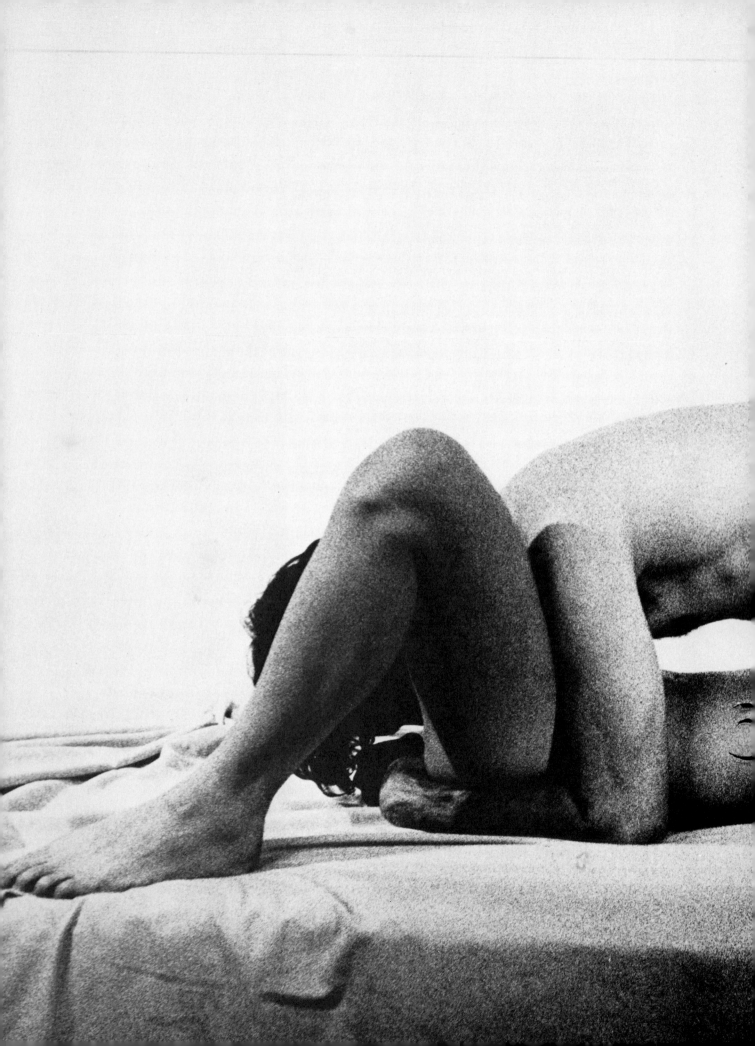

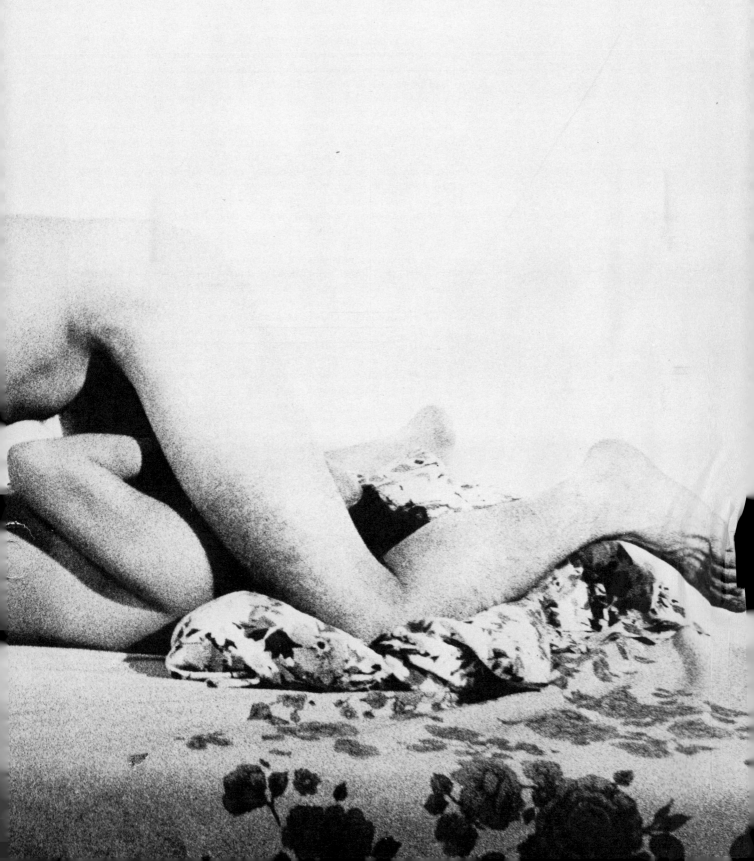

GENITAL INTERCOURSE

Genital intercourse is here defined as involving sexual contact between the sex organs of two persons.

The sex organs are the most sensitive erogenous zones of the human body, and for the great majority of men and women genital contact is therefore the favorite form of sexual intercourse. Furthermore, anatomically penis and vagina are easily joined together. Indeed, throughout most of human history it was only this joining (Latin: *copulatio*) of the male and female bodies that made the conception of new human life possible. (Today, a woman may also conceive by means of artificial insemination.)

In our Judeo-Christian culture, sex has traditionally been tied to the purpose of procreation. Thus, for a very long time the union of penis and vagina was declared to be the only natural form of sexual intercourse. Manual and oral stimulation was sometimes permitted, as long as the partners intended it to lead up to coitus. Without this intention, however, such sexual contact was always considered sinful. Moreover, in most Western countries the sin was also punished as a crime.

When, during the 19th century, psychiatrists started to focus their attention on human sexual behavior, they first did not dare to question the conventional sexual morality. While their vocabulary was new and different, the message was still the same: All noncoital sex was wrong. However, instead of damnation after death they now threatened immediate suffering in life. Masturbation, "oralism," and "analism" turned from religious offenses into psychiatric disorders, and thus the sinners found themselves suddenly transformed into the mentally ill.

Still, in the course of time, a growing number of psychiatrists began to examine the unquestioned general assumptions about the purpose of sexual behavior, and, as a result, they became much more cautious in their pronouncements. Much of what at first had been labeled as "perverse" and "aberrant" was now simply called "immature," and it was no longer always seen as a symptom of illness. As a matter of fact, masturbation and oral intercourse began to be widely accepted as healthy and therapeutic. It is true that even today some traditional psychiatric texts still define the regular preference for noncoital sex as a "perversion" which must be corrected, but the majority of modern psychiatrists no longer share this formalistic approach. Instead, they are more interested in the subjective and objective effects of sexual activity. There is now a consensus among most professionals that labels like illness, perversion, disorder, and abnormality should be strictly reserved for those cases where sexual acts cause distress in the person who performs them, or where they are clearly harmful to others. According to this view of human sexuality, noncoital sex as such need never cause anybody's concern. On the other hand, in certain cases such as rape, coitus itself may very well become a psychiatric problem. (For details, see "Compulsive and Destructive Behavior.")

There is, of course, every reason to believe that genital intercourse will never become unpopular. In the past, it has always been the preferred form of lovemaking for most people, and it will certainly remain so in the future. However, in our own society, which is only now emerging from a long period of sexual repression, many couples may still have to learn how to make the most of it. (See also "Sexual Inadequacy.")

Apposition of Sex Organs

When unmarried teenagers first begin to experiment with sexual intercourse, they often avoid the insertion of the penis into the vagina because they fear an unwanted pregnancy, or because the girl wants to preserve her "virginity" (see "Adolescence"). However, since at least the boys usually become highly aroused during their loveplay, girls sometimes allow them to reach orgasm by "heavy petting." For example, a girl who does not feel very excited herself may encourage her boyfriend to go through the motions of coitus while lying fully clothed on top of her. Most boys easily reach orgasm this way, and, among themselves, they refer to the experience as "dry humping."

As their girl friends gradually allow them more liberties, they may remove some or most of their clothing, and eventually the couple may even decide to continue their experiments in complete nudity. Nevertheless, the girl may, for a while, still fear a conception or want to keep an unbroken hymen (the thin membrane that stretches across the vaginal opening). She may also worry about bleeding and pain, or an infection with a venereal disease. Still, she may gladly permit her boyfriend to rub his penis against her vulva, as long as he does not try to insert it. Indeed, such an apposition of the male and female sex organs can be quite pleasant for both partners, and, with some practice, both of them may very well become able to reach orgasm through this technique. (After all, the penis is stimulated directly, and, as it pushes against certain areas of the vulva, it can indirectly stimulate the sensitive clitoris and the minor lips.) Even couples who normally engage in coitus may sometimes enjoy this simple form of sexual intercourse, if the woman's internal sex organs become too sensitive because of some injury or disease. (See "Pain During Sexual Intercourse.")

However, it is perhaps unwise to think of the apposition of sex organs only as a substitute for coitus. Some men and women may see it as a valuable experience in its own right, and they may find their own ways of making it especially exciting. Thus, they may regularly engage in it after cunnilingus, when the vulva is well drenched in saliva and vaginal lubrication, or they may use special lubricants which protect their sex organs against irritation and which enhance their mutual sensitivity.

Coitus

The terms "coitus" and "coition" (from Latin *coire*: to go together) refer to the insertion of the penis into the vagina—probably the most common form of sexual intercourse. (It is also the only kind of sexual intercourse that can lead to the conception of a child.)

There have been human societies where sexual contact between males and females was restricted to coitus without any preliminaries, variations, or improvisations. Such societies usually put a heavy emphasis on the procreative function of sex and discouraged all sexual pleasure, especially in women. Indeed, there are still some men even in our own culture who are interested only in the union of penis and vagina, and for whom any other loveplay is a ridiculous nuisance. Moreover, their coitus may never last more than a few seconds, and thus, apart from a quick orgasm, these men may find little sexual enjoyment. Their female partners, on the other hand, often remain completely frustrated. However, there are also some couples who turn their sexual intercourse into a slow, elaborate, and highly varied ritual. They may see coitus as only one among many ways of satisfying each other, but when they engage in it, they may do so for several hours at a time.

In recent decades, the invention of reliable contraceptives has freed many men and women from the fear of an unwanted pregnancy. This, in turn, has increased their enjoyment of coitus. More and more women insist on their right to sexual satisfaction and are no longer content with simply playing the role of a "sex object." They not only like to receive pleasure, but also to give it, and instead of just waiting to be aroused, they become truly equal sexual partners. Many couples now realize that coitus is not something that has to take place between an "active" male and a "passive" female, but that it is most satisfying when they both really "go together" or when they let the initiative shift back and forth between them. Thus, coitus has gained a new importance as a means of human communication.

It is easy enough to start coitus, but, as with all other forms of sexual intercourse, complete mutual satisfaction is almost always the result of practice and experience. Young people especially often tend to expect too much too soon. Most boys and girls think, dream, and even talk about their first coitus long before it actually occurs, and their hopes, fears, and fantasies can turn the eventual real experience into something of an anticlimax. A good example is the great significance that is usually attributed to a girl's "deflora-

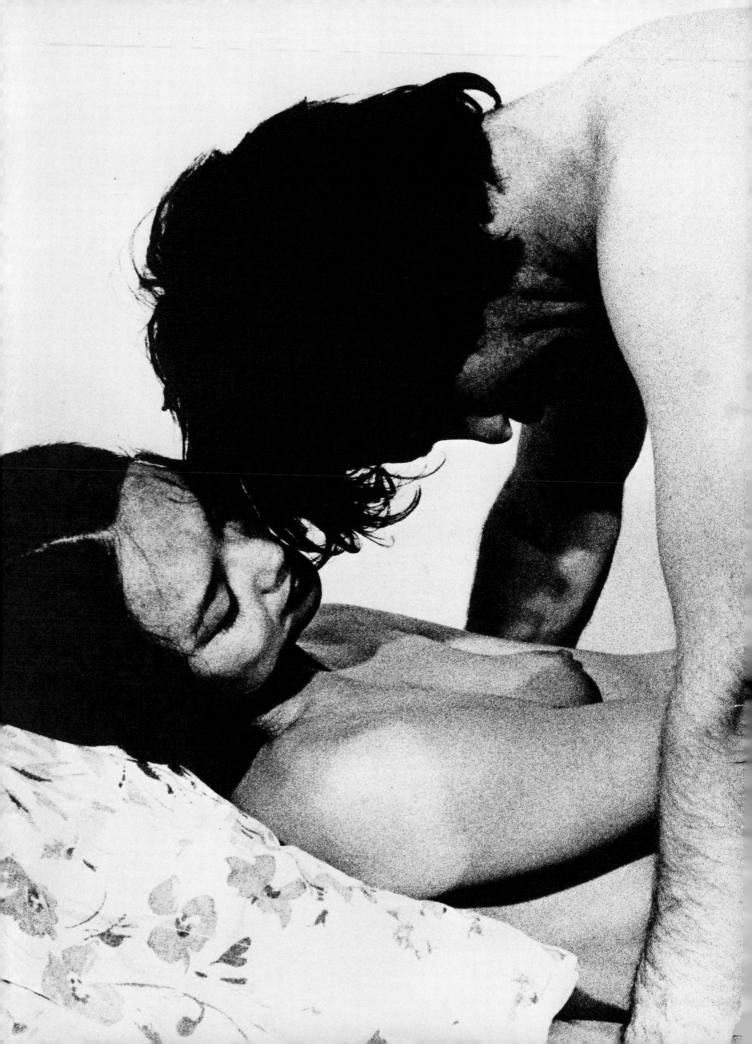

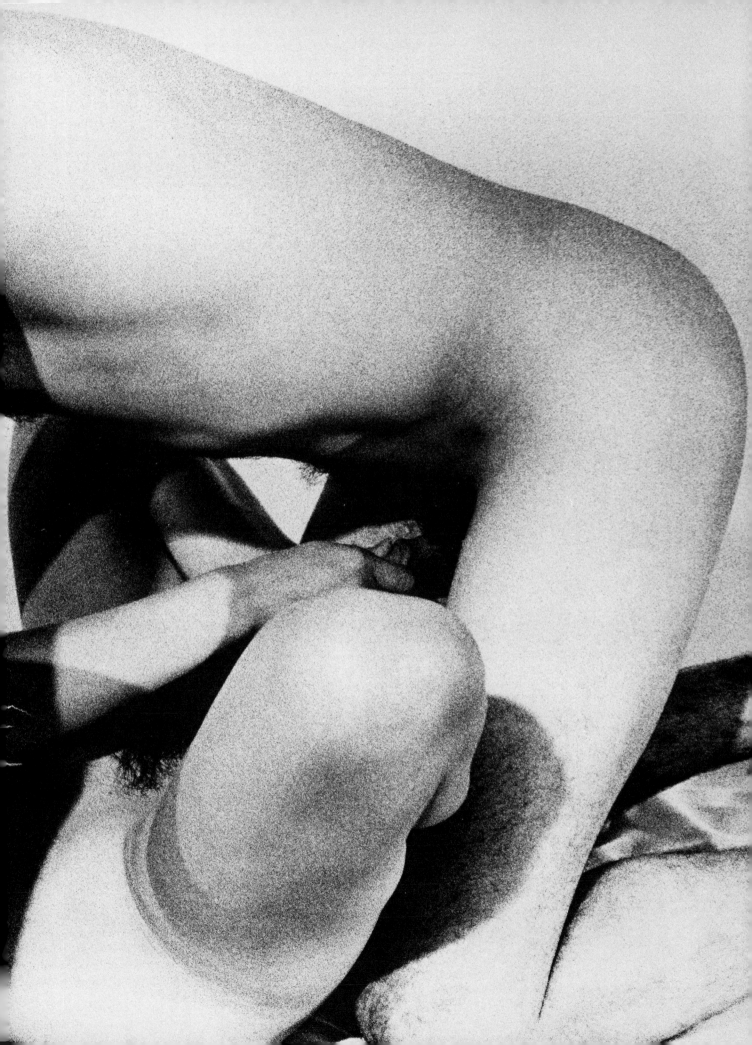

tion," i.e., the rupturing of her hymen (the thin membrane that stretches across the vaginal opening). The hymen may, of course, be ruptured by the use of tampons, by masturbation, or as a result of certain athletic activities. Still, in most females it remains more or less intact until that moment when a penis is first inserted into the vagina. Many adolescents have exaggerated and unrealistic ideas about this moment and may, in fact, worry about it years in advance. Thus, a boy may wonder if his penis will ever be hard enough to penetrate the hymen, and a girl may anticipate some painful physical injury. However, none of these worries are justified. There is no need for males to be tough and brutal because the hymen normally ruptures very easily. Indeed, a gradual, slow, and gentle approach is best. Females, on the other hand, may experience some discomfort and slight bleeding, but they need not fear any great pain. Only in very rare cases does the hymen prove to be too thick for penetration, but then a physician can easily solve the problem in his office by a simple surgical procedure.

In general, couples are well advised not to begin coitus suddenly and hastily, but to take their time working up to it in a deliberate fashion. For instance, they may greatly heighten their pleasure by first engaging in some kind of manual or oral intercourse. (This way a woman may even enjoy one or several orgasms before coitus.) At any rate, coitus should be attempted only when the vagina has produced enough of its own natural lubrication. As a woman becomes sexually excited during her loveplay, the vaginal walls begin to secrete a clear fluid which protects them against irritation and which makes the smooth insertion of the penis possible. Without such lubrication coitus can be painful for both partners. (It is only with advancing age that the natural vaginal lubrication may become insufficient in some women. The condition can usually be improved by hormone therapy. There are also some prelubricated condoms on the market which may prove helpful in such cases. However, certain artificial household lubricants, such as Vaseline which can be used in manual and anal intercourse, should not be introduced into the vagina.)

Once the woman's vagina is sufficiently lubricated, the man can gradually insert his penis. There is no need to penetrate very deeply right away, because, in spite of her sexual excitement, the woman may still feel a little tense for a while. In this case, the man can often help her relax by slowly moving just the tip of his penis back and forth in the outer part of the vagina. Then, when she feels like it, she can deepen the penetration by her own pelvic thrusting. Pelvic thrusting during sexual intercourse comes "naturally" to all mammals and can, in fact, already be observed in human infants when they begin to discover and enjoy their sexual responses (see "Infancy and Childhood"). However, instinctual as this behavior may be, it can be greatly improved upon by experienced lovers.

Men with limited sexual experience may believe that unvaried, deep, and quick thrusts are the most effective, but in actual fact this is rarely the case. At least at the beginning of coitus, a man can give and receive much more pleasure by moving slowly and keeping the penetration shallow. Indeed, he may learn a great deal by first leaving the initiative to the woman. In most cases, she will prefer long and deliberate movements in which the tip of the penis is withdrawn toward the vaginal opening before each new deep penetration. The reason for this is simple: With mounting sexual excitement, the inner portion of the vagina widens while the outer third narrows as it becomes congested with blood. In other words, it is the outer third of the vagina (the so-called orgasmic platform) which provides the greatest stimulation for the penis. (For details, see "The Female Sexual Response.")

At this point, it should also be mentioned that many women learn to control the interior muscles surrounding the vaginal entrance. Thus, they keep a firm grip on the penis and increase the mutual stimulation even further. (Women who have a wide and slack vaginal entrance, who are unaware of their vaginal muscles, or who find them underdeveloped, can improve their condition by appropriate exercises. (See "Sexual Inadequacy in Women—Absence of Orgasm.")

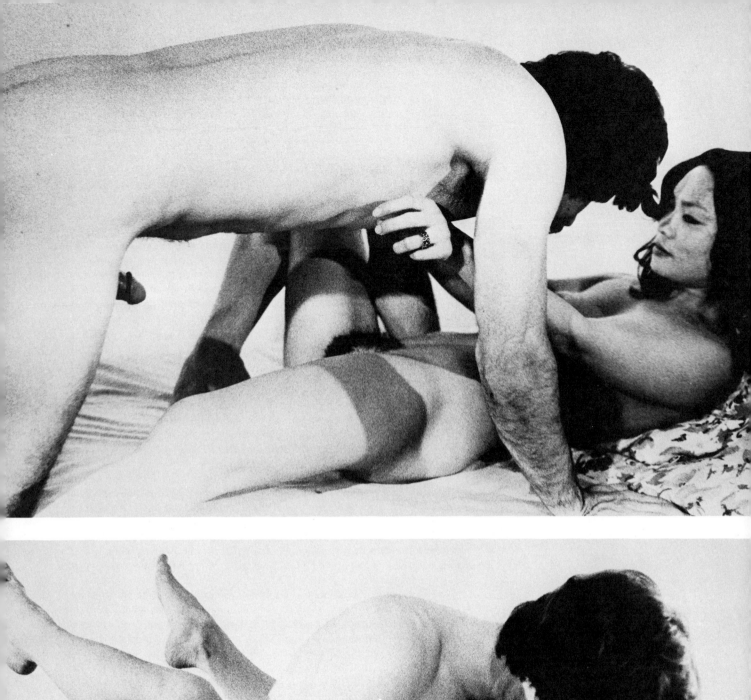
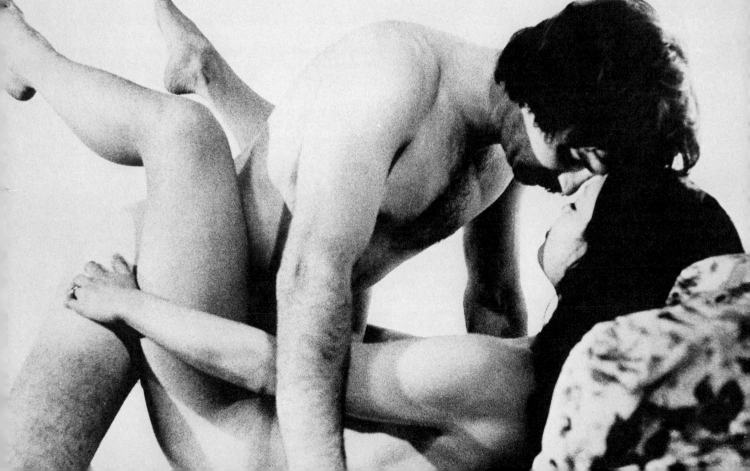

As man and woman continue their coitus, they usually accelerate their pelvic thrusting and aim for a deeper penetration of the vagina. Sometimes only one partner executes all these movements, while the other remains relatively passive; at other times, both partners move together. Furthermore, within their general rhythmic pattern, they may greatly vary their thrusts from deep to shallow, and they may also let the penis rotate deep inside the vagina by a circular forward and back motion of their hips.

Only experience can teach a particular couple how to derive the greatest pleasure from coitus, but if they are sensitive to each other's reactions, they will soon learn how to satisfy each other best. After all, coitus is, above everything else, an intimate interaction of two individuals, and no expert technical advice can ever help them as much as direct and open communication. The woman especially should never be afraid to tell the man exactly how she likes to be stimulated, and she should realize that she acts in their mutual interest when she abandons herself to her own sexual feelings. While a man may want to retain some control over the timing of his orgasm, a woman never needs to hold back. She can continue to have orgasms as long as he can keep his erection.

Unfortunately, many men and women diminish their enjoyment of coitus by an overconcern with orgasm. Since men know that they can reach orgasm relatively quickly, they may wonder whether they will last long enough to satisfy their partners. Women, on the other hand, may fear that their orgasm will not come soon enough, or that they will have no orgasm at all. Needless to say, such secret worries can seriously interfere with a couple's communication and even make normal sexual functioning impossible.

It seems that most couples would find greater sexual happiness if they concentrated more on the process of coitus itself and less on its possible outcome. There is no law that says orgasm has to be the goal of every sexual encounter. Indeed, when it comes to making love, people do themselves a disservice if they strive for any specific goal at all. It is the shared experience of physical pleasure, not its "climax" or "successful" finale, that makes coitus worthwhile. Thus, for experienced lovers the artful build-up of tension is more important than its eventual release. Orgasm is simply something that happens involuntarily at the height of sexual stimulation; it is not a prize that has to be fought for and won.

In some older marital guides, couples were urged not only to strive for orgasm, but also to reach their orgasms simultaneously. As a reward, they were promised an experience of total ecstasy. In actual fact, however, this curious advice did more harm than good, and it is easy to understand why. First of all, it put the emphasis not on the sexual act, but on its result. Secondly, it forced both partners to adopt a cold and detached attitude that would allow them to remain in control at all times. Such an attitude then often prevented them from having any orgasm at all. Finally, those men and women who failed to synchronize their responses were made to feel inadequate.

It is fortunate that this mechanistic approach to coitus has gone out of fashion. In the meantime, most "sex experts" have become more realistic and therefore see simultaneous orgasms no longer as proof of a perfect relationship. As a matter of fact, there is now a growing realization that it is better to stop worrying about orgasms altogether. Instead, couples learn to savor every moment of intimacy for its own sake without trying to achieve or prove anything in particular. Paradoxically, it has turned out that it is this nondemanding, leisurely loveplay that provides the deepest satisfaction. It often helps to unblock long inhibited sexual responses and thus increases a person's erotic capacities. Naturally, it also leads to more orgasms. (For details, see "Sexual Inadequacy.")

In the past, most Christian Western cultures expected the faithful to have coitus in only one position: face-to-face, with the woman lying on her back and the man on top of her. (The less inhibited "heathens" of Africa, Asia, and the Pacific Islands used to ridicule it as the "missionary position.") However, with the increase of cross-cultural contact in the 19th century, Europeans and Americans realized that their approach to sex was unnecessarily rigid. They began to search ancient Greek vase paintings, Roman murals, Chinese scrolls, Japanese woodcuts, and Indian love manuals for new, exciting coital positions, and their discoveries soon led them to believe that they had found the long lost secrets of true sexual fulfillment.

However, while rigidity and routine in sexual matters are undoubtedly bad, there is no special magic in ever-varying athletic contortions. Nor is there such a thing as the ultimate, superior, or even natural or normal position for coitus. It is for this reason that the most recent Western marital guides no longer devote much space to the description of coital positions. After all, imaginative sexual partners who try to satisfy all of their needs and desires will vary their approaches spontaneously as the circumstances require, and thus they will continue to find new coital positions on their own. Detailed descriptions of such positions are unnecessary and may even be harmful because they tend to encourage a mechanistic view of coitus.

Indeed, it is perhaps unwise to list any distinct and clearly defined coital positions at all. Coitus always involves a series of movements which form a continuous whole, and most partners shift from one position to another without any advance planning or conscious effort. It seems pedantic to single out 10, 12, 20, or more particular postures and to ascribe to each of them some special meaning. One can, of course, differentiate between a few basic approaches to coitus, but their number is really quite limited: the partners may stand, sit, or lie down; they may face each other, or the woman may turn her back to the man; either partner can be on top, or they can both lie on their sides.

It used to be believed that certain coital approaches were especially effective because they made it possible for a man to stimulate a woman's clitoris with his penis. By the same token, certain other approaches were considered inferior because they allowed the penis to leave the clitoris completely unstimulated. Modern sex research has shown that both assumptions are false. As repeatedly mentioned in this book, with mounting sexual excitement the clitoris withdraws under its hood and thus becomes inaccessible to any direct stimulation. However, it is stimulated indirectly by the movements of this hood which are caused by the pushing and pulling of the attached minor lips as the penis moves back and forth inside the vagina. This indirect stimulation is almost always assured. It does not matter all that much from which direction or at what angle the penis is inserted.

However, there is one approach that many women find particularly satisfying, because it gives them almost complete control over the coital movements: straddling the man who lies passively on his back. This approach was also very popular among the ancient Greeks and Romans and was, in fact, considered "normal" by them. Today, it is often recommended by sex therapists because it seems to help both men and women to overcome sexual inadequacies. (For details, see "Sexual Inadequacy.")

There are also women who prefer to remain rather passive themselves, and who enjoy lying on their backs while carrying the weight of a man's body. For them, the "missionary position" (man on top of woman, facing her) may indeed be the most rewarding. Furthermore, if they flex their legs in this position they make it possible for the penis to penetrate very deeply into the vagina, thus increasing the chance of a pregnancy. (The ejaculated semen forms a so-called seminal pool close to the cervix, and a woman can favor a fertilization simply by remaining on her back for a while after coitus.) Furthermore, the deep penetration itself may be sexually rewarding for many women, and thus they may spontaneously shift to coital positions which make this possible.

Finally, it remains to be stated that people who are obese or weak usually find it most comfortable to have coitus while lying on their sides. Indeed, a rear entry approach in this position may be the least stressful of all. It naturally also recommends itself to women in the later stages of pregnancy.

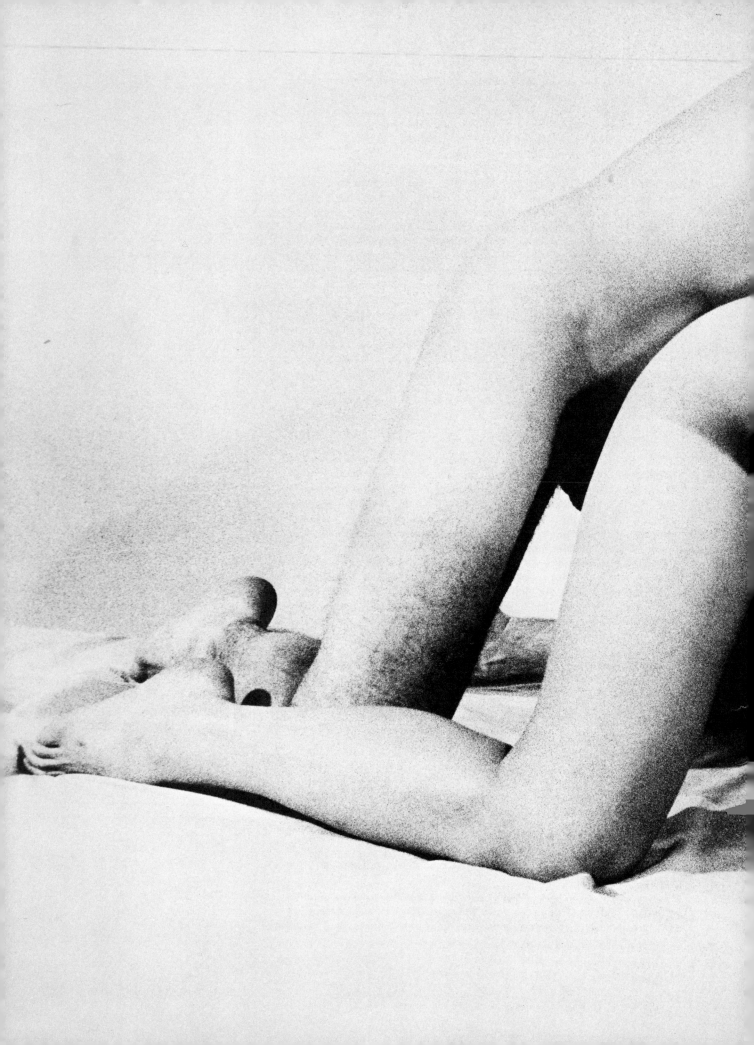

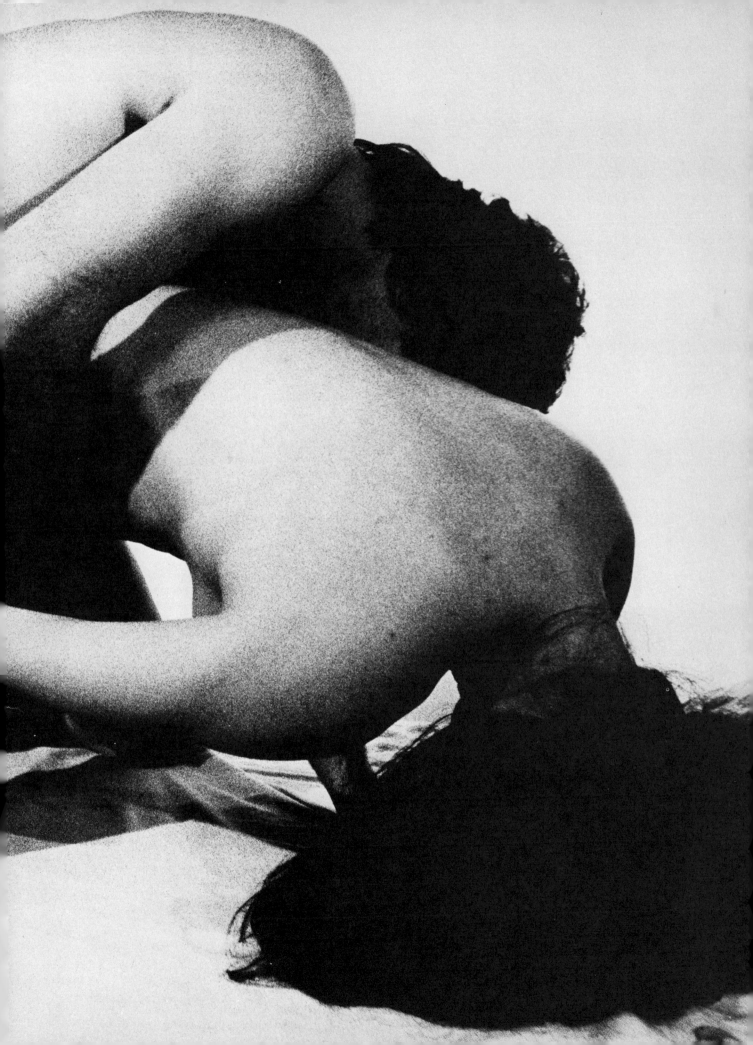

ANAL INTERCOURSE

Anal intercourse is here defined as involving sexual contact between the sex organs of one person and the anus of another.

In most individuals, the anus is highly sensitive to the touch and is, in fact, one of the most important erogenous zones. It is therefore hardly surprising that many people enjoy some form of anal stimulation during their sexual activity. For example, they may insert their fingers or some cylindrical object into their anus while they masturbate, or they may like some anal manipulation during oral and genital intercourse. Some men and women also like having the anus licked or kissed, and their partners may be quite happy to oblige. (In professional language, this practice is known as anilingus (from Latin anus: the rectal opening and linguere: to lick). However, it should be pointed out that without the most scrupulous cleanliness, this practice can, in some cases, lead to an infection with hepatitis.

Finally, it should be mentioned that some men enjoy placing their penis between a woman's buttocks and then moving it back and forth until they reach orgasm. Although in this case there is no penetration or insertion, the woman may nevertheless also experience some pleasure.

It is, of course, also possible for a man to insert his penis into a woman's anus, and there are women who find great pleasure in such anal intercourse. However, unlike the vagina, the anus does not provide its own natural lubrication, and therefore some saliva or artificial lubricant, such as KY or Vaseline, has to be used. The lubricant is best applied to the anus itself. This also offers the opportunity for a gentle massage of the anal sphincter or even the insertion of a finger. After this preparation, the penis can be inserted. The insertion itself should be very slow, and, once inside, the penis should not be moved for a while until the anal sphincter is completely relaxed. Then one or both partners can begin some cautious pelvic thrusting.

A woman who is not used to it may, at first, find the insertion of the penis into her anus unpleasant or even painful. However, after several gentle attempts, she may begin to enjoy it even if she does not reach orgasm herself. Her partner can, of course, masturbate her during anal intercourse, and if she does have one or several orgasms, the resulting contractions of her anal sphincter will provide a most pleasant additional stimulation for his penis. (See "The Female Sexual Response.")

Obviously, anal intercourse can be performed in many different positions. In most cases, however, the woman simply lies on her stomach while the man approaches her from behind, or she lies on her back with her knees raised to the sides of her chest while he approaches her face-to-face.

While anal intercourse cannot lead to pregnancy, and while it may be very satisfying to both partners, it is not as common as one might suppose. After all, for centuries it was denounced as sinful and perverse in our culture. Indeed, in many states of the United States today it is still defined as "sodomy" or a "crime against nature" which may carry a penalty of many years in prison. (For a discussion of American sex laws, see "Conformity and Deviance.") Furthermore, many people in our society are conditioned to consider the anus filthy and repulsive because of its excretory function. (To a lesser extent, the sex organs are also seen as disgusting because of their association with the release of urine.) However, as long as the organs of excretion are kept scrupulously clean, there is no valid reason for this attitude. Outside the United States the revulsion against anal intercourse is not always as great as it is here.

Anal intercourse can very well be a healthy experience if both partners want it and truly enjoy it. There is only one important health rule that must be observed: A couple should never switch from anal intercourse to coitus without a thorough washing of the penis in between. Otherwise, rectal bacteria may be carried into the vagina where they can cause infections. Such problems can be prevented by washing the penis with soap and water immediately after withdrawal from the rectum and before resuming any other form of sexual intercourse.

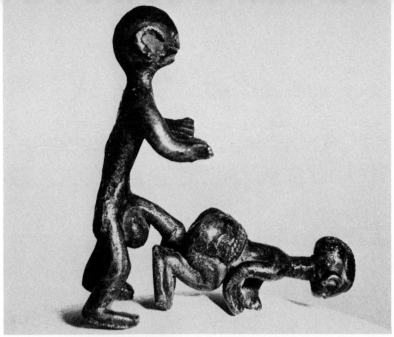

HETEROSEXUAL
INTERCOURSE IN ART
Throughout history, sculptors and painters all over the world have depicted human sexual activity. Sometimes these works of art had a religious purpose, sometimes they served as means of instruction, but quite often they were simply meant to please, arouse, or entertain the viewer. Today, the erotic art of different societies offers us excellent clues as to their sexual attitudes.

EROTIC ART IN AFRICA
The pictures show two bronze figures from the Ivory Coast which can be put together in various combinations, showing many forms of sexual intercourse.

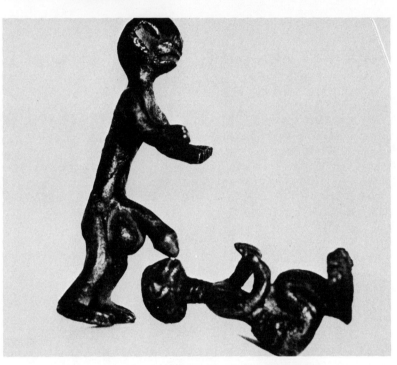

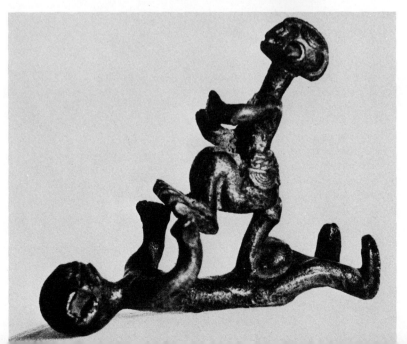

EROTIC ART IN ANCIENT GREECE
The ancient Greeks and Romans did not restrict themselves to a single position for coitus. However, they usually preferred a position with the female above the male. The three vase paintings on the right show some typical approaches.

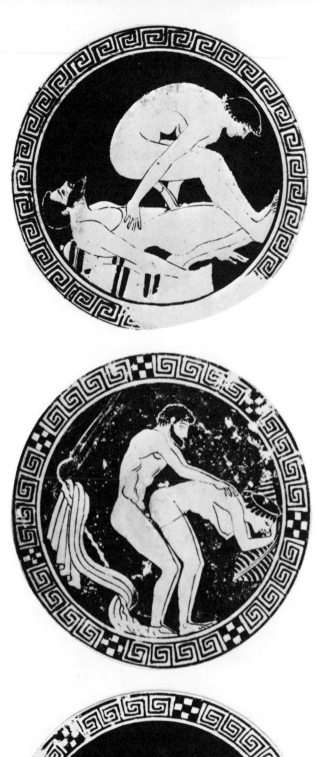

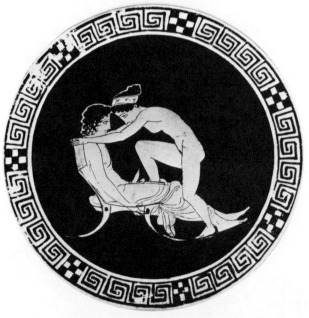

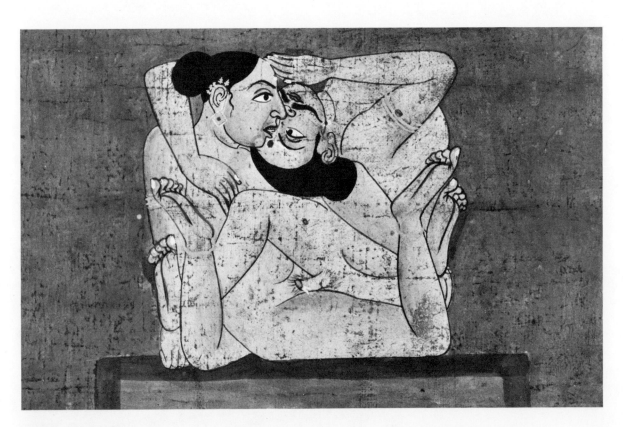

EROTIC ART IN INDIA

(Top) Many Indian artists painted series of elaborate coital positions. This 18th century painting shows a particularly involved position which is designed to affect the pattern of energies in the spinal column.

(Bottom) An 18th century painting showing a European man having sexual intercourse with an Indian woman in the "missionary position".

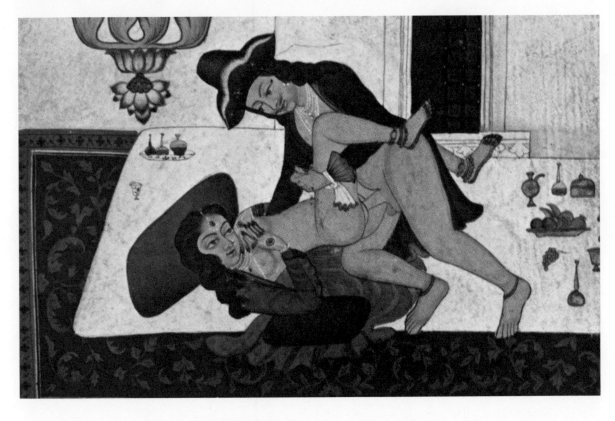

EROTIC ART IN CHINA

Chinese artists usually stressed the deliberate and gentle aspects of sexual intercourse and did little to emphasize the anatomical differences between men and women. Thus, Chinese erotic paintings often have a quiet and delicate character. The depiction of passion is relatively rare.

(Top) Scene from a painted album showing a man engaged in coitus with one woman while he is masturbating another with an artificial penis. (Late Ming dynasty)

(Bottom) An unusual picture of sexual vehemence from an album showing the sexual adventures of Mongol horsemen. (Late Ming dynasty)

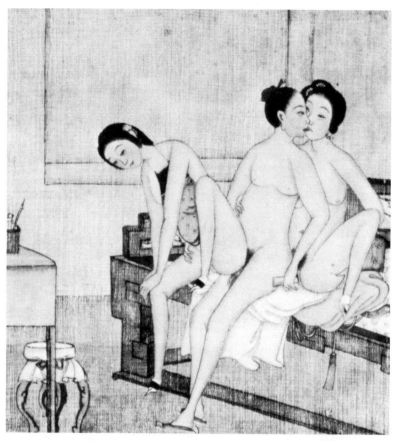

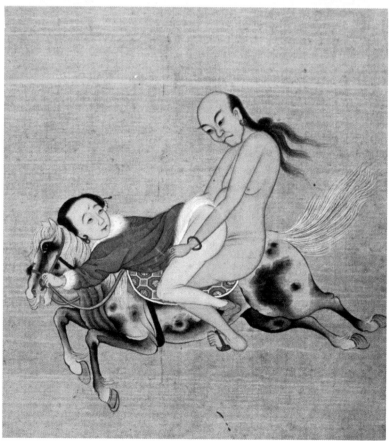

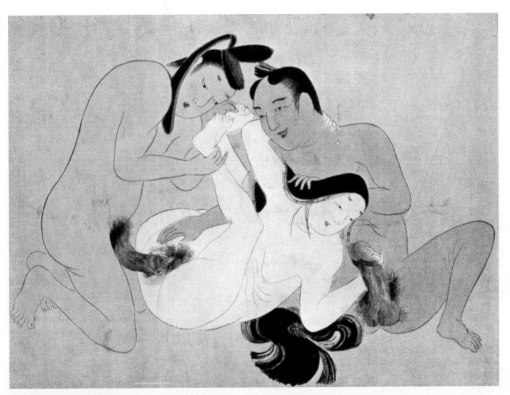

EROTIC ART IN JAPAN

In many traditional Japanese scrolls sexual intercourse is depicted as a passionate and even violent struggle. Japanese artists usually also over-emphasized the male sex organs, giving them a somewhat frightening appearance.

(Top) Scroll painting showing a woman having sexual intercourse with two men simultaneously.

(Bottom) Scroll painting showing a man with a resisting young prostitute-in-training who is being held down by an older woman.

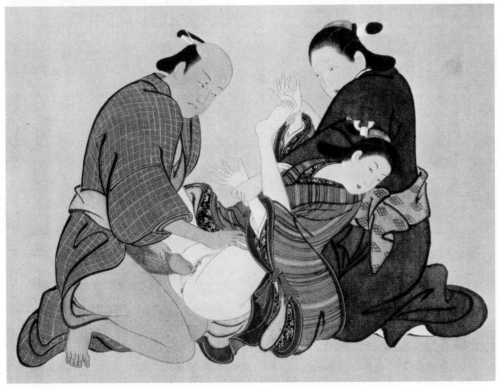

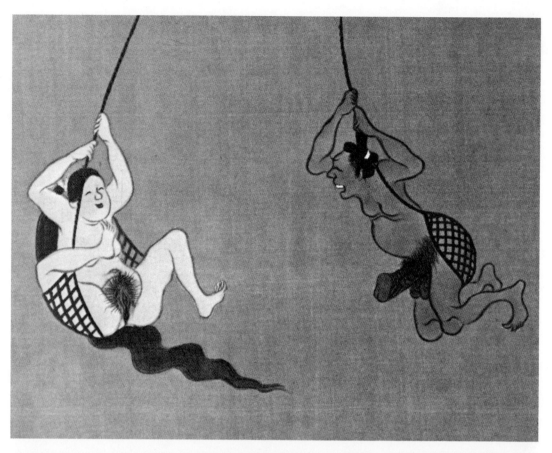

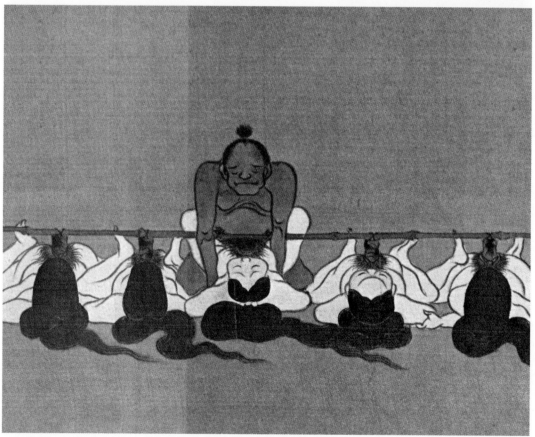

226 HUMAN SEXUAL BEHAVIOR

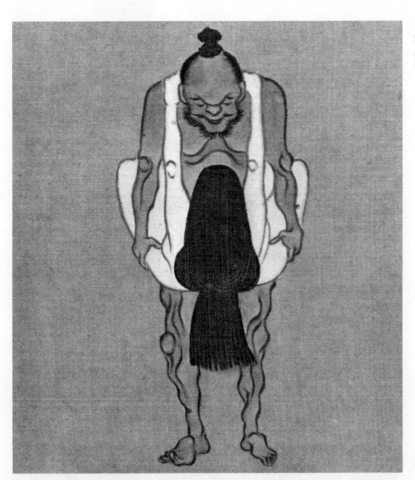

EROTIC ART IN JAPAN
Scenes from a humorous
painted silk scroll by
Katushika Hokusai (1760-1849)

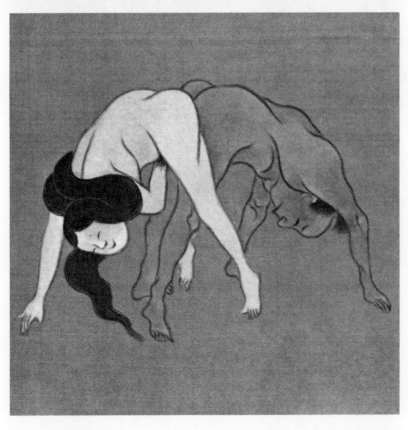

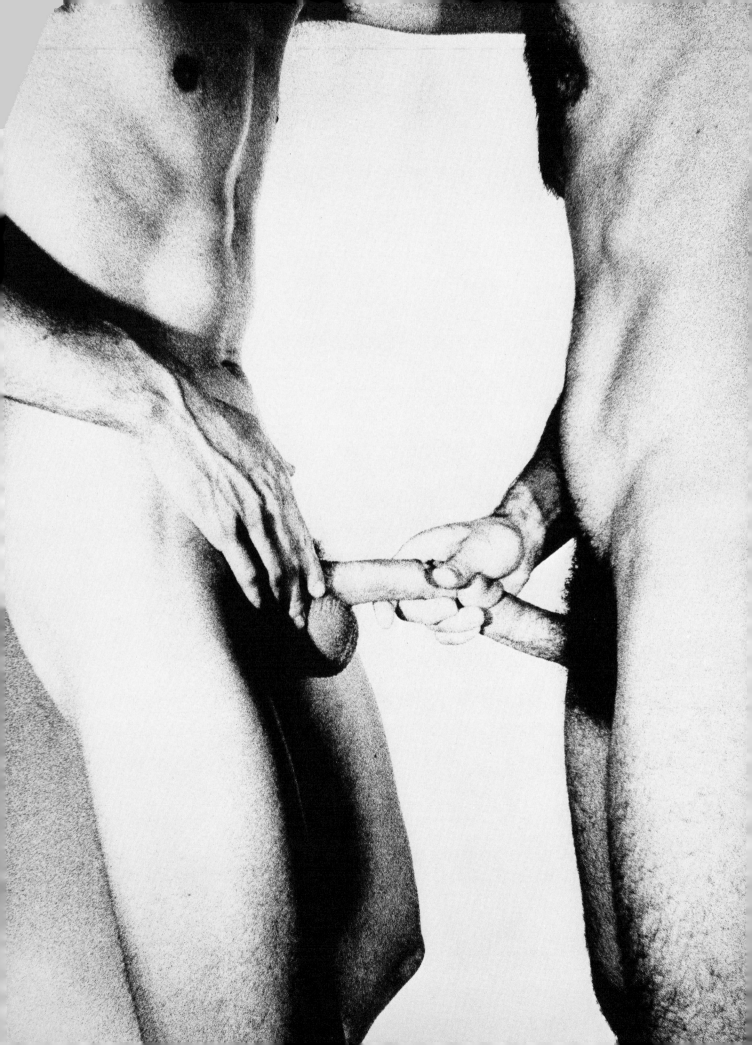

HOMOSEXUAL INTERCOURSE

Human beings, like all other mammals, may have sexual intercourse not only with partners of the other sex, but also with those of the same sex. In other words, males and females may engage in both heterosexual and homosexual intercourse. (The prefixes *hetero-* and *homo-* simply mean "different" and "same" in Greek.)

As mentioned earlier in this book, same-sex behavior is quite common in childhood and is not at all unusual in adolescence. (See "Infancy and Childhood" and "Adolescence.") Indeed, in the years before puberty people in our culture may have more sexual contact with members of their own than with those of the other sex. During this period, they are often actively discouraged from playing heterosexual games while their homosexual activity attracts little or no attention. It is only later that the situation reverses itself. Once they have reached their teens, boys and girls are expected to develop exclusively heterosexual interests, and any homosexual exploration is strongly condemned. Nevertheless, many individuals continue to have homosexual contact well into their old age. For some of them, these contacts represent nothing more than isolated incidents in an otherwise predominantly heterosexual life. For others, they become a frequent, if sporadic, experience, and for still others they are the preferred or even the only form of sexual expression.

In their two monumental studies on human sexual behavior, Alfred C. Kinsey and his associates used a very practical method of clarifying the matter. They devised a seven-point rating scale (with categories ranging from 0 to 6) which measured the balance of heterosexual and homosexual behavior in the population as a whole. At the one end of this scale (in category 0), they placed those whose experiences are exclusively heterosexual, and at the other end (in category 6) they placed those whose experiences are exclusively homosexual. Between these two extremes are those who have both heterosexual and homosexual experiences in various degrees (categories 1–5). Thus, the exact breakdown is as follows:

0. Exclusively heterosexual behavior.
1. Largely heterosexual, but incidental homosexual behavior.
2. Largely heterosexual, but more than incidental homosexual behavior.
3. Equal amount of heterosexual and homosexual behavior.
4. Largely homosexual, but more than incidental heterosexual behavior.
5. Largely homosexual, but incidental heterosexual behavior.
6. Exclusively homosexual behavior.

(See also chart on page 231.)

There is, of course, nothing new or revolutionary about these categories as such. It has always been known that there are people who engage only in heterosexual intercourse, and that there are others who engage only in homosexual intercourse. It was also well understood that some individuals have intercourse with members of both sexes. Thus, theoretically Kinsey's rating scale could very well have been developed hundreds or even thousands of years ago. In fact, long before Kinsey the basic idea must have occurred to many others. However, at least in our Judeo-Christian culture this idea never found any acceptance because of an unquestioned general assumption: It was simply assumed that the percentage of people with exclusively heterosexual histories was so great and the percentage of all others so small that any scale would have been hopelessly out of balance. In other words, before Kinsey undertook his vast statistical survey, homosexual acts were believed to be so rare as to represent nothing more than "unnatural" and freakish exceptions.

Kinsey showed that this traditional view was quite mistaken. For example, his statistics revealed that, by the time they reach middle age, about 50% of all males (and 20% of all females) have had some sort of overt erotic experience with members of their own sex. This accounts for every second man and every fifth woman in the country. Indeed, 37% of all males (and 13% of all females) have at least one homosexual experience to the point of orgasm between adolescence and old age. This applies to nearly two males out of every five and to more than one female out of every eight. Finally, according to Kinsey's findings, 4% of all males (and about 2% of all females) are exclusively homosexual in their behavior throughout their lives.

When these statistics were first published, they caused a great deal of public consternation. First of all, many people simply refused to accept the great number of reported homosexual acts. Indeed, even now various experts continue to challenge the figures as inflated and unrepresentative. Nevertheless, so far there has been no other research extensive enough to support these challenges. Kinsey's work may contain some errors and it may be dated, but it still provides the best information available. For all we know a new study undertaken today might very well show an even greater incidence of homosexual behavior, especially among females.

By far the greatest shock for the public, however, was the conclusion which Kinsey drew from his discoveries. Before Kinsey, it had been customary to think of "heterosexuals" and "homosexuals" as two distinct groups of people. Indeed, "homosexuals" were sometimes referred to as "contrasexuals," "sexual inverts," "psychosexual hermaphrodites," or even "the third sex." It was believed that they were afflicted with a special condition called "homosexuality," and that this condition clearly set them apart from the rest of mankind. (A person who had sexual intercourse with both men and women was regarded as a "homosexual" who somehow managed to "fake it.") Now all of these stereotypes simply collapsed in face of the evidence. The statistics proved that "heterosexuality" and "homosexuality" are not clear-cut, separate, and irreconcilable entities, but rather matters of degree. In Kinsey's own words, it is wrong to distinguish between "two discrete populations, heterosexual and homosexual. The world is not to be divided into sheep and goats. Not all things are black nor all things white. . . . Nature rarely deals with discrete categories. Only the human mind invents categories and tries to force facts into separated pigeon-holes. The living world is a continuum in each and every one of its aspects. The sooner we learn this concerning human sexual behavior the sooner we shall reach a sound understanding of the realities of sex."

Kinsey also spelled out the logical implications of his new approach: "It would encourage clearer thinking on these matters if persons were not characterized as heterosexual or homosexual, but as individuals who have had certain amounts of heterosexual experience and certain amounts of homosexual experience. Instead of using these terms as substantives which stand for persons, or even as adjectives to describe persons, they may better be used to describe the nature of the overt sexual relations, or of the stimuli to which an individual erotically responds."

The point is well taken, because much of the "homosexual problem" is indeed caused by the sloppy thinking and the confused language of those who talk about it. To give only one example, in the armed forces, in prison, and in mental hospitals, people may be labeled homosexual when they are discovered to have had a single homosexual experience. It never occurs to those who apply this label that, by the same logic, every person with a single heterosexual experience would have to be called heterosexual.

Unfortunately, this is not just a matter of semantics. There are real human lives involved. In many states of the United States, a man may go to prison, lose his job or professional license, and be officially registered as a "sexual psychopath" on the basis of one isolated and never repeated homosexual contact. Adolescents who are caught in an act of homosexual experimentation may be called "queer" by their friends and families and thus be pushed

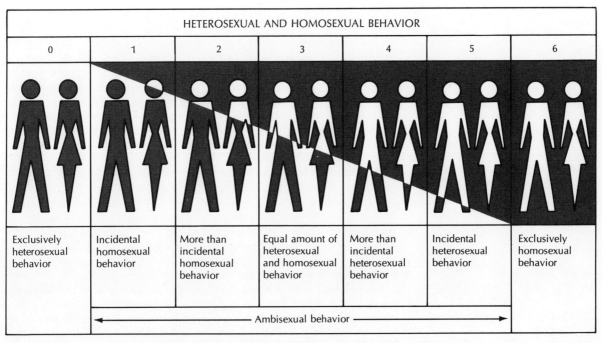

HETEROSEXUAL AND HOMOSEXUAL BEHAVIOR						
0	1	2	3	4	5	6
Exclusively heterosexual behavior	Incidental homosexual behavior	More than incidental homosexual behavior	Equal amount of heterosexual and homosexual behavior	More than incidental heterosexual behavior	Incidental heterosexual behavior	Exclusively homosexual behavior

◄——————————— Ambisexual behavior ———————————►

HETEROSEXUAL-HOMOSEXUAL RATINGS (AGES 20-35)						
0	1	2	3	4	5	6
Single M = 52-78% F = 61-72%						M = 3-16% F = 1-3%
					M = 5-22% F = 2-6%	
Married M = 90-92% F = 89-90%				M = 7-26% F = 3-8%		
			M = 9-32% F = 4-11%			
Previously Married F = 75-80%		M = 13-38% F = 6-14%				
	M = 18-42% F = 11-20%					

HETEROSEXUAL-HOMOSEXUAL RATING SCALE. Scale and figures adapted from Kinsey's data for males (M) and females (F) published in 1953. The ranges of percentages result from different ratios in various subgroups within the seven categories. These categories themselves are somewhat arbitrary, and the whole scale should therefore be read as a continuum. (Kinsey et al. *Sexual Behavior in the Human Female*, p. 488)

into the role of sexual and social misfits. As a result, they may be deprived of any chance to develop their heterosexual potential. A happily married "family man" who, in a moment of alcoholic sentimentality, is found in a compromising situation with another male may be branded as "one of those" by his community, and his marriage may break up.

Apart from being socially destructive, such labeling is also logically indefensible. As already pointed out, it is never applied in the reverse (i.e., a single heterosexual experience is never considered sufficient to qualify anyone as a "heterosexual"). Moreover, this biased usage defeats its own purpose by needlessly raising the number of "homosexuals" and thus revealing "homosexuality" as a very common "condition." (As mentioned above, about half of the male and one-fifth of the female population have at least some sort of overt erotic experience with members of their own sex.)

On the other hand, it does not help to restrict the term "homosexual" to those few individuals who respond exclusively to their own sex (category 6 on Kinsey's rating scale). In this case, logic would demand that the term "heterosexual" be applied only to those who respond exclusively to the other sex (category 0 on Kinsey's scale). This would make no allowance for the great number of people who respond to both sexes (categories 1–5 on Kinsey's scale).

Finally, we have to realize that even in one and the same individual the heterosexual-homosexual balance may shift over a period of time. There are men and women whose behavior is exclusively heterosexual at one time in their lives and exclusively homosexual at another time. Some engage in both types of behavior but with varying degrees of intensity. Others begin with an equal erotic interest in both sexes and only gradually develop a clear preference for one or the other. However, this preference may not always remain permanent. In short, a person's position on Kinsey's rating scale may change several times over the years.

Therefore, if it is wrong to divide the population as a whole into "heterosexuals" and "homosexuals," it is just as wrong to call any particular individual a "heterosexual" or a "homosexual." By the same token, it is impossible to determine how many people are "heterosexual" or "homosexual." It is only possible to determine how many people belong, at any given time, to each of the categories on a heterosexual-homosexual rating scale. Questions like "How many homosexuals are there?" or "Am I a homosexual?" do not have a scientifically meaningful answer.

Nevertheless, it remains a fact of life that our society does not approach the issue in a logical and systematic fashion. The old way of thinking is too deeply ingrained. In actual practice, people are still called heterosexuals or homosexuals, and, so far, few of them seem to object. Indeed, for the sake of communication many professionals also continue to use these terms, although each of them may define them a little differently.

Thus, if we do not want to cut ourselves off from the general discussion, we have to adopt some sort of compromise in the present book. After all, imprecise as it may be, the common usage also has its advantages. For instance, it often helps to simplify certain arguments and to articulate urgent social problems. In other words, as long as its arbitrary character is clearly understood, the traditional terminology can very well serve some useful purposes.

It is in this spirit that we now make the following suggestions:

- The term **heterosexual** may be used to describe someone who has a clear erotic preference for partners of the other sex (categories 0–2 on Kinsey's rating scale).
- The term **homosexual** may be used to describe someone who has a clear erotic preference for partners of the same sex (categories 4–6 on Kinsey's rating scale).
- The term **ambisexual** may be used to describe someone who is erotically attracted to partners of both sexes (categories 1–5 on Kinsey's rating scale).

It will be observed that the third of these definitions partly overlaps with each of the other two. That is to say, the classification "ambisexual" (from Latin *ambo:* both) includes some "heterosexuals" (those in categories 1 and 2) as well as some "homosexuals" (those in categories 4 and 5). This inconsistency is unavoidable unless one wants to call only those persons ambisexual whose erotic interest is evenly divided between the sexes (category 3). However, such a usage has never been widely accepted. We therefore have to live with the fact that certain persons may be referred to as "heterosexual" (or "homosexual") in one context, and as "ambisexual" in another.

Since we have linked our terms to Kinsey's rating scale, we also have to point out once again that this scale is not based on the amount of sexual activity, but on the balance between heterosexual and homosexual experiences. This means, for example, that individuals who have the same amount of homosexual experience may be assigned to different categories. Thus, a person who has had 10 homosexual experiences and only 5 heterosexual experiences will be considered a homosexual, while another person who also has had 10 homosexual experiences but 50 heterosexual experiences will be considered a heterosexual. (Depending on the context, both of them may, of course, also be called ambisexuals.)

Finally, it has to be understood that the term "experience" as used here refers not only to overt acts, but also to psychological responses that do not lead to any direct physical contact. In other words, a man whose overt sexual activity is entirely heterosexual may nevertheless be called a homosexual if psychologically he responds much more often to men than to women. For the same reason, the term "homosexual" may also be used for someone who does not engage in any overt sexual activity at all. (In older books these latter cases were sometimes described as examples of "latent homosexuality" [from Latin *latere:* to hide]. Unfortunately, this curious expression always covered much more than just unfulfilled or concealed desires. It was also meant to refer to subconscious, unrecognized, and unrealized homosexual tendencies. However, since such tendencies exist in virtually every human being, the term "latent homosexual" makes no more sense than terms like "latent smoker," "latent gourmet," or "latent insomniac.")

Naturally, all of these explanations and qualifications also have to be kept in mind when one talks about "homosexuality" as a sexual orientation. Indeed, the very fact that they are necessary only confirms what we have pointed out earlier in this book: The sexual orientation of men and women is best understood not in absolute but in relative terms, just as their biological sex and their gender roles. In short, we have already learned from the observation of human sexual development that maleness and femaleness, masculinity and femininity, heterosexuality and homosexuality are matters of degree. (For details, see the introduction to "The Development of Sexual Behavior.")

There is, however, one other important point that now has to be considered: In our particular culture, the word "homosexual" is never just a neutral technical term, and there is always more involved in its use than mere logic. No matter how cautiously it is applied, it evokes a certain image and triggers very definite social responses. In actual practice, people are called homosexuals not for some abstract statistical reason, but because they seem to fit a general concept of what homosexuals look like and how they behave. Most often this concept is quite unrealistic. For instance, there is a widespread belief today that homosexuality is caused by the adoption of an inappropriate gender role. It is simply assumed that male homosexuals tend to act like women and that female homosexuals try to imitate men. The false assumption then leads to the wrong conclusion: Parents who prevent their sons from becoming "sissies" and their daughters from becoming "tomboys" thereby prevent them from becoming homosexuals.

Curiously enough, historical and cross-cultural studies have shown that this particular notion arises only in certain societies and not in certain others. In some of the ancient Greek city states, for example, male homosexuality was associated not with weakness and effeminacy, but with virility, bravery, and heroism. As a matter of fact, the most famous of all Greek military elite troops, the "sacred band" of Thebes, which was finally defeated by Philip of Macedonia, is said to have consisted entirely of male lovers.

This example shows that the social stereotype of the "homosexual" may vary considerably from one time and place to another. It also demonstrates once again that there is no such thing as a "typical" homosexual, and that it makes no sense to speak of a "homosexual personality." The very fact that different cultures can develop different and even contradictory concepts of homosexuality indicates that it is not an objective condition with distinct, unchangeable, and unmistakable "symptoms." Homosexuals are not defined by any intrinsic qualities of their own, but by the image that people have of them.

This is also the reason why Kinsey had no choice but to treat the subject in a nonjudgmental, purely descriptive manner. He was forced to realize that a great number of people can and do engage in homosexual intercourse and that only a fraction of them are ever regarded as homosexuals. Kinsey understood that the decision as to who shall be so regarded can only be arbitrary and that it depends entirely on social conventions. Naturally, these conventions also determine whether homosexuality stands for weakness or strength, sin or righteousness, heresy or orthodoxy, mental illness or mental health. In short, homosexuality as such is neither a moral nor a legal nor a medical condition, but a conferred status. It is a social category or label that is applied to certain persons in certain situations. To be a homosexual means to play the role of the homosexual as it is understood in a particular society.

It is interesting to note that in some societies there is no role for "homosexuals," although there may be a great deal of homosexual behavior. Indeed, unless such behavior is singled out and classified as special, it may never become an issue for either the individual or society. For example, we know of various "primitive" societies, such as the Siwans in Africa, the Aranda in Australia, and the Keraki in New Guinea, where virtually all males engage in both heterosexual and homosexual intercourse. Obviously, in these societies one cannot distinguish between heterosexuals and homosexuals, not even as a matter of terminological compromise. Kinsey's rating scale could, of course, still be applied, but, at least for males, it would show only varying degrees of ambisexual behavior (categories 1–5). There simply would not be anything to record for the heterosexual and homosexual extremes of the scale (categories 0 and 6).

There is some reason to believe that even in our own Western civilization the lines have not always been drawn as sharply as they are today. In ancient Greece, for instance, homosexual behavior was widely accepted as a normal part of a man's sexual activity, and it was never considered an obstacle to marriage or fatherhood. The very word "homosexuality" was unknown. Instead, people spoke of *paiderastia* (literally, love of boys, from *pais*: boy, or rather here male adolescent, and *eran*: to love) which was cultivated as a socially beneficial and laudable custom. However, neither the older lover (called "the inspirer") nor the younger beloved (called "the listener") was ever assumed to be incapable of relationships with women. In short, the modern term "homosexual" would hardly do justice to the ancient Greeks. If a modern classification has to be used at all, "ambisexual" seems to be more accurate than any other.

Even in medieval Europe, where homosexual acts were condemned as sinful, they were not necessarily seen as manifestations of a "homosexual condition." When people were punished for "sodomy" (after the biblical city of Sodom) or "buggery" (after a heretical sect in Bulgaria), it was always assumed that they were very well capable of "proper" heterosexual behavior. We also have to remember that the punishment applied only to a few very specific acts, such as anal and oral intercourse. Other expressions of love and tenderness between men attracted no special attention.

It was only in the Modern Age that persons who engaged in same-sex behavior began to be viewed as fundamentally different from everyone else. By the same token, the average man and woman came to be seen as incapable of erotic responses toward members of their own sex. Such responses could result only from an inborn abnormal condition. Psychiatrists began to concern themselves with this alleged condition, and they referred to it by various exotic names until, toward the end of the 19th century, the new term "homosexuality" was invented. This term (as well as its antonym "heterosexuality") soon found wide acceptance and thus entered all European languages. (The word "homosexuality" was reluctantly introduced into English in 1897 by Havelock Ellis because it had become popular on the continent as *Homosexualität* [German] and *homosexualité* [French].)

A modern reader who knows nothing about the origin and the history of these words is likely to misunderstand the phenomena they are meant to describe. Today, we speak all too glibly of homosexuality and heterosexuality, and everyone seems to know immediately what we mean. However, we would do well to realize that, from the very beginning, these mutually exclusive categories oversimplified and prejudged the issue. Indeed, they could

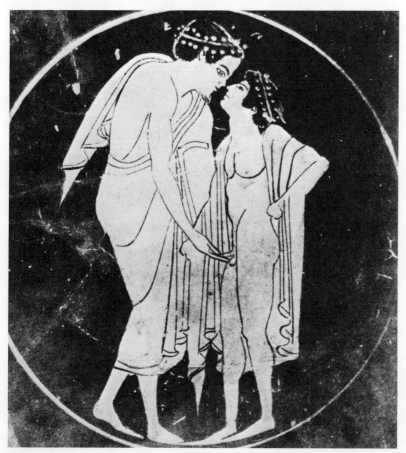

PEDERASTY
Many ancient Greek city states cultivated the custom of paiderastia *(pederasty) i.e. an educational love relationship between a man and a male adolescent. While such a relationship often involved sexual intercourse, it was never regarded as an obstacle to marriage and fatherhood. In the vase painting shown here we see a youth being caressed by his older lover.*

originate only in a repressive culture where the full range of human sexual capacities was no longer accepted. Any culture that draws an artificial dividing line between homosexuals and heterosexuals thereby betrays a highly peculiar and very narrow view of human nature. It is a view that has become blind to the gradual character of human differences, to the shades and nuances of human behavior, in short, to the natural variety of life.

In the absence of negative training, psychological pressure, and social sanctions, human beings are capable of sexual responses toward members of both sexes. People whose erotic interest is restricted to one sex can be produced only by cultural conditioning. As a matter of fact, one might say that men and women who are completely unaware of their homosexual leanings are just as much creatures of their education as those who are totally incapable of responding to heterosexual partners. Obviously, this does not mean that, in an ideal world, everybody would lead an ambisexual life. Strong sexual preferences and, indeed, a certain exclusivity of sexual interests are likely to develop in any case. Furthermore, as we have mentioned elsewhere, in most men and women these interests can be expected to become predominantly heterosexual. (See introduction to "Types of Sexual Activity.") There is no valid reason why this should be deplored. What must be deplored, however, is the fact that many people become oblivious to their own neglected capacities and then set themselves up as models or norms for their fellow human beings. Deplorable are the narrow-mindedness and intoler-

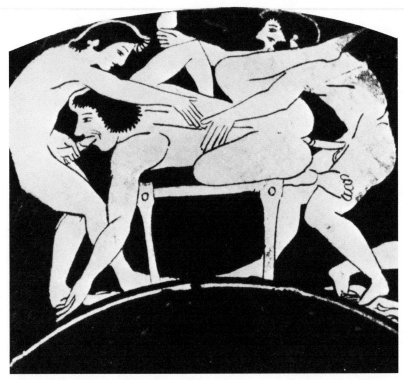

MALE HOMOSEXUALITY IN GREEK ART
The picture is part of a larger vase painting showing both heterosexual and homosexual intercourse. In this particular section we see three men engaged in oral and anal intercourse.

ance with which such "one-sided" individuals treat everyone else who is different.

Yet we know that in our own culture there are many exclusive "heterosexuals" and "homosexuals" who view each other with open hostility. The former are, as a rule, proud of their exclusive sexual orientation. They may even boast of it or, in some cases, insist on it with such desperate determination as to invite the ridicule of their opponents. These, the exclusive homosexuals, on the other hand, are usually expected to be downcast and apologetic. After all, as sinful, criminal, or sick "deviants," they are routinely treated as second-class citizens. It is hardly surprising, therefore, that, in the past, they have often had a low opinion of themselves. It is only recently that many of them have developed a positive self-image. Calling themselves "gay and proud," they now challenge the official value system and claim their long denied civil rights. This latter development is, of course, in many respects healthy and good. Still, necessary as it may be, it also has a disturbing side because it tends to accentuate the existing unfortunate division of people into two camps: "gay" and "straight." An increasingly militant "gay" (i.e., homosexual) world may eventually win concessions from the "straight" (i.e., heterosexual) world, and thus both worlds may arrive at a state of "peaceful coexistence," but, by the same token, they may also learn to forget that the divisions between them are, and have always been, artificial. In actual fact, both "gays" and "straights" are part of only one world, and without this realization they will continue to misunderstand themselves and each other.

In the past, it was mainly the socially dominant heterosexual population which created its homosexuals by so labeling certain persons who did not conform to its narrow sexual standards. Needless to say, this kind of labeling continues as before. However, under the influence of the homosexual civil rights movement, many men and women now also take the initiative and label themselves as "gay." They develop a "gay identity" and then "come out (of the straight closet)" into the open as confirmed "homosexuals." They do so because they are "tired of leading a double life" and because they feel

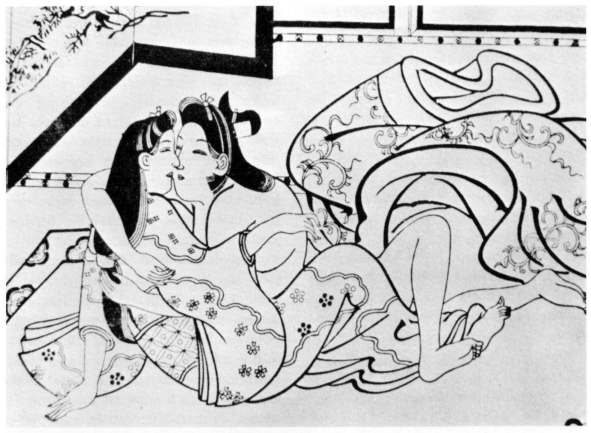

FEMALE HOMOSEXUALITY IN JAPANESE AND FRENCH ART
Many artists in many cultures have enjoyed depicting women in loving embrace. Shown here are a woodcut by Suzuki Moronoba (17th century) and a painting by Gustave Courbet (19th century).

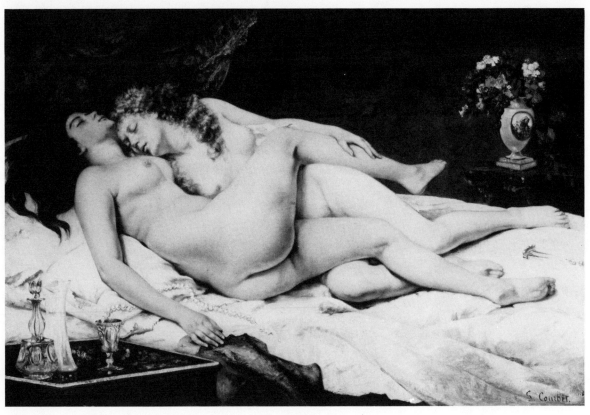

they must "clear the air." They also believe that they must "stand up and be counted" in the struggle for legal equality. In short, in our present social situation people experience a great deal of psychological pressure from both the "straight" and "gay" worlds to "choose sides" and to be "either one or the other."

Nevertheless, in the case of "homosexuals" such self-identification may come about very slowly. While someone who has been officially branded as homosexual (perhaps after the discovery of some minor homosexual episode) may have no choice but to accept the label quickly, the "hidden" individual with homosexual interests may take many years before he can see himself as "gay." At first, he may not attach much significance to his inclinations and may be reluctant to consider himself different from his "straight" friends. Indeed, as we have seen, this reluctance is well justified. It does not spring from his lack of insight, but rather from his natural revulsion against being pigeonholed or stereotyped. This revulsion may even turn into outrage if he is shown certain "typical" homosexuals with whom, as he knows, he has nothing in common. The process of "coming out" may therefore be rather complex and involved, with many psychological detours, dead ends, false starts, and reversals. Actually, as we have noted earlier, most people with homosexual inclinations never "come out" at all. Some simply renounce all sexual contact, some cultivate such modest heterosexual interests as they may have, others carry on both heterosexual and homosexual relationships, but define themselves as basically straight, and still others engage exclusively in homosexual intercourse while telling themselves that they do so only for nonsexual, "legitimate" reasons (such as earning some money as male prostitutes).

In present day America, many of those who end up defined as homosexuals (either by themselves or by others) adopt a "gay life-style," i.e., they become part of a gay subculture which offers them various ready-made role models, ideologies, tastes, fashions, and patterns of social interaction. This life-style, in turn, becomes synonymous with "homosexuality" for the society at large. However, in view of everything we have said before, it should have become clear by now that the issue cannot really be understood on these superficial terms. Instead, if we want to discover the truth about the "homosexuals" in our midst, we have to look at ourselves and our culture in its totality.

Finally, it remains to be stated that, at least in the United States, the aforementioned social, legal, and psychological problems are quite different for male and female homosexuals. It is for this reason that many female homosexuals in America prefer the name "lesbians" (after the island of Lesbos, home of the homosexual ancient Greek poetess Sappho). Words like "lesbian" and "lesbianism" are meant to show that homosexual females do not necessarily identify with every concern of homosexual males and that, in many respects, their situation is unique. This question (and the relative merits of a separate label) are discussed in more detail elsewhere (see "The Sexually Oppressed—Homosexuals").

The following pages briefly summarize the various forms of homosexual intercourse. The term "sexual intercourse" is, of course, used here in the same sense as in the preceding section. (For details, see the introduction to "Heterosexual Intercourse.") After all, as will soon become obvious, the sexual techniques of homosexuals and heterosexuals are essentially the same. People who ask, "But what do homosexuals *do*?" only reveal by that question that their own heterosexual relationships suffer from a lack of imagination. This kind of restrictedness demonstrates once again how people can become totally alienated from the erotic potential of their own bodies. It is another indication of the sexual barbarism that oppresses both "heterosexuals" and "homosexuals" in our society.

The social attitudes toward homosexual behavior are discussed more fully in the third part of this book, "Sex and Society." (See especially "Conformity and Deviance").

Manual intercourse is here defined as involving sexual contact between the sex organs of one person and the hand(s) of another.

Both male and female homosexual couples may enjoy manipulating each other's sex organs either as an end in itself or as a means of stimulation before they proceed to other forms of sexual intercourse. Obviously, the practice can be very rewarding because anybody who masturbates a partner of the same sex knows from personal experience how to provide the greatest amount of satisfaction. In any case, manual intercourse is probably the simplest and most common form of homosexual activity.

Males who engage in mutual masturbation usually find it practical to apply some saliva or artificial lubricant to their penises in order to increase their pleasure and to avoid hurting sensitive penile areas. The best known of these lubricants are Vaseline and KY jelly. If enough lubrication is provided, the partners can easily switch to genital intercourse. (For details, see below.) Indeed, many men like to take their own penis and that of their partner into one hand and then masturbate both penises together. Naturally, if they feel like it, the partners can alternate several times trying this technique before they reach orgasm. However, there are also many males who simply enjoy being masturbated without reciprocating themselves.

Manual intercourse between females is rather similar to that between males. Of course, it should be remembered that women normally love to be touched and caressed all over their bodies, and that they are not necessarily as eager as men to proceed to the manipulation of their sex organs. Still, when they do masturbate each other they can very well reach orgasm. Women know best what gives women pleasure, and thus they have little difficulty satisfying their female partners. Furthermore, since sexual excitement in women produces natural vaginal lubrication, no artificial lubricants are needed. Contrary to what many men imagine, women usually do not insert anything into their vaginas when they masturbate, but simply touch and stroke the external sex organs such as the shaft (not the glans) of the clitoris, the minor lips, and the vaginal opening. They may also stimulate these areas very effectively with an electric vibrator. Two women can, of course, use two of these vibrators on each other or take turns using only one. (For details on electric vibrators, see "Sexual Self-stimulation" and "Sexual Inadequacy in Women—Absence of Orgasm.")

Oral intercourse is here defined as involving sexual contact between the sex organs of one person and the mouth of another.

The sex organs and the mouth are the two most easily stimulated erogenous zones of the body, and it is therefore only natural that they should sometimes be brought into direct contact. Indeed, such behavior is quite common in nearly all mammals, and, from a biological standpoint, there is no reason why human beings as the most highly developed and most sensitive mammals should be an exception. However, in some human societies and historical periods oral intercourse was considered sinful, criminal, or sick, and people who engaged in it were severely punished. As a matter of fact, in many states of the United States today oral intercourse is still defined as a "crime against nature" which may carry a penalty of many years in prison. (For a discussion of American sex laws, see "Conformity and Deviance—Legal–Illegal.")

Still, in spite of its traditional religious, legal, and psychiatric condemnation in our culture, oral intercourse is widely practiced by both heterosexual and homosexual couples. The techniques employed are, of course, also the same in both cases.

Fellatio

The term "fellatio" (from Latin *fellare:* to suck) is used to describe the licking or sucking of the male sex organs.

Obviously, when two males have sexual intercourse, they may very well

MANUAL INTERCOURSE

ORAL INTERCOURSE

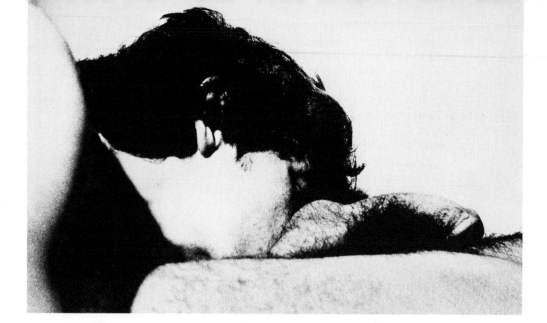
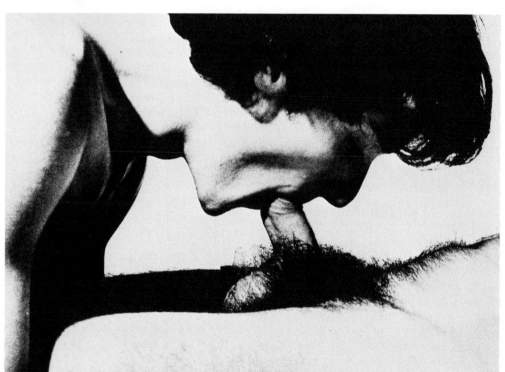
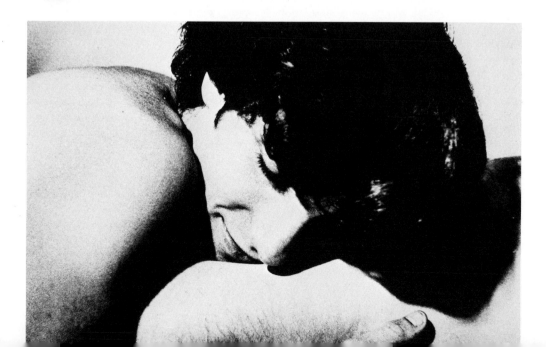

fellate each other. In some cases, a man may prefer having his own penis sucked to sucking that of his partner. In other cases, the preference is reversed. Most men who engage in homosexual oral intercourse, however, have no clear preference either way, but simply change their approach according to the circumstances. Naturally, two men can also engage in simultaneous mutual oral intercourse. (See "69" below.) Men may engage in fellatio as a means of stimulation before they proceed to other forms of sexual intercourse, or they may enjoy it for its own sake and continue it through orgasm. Indeed, not only women, but also many men learn to love the taste of warm semen in their mouths. (Semen is a clean, harmless substance which can be swallowed without any ill effects. The only exception is the contaminated semen of a man who is suffering from a venereal disease.)

In the past, certain people tried to distinguish between "active" and "passive" partners in fellatio. According to this curious distinction, the "active" fellator was playing a female role, while the "passive" man who was being fellated remained true to his role as a male. This line of reasoning (which, by the way, completely reversed the usual stereotype of the active male and passive female) then led to the bizarre claim that only the "active" partner was a true homosexual, while the "passive" partner somehow preserved his heterosexuality. (In another version of the same argument, a receptor [i.e., in this case the man receiving the penis in his mouth] is, by definition, always playing a female role, while the role of an inserter [i.e., the man inserting his penis] is always male. Without any further explanation, the "female role" is then again defined as homosexual, the "male role" as heterosexual.)

Not surprisingly, many guilt-ridden ambisexual men and male prostitutes used this kind of contorted logic to rationalize their homosexual behavior. They always insisted on the "passive" role, avoided any bodily movement of their own, and tried to appear as cold and aloof as possible. They then claimed that they were not really doing anything "queer." Of course, they fooled nobody but themselves. The fact of the matter is that activity and passivity have nothing to do with either biological sex or sexual orientation. Moreover, anybody who can be brought to orgasm by a man is sexually fully responsive to him, and no amount of sophistry can explain this simple fact away.

Cunnilingus

The term "cunnilingus" (from Latin *cunnus:* vulva and *linguere:* to lick) is used to describe the licking and sucking of the female sex organs.

Many women enjoy having their sex organs licked, and, if they have sexual intercourse with another woman, they may very well like to return the favor. Naturally, women can also engage in simultaneous mutual oral intercourse. (See "69" below.)

Women may try cunnilingus just as a means of stimulation before they proceed to other forms of sexual intercourse, or they may practice it for its own sake and continue it through orgasm. Since a woman knows from experience what gives her the greatest pleasure, she usually has little difficulty providing the most effective oral stimulation for her female partner. Thus, cunnilingus between two females can be completely satisfying to both of them.

"69"

The slang term "sixty-nine" (or French *soixante-neuf*) is used to describe a form of oral intercourse in which the sexual partners simultaneously lick each other's sex organs. In doing so, the position of their bodies in relation to each other is similar to that of the inverted numerals in the number 69.

Obviously, both male and female homosexual couples can engage in this practice, and it can be equally satisfying to men and women. Simultaneous mutual oral intercourse can be used just as a means of stimulation, but it can also be continued through orgasm, particularly if the partners take their time and assume a comfortable position lying on their sides.

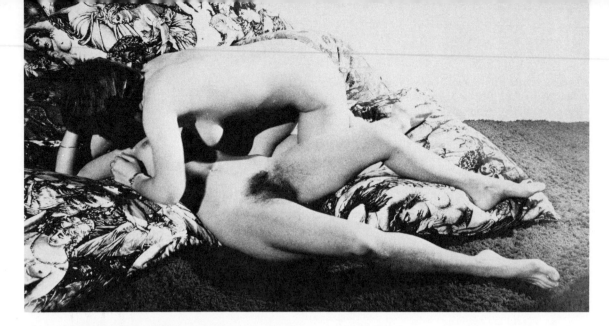

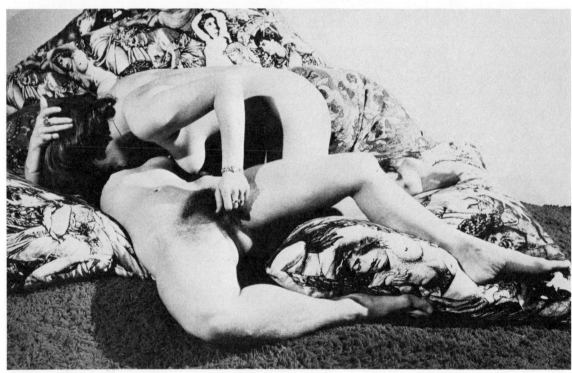

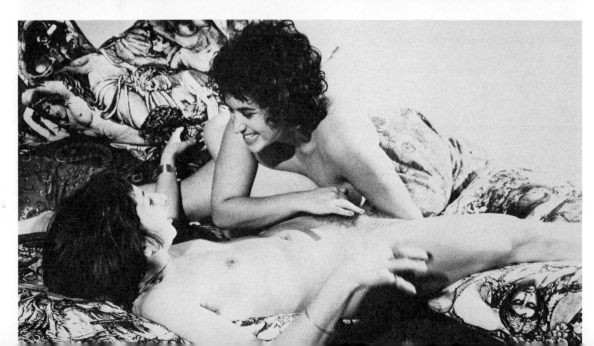

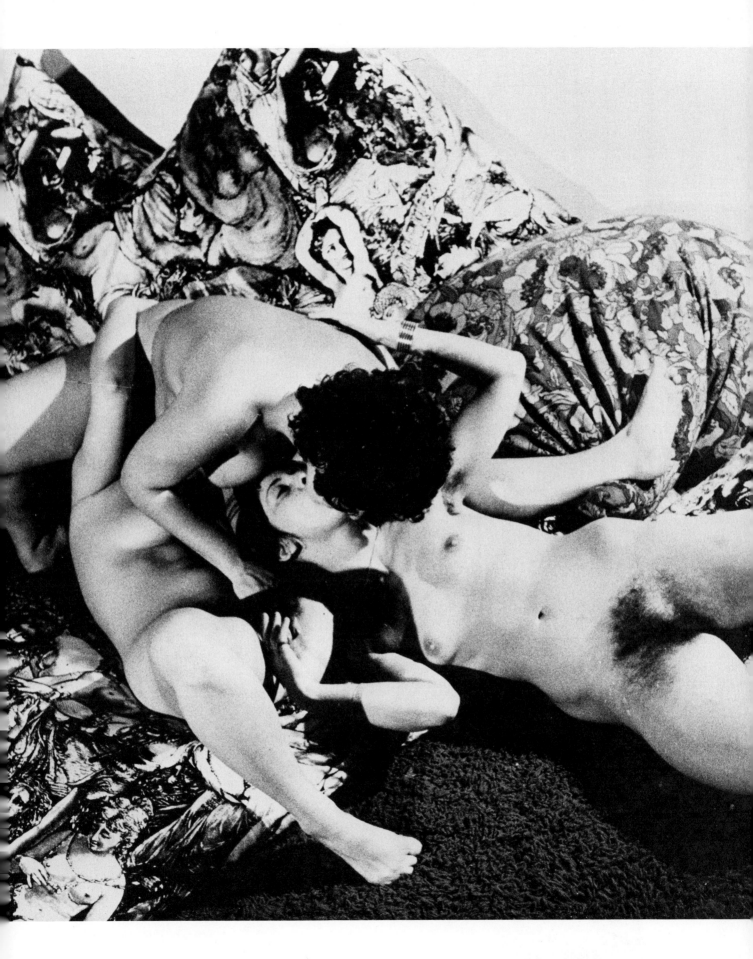

GENITAL INTERCOURSE

Genital intercourse is here defined as involving sexual contact between the sex organs of two persons.

According to Freud and his followers, the goal of a person's sexual development is "genital maturity," and genital intercourse is therefore the one truly "mature" form of sexual expression. However, this claim is made only for heterosexual couples. Homosexuals are said to have deviated so far from the norm in any case that it makes little difference how they satisfy each other. Indeed, whether one accepts the psychoanalytic view or not, it seems absurd to restrict male or female homosexual couples to genital intercourse. After all, since two men or two women cannot procreate, contact between their sex organs cannot serve any ulterior biological purpose, and they may very well find much more pleasure in other forms of lovemaking. Still, homosexual men and women do sometimes engage in genital intercourse, and they can find complete sexual satisfaction this way. This is easily understandable because both the male and the female sex organs are highly sensitive to tactile stimulation. Obviously, for anatomical reasons, genital intercourse between partners of the same sex is somewhat different from that between a man and a woman. However, this difference is less pronounced than some people might be willing to admit at first glance.

Apposition of Sex Organs

Both male and female homosexual couples may embrace very closely and thus bring their sex organs into direct contact. Rhythmic pelvic movements can then provide very effective mutual stimulation.

Males who bring their penises together in this fashion often find it practical to use a lubricant in order to enhance their pleasure and to prevent the chafing and chapping of sensitive penile areas. Vaseline, KY, and simple saliva are the most popular of these lubricants. (Without some protective lubrication, the glans of the penis may soon begin to hurt as it rubs against the partner's pubic hair.) Many males also enjoy taking both penises into one hand and then masturbating to orgasm. This practice can, of course, also be described as manual intercourse.

For two females, the apposition of their sex organs may also be very satisfying, and may, in fact, allow both of them to reach orgasm. As pointed out earlier, even during heterosexual coitus the main areas of female sexual stimulation are the clitoris, the minor lips, and the entrance of the vagina. These same areas can be effectively stimulated by rubbing them against the body of another female. Still, there are some women who find a particular satisfaction in deep vaginal penetration. Such women may very well engage in homosexual intercourse, but they may also find its physical pleasures somewhat inferior to coitus.

Simulated Coitus

It is possible for two females to simulate coitus if one of them straps an artificial penis to her body. Indeed, many males enjoy contemplating such female activity, and the necessary special artificial penises are available by mail order or in some "sex stores." However, in actual fact, only very few women ever make the attempt. If they do, it may be less a matter of pleasing themselves than of entertaining some male spectator. As already mentioned, when women begin sexual intercourse, they usually first like to be caressed in a rather general way. Then, once they have reached a certain level of excitement, they enjoy, above all, the uninterrupted stimulation of the external sex organs. (Also see "Sexual Self-stimulation" and "Heterosexual Intercourse.")

ANAL INTERCOURSE

Anal intercourse is here defined as involving sexual contact between the sex organs of one person and the anus of another.

Since the anus is one of the more sensitive erogenous zones of the body, many men and women enjoy some form of anal stimulation during their sexual activity. (Also see "Heterosexual Intercourse.") As a matter of fact, some individuals insert a finger or some cylindrical object into their anus when they masturbate in order to heighten their pleasure. It is therefore hardly surprising that, during sexual intercourse between males, the anus of one partner and the penis of the other should sometimes be brought into direct contact.

It is very well possible for a man to insert his penis into his partner's anus. However, since the anus, unlike the vagina, does not provide its own natural lubrication, some artificial lubricant has to be used. Vaseline and KY jelly (sometimes also simple saliva) are the most popular of these lubricants, and they are best applied gently and deliberately to the anus itself. This offers the opportunity for a relaxing massage of the anal sphincter, or even for the insertion of a finger. After this preparation, the penis must be inserted very slowly and, once inside, it should remain motionless for a while until the sphincter is completely relaxed. Then one or both of the partners can begin pelvic thrusting. Many men enjoy being masturbated by their partner while they have his penis in their rectum. He, in turn, may be glad to oblige because he knows that the anal sphincter will contract during orgasm and thus provide additional stimulation for his penis. (Also see "The Male Sexual Response.")

Anal intercourse can, of course, be practiced in many different positions. Most often, however, one of the partners lies on his stomach while he is approached from behind, or he lies on his back with his knees raised to the sides of his chest while he is approached face-to-face. There are also some men who avoid the insertion of the penis into their partner's anus, but instead enjoy rubbing it between his buttocks until they reach orgasm.

While anal intercourse can be highly satisfying for both partners, it is not nearly as common as is often believed. After all, most people in our culture are conditioned to consider the anus filthy and repulsive because of its excretory function. (To a lesser extent, the sex organs are also seen as disgusting because of their association with the release of urine.) In addition, there are strong religious, social, and legal taboos against contact between anus and penis. Indeed, in many states of the United States today anal intercourse is still defined as a "crime against nature" which may carry a penalty of many years in prison. (For a detailed discussion of American sex laws, see "Conformity and Deviance—Legal-Illegal.")

Under the circumstances, it is hardly surprising that some homosexual men object to anal stimulation just as vehemently as many heterosexuals do. Others object only to becoming the "passive" partner in anal intercourse (the one receiving the penis), but have no scruples about being the "active" partner (the one inserting the penis). The curious distinction between "active" and "passive" partners in anal intercourse is quite similar to that already discussed under "Oral Intercourse." There is only one difference: In the case of anal intercourse, it is the "passive" partner who is seen as playing a female role, while the "active" partner is said to play that of the male. Nevertheless, the argument here also implies that only the former is a "true" homosexual, while the latter somehow preserves his heterosexuality.

This kind of nonsense seems particularly appealing to guilt-ridden and insecure ambisexual men who try to justify their homosexual acts. For instance, in prison such men may regularly rape other male inmates while telling themselves that they are not really doing anything "queer." Naturally, they are not fooling their victims. However, the fact that some men would even feel the need for such self-delusions reflects the all-pervading and continuing sexism of our society.

The truth of the matter is that activity and passivity have nothing to do with either biological sex or sexual orientation. Thus, most homosexuals who enjoy anal intercourse switch freely back and forth between the inserter and receptor roles without ever suffering any confusion about their sexual identities.

In this context, it should perhaps also be mentioned that some men enjoy having their partners insert long and hard objects or even the whole hand into their rectum (''fistfucking''). One can only assume that these men are unaware of the dangers of this practice. First of all, there is a great likelihood of infection through scratches and dirt accumulated under the fingernails. Furthermore, while the anal sphincter muscle can adjust to a slowly inserted normal penis without being torn or losing its elasticity, it is likely to be overstretched by a fist or other object of comparable size. In other words, while anal intercourse as such poses no problem, ''fistfucking'' can lead to serious injuries, particularly if it becomes a habit. There have been cases where the anus became completely dysfunctional and had to be sewn up by a surgeon who then had to create an artificial opening in the abdominal wall for the elimination of waste.

Finally, it remains to be stated that, for anatomical reasons, there can be no anal intercourse between females. The only exception would be a female who wears an artificial penis strapped to her body. However, this possibility is more theoretical than real, since virtually all homosexual women are content with other forms of sexual stimulation.

SEXUAL CONTACT WITH ANIMALS

The myths and folk tales of many cultures contain references to sexual intercourse between human beings and other species of animals, such as bears, wolves, horses, snakes, and crocodiles. Very often these animals are objects of sudden human passions, but ancient Greek and Roman writers also tell of some cases in which an animal takes the initiative. For example, in a famous story by Aelian, a dolphin falls in love with a beautiful boy and, after an intense courtship, makes him his lover. The Greeks also believed that Zeus, their highest God, occasionally assumed the form of an animal in order to win the sexual favors of an otherwise inaccessible human female. Thus, he approached Europa as a bull and Leda as a swan. Greek mythology further tells us that Pasiphaë, the queen of Crete, had intercourse with a bull and then gave birth to the Minotaur, a human monster with a bull's head. Similar tales were told by various ''primitive'' peoples in Asia, Africa, and the Americas. For instance, a certain Eskimo tribe believed that the white human race resulted from sexual intercourse between a woman and a dog.

To this day, human sexual contact with animals has also held great interest for painters and sculptors. In fact, some of the greatest masterpieces in the history of art are devoted to this subject. It is interesting to note, however, that in the overwhelming number of cases the artists have chosen to depict the human participant in the act as a woman. Artistic representations of men having sexual contact with female animals are quite rare. The same is true for live stage shows that can be seen in some countries. They usually present women having sexual intercourse with dogs, pigs, or even donkeys or horses. Comparable public displays with men are practically unknown. It seems that such shows (as well as the paintings and sculptures) are created largely to satisfy certain male fantasies, and not to answer any genuine female needs.

In our Judeo-Christian culture, even the criminal law has often concerned itself with sexual activity between humans and animals. As we can read in the Bible, the ancient Hebrews expressly prohibited such activity under the penalty of death (Leviticus 20). The Talmud did not even allow a widow to keep a pet dog for fear that she might use it for sexual purposes (Abodah Zarah 22b; Baba Metziah 71a). These negative Jewish attitudes were later adopted by the Christian churches which, in turn, influenced the secular law

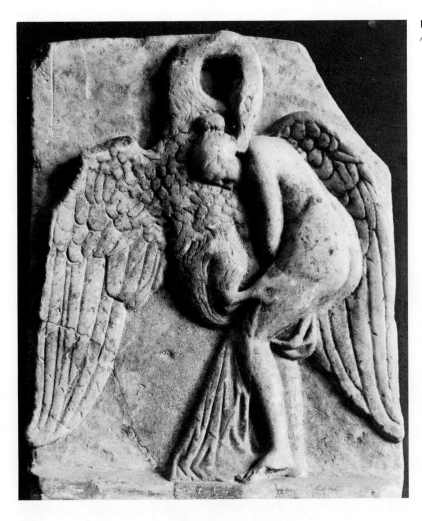

LEDA AND THE SWAN
Ancient Greek sculpture

in most Western countries. Indeed, in a deeply ironic turn of history, these laws were eventually used against the Jews themselves. Some medieval theologians declared that a Christian's sexual contact with a Jew or Moslem was the moral equivalent of "unnatural" intercourse with an animal "inasmuch as such persons in the eyes of the law and our holy faith differ in no wise from beasts." The crime was considered very serious. Throughout the Middle Ages, and even well into modern times, men and women were buried alive, burned at the stake, or hanged for having had sexual contact with animals. In some cases, the animals were executed along with them.

Today, very few people would still approve of such drastic punishment. In fact, recent decades have seen the complete abolition of laws against sexual contact with animals in several European countries and some states of the United States. Nevertheless, most states still have such laws, and the prescribed penalties may be very severe. (In some states, the possible maximum sentence is life imprisonment.)

For a long time, these religious and legal traditions were also reflected in Western medical thinking. Thus, behavior that appeared sinful and criminal to clergymen and legislators was readily denounced as sick by psychiatrists. Innumerable psychiatric texts devoted considerable space to sexual intercourse with animals, which was labeled as a symptom of a "disorder," "aberration," "abnormality," or "perversion." What the church and the state had called "sodomy" and a "crime against nature," psychiatry hastened to condemn as "zoophilia" or "bestiality." People who engaged in such behavior were to be considered mentally ill. (See also "Conformity and Deviance.")

TWO MEN COPULATING WITH ANIMALS
Detail from an Indian painting (19th century)

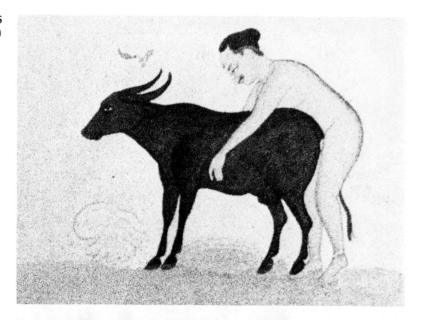

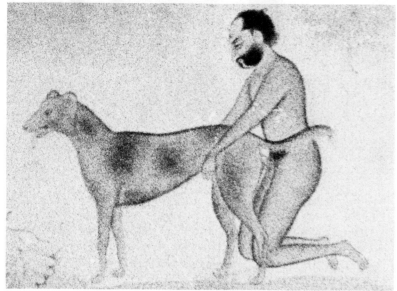

Today, after exhaustive studies of the statistical frequency of human sexual contact with animals, it seems rather odd that eminent religious, legal, and psychiatric authorities should ever have bothered to pay any attention to it. We now know that this type of sexual activity is actually very uncommon. It is quite rare among men, and even rarer among women. In short, it is of no real social significance. We therefore have to assume that its strong social condemnation originally served only certain symbolic religious purposes.

In modern Western countries, human sexual contact with animals occurs, if at all, mostly in rural areas. For instance, boys who grow up on farms may observe the mating of cattle and thus become tempted to engage in some sexual experimentation of their own. They may attempt coitus with calves, ponies, sheep, pigs, dogs, and even ducks or chickens. Usually these attempts are not repeated more than a few times, although in some exceptional cases a boy may, for a while, establish a regular sexual relationship with a particular animal. Coitus is, of course, not the only possible form of sexual contact. Some boys simply masturbate the animal (as farmers may do in order to obtain semen for artificial inseminations), or they let the animal lick their penis or their anus. Corresponding techniques are also used by girls or women, although, as already mentioned, for females sexual contact with animals is even rarer than for males.

If sexual intercourse between humans and animals is relatively rare, it is not so very unusual between animals of different species. In some cases (horse and donkey, or lion and tiger), such interspecific mating may even produce offspring (mules, "ligers"). The human animal has, of course, no really close relative among the other mammals, and this may be reason enough to limit sexual contact with them. Obviously, such contact can also never lead to either a human or an animal pregnancy.

It is likely that, in the future, the legal and medical authorities in our society will be much less preoccupied with sexual contact between humans and animals. After all, as long as the animal is not hurt or mistreated, there is no need for social interference. It is also unreasonable to attach psychiatric labels to isolated attempts at such contact. Only men and women who always prefer animals to human partners can really be considered sexually maladjusted. In this case, as in all other cases of exclusive or compulsive sexual behavior, professional help may very well be recommended. (Also see "Sexual Maladjustment—Compulsive and Destructive Behavior.")

Reference and Recommended Reading

Churchill, Wainwright. *Homosexual Behavior Among Males: A Cross Cultural and Cross Species Investigation*. Englewood Cliffs, N.J.: Prentice-Hall, 1971.

Comfort, Alex, ed. *The Joy of Sex*. New York: Crown, 1972 (cloth); New York: Simon & Schuster, 1974 (paper).

———*More Joy*. New York: Crown, 1974 (cloth); New York: Simon & Schuster, 1975 (paper).

Ford, Clellan S., and Beach, Frank A. *Patterns of Sexual Behavior*. New York: Harper & Row, 1951 (cloth); 1970 (paper).

Kinsey, Alfred C., *et al. Sexual Behavior in the Human Female*. Philadelphia: Saunders, 1953 (cloth); New York: Pocket Books, 1965 (paper).

Tripp, C.A. *The Homosexual Matrix*. New York: McGraw-Hill, 1975 (cloth); New York: New American Library, 1976 (paper).

8. SEXUAL MALADJUSTMENT

In our society, the word "maladjustment" is easily misused. All sorts of individualistic, energetic, enterprising, curious, critical, and creative people are called maladjusted by conformist dullards who are afraid of any sign of spontaneity. In fact, very often the so-called well-adjusted person who passively accepts oppressive living conditions is the one with the problem. In some situations, maladjustment is the only proper response.

This is especially true in regard to sexual oppression. People who have no difficulty renouncing their sexual interests, who readily adapt to narrow sexual roles, and who never question the official sexual morality hardly seem human and (if indeed they exist) may very well be unfeeling, dangerous characters. Actually, and perhaps fortunately, in real life this kind of total adjustment is rare. After all, not even the most righteous New England Puritans were always free of temptation. No matter how hard they tried to conform to their rigid culture, they never succeeded for long. Thus, by their own unrealistic standards, they were sexually maladjusted, but actually they had little reason to feel guilty.

Our own present culture still contains many puritanical elements, although to the superficial observer it may seem that we have freed ourselves from most of the traditional fetters. However, our moral values, criminal laws, and medical standards still reflect an arbitrary and very restrictive sexual ideal. Thus, now as before, a certain amount of maladjustment is unavoidable. In other words, under the present circumstances only very few people can claim to be perfectly happy in their sexual lives.

On the other hand, it remains an open question whether complete sexual liberation is even possible. To some extent, sexual misery may simply be part of the human condition. Or perhaps it is a price we have to pay for being civilized creatures. At any rate, it seems childish and insolent to insist at all times on total gratification. A mature person can live with some disappointment and does not always expect to be in harmony with his surroundings. Where he sees room for improvement, he readily works for it, but he also learns to accept what he cannot change.

Therefore, given the general imperfection of the world, and taking into account the inevitable frustrations of our particular civilization, we should not become disturbed by every instance of sexual maladjustment. After all, very often it is merely a sign of life. Indeed, both the ready suppression of all personal sexual desires and the stubborn insistence on their complete satisfaction seem to merit much greater concern. Most human beings spontaneously try to find a reasonable balance between these two extremes. They may very well be maladjusted, but they neither want nor need professional help.

It seems necessary to repeat these truisms here because otherwise the following remarks could easily be misunderstood. When we now proceed to discuss various specific forms of sexual maladjustment, we do not necessarily imply that they represent "unnatural" conditions, moral transgressions, crimes, or diseases. We simply recognize that in some men and women the "normal" lack of sexual conformity or contentment can become aggravated to the point where it seriously interferes with their ability to maintain simple personal relationships. Or, stated in another way, certain people are sexually so ill at ease that some outside intervention seems justified and desirable, either in their own interest or in that of their partners.

We are, of course, not talking about physical shortcomings, malformations, or handicaps, or about illness in the usual sense of the word. These are discussed in detail elsewhere in this book (see "Some Physical Problems"). Instead, we are referring to persons whose bodies are perfectly healthy, and whose sexual problems are of a psychological nature. For example, some men and women suffer from a psychological impairment of their sexual response. They are, to use a current professional term, "sexually inadequate." However, many of them can be helped by some special sex therapy. Others are so helplessly inflexible in their sexual behavior that they become unhappy with themselves and inconsiderate of others. Their sexual acts either constitute some frustrating and self-defeating ritual or turn into outright assault. Therefore, they can only be described as compulsive and destructive. In extreme cases, such individuals have to be restrained by the law. Very often, however, they can also profit from some form of psychotherapy.

Finally, there are some persons who are maladjusted to their very anatomies. Through no fault of their own, they have developed a gender identity that is contradicted by their biological sex. They feel that they are trapped in the wrong body, and therefore they cannot be truly happy until the mistake is corrected. Only a "sex change" will eventually bring them full peace of mind. Obviously, these so-called transsexuals appreciate any professional intervention which can bring them closer to their goal.

The following pages provide some basic information about the problems of sexual inadequacy, compulsive and destructive sexual behavior, and transsexualism. The social implications of some of these behaviors are discussed more fully in the third part of this book, "Sex and Society."

SEXUAL INADEQUACY

As we have seen in a previous section, some men and women are restricted in their sexual expression by physical malformations, handicaps, diseases, or injuries (see "Some Physical Problems"). However, there are also physically healthy individuals who cannot fully enjoy sexual intercourse because their sexual responses have become weakened, inhibited, or even completely blocked for psychological reasons. Today, such a person is usually said to suffer from "sexual inadequacy" or "sexual dysfunction."

Obviously, the distinction between physical and psychological causes of sexual inadequacy is, to a certain extent, arbitrary, since body and mind are so closely interrelated that a sharp dividing line between them cannot be drawn. Furthermore, it may be an oversimplification to speak of sexual inadequacy in any individual, because, as a rule, it manifests itself only in relation to another individual. Indeed, in many cases it may be more useful to speak of an inadequate sexual relationship between two persons. At any rate, sex therapists today often act on the assumption that it is less the individual than the couple who has a problem. Consequently, they insist on treating both partners together.

It has recently been estimated that in more than half of all American marriages at least one partner suffers from some form of sexual inadequacy. Needless to say, this, in turn, is bound to affect the other sexually adequate partner, and thus both of them spend their lives in sexual frustration. In some marriages, this frustration is, of course, due to permanent physical handicaps, although even in these cases realistic counseling can sometimes increase sexual options and thereby restore a reasonable minimum of satisfaction. Most often, however, the problems are of a psychological nature and could be completely eliminated by modern sex therapy. Following the pioneering work of William H. Masters and Virginia E. Johnson in the 1960s, a variety of new therapeutic techniques have been developed which are now being used successfully in many parts of the United States.

Curiously enough, the very success of sex therapy and the growing demand for it have underlined the general need for new sexual attitudes. Sexual misery seems to be widespread, and while one can argue about precise figures, the importance of the problem is no longer in doubt.

In the past, a man's sexual inadequacy was often ascribed to witchcraft or some evil curse (if he was believed to be innocent) or to "degeneracy," "self-abuse," "immorality," and "excess" (if he was held responsible for his condition). Today, we have learned, however, that both kinds of explanation are false, and that the real causes lie elsewhere. In fact, as sex therapists have shown, people become sexually inadequate mainly because of a rigid upbringing, traumatic sexual experiences, ignorance, narrow religious beliefs, and bad advice from ill-informed clergymen, marriage counselors, doctors, psychotherapists, and other professionals. All of these different causes, in turn, can be traced to the sexually oppressive character of our civilization.

The sexual oppression under which all of us live has many aspects, and most of them are discussed in various other sections in this book. However, with regard to human sexual functioning, we can point to one specific negative factor which seems to be more significant than any other—the nearly exclusive concern, indeed the obsession, with the male and female sex organs. The exaggerated importance ascribed to the sex organs has blinded not only the average person, but even certain theoreticians of sex to the full range of human sexual capacities. "Genitality" still reigns as the supreme sexual ideal, and, as a result, the sexual relationships in our society suffer a triple distortion:

- An overemphasis on the male initiative (at the expense of the female initiative),
- an overemphasis on coitus (at the expense of other forms of sexual intercourse), and
- an overemphasis on orgasm (at the expense of leisurely sensual enjoyment).

Therefore, we now find countless men and women who are sexually inadequate. Fortunately, in recent years we have learned that many of them can be helped simply by redirecting the emphasis and restoring a more balanced sexual approach. For example, the stereotypes of the sexually active male and the passive female, after which men and women try to model themselves, are often too confining. A man who is always expected to initiate coitus, and who is never allowed to "take it lying down," may begin to worry about his continued ability to perform. In fact, eventually this worry is likely to grow into an outright fear of failure. This fear, in turn, then blocks his natural sexual responses, and thus he becomes unable to satisfy his partner. A woman, on the other hand, who is told that taking the initiative is unfeminine may try very hard to restrain herself and become so frustrated in her artificial passivity that sexual intercourse becomes unpleasant and unrewarding. Not surprisingly, she then also becomes dysfunctional. The solution in both of these cases is obvious: A conscious temporary reversal of attitudes relieves anxiety and frustration, and the inhibited sexual responses are set free again. As the following detailed discussions will show, modern sex therapy often involves specific exercises which shift the initiative to the female.

Secondly, the overemphasis on coitus causes many men and women to neglect other forms of lovemaking and thus to fall victim to boredom and rigidity. Even worse, by focusing only on their genital contact, they may gradually desensitize other erogenous zones. This, in turn, leads to a situation where the sex organs alone "carry the entire responsibility" for sexual satisfaction, while the rest of the body remains "uninvolved." However, the sexual response is not to be restricted, divided, or compartmentalized in this fashion, and, in the long run, it may therefore become seriously impaired. On the other hand, it is truly remarkable how the sexual response often regains its full strength as soon as a couple turns to noncoital forms of sexual intercourse. It is for this reason that many modern sex therapists instruct their clients to practice manual and oral intercourse as a means of rebuilding sexual self-confidence. It is also worth noting that homosexual couples, who cannot engage in coitus, rarely suffer from the severe dysfunctions so common among heterosexuals. Both male and female homosexuals take it for granted that sexual satisfaction can be obtained in many different ways, and therefore they are used to making the best of any sexual situation. There is no doubt that many "straight" couples could profit from adopting the same attitude. It is ironic, however, that in many states of the United States noncoital forms of sexual intercourse (even between husband and wife) are legally defined as "crimes against nature," and that offenders can be sentenced to long prison terms. This, perhaps more than anything else, shows the barbarity of our official sexual standards (for details, see "Conformity and Deviance—Legal-Illegal").

Finally, the overemphasis on orgasm robs men and women of much sexual pleasure by shortening the duration of their sexual intercourse and by turning it into a goal-oriented task. Thus, sex becomes work and, as such, still another testing ground for personal success or failure. At the same time, the successful finale, the "climax" of sexual intercourse, not the intercourse itself, becomes the major concern. In other words, it is no longer the process but the product which now commands all the attention. Unfortunately, this narrow fixation on the possible outcome tends to diminish the real pleasures of the moment. Indeed, it may seriously interfere with the normal sexual response. As a result, males may reach orgasm much too quickly for their own satisfaction, and women may not reach any orgasm at all. Modern sex therapists have shown, however, that these sexual dysfunctions (just as the others mentioned above) may disappear when the partners adopt a different attitude. Indeed, in therapy programs both the man and the woman are now often asked to deliberately avoid orgasm in their sexual intercourse. For example, the couple may be told to engage in extended mutual pleasuring, but to interrupt their physical contact as soon as either of them approaches orgasm. Some therapists even go so far as to prohibit their clients from reaching orgasm while at the same time ordering them to touch and caress each other for several hours every day. This simple regimen often produces dramatic results. Relieved of their "duty to perform," both partners may, for the first time in their lives, abandon themselves to sexual pleasure, and therefore they may change their whole attitude toward each other. This new attitude then becomes the source of a greatly increased orgasmic potential. Finally, after a few weeks, when the sexual response has been restored and the therapist has lifted the prohibition, orgasm becomes a regular, welcome experience, and its timing is no longer a problem. By the same token, however, this experience has now turned from an obligation into an option. Orgasm is nothing more and nothing less than a delightful interruption of an otherwise continuous process of generating pleasurable sensations. Most importantly, the partners have learned that they do not have to reach orgasm simultaneously or in every sexual encounter. An occasional lack of orgasm need not diminish their happiness. After all, making love is neither a battle nor an athletic competition. Notions of success or achievement have no place in a happy sexual relationship.

It seems that sexual dysfunctions of one kind or another have plagued many people in many societies since the dawn of history. We know, for example, that ancient and medieval physicians studied the problem and sought various medical remedies. However, it also seems that these dysfunctions have become more severe and widespread in modern times. In the 19th and 20th centuries, they were often treated by psychiatrists, and the rate of "cure" was not always encouraging. Today, we can see that this could hardly have been otherwise, since the physiological processes involved in sexual functioning were still poorly understood. (For details, see "Conformity and Deviance—Healthy-Sick.")

It was only the specific research of scientists like Masters and Johnson which finally allowed therapists to approach sexual dysfunctions directly, instead of treating them as symptoms of something else. Masters and Johnson themselves established a clinic for sexual therapy, and their success soon encouraged others to follow their example. Masters and Johnson also pioneered the male-female "dual team" of therapists and treated couples rather than individuals. These couples were either husband or wife or single men and women who brought along their (heterosexual or homosexual) partners. Some persons who did not have partners of their own were supplied with "surrogate partners" for the duration of the therapy. These and many other features of Masters' and Johnson's approach have, in the meantime, been copied widely. Today, there are many competent sex therapists in the United States and other Western countries who are increasingly successful in helping their clients.

An interesting new program of sex therapy has also been developed by the National Sex Forum in collaboration with the University of California Medical Center in San Francisco. This program, known as SAR (Sexual Attitude Restructuring) involves the use of films and various other visual aids.

Unfortunately, at the present time there are also still many unqualified people who call themselves sex therapists and who exploit their clients doing more harm than good. It is to be hoped, therefore, that in the future sex therapy will become a licensed profession. In this important field, nobody should be allowed to practice without having demonstrated the necessary knowledge and experience.

The following pages briefly summarize the most successful current techniques of sex therapy, especially those used by Masters and Johnson. However, upon closer examination, it has seemed advisable to replace several of their professional terms with simple English expressions.

SEXUAL INADEQUACY IN MEN

Most books on human sexuality today distinguish between three male sexual dysfunctions: "impotence," "premature ejaculation," and "ejaculatory incompetence." Unfortunately, the average layman is not likely to find these strange Latin terms very helpful. Indeed, if he ever takes the trouble to consult his dictionary for their literal meaning, he is bound to be thoroughly confused.

The term "impotence" (literally, lack of power, from Latin *impotens:* powerless) sounds somber and threatening, but is also curiously vague. The term "premature ejaculation" seems to imply that there is an objective standard for timing ejaculations or, in other words, that there is such a thing as a "mature ejaculation" which occurs only after a fixed period of time. Finally, the expression "ejaculatory incompetence" seems to suggest that, when it comes to ejaculating semen, some men are more competent than others. However, in actual fact, competence has nothing to do with it. An ejaculation, like a sneeze, is a purely involuntary response. It may not occur at all, but when it does, nobody can suppress, delay, control, or modify it in any way. Furthermore, it must be remembered that ejaculations are only incidental to orgasms, and that a male can very well have an orgasm without ejaculating anything. Obviously, it would be foolish to consider such a male sexually inadequate. In other words, it is not the absent ejaculation but the absent orgasm which actually creates the problem. (For details, see "The Male Sexual Response.")

The traditional terminology has still another drawback: The terms used for male and female sexual problems are entirely different. As a result, many people are under the false impression that the physical reactions of men and women cannot really be compared. However, modern sex research has clearly demonstrated that such a comparison makes a great deal of sense. Indeed, we are now beginning to realize that, just as the sexual responses of males and females are quite similar, so are their sexual inadequacies. We therefore need new special terms that can be applied to both sexes. Both the male and the female sexual responses can be inadequate in three ways:

1. Coitus cannot begin because the sex organs do not show the necessary initial reaction (lack of erection, vaginismus).
2. Coitus is frustrating because, in the opinion of one or both partners, orgasm occurs either too early or too late (unsatisfactory timing of orgasm).
3. No orgasm is reached at all (absence of orgasm).

The following pages deal with these three basic inadequacies as they affect men.

Lack of Erection

A chronic lack of erection can, of course, be caused by a variety of bodily injuries, diseases, and disorders, from a severing of nerves to diabetes. Such cases must be treated by a physician. There are now several promising treatments (including silicone and inflatable prosthesis implants) which can greatly improve the condition. However, since these are strictly physical problems, they are not discussed in this section.

There are some physically healthy men who never in their lives had an erection of the penis when they attempted coitus. That is to say, their natural sexual response is so completely inhibited that they despair of ever finding satisfaction with a sexual partner. This depressing condition can have several possible causes. Usually, however, it is brought about by a combination of unfortunate circumstances. For example, a male may be raised by a possessive and highly seductive mother who just does not allow him to "be his own man," or he may learn to think of all sexual activity as sinful, dirty, or dangerous. If such a male then fails the first time he tries coitus, he may forever remain unable to overcome his negative conditioning. Another male may have strong homosexual tendencies, but may fear to come to terms with them. The unresolved inner conflict may then prevent his body from functioning properly. Obviously in these and similar cases, a man needs more help than he is likely to get from his girl friend or wife alone. Indeed, his best hope is intensive sex therapy.

Such therapy may also become necessary for a second much larger group of men—those who have been capable of coitus at some time in their lives, but who seem to have lost much or all of this capability. They either no longer have any erections at all, or fail to have them a great deal of the time. It has to be remembered, of course, that an occasional lack of erection is perfectly normal. After all, men are not machines. Sometimes, when they are tired, worried, distracted, or drunk, they may feel amorous, but their bodies simply refuse to respond. In such a case, frantic efforts, will power, or special acrobatics lead nowhere. Instead, the couple is well advised to accept the situation and to make the best of it. For instance, they might remember that a man does not need an erection to satisfy his partner. A limp penis can be "stuffed" into the vagina by hand and even if it then remains limp, the couple can go through some motions of coitus. It is not at all impossible for a woman to reach orgasm in this way. Furthermore, the man can also make love with his hands, lips, and tongue (see "Manual Intercourse" and "Oral Intercourse"). In any case, he can rest assured that, at another time when conditions are more favorable, the penis will easily become erect again.

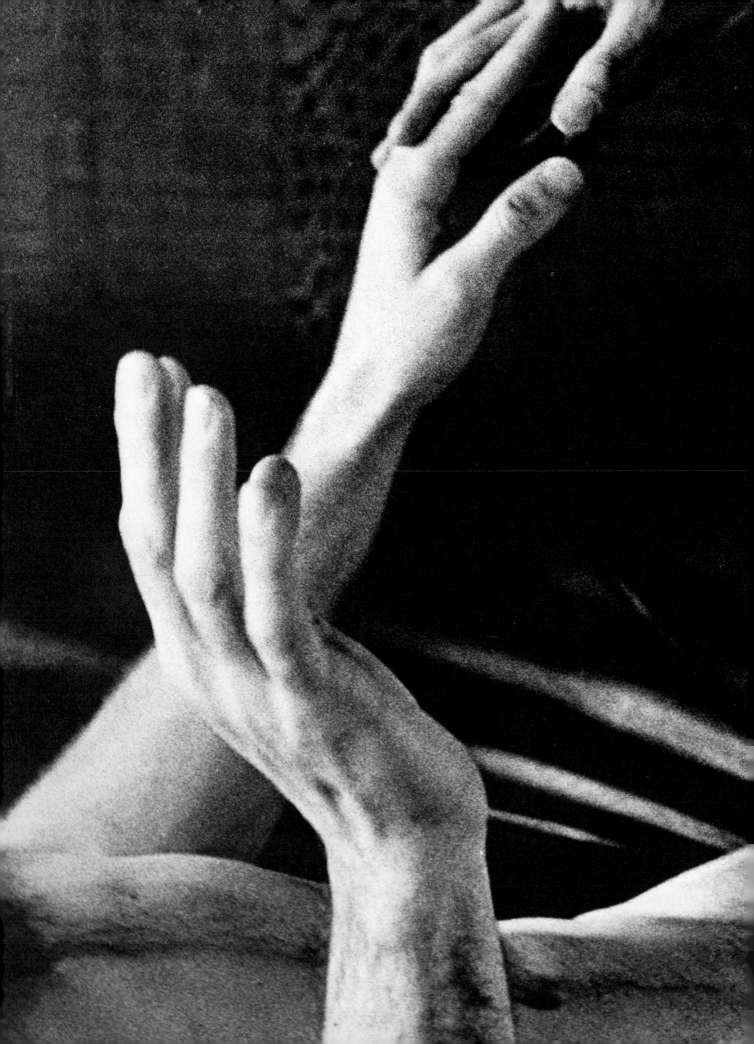

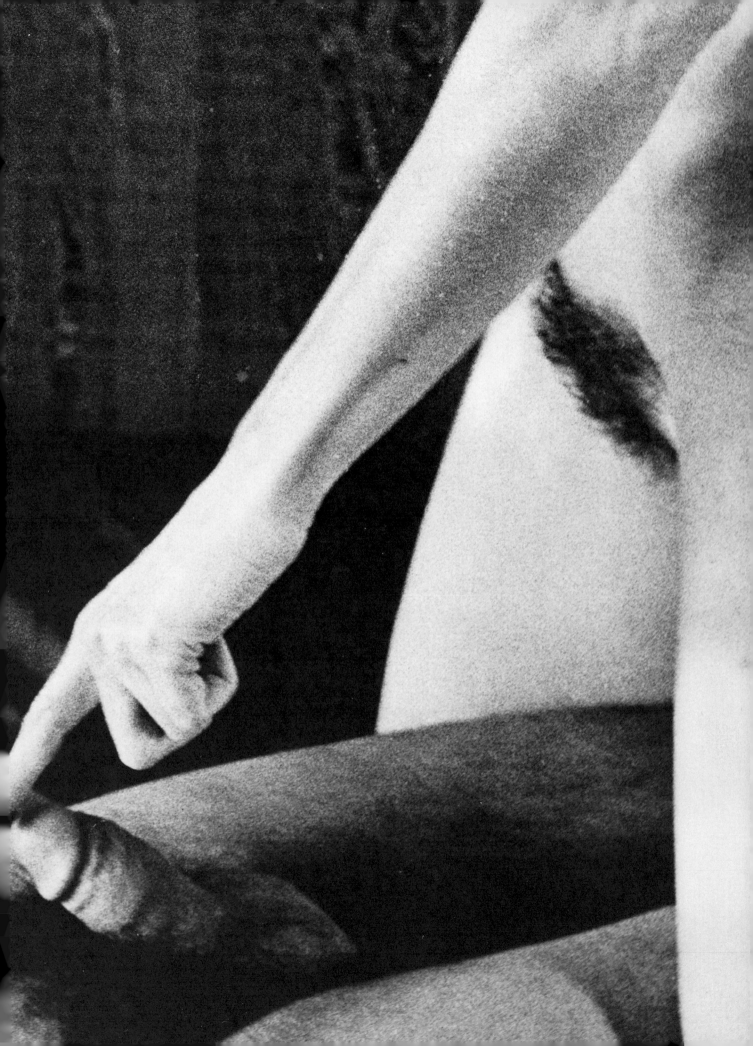

However, some men are so insecure that they develop a fear of failure. Others just demand too much of themselves and begin to put their own responses to the test, thus turning every sexual encounter into a win or lose battle. Still others try to "stiffen their resolve" by drinking. Naturally, these stratagems only invite defeat, and thus the occasional problem turns into a chronic condition. The same fate may befall a man whose orgasm always occurs much sooner than that of his partner. (For details, see "Unsatisfactory Timing of Orgasm" below.) There are also some men who are unable to free themselves emotionally from the domination of one or both of their parents, and there are those whose puritanical upbringing has left them uncomfortable with their sexual feelings. Furthermore, certain men may have difficulty starting coitus because of homosexual interests, and others are simply overwhelmed by their sexual inexperience. All of these men may eventually find themselves unable to have or hold an erection that would allow them to engage in coitus. As a matter of fact, as soon as they regularly fail more than one-fourth of the time, their problem is serious enough to demand special therapy.

Treatment programs, such as that developed by Masters and Johnson, have been quite successful in restoring a man's normal sexual responses. This success depends, however, largely on the cooperation of both sexual partners. A woman whose male partner regularly fails to have an erection is bound to be negatively affected too, and it is therefore the whole sexual relationship that has to be treated.

The first therapeutic step usually consists of a couple's sexual reeducation. For example, they have to understand once and for all that an erection is an involuntary response. No man can will an erection; he can only allow it to happen. He can be certain, however, that it will happen if there is some sexual feedback between him and his partner, and if he is relaxed enough. Anxiety and apprehension, on the other hand, are likely to block his responses. In short, the couple learns that they have "nothing to fear but fear itself." Naturally, the underlying reasons for such fear have to be discussed also, and if one or both of the partners have negative and unrealistic attitudes toward sex in general, they must be corrected. In addition, the nonsexual aspects of the couple's relationship have to be considered. In the final analysis, it is the full human communication between man and woman that leads to their mutual happiness.

In order to further this communication, sex therapists have devised some simple exercises that the couple can practice together in the privacy of their bedroom. First, both the man and the woman have to learn to give and receive pleasure simply by touching each other's bodies. At that stage, they are not allowed to have coitus or even to try reaching orgasm any other way. Instead, they are encouraged to pleasure each other with gentle strokes and caresses. They are also told how to increase their pleasure by slowly guiding each other's hands. Often the use of some lotion or body oil is recommended. However, there is no specific area to be singled out, no specific goal to be reached, and thus there is no pressure to perform. Once the partners have practiced such pleasuring a few times, they usually begin to relax, lose their self-consciousness, and abandon themselves to their sexual feelings.

After several days of these exercises, the partners may concentrate their caresses on the sex organs and the woman's breasts. Again, guiding each other's hands can be very helpful. Both partners should also let each other know exactly how they like to be masturbated, and especially the man must tell the woman how he wants her to hold and stroke his penis. This kind of openness truly enables the partners to give each other pleasure. However, they still remain under the therapist's firm instruction not to aim for coitus or even for orgasm. If an erection of the penis occurs, the partners just stop playing for a while until it goes down. Then the man can allow himself to be masturbated again until he has another erection which he loses again, and so forth through several repetitions. This simple "teasing" of the penis will

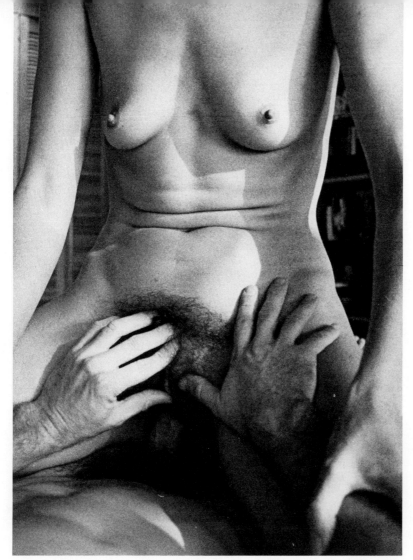

assure him that there is nothing frightening about losing an erection, and that he can always get it back.

About a week later, when the man has overcome his fear of failure and has begun to have confidence in his responses, the couple may proceed to coitus in a deliberate and nondemanding fashion. Again, the woman takes the initiative. While the man remains passive lying on his back, she sits on top of him and masturbates him until he has an erection. She then lowers herself onto the erect penis and inserts it into her vagina. After the insertion, she remains still for a while, so that the man can get used to the feeling of being inside her. Within a few minutes, she begins to move slowly, thus stimulating the penis and keeping it erect. Should the erection be lost, she simply moves off the penis and masturbates it again until it is hard. Usually, however, the man will be able to keep his erection as long as the woman avoids quick and vigorous movements.

Eventually, part of the initiative may be shifted to the man. That is to say, the woman remains in a position above her partner and she still inserts his penis into her vagina, but, after a while, she stops her gentle thrusting and allows him to move back and forth inside of her. Both partners stay under orders, however, not to aim for orgasm. When either of the partners does have an orgasm, it should be regarded as a pleasant surprise. Once a couple has learned to relax in this manner, they are usually also delighted to find that the penis can stay erect inside the vagina as long as either of them may wish. Finally, with their confidence strengthened, they are ready to make the most of each coitus and also to experiment freely with different coital positions.

Unsatisfactory Timing of Orgasm

Masturbation and sexual intercourse are among the greatest pleasures of life, and it is therefore only natural that people should try to enjoy them as often as they can. It is also understandable that they should want to make them last as long as possible.

In this latter respect, a woman has a certain advantage over a man. She can experience many orgasms in quick succession and thus can continue sexual intercourse as long as her partner is able to keep up with her. A man, on the other hand, can usually have only one orgasm at a time, after which his body needs a period of rest. (See "The Male Sexual Reponse" and "The Female Sexual Response.") In other words, in contrast to women, men who want to make their sexual activity last longer can do so only by delaying their orgasms.

In their younger years, men may not be much interested in such a delay because then they are often also capable of multiple orgasms. As a matter of fact, it is not unusual for adolescent boys to engage in masturbation contests in order to find out which member of their group can reach orgasm first. The "winner" of such a contest is usually much admired and even envied for his virility. It is only later, when the boy attempts coitus with a girl, that the speed of his sexual response suddenly turns into a disadvantage. He may then reach orgasm much sooner than she and thus leave her unsatisfied. When this happens, the boy may develop serious doubts about his sexual abilities, and eventually he may even become unable to have an erection in the girl's presence.

Fortunately, this problem can almost always be solved, if both partners are willing to cooperate. Indeed, it may already help them a great deal if they approach the matter with a little common sense.

First of all, the fact that the man reaches orgasm before the woman is, in itself, no reason why he should not continue sexual intercourse. All he has to do is switch from coitus to other forms of sexual stimulation. In other words, once his penis has lost its erection he can still use his hands or his mouth to bring the woman to orgasm. (See "Manual Intercourse" and "Oral Intercourse.") Once both partners realize that the man's "premature" orgasm does not have to deprive the woman of hers, much of their anxiety and frustration is bound to be relieved.

Secondly, it should be obvious that the ability to control the timing of one's orgasm is a matter of practice and experience. For example, males who enjoy masturbating in their adolescence often train themselves to delay their orgasms by interrupting or slowing down their movements. Girls, on the other hand, can learn through masturbation how to reach orgasm quickly. People first have to become familiar with their own sexual responses before they can gain some control over them.

Finally, it should be remembered that there is no such thing as an ill-timed orgasm for people who are alone. The problem arises only in relation to another person, and it can therefore always be defined from two different points of view: 1. "The man's orgasm comes too soon," and 2. "The woman's orgasm comes too late." Thus, a woman may find the timing of a man's orgasm unsatisfactory because it occurs several minutes before she herself is satisfied. However, the same man may very well be able to satisfy another woman with quicker responses. (Also see "Sexual Inadequacy in Women.")

All of these observations point to the same conclusion: The timing of orgasms is basically a matter of a couple's mutual adjustment, and, in many cases, it may well be the woman who can contribute most toward this goal. At any rate, she should know that, with her help, practically every man can learn to delay his orgasm as long as either of them want it delayed.

In recent years, sex therapists have developed some simple exercises which can help men and women make their sexual intercourse last longer. Occasionally, an especially frustrated and maladjusted couple may need professional guidance in learning and practicing these exercises. Still, many couples may also be able to make the adjustment on their own. The most

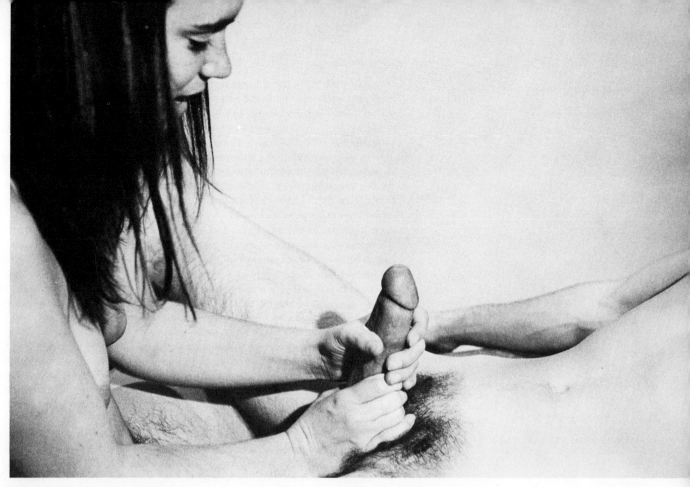

LEARNING TO DELAY ORGASM

Men who want to gain more control over the timing of their orgasms can practice some simple exercises with their partners. Shown here is the "squeeze technique".

(Top) The woman masturbates the man until he is close to orgasm. (Bottom) Just before the man reaches orgasm, the woman applies the "squeeze". (Note the exact position of her fingers.) For a detailed description see next page.

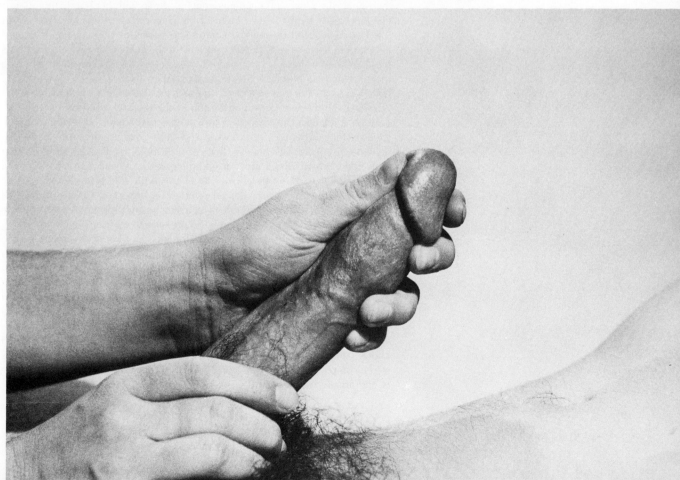

important technique to be learned is the so-called "squeeze," which should be practiced in the following way: The man lies on his back with his legs spread apart. The woman sits between his legs with her feet on each side of his torso. This position gives her hands free access to his sex organs. Using some massaging oil or body lotion, she then gently strokes his penis until he gets an erection. While the man remains relaxed and passive throughout, the woman continues to masturbate him until he approaches orgasm. (In order to do this properly, she should ask the man for instructions as to tempo and firmness of grip. Some men are more easily excited by slow, firm strokes; others like them light and quick. Also, as arousal progresses, the man may want a change of rhythm. Open and explicit verbal communication between the partners is therefore essential.) As the man comes closer to orgasm, and just as he reaches his "point of no return," he signals the woman to apply the "squeeze." She then squeezes the penis firmly for 4–6 seconds by placing her thumb just below the glans on its underside and her first and second fingers above and below the ridge of the glans on its upper side. (See illustration on page 261.) There is no need to fear that the penis will be hurt because it is relatively tough when it is hard. However, if the man should find a firm squeeze uncomfortable, the woman can squeeze more gently for 8–15 seconds. In both cases, the effect is the same—no ejaculation occurs, and the man begins to lose his erection. Once the penis has become soft, the woman repeats the stimulation and the squeeze three or four more times, each time bringing the man close to orgasm, but preventing it at the last moment by the pressure of her fingers around the ridge of the glans. This whole exercise should then be repeated in at least two more special sessions.

After three or four sessions devoted to the squeeze technique, the couple may proceed to the next step, the so-called stuffing exercise. In this session, the woman first repeats the squeeze technique as practiced before. However, after the first squeeze, when the man loses his erection, she leans forward and stuffs the limp penis into her vagina. Doing so, she sits on top of the man who remains completely passive lying on his back. She then remains still while he gets used to being inside her. After a few minutes, she slowly begins to move, thus giving him an erection. As he approaches orgasm, he gives her the signal, she moves off his penis, reaches down with her hand, and applies the squeeze as before. Once he loses his erection, she stuffs his penis again into her vagina and repeats the exercise. This stuffing and squeezing should also be repeated several times in at least three special sessions. As soon as these techniques have been mastered, the couple should continue to practice them regularly until they feel confident that they can control the timing of the man's orgasm. For the first few weeks, it is advisable to retain the coital position with the woman sitting on top of the man who lies on his back. In case of a relapse, they simply return to the first squeezing exercises. (The squeeze technique does not always work if the man applies it to himself.)

Some sex therapists believe that, during their practice sessions, neither man nor woman should aim for complete sexual satisfaction. Others think that an ejaculation can be allowed to occur at the end of a session, as long as it happens without any special effort. It is important for the success of these exercises that they should take place in an atmosphere of complete relaxation. There must be absolutely no pressure to perform. Another training program for men who want to "last longer" has been developed at the University of California School of Medicine in San Francisco. This program does not necessarily rely on the "squeeze technique." Instead, the man learns to delay his orgasm for 15 minutes masturbating himself (first without and then with lubrication). Once he has successfully completed these initial steps, he lets himself be masturbated by his partner (again first without and then with lubrication) until he can delay his orgasm for 15 minutes. Thereafter the couple can proceed to the undemanding coital forms described above. The "squeeze" may or may not be used. The man simply proceeds step by step until he can "last" 15 minutes in each case. The whole training is undramatic, but seems to work well.

Absence of Orgasm

Virtually all men who achieve an erection of the penis also achieve orgasm. That is to say, in contrast to many women who have difficulty going beyond the plateau phase, men can normally count on completing their sexual response cycle. (See "The Male Sexual Response" and "The Female Sexual Response.") However, there are some rare cases where men can reach orgasm only through masturbation or certain specific forms of sexual intercourse. For example, a man may be unable to have an orgasm as long as his penis is inside a woman's vagina or in her mouth. Thus, a woman who wants to become pregnant or who enjoys swallowing semen may find herself disappointed. Her partner can easily maintain an erection, but he reaches orgasm (and therefore ejaculates) only after he has either withdrawn from her body or completely removed himself for her presence. Quite obviously, this curious condition is caused by some mental or emotional block that prevents the man from letting himself go when he should. For instance, he may suffer from an overpowering and irrational fear of making the woman pregnant, or he may dislike her so much that he takes pleasure in frustrating her. In another case, the man may be the victim of a traumatic early experience. Thus, a boy who is punished by his parents for masturbating or having a "wet dream" may later find himself unable to have an orgasm during coitus. In still other cases, this inability is brought about late in life by an unpleasant sexual encounter in which the woman's vagina or mouth somehow appeared unclean or disgusting.

Like other sexual dysfunctions, this problem can be overcome by a nondemanding attitude of the partners toward each other, by full communication of their needs, wishes, and fears, and by appropriate exercises. For example, a woman who gradually manages to masturbate the man to orgasm may thereby succeed in breaking his phobic behavior pattern. As he begins to associate his sexual release with her presence, he may become able to accept the idea of ejaculating close to or even inside of her body. Here again, the joyful appreciation of noncoital forms of sexual intercourse can do much to put the partners at ease. In some cases, professional sex therapy may be advisable.

Still, it should be pointed out that not all couples confronted with this phenomenon feel the need for treatment. After all, a man who is simply unable to ejaculate into a woman's vagina or mouth can still bring her to orgasm. Once she is sexually satisfied, he can then reach orgasm himself by masturbating or by any other method that suits him. Thus, both partners can have a satisfying sexual relationship, and they may even enjoy the advantage of never having to worry about contraception. If, on the other hand, they decide to have a child, they can always resort to artificial insemination. (See "Infertility.")

It should perhaps also be mentioned that certain religious groups of the past actively encouraged men to practice coitus without ejaculation. This kind of coitus (also known as karezza or coitus reservatus) was often supposed to last many hours and to further a couple's spiritual growth. Needless to say, for such a couple the absence of the man's orgasm was never a problem.

There was a time when men used a single word to describe all possible female sexual dysfunctions: frigidity (literally, coldness, from Latin frigidus: cold). Today, we know that this vague and derogatory term is no longer acceptable. After all, just as the sexual responses of males and females are quite similar, so are their sexual inadequacies. We therefore need a terminology that can be applied to both sexes.

Modern sex research has shown that both the male and the female sexual response can be inadequate in three ways:

1. Coitus cannot begin because the sex organs do not show the necessary initial reaction (lack of erection, vaginismus).

SEXUAL INADEQUACY IN WOMEN

2. Coitus is frustrating because, in the opinion of one or both partners, orgasm occurs either too early or too late (unsatisfactory timing of orgasm).
3. No orgasm is reached at all (absence of orgasm).

The following pages deal with these three basic inadequacies as they affect women.

Vaginismus

The lack of penile erection in men is physiologically equivalent to the lack of vaginal lubrication in women. However, for a woman this inadequacy is less upsetting than for a man because it is easily overcome by the use of artificial lubricants. Thus, unlike a man with a limp penis, a woman with an unlubricated vagina can still easily begin coitus, if she so chooses. Nevertheless, women, like men, may also find themselves in a condition which denies them his choice:

There are some women who cannot engage in coitus because of involuntary muscular spasms which close the opening of the vagina. As a result, the insertion of a man's penis becomes extremely difficult or even impossible. The condition is known as vaginismus. In a few rare cases, vaginismus develops as a protective reaction against previously experienced pain during sexual intercourse which, in turn, was caused by some injury or disease of the internal sex organs. Obviously, in such a case, the underlying physical cause must be treated. (See "Pain During Sexual Intercourse.")

However, very often the causes of vaginismus are entirely psychological. For example, a woman whose husband is unable to have or hold an erection may become so frustrated and apprehensive about his futile attempts at coitus that her vagina tightens involuntarily. On the other hand, even a man with normal sexual responses may eventually become dysfunctional if he always finds the woman's vagina too tight for penetration. Thus, a couple may enter a vicious circle of mutual disappointment. It then makes little difference how the problem began. Both the man and the woman need treatment. Another possible cause of vaginismus is a strict and puritanical upbringing that teaches a girl to consider sex dirty or evil. Such negative attitudes can very well prevent her from functioning sexually at all. In other cases, a woman's vaginismus can be traced back to a particular traumatic experience, such as rape or coitus with an inconsiderate partner.

Whatever its cause, vaginismus can always be treated successfully if the couple is willing to cooperate. The first and most important therapeutic step is simply an educational one. A sex therapist explains the phenomenon in detail and then demonstrates it physically by placing the woman on the examining table. As soon as he tries to insert a finger into her vagina, the involuntary spasm closes the opening. The woman's sexual partner is then asked to put on a rubber examining glove and to feel the constriction himself. Once both partners realize that they are indeed dealing with a clear physical obstacle to coitus, they are ready to take the appropriate practical steps. The therapist gives them several special vaginal dilators in graduated sizes which they can use in the privacy of their bedroom. There, under the woman's direction, the man begins by inserting the smallest dilator into her vagina. As she becomes more relaxed, he is able to use the larger dilators, and, after a few days, the woman is asked to keep a fairly large dilator in her vagina for several hours during the night. Eventually, the man can attempt to insert his own penis instead of the mechanical device. If the dilators are used every night, the vaginal spasms usually disappear within less than a week, although, in rare cases, the dilators may still be needed before coitus for a month or so.

The successful physical therapy is usually followed by some psychological counseling. This is the best time for the therapist to build the confidence of his clients and to relieve them of any remaining tensions and misconceptions.

It should perhaps also be mentioned in this context that, according to a popular belief, vaginal spasms can occur not only before, but also after the insertion of a penis, thus trapping it inside the woman's body. However, among humans, this is impossible. (The phenomenon, also known as *penis captivus* [Latin: trapped penis], is found only in certain animals.)

Unsatisfactory Timing of Orgasm

There are women who are much slower in reaching orgasm than most men. As long as such women engage only in "solitary sex," they have no reason to feel inadequate. It is only when they begin sexual intercourse that they may find themselves at a disadvantage. Their male partners may reach orgasm much sooner than they and therefore leave them unsatisfied.

In the past, it was customary to define this problem exclusively in terms of male failure. Today, however, we understand that it is more helpful and realistic to see it as a problem of male-female adjustment. After all, given the proper stimulation, the average female can respond just as quickly as the average male. Many women can also train themselves through masturbation to speed up their sexual responses. (See "The Female Sexual Response.") Still, a woman may feel that there is little virtue in such efficiency, and that leisurely lovemaking is preferable to a race for orgasms. She may also enjoy having more than one orgasm during coitus, and this may be reason enough to wish for a better sexual adjustment with her partner.

Fortunately, such an adjustment can almost always be achieved if both partners are sufficiently motivated. Modern sex therapists have developed some simple exercises that can help men and women make their sexual intercourse last longer. Indeed, using these exercises, a woman can train any man to delay his orgasm for as long as either of them may wish. As a result of his improved sexual abilities, she may then also become more responsive herself. In short, the unsatisfactory timing of orgasm need not be a problem for either sex. (For a detailed description of the exercises, see the corresponding section under "Sexual Inadequacy in Men.")

Finally, it should perhaps also be mentioned that, according to a popular belief, sexual perfection requires both partners to reach orgasm at the same time. However, the pursuit of such an ideal can do more harm than good. It forces the partners to observe and control their own responses at all times and thus kills their spontaneity. It is better to think of simultaneous orgasms as agreeable coincidences. There is no point in considering them in any way superior.

Absence of Orgasm

While virtually all men easily reach orgasm, many women find it difficult to achieve this simple goal. There may be many different reasons for this, but the most important reason is undoubtedly the negative attitude toward sexual pleasure that women in our society learn to adopt early in their lives.

It has often been observed that our Western culture does not encourage girls to develop sexual needs, to be proud of themselves as sexual beings, and to feel entitled to sexual activity. On the contrary, from their earliest childhood, girls are taught to be "nice," "good," "decent," "proper," and "respectable." They are asked to control, hide, or deny their sexual urges and are discouraged from actively exploring their bodies. They may be allowed to entertain some vague romantic fantasies, but are prevented from having any practical sexual experiences. In fact, they are told that girls who seek such experiences are worthless, despicable creatures. At the same time, they are warned against the base and animalistic instincts of men who are "all after only one thing" and who use and abuse women as sexual objects. It is never admitted that women might have the same instincts or might be able to reciprocate.

As a result of this negative conditioning, many women develop unrealistic and very restrictive sexual values. They feel that they need some special permission to be sexual, and that they can grant themselves this permission only under very unusual, almost ideal circumstances. Unfortunately, these ideal circumstances may never be found in real life, and thus the women may never become relaxed enough to enjoy their sexual capacities to the fullest.

Apart from this general handicap, women may, of course, also have individual reasons of their own for being nonorgasmic. For example, a woman may have been raised with especially rigid religious views about sex and may therefore be unable to enjoy it. In another case, the woman may have a partner whom she does not really like very much. Consequently, she never allows herself to "get carried away" with him. In still another case, the partner himself is sexually inadequate in some way and therefore makes the woman apprehensive and frustrated. There are also some women with homosexual tendencies who just do not like heterosexual intercourse, but would be responsive with a female partner. Finally, one has to concede the possibility that some individuals are simply not very interested in sex.

There are women who have never had an orgasm in their lives, and there are others who just fail to have orgasms a great deal of the time. However, today most of these women can be helped by appropriate sex therapy. So far the best known of these therapies is that devised by Masters and Johnson. In their intensive short-term program, they treat nonorgasmic women together with their partners by means of intensive counseling and indirectly supervised exercises. The counseling aims at restructuring the couple's approach to sex and to each other. The exercises are specifically designed to unblock the inhibited natural sexual responses.

Obviously, there is no substitute for individual personal treatment, and, in this book, we cannot attempt to offer anything like a do-it-yourself sex therapy program. However, for the sake of general information, we can at least describe some of the physical exercises that therapists recommend for nonorgasmic women.

The first of these exercises consists simply of touching and stroking the body in a relaxed and nondemanding way. This allows the couple to discover their erogenous zones and to feel sensual pleasure without any pressure to perform. When pleasuring each other in this fashion, the partners can gently guide each other's hands in order to increase their enjoyment. In addition, they are often encouraged to use some massaging oil or body lotion which may help the woman overcome her fear of sex as "wet" and "messy."

After a few days of these exercises, the couple can begin to concentrate on stimulating the female sex organs. The best way to do this is for the man to sit directly behind the woman who spreads her legs by throwing them over his thighs. This position enables the man to hold the woman reassuringly close while he manipulates her breasts and her vulva. The woman, in turn, can guide the man's hands to those areas of her body that give her the greatest pleasure. At the same time, she can teach him to avoid stroking the sensitive glans of her clitoris directly and to caress instead the general area of the clitoris and the minor lips (labia minora). As she becomes sexually excited, her vagina begins to lubricate naturally, and this lubrication can then be spread to the clitoral area to reduce the possibility of irritation. Both partners are warned, however, not to strive for orgasm. Instead, they are encouraged to relish their sexual feelings and to abandon themselves to the pleasures of the moment.

Once the partners have learned to perform and enjoy these simple exercises, they are ready for the next step: coitus in the female-superior position. That is to say, while the man lies passively on his back, the woman straddles him and then lowers herself on his erect penis. However, once it has entered her vagina, she remains motionless in order to get used to the feeling. A few minutes later she begins to move very slowly without any particular aim other than simple enjoyment. Eventually, the man may respond to her movements with some slow pelvic thrusting of his own. Still, both partners are asked not to aim for orgasm but to enjoy the stimulation for its own sake. If orgasm does occur, it should be regarded as a pleasant surprise.

It is often useful for a couple to interrupt this kind of coitus when it becomes too demanding and to relax again in each other's arms. Some simple pleasuring can then lead to new arousal and to a new insertion of the penis. Finally, when both the man and the woman have learned to control their sexual impatience and are comfortable with each other's sexual responses, they can try coitus in a side-by-side position. The change from the female-superior position is easy; the man remains lying on his back, raising one knee. The woman stretches out on top of him with one leg between his legs. Then both partners roll slightly over to one side.

If all of these exercises are done properly, they sooner or later free the woman from her inhibitions and thus allow her to reach orgasm. Nevertheless, there are some cases that may require additional therapy. For example, sometimes the female sexual response during coitus is impaired by a wide and slack vaginal entrance. In other words, the muscles inside the woman's body which surround the vagina are in such poor condition that there is not enough friction between the penis and the vaginal walls. Indeed, neither of the partners may even feel very distinctly whether the insertion has taken place or not.

The main muscle that needs to be strengthened in this case is called the pubococcygeus. It can be described as the master sphincter of the entire pelvic area, and it runs from the pubic bone in the front all the way to the coccyx, or end of the spine, in the back. A few decades ago, a gynecologist by the name of Arnold H. Kegel developed some exercises for this particular muscle which can be practiced by any woman at any time anywhere. Naturally, first she must learn how to identify the muscle for herself. In order to do this, she is advised to sit on the toilet with her legs spread as far apart as possible. If she then starts and stops the flow of urine, she becomes aware of the pubococcygeus because it is the only muscle that can stop urine under this circumstance. Once the muscle is identified, the woman can practice contracting it repeatedly whenever she has the time. She simply flexes this muscle ten times in a row three to five times a day until it is firm. As a result, coitus becomes much more enjoyable for both partners because the contact between penis and vagina is closer. While it is true that the vaginal walls themselves contain hardly any nerve endings and therefore no feeling, the muscles surrounding the vaginal barrel do contain nerve endings, and, if these muscles are firm, their stimulation can be felt and enjoyed. In any case, the ability to control her vaginal muscles is bound to be welcomed by any woman who wants to make the most of her sexual relationships.

Still another way in which a woman can increase her sexual responsiveness involves the use of an electric vibrator. There are basically three types

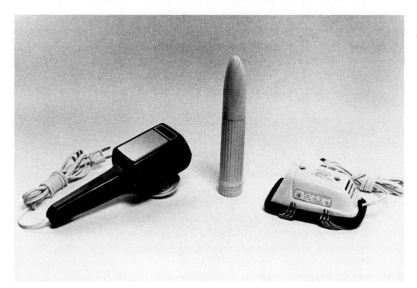

THREE COMMON TYPES OF ELECTRIC VIBRATORS
(The one in the middle is battery-operated)

of such vibrators available in drugstores and large department stores. The best known is perhaps the battery-operated, penis-shaped model that sells for about five dollars. However, it is also the one that is least effective. More useful is a model that consists of a small electric motor encased in plastic which is held in the hand, and which has a vibrating rubber cup. It costs between ten and twenty dollars. Finally, there are some rather expensive models, priced between fifteen and sixty dollars, which consist of a small motor that is held on the back of the hand with an elastic strap. The motor's vibrations are thus transmitted through the hand itself.

The woman or her sexual partner places the vibrator (or the vibrating hand) over those areas near her vaginal opening or her clitoris where it causes the greatest pleasure. As a result, she usually becomes aroused and reaches orgasm very quickly. It is important, however, that the vibrator be removed soon thereafter because otherwise the woman may become insensitive to its use. Women who decide to use a vibrator should also remember that it cannot be guaranteed to produce an orgasm every time. Still, if the woman is relaxed enough, it is often remarkably effective.

COMPULSIVE AND DESTRUCTIVE BEHAVIOR

History knows of some human cultures which accepted nearly all forms of sexual behavior as divinely inspired and therefore natural. These cultures were not necessarily liberal or permissive in the modern sense, but they had room for many different erotic tastes. Individuals were usually left alone to pursue their personal sexual interests and were punished only when they violated the rights of others.

However, our own Judeo-Christian culture is built on quite another tradition. The ancient Israelites as well as the early and medieval Christians believed that the only natural purpose of sex was procreation, and therefore they were extremely intolerant of any nonprocreative sexual activity. For example, the Bible reports that in Israel male homosexual intercourse and sexual contact with animals were punished by death, a custom which survived for more than a thousand years in Christian Europe. Even today, many states in the United States continue to treat these harmless behaviors as crimes.

The traditional Christian doctrine was summarized in the 13th century by the theologian Thomas Aquinas who declared that God allowed sexual intercourse only

- for the right purpose (i.e., procreation),
- with the right person (i.e., the marriage partner), and
- in the right way (i.e., by means of coitus).

Any sexual activity that did not meet this triple standard was "unnatural" and sinful.

In modern times, when the church lost much of its influence to the state, theologians were replaced by psychiatrists as the new experts on sexual behavior, but the old doctrine persisted. It was merely translated from religious into medical language. What once had been called unnatural was now described as unhealthy, and sin became sickness. In the 19th century, psychiatrists introduced the concept of "sexual psychopathology" (i.e., sexual sickness of the mind) and began to speak of sexual "deviations," "aberrations," and "perversions."

Obviously, the terms "deviation," "aberration," and "perversion" imply the violation of some undisputed norm, a wandering from the correct course, a turning away from the proper path, a corruption of what is right. Indeed, centuries before they were introduced into psychiatry, all three of these words had already been used by Christian moralists to denounce heresy and disbelief. It is hardly surprising, therefore, that the new sexual deviations, aberrations, and perversions turned out to be the same sexual heresies that had already been condemned in the Middle Ages. Even for modern psychiatrists the sexual norm was still the "right" kind of coitus with the "right" person. Every other form of human sexual expression was termed pathological and perverted. However, if there was no difference in substance, there was a difference in style. The various "psychopathologies" and "perversions" were now methodically listed and categorized under fanciful new names, and this gave the whole enterprise an aura of scientific objectivity. The following abbreviated catalogue may serve as an illustration.

Just as before, people could deviate from the norm of "approved" coitus mainly in two ways:

1. By choosing the "wrong" sexual object.
2. By choosing the "wrong" sexual activity.

For example, a male was sexually "perverted" if, instead of choosing a nonrelated female of his own age, he chose

- himself (autoeroticism),
- another male (homosexuality),
- two or more females at the same time (troilism),
- a close relative (incest),
- a child (pedophilia)
- an old woman (gerontophilia),
- an animal (zoophilia or bestiality),
- a dead body (necrophilia),
- a statue (pygmalionism),
- an inanimate object (fetishism).

Needless to say, these "perversions" became aggravated when they appeared in combination, as for instance when a young man chose a boy (homosexual pedophilia), or when he chose the dead body of an old woman (gerontophilic necrophilia). However, even if a man chose the "right" sexual object, he could still prove to be perverted if, instead of engaging in simple coitus, he derived his sexual satisfaction mainly from

- observing nudity and sexual activity in others (voyeurism),
- exposing his own sex organs (exhibitionism),
- rubbing his body against that of his partner (frottage),
- engaging in oral intercourse (oralism),
- engaging in anal intercourse (analism),
- hurting or humiliating his partner (sadism),
- being hurt or humiliated by his partner (masochism),
- wearing clothes of the other sex (transvestism),
- stealing something (kleptolagnia),
- setting fires (pyrolagnia),
- playing with his own or his partner's urine (urolagnia),
- playing with his own or his partner's excrement (coprophilia).

Again, these perversions were aggravated in combination, as for instance when someone preferred anal intercourse while inflicting pain on his partner (sadistic analism), or when he liked to be insulted while playing with his partner's urine (masochistic urolagnia).

By the same token, the height of sexual perversion was reached when someone preferred the "wrong" sexual activity with the "wrong" sexual object. This was the case, for example, when a man engaged in oral intercourse with several women at the same time (oralistic troilism), or when he masturbated into the soiled diapers of his baby sister (coprophilic incestuous pedophilic fetishism). Finally, all of these perversions and possible combinations of perversions could be rendered even more serious by an "excessive" sexual urge, called "satyriasis," in males and "nymphomania" in females, or "erotomania" in both sexes.

As we have already mentioned, the above catalogue or system of perversions is by no means complete. Different psychiatrists usually had different lists of their own, and these were often much more extensive. Moreover, their terminology was not always consistent and uniform. Thus, "homosexuality" was sometimes also called "contrasexualism," or "psychosexual hermaphroditism," or "uranism," or "inversion." Sometimes a distinction was made between male and female homosexuality, the former being called "pederasty" and the latter "sapphism," or "tribadism." On the other hand, some psychiatrists disapproved of too many distinctions. Consequently, they did not recognize certain special perversions, such as "pygmalionism" or "transvestism," but simply subsumed them under the more comprehensive term "fetishism." After all, as they pointed out, statues and clothing are inanimate objects and therefore "fetishes."

It must further be noted that not all perversions were considered equally bad. For example, "fetishism" was more easily tolerated than "homosexuality" which, in turn, was more acceptable than "incest." However, there was never a lasting consensus as to what constituted the worst perversion, i.e., the most frightful sexual psychopathology. At times, "autoeroticism" was seen as the greatest evil; at other times, "troilism" generated the strongest disgust. One day, "exhibitionism" seemed the most dangerous affliction; the day after that "analism" was regarded as the ultimate sexual depravity. And then, of course, there were those perversions that directly harmed other people, such as "pedophilia" (child molestation), "sadism" (lust murder), "kleptolagnia" (theft), and "pyrolagnia" (arson).

Still, whatever the level of his pathology or its potential for harming others, it was mainly the "pervert" who needed professional help. Indeed, this view followed logically from the very concept of perversion as a sickness. If perverts were sick, they could not really be held responsible for their actions. The proper social response to "abnormal" sexual behavior was therefore not moral condemnation or criminal punishment, but medical treatment.

On the other hand, as soon became clear, almost everyone suffered from some form of perversion, if only to a very moderate extent. Millions of men and women masturbated or fantasized about sexual orgies. Countless people had homosexual impulses or incestuous wishes, and a great number treasured some love letter, hair, handkerchief, or piece of clothing obtained from a beloved person. Many also enjoyed looking at nudity or displaying their own bodies, became aggressive or submissive in their sexual encounters, were fascinated by bathrooms, and loved "dirty" words.

These observations finally suggested that sexual perversions were not bizarre special diseases, but rather exaggerations of "normal" tendencies, i.e., matters of degree. Therefore, more and more psychiatrists came to believe that only exclusive or nearly exclusive wrong sexual choices deserved to be called perverse. Someone who chose the wrong sexual object or activity only occasionally, and who otherwise remained capable of enjoying "healthy" coitus, was not a true pervert. As a matter of fact, some psychiatrists demanded a drastic reduction of the old catalogue claiming that, even in their exclusive forms, such behaviors as "autoeroticism," "homosexuality," "troilism," "gerontophilia," "oralism," "analism," and "transvestism" were not perversions at all. They could perhaps be described as narrow personal habits, but they were clearly outside the province of medicine.

At any rate, in the course of time it was understood that the so-called sexual deviations, aberrations, or perversions were a rather mixed assortment. There were rare and outlandish as well as very common behaviors, blindly compulsive as well as deliberate, harmless as well as dangerous activities, and people began to wonder whether it was really justified to lump them together. Moreover, the notion that they all represented different "psychopathologies" or illnesses seemed increasingly questionable. In short, most critical observers soon felt the need for a thorough theoretical reassessment.

This reassessment was provided by Sigmund Freud with his psychoanalytic theory. Freud described the sexual perversions as manifestations of a "fixated" or arrested "psychosexual development." That is to say, in his view children were born with a powerful sexual instinct, but could not yet give it normal expression. Instead, they were all "polymorphous perverts" (literally, multiform perverts, or perverts of various shapes or stages). Their eventual proper sexual behavior was the result of a gradual, largely unconscious psychological process. However, an interference with this process could lead to a "fixation,' and thus the later adult behavior remained immature, i.e., "perverse." (Also see the introduction to "The Development of Sexual Behavior.")

The psychoanalytic view, although originally controversial, gained wide acceptance within a few decades and had a considerable influence on child-rearing practices in Europe and America. Still, many sex researchers also continued to voice their doubts. To them, the whole notion of a "correct" sexual urge which could be "perverted" seemed unscientific and presumptuous. Thus, when in the 1940s and 1950s Alfred C. Kinsey and his associates presented their massive findings on human sexual behavior, they found no use for the concept of perversion at all. In the meantime, Kinsey's sober approach has been followed by many others, and among most American scientists today the words "sexual perversion," "aberration," and "deviation" have fallen into disrepute. There is some discussion of "sexual deviance," but the implications of this term are quite different. (For details, see "Conformity and Deviance.")

Of course, by adopting a more objective and less dogmatic attitude, modern sex researchers do not mean to imply that all sexual norms or standards should be thrown overboard. When it comes down to cases, there is, in fact, considerable agreement that some forms of sexual behavior give cause for concern. This applies especially to behavior that is

- compulsive,
- destructive,
- exclusive, or
- distressing to the individual.

Clearly, any sexual activity that distresses those who engage in it deserves to be changed. Narrow, rigid, and exclusive behavior patterns which prevent people from fully enjoying themselves cannot be considered ideal. Destructive behavior, quite apart from its subjective effects, can become harmful to other people and must therefore be stopped. Sexual compulsions, even if they harm no one else, lead to unhappiness and frustration.

In many of these cases, the negative behavior can be changed or at least improved by some form of psychotherapy. However, in order to succeed, such therapy must be based on the voluntary consent, or even better, the expressed desire of the maladjusted person. In this area, there is little to be hoped from involuntary treatment. Moreover, any involuntary modification of human behavior raises the most serious ethical questions. Except in truly extraordinary and extreme cases, it does not seem morally justified.

Another question is the criminal prosecution and punishment of destructive behavior which has harmed unwilling victims. Legal protection against sexual assault in all its forms is one of the elementary duties of government. (Whether convicted offenders can or should be treated by psychiatrists is a complex issue beyond the scope of this book.)

By the same token, unconventional sexual behavior without clearly identifiable complaining victims should not be criminalized. Persons with otherwise harmless specialized sexual interests can reasonably demand to be left alone by the police. Their persecution is unfair and ill-advised. (For details, see "The Sexually Oppressed.")

SOME EXAMPLES OF COMPULSIVE AND DESTRUCTIVE SEXUAL BEHAVIOR

Human sexual activity does not always bring joy and happiness. Indeed, in many people sexual urges turn into outright compulsions, and in some cases they lead to brutality and violence.

Compulsive sexual behavior, like any other compulsive behavior, is, by definition, distressing and ultimately unsatisfying to the individual. Destructive or socially harmful behavior obviously calls for criminal punishment. There is no question, therefore, that both kinds of behavior are undesirable.

Sexual compulsions can take many forms, and so can sexual aggression. It is debatable whether all of these forms should be differentiated and listed under separate labels as "perversions" or "sexual psychopathologies." At any rate, in recent years such psychiatric labeling has become increasingly cautious. Nevertheless, some of the traditional labels are still widely used today, and since they can simplify the discussion, it seems appropriate here to offer a few examples.

Exhibitionism

Exhibitionism (from Latin *exhibere*: to present, to offer) means the unwelcome exposure of the sex organs to others, usually strangers, in order to obtain some sexual or emotional satisfaction. This behavior is quite often compulsive. Most exhibitionists are males.

It seems that exhibitionists are often sexually timid or unsatisfied. By their actions they try to provoke surprise, shock, or disgust, which gives them some relief from their psychological tension. By the same token, a calm reaction or ridicule leaves them frustrated and humiliated. As a rule, they do not attack or even come close to their "victims," but flee immediately after the exposure. Some may become highly aroused and then masturbate.

The causes of exhibitionism are not clear. It is known that some senile and mentally retarded persons expose themselves. The behavior may also occur as a result of certain brain diseases. It is further known that some animals expose their sex organs in a gesture of warning or aggression. Among otherwise healthy human beings, however, exhibitionism often seems tied to some psychological conflict or faulty learning.

While exhibitionism may not be as dangerous as was once believed, there is no question that it remains an unacceptable nuisance and cannot be tolerated in a civilized society.

Voyeurism

The term "voyeurism" (from French *voir*: to see) refers to the compulsive observation of nudity or sexual activity. The "victims" are usually unaware that they are being watched, and, when they suddenly realize it, they are understandably upset. The "voyeur" or "Peeping Tom," on the other hand, is often a sexually frustrated individual who feels too inadequate to establish a regular sexual relationship. His "peeping" provides him with some substitute for complete fulfillment. However, he may sometimes be helped to break with his confining and risky habit by some form of psychotherapy.

Voyeurism may not be the worst sexual crime, but since it constitutes an intolerable invasion of privacy, it is properly prohibited.

Transvestism

In the past, the term "transvestism" (from Latin *trans*: across and *vestis*: dress) was used very broadly for all cases of gender cross-dressing. In other words, every man and every woman who habitually wore clothing of the opposite sex was called a transvestite. Sometimes the word was also used for anyone who preferred to disguise himself in some fashion during sexual intercourse or whose sexual excitement depended on assuming some strange role, such as that of a baby, a toy, or an animal.

However, in recent years the word "transvestite" has been used more restrictively only for those persons who find sexual stimulation in cross-dressing, a condition which has also been called "fetishistic cross-dressing." This transvestism is more common among males than among females. Contrary to popular belief, most transvestites are heterosexual in orientation. Many of them are, in fact, married and pursue their sexual interest at home with the consent of their spouse. There are some male and female homosexuals who like to wear "drag" (i.e., clothing of the opposite sex). However, many of them do not depend on it for sexual excitement, and thus it is inappropriate to call them transvestites in the above sense.

The same applies to certain male entertainers who work as female impersonators. They may neither have a fetishistic attachment to their dresses nor be homosexual in orientation. Instead, they may simply find it rewarding to play a feminine role. (See introduction to "The Development of Sexual Behavior.")

Finally, there are some men and women who identify completely with a gender role inappropriate to their biological sex. In their case, the very term "cross-dressing" would be misleading because they dress according to their honest self-perception, even if it is contradicted by their anatomy. These persons are not transvestites, but transsexuals. (For details, see "Transsexualism.")

Pedophilia

Pedophilia (from the Greek *pais*: boy or child and *philein*: to love) in the strict sense is the psychological inability of adults to have sexual relationships with other adults and their resulting urge to seek such relationships with children. Obviously, by no means all adults who have sexual contact with children can be called pedophiles in this sense.

In some rare cases, pedophiles are inconsiderate or even violent, but most often they are fairly gentle, highly moralistic people who suffer from loneliness or a loss of self-esteem. In many cases, they are well known to the children as grandparents, uncles, neighbors, or friends of the family. The children, in turn, may not always feel molested, but may be willing and active participants. Most pedophiles are heterosexual in orientation. Among homosexuals, pedophilia is rare.

The issue of sexual contact between adults and children is a difficult one, and in the United States it is further complicated by the divergent legal definitions of the "age of consent" in state penal codes. In some states, this age is unreasonably high, and thus some people may be declared to be pedophiles or child molesters who would not have any problem in another state or another country. A person who seeks out sexually mature adolescents should never be called a pedophile. This term is appropriate only if the preferred sex objects are children who have not yet reached puberty.

Children are of course, expecially vulnerable to sexual exploitation. Persons who compulsively make sexual advances to children must therefore be restrained, if necessary by force. Sexual assault on children must be punished as a serious violent crime. In some cases, some form of psychotherapy may be helpful in rehabilitating the offender.

Sadism and Masochism

The term "sadism" (after the 18th-century French writer de Sade) refers to the tendency of some people to hurt or humiliate their sexual partners. The term "masochism" (after the 19th-century Austrian writer von Sacher-Masoch) denotes the reverse—a desire to be hurt or humiliated by one's sexual partner. There is also a single term "sadomasochism" (s/m for short) which refers to both sexual attitudes.

As mentioned earlier, to a certain extent such attitudes are quite common. They may even have some biological basis, since it is well known that the mating of certain animals is quite violent or even ends with the death of one of the partners. Still, among human beings strong sadistic or masochistic urges must be considered unusual, and they can very well become rather unsettling for those who feel them. Needless to say, sadism can also be socially harmful because in some instances it may lead to sexual assault or even murder.

However, professionals today usually make a distinction between forced and consensual acts of sadomasochism. It is not uncommon for either heterosexual or homosexual couples to form sadomasochistic relationships, with one partner inflicting pain and abuse on the fully consenting other. Indeed, sometimes it is the masochist who provokes and controls the sadism of his partner. At any rate, such voluntary relationships can become very finely tuned and quite close. In these cases, no outside interference, either legal or psychiatric, seems warranted.

However, there can be no argument that involuntary victims of sadism deserve every protection. Any form of sadistic assault on ordinary men and women who abhor such practices must therefore be promptly punished by the state.

Rape

Rape (from Latin *rapere:* to seize) is serious sexual assault or sexual intercourse against the will and over the objections of the partner. It is usually accompanied by force or the threat of force. Rape is not so much a sexual act as an act of hostility and aggression.

From the psychological point of view, the specific form of the assault makes little difference. More important is its severity. Thus, unlike lawyers, psychologists and psychiatrists regard not only forced coitus as rape, but also all forced manual, oral, and anal intercourse. Therefore, according to this usage, both females and males can be raped. (The rape of males occurs particularly often in prison.)

Some rapists have a sadistic streak, but often they are just brutish and insensitive individuals with delinquent or criminal backgrounds. Some rapists are seriously disturbed, but a few may also be rather normal people who act on a sudden impulse or misjudge the reactions of their partners.

It follows from these observations that, as a group, rapists do not present a uniform picture. The problem of their possible psychiatric treatment is therefore complex. Seen from a criminological standpoint, rape is essentially a crime of violence which demands swift and severe punishment.

TRANSSEXUALISM

As we have pointed out earlier in this book, human sexual development has at least three major aspects: biological sex, gender role, and sexual orientation. (See "The Development of Sexual Behavior.") We have also mentioned that some individuals may totally identify with a gender role that contradicts their biological sex. In other words, there are persons with male bodies who consider themselves females, and there are persons with female bodies who consider themselves males. Particularly after puberty, such people become very uncomfortable with their anatomical appearance and therefore try everything in their power (including a "sex change" operation) to make the body conform to their self-image. Their condition is called transsexualism (from Latin *trans*: across and *sexualis*: sexual).

The causes of transsexualism are not yet fully understood. We only know that gender roles are established at a very early age and that, after a certain critical time has passed, a person's sexual self-identification is irreversible. Thus, a hermaphroditic boy whose sex is misdiagnosed at birth may be brought up as a girl by his parents. When they finally discover their error, it may be too late to correct it, and the boy may continue to consider himself female. Unfortunately, there are also some rare cases where parents simply refuse to accept the biological sex of their child. (One example is the mother who deliberately forces her infant daughter into the role of the son she had

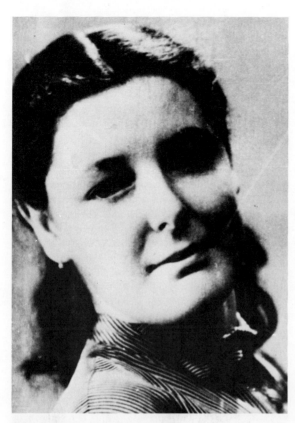
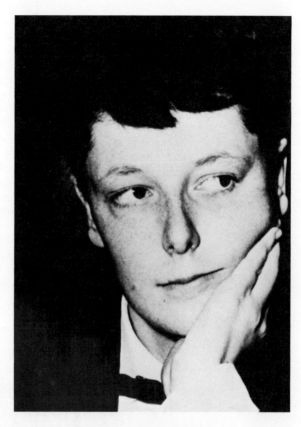

TWO CASES OF TRANSSEXUALISM

From Female to Male *Annie M. on her sixteenth birthday (left) and four years later after a "sex change operation" (right).*

From Male to Female *The English writer James Morris (left) became Jan Morris (right), remaining equally successful after a "sex change operation".*

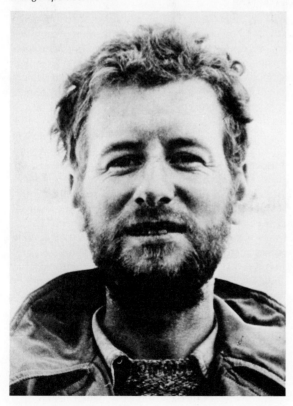
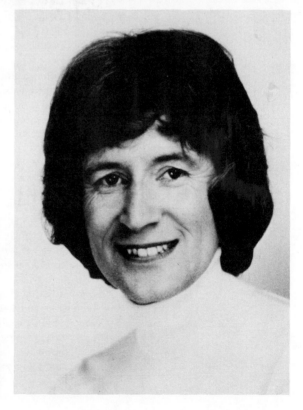

really wanted.) However, in other cases children seem to adopt an inappropriate gender role all on their own and in open defiance of clear parental suggestions. In view of these facts, many sex researchers today believe that transsexualism may be caused by a combination of biological and social factors, and that some children may develop a transsexual disposition even before they are born.

As far as we know, transsexualism is as old as mankind itself, although transsexuals have been treated very differently in different cultures and historical periods. In ancient times a sex change was often seen as a religious mystery which inspired respect and awe. An ancient Greek myth, for example, tells of the blind prophet Teiresias who, as a young man, was miraculously changed into a woman and then, several years later, back into a man. Thus, he knew the sexual response of both males and females from personal experience, a fact which added to his authority. We also know that in some societies of the past (including some American Indian tribes) certain males were allowed or even encouraged to adopt a feminine gender role and live as "shamans," "alyhas," or "berdaches." They wore female clothes, married some great warrior or other important man in the community, and took care of his household. Very often they also enjoyed great prestige themselves because they were believed to possess magical powers. (Obviously, this social arrangement provided a convenient outlet not only for transsexuals, but also for other sexual minorities, such as hermaphrodites, transvestites, and effeminate homosexuals. More virile homosexuals, on the other hand, could find sexual fulfillment within their masculine role by marrying a berdache.)

The sexually intolerant modern Western societies have never offered a comparable simple solution. On the contrary, our Judeo-Christian culture has always been characterized by the fanatical oppression and persecution of sexual deviants, and thus, for a very long time, the approach to transsexualism was also mostly punitive. However, it is now recognized that verbal threats, criminal sanctions, physical force, and electroshock or aversion therapies can do nothing to change the condition.

Today, many professionals feel that transsexuals should be helped to achieve, or at least approach, their goal. Or, as a distinguished physician once put it: "If the mind cannot be changed to fit the body, then perhaps we should consider changing the body to fit the mind." Modern hormone therapy and new surgical techniques have now made it possible to alter a person's anatomical appearance considerably. Thus, with hormonal treatment and a so-called "sex change operation," a man may acquire so many female physical characteristics (including breasts and an artificial vagina) that he can generally pass for a woman. (To a lesser extent, the reverse is also possible. Still, it is easier for a surgeon to construct a vagina in a male than a penis in a female.) There are now a number of gender identity clinics in various parts of the country where transsexuals can find help. These clinics are usually associated with a university or a medical school. However, in recent years many private physicians and surgeons have also begun to specialize in this field. (In the last six years about 500 persons have undergone "sex change" surgery in America, and several hundred more have applied for it.)

The "sex change" itself may extend over several years. It begins with hormone therapy (reversible) and eventually leads to the operation (i.e., irreversible corrective surgery). Even after surgery, the patient is usually asked to appear periodically for follow-up interviews in which the therapeutic results and the adjustment to the new life-style can be discussed.

Professional advice and assistance are important every step of the way. For instance, transsexuals who are being prepared for their sex reassignment surgery will, at some point, have to start wearing the clothing of their new sex. Unfortunately, in some parts of the country they may thereby violate certain state laws or local ordinances against cross-dressing. Sometimes, a special letter from the physician attesting to the treatment can ease the problem. Many county departments of medical services (mental health division) and state departments of health (bureau of special health services) also confirm such treatment on official letterhead. Once the treatment is completed, many other legal details still have to be worked out. Among other things, the "new" man or woman may need a new name, birth certificate, driver's license, social security card, and passport. In some cases, relocation and vocational rehabilitation may also be necessary. In countries outside the United States, especially in Europe, sex changes are often denied recognition by the law. The results of this official cruelty for the transsexual are devastating. It can only be hoped that the legislatures and judges in these countries will soon be better educated in regard to this problem.

Readers who want more practical information on these and other aspects of transsexualism may contact the Erickson Educational Foundation, 1627 Moreland Avenue, Baton Rouge, La. 70808. This nonprofit organization has published some useful pamphlets dealing with various problems confronting the transsexual. In addition, it keeps on file an extensive list of medical and other professionals involved in the treatment of transsexualism. Finally, the foundation also issues special ID cards for transsexuals undergoing treatment.

Reference and Recommended Reading

Annon, Jack S. *The Behavioral Treatment of Sexual Problems: Brief Therapy.* New York: Harper & Row, 1976.
———— *The Behavioral Treatment of Sexual Problems: Intensive Therapy.* Honolulu, Hawaii: Enabling Systems, 1975.
Belliveau, Fred, and Richter, Lin. *Understanding Human Sexual Inadequacy.* Boston: Little, Brown & Company, 1970 (cloth); New York: Bantam, 1970 (paper).
Benjamin, Harry. *The Transsexual Phenomenon.* 2nd ed., New York: Warner, 1977 (paper).
Feinbloom, Deborah. *Transvestites and Transsexuals.* New York: Delacorte Press, 1976 (cloth); New York: Dell, 1977 (paper).
Green, Richard, *Sexual Identity Conflict in Children and Adults,* New York 1974: Basic Books, 1974.
Hartman, William E., and Fithian, Marilyn A. *The Treatment of Sexual Dysfunction: A Bio-Psycho-Social Approach.* Long Beach, CA.: Center for Marital and Sexual Studies, 1972.
Kaplan, Helen Singer. *The Illustrated Manual of Sex Therapy.* New York: Quadrangle, 1975 (cloth); New York: A & W Visual Library, 1976 (paper).
Masters, William E., and Johnson, Virginia. *The Pleasure Bond.* Boston: Little, Brown & Company, 1975 (cloth); New York: Bantam, 1976 (paper).
Morris, Jan. *Conundrum.* New York: Harcourt Brace Jovanovich, 1974 (cloth); New York: New American Library, 1975 (paper).
The National Sex Forum. *SAR Guide for a Better Sex Life.* San Francisco, CA: The National Sex Forum, 1975.
Stoller, Robert J. *Sex and Gender, Volume II: The Transsexual Experience.* New York: Aronson, 1976.

SEX AND SOCIETY

Human beings are "social animals," and their habits, desires, hopes, fears, and beliefs are shaped by the various societies into which they are born. This is also true of their sexual attitudes and behaviors. People are born with a certain potential for sexual expression, but this potential can be realized in a great variety of ways. Indeed, in sexually repressive societies it may well remain partially or completely unrealized.

The point is perhaps best illustrated with the often-used analogy of language: All children are born with the potential for speech, but they are not programmed for any particular language. In England, they will grow up to speak English, in China, Chinese. Some societies have different "secret" languages for males and females, and children will learn these too, according to their sex. Furthermore, if they have intelligent parents and good teachers, they may learn to speak exceptionally well. By the same token, harsh and ignorant parents may keep their children mute or inarticulate, or may cause them to stutter. On the other hand, some mistreated children may develop a "loose tongue" and use it to vent their hostility; others, who are more fortunate, may choose their words carefully to express only love and devotion. Finally, some people may voluntarily give up the pleasures of speech and, for some religious or moral reason, take a vow of silence.

Human sexual behavior develops in a very similar fashion. Children learn to adopt that behavior which is acceptable to their particular culture. They also acquire different masculine and feminine qualities according to their sex. If they have tolerant parents, their erotic capacities will grow, but a puritanical education will make them feel guilty and block or cripple their sexual responses. On the other hand, some frustrated children develop "loose morals" and use sex mainly to express their hostility; others, who are well satisfied, choose their sexual partners carefully and shower them with affection. Finally, some people decide to give up the pleasures of sex and, for some religious or moral reason, take a vow of chastity.

However, the comparison need not restrict itself to this individual level, i.e., to personal idiosyncrasies, failures, or successes. Human sexuality and language are also comparable on a general level and can be examined for their collective implications. After all, as every linguist knows, different languages express different basic philosophies. They paint different pictures of reality and reflect different approaches to life. In short, every language preforms the perceptions of those who grow up with it. Quite apart from specific personal opinions, large groups of people together learn to view the world differently according to their different "native tongues."

This is also true of "native" philosophies of sex. The sexual behavior of men and women reflects not only their personal tastes, but, to a large extent, also the basic values of the society or social group to which they belong. No matter how much they may differ as individuals, their moral sense is always shaped by the underlying assumptions of their whole culture. In hedonistic and tolerant cultures, most people are likely to be joyful and sensuous; in puritanical and repressive cultures, they tend to be anxious and inhibited. In the first case, they will celebrate sex as a source of happiness; in the second case, they will deplore and conceal it as a source of shame. Therefore, when we study the sexual attitudes of any individual, we are actually dealing with two separate sets of questions. We ask not only: "How well does this man or this woman conform to the sexual standards of his or her society?" but also: "What is the basis of these standards? What does this society believe about the ultimate purpose, or meaning, or 'nature' of sex?"

In most societies, of course, the meaning of sex, as the meaning of anything else, is revealed by religion. At least this has always been the case in societies of the past, and even in modern, secular societies the sexual standards often remain tied to older religious doctrines. There can be no doubt, for example, that the sexual standards of our own society are still influenced by our Judeo-Christian heritage. However, cross-cultural studies reveal that this heritage has always been highly peculiar. The ancient Israelites saw the nature of sex in reproduction and condemned any sexual behavior that did not promote this goal. The early Christians adopted this narrow view and even restricted it further by treating sex as a necessary evil and extolling the virtues of sexual abstinence. Since they expected the second coming of Christ and the end of the world in their lifetimes, they did not think very much of sexual pleasure. Instead, they became susceptible to the various ascetic philosophies of their time and incorporated them into their own religion. When Christ failed to return, and the world went on as before, they became a little more tolerant, but their basic belief did not change: Sexual activity was acceptable only when it could lead to pregnancy within marriage, and even then it was something of an embarrassment.

Needless to say, the Christian sexual philosophy did not seem arbitrary or accidental to its proponents. On the contrary, to them it appeared as the objective, eternal, and universal truth. Indeed, wherever they looked, they found this truth confirmed by factual observations. Did not respectable men and women cover their bodies with clothing, and did this not prove that they had an "inborn sense of modesty?" Did not people avoid discussing their sexual fantasies openly, and did this not prove that they felt uneasy about them? Did not parents hide the intimate side of their marriage from their children, and did this not prove that there was something wrong with sexual intercourse? In short, did not nature itself demonstrate everywhere that sex was inherently base and humiliating? Thus, the North African bishop and "church father" Augustine wrote dogmatically of the "shame which attends all sexual intercourse" in his book *The City of God* (Book XIV, Chapter 18):

> Sexual intercourse is always performed with lust and therefore needs to be hidden. . . . Indeed a natural sense of shame ensures that secrecy is provided even in brothels. . . . Fornication is called shameful even by shameless men, and though they are fond of it, they dare not display it. . . . Even conjugal intercourse, respectable and legitimate though it be, does it not always require a private room and the exclusion of witnesses? Before the bridegroom caresses his bride, does he not turn away all the attendants . . . and even those relatives that had been admitted to the bridal chamber? . . . And why so, if not because that which is by nature fitting and proper is so done as to be accompanied by the penalty of shame?

In accordance with this opinion, Augustine referred to the male and female sex organs as *obscoenae partes* (obscene parts) and viewed all "carnal" desire with barely concealed disgust. Moreover, he was convinced that all decent people everywhere felt the same way. Yet, in actual fact, his attitude was not universally shared even in his own time. There were still tribes in distant parts of the Roman empire who preserved their old "pagan" customs and delighted in group sex and various sexual displays. Thus, Augustine's statement about the "shame attending all sexual intercourse" was not really true. It was only much later, and only through Christian influence, that it became true for most Europeans. Outside of Europe, however, many societies developed very different sexual values. When, after centuries of isolation, Christian explorers finally discovered such societies, they were amazed and incredulous. For example, when Captain Cook came to Tahiti he was greatly surprised to find that the Tahitians had sexual intercourse in public and "gratified every appetite and passion before witnesses." Thus, he reported in his *Account of a Voyage Around the World* (1769):

> A young man, nearly six feet high, performed the rites of Venus with a little girl about 11 or 12 years of age, before several of our people and a great number of natives, without the least sense of its being indecent or improper, but, as appeared, in perfect conformity to the custom of the place. Among the spectators were several women of superior rank who . . . gave instructions to the girl how to perform her part, which, young as she was, she did not seem much to stand in need of.

In spite of his consternation, however, Captain Cook apparently kept his composure and did not try to stop the performance. After all, he was not a moral crusader, but a practical Englishman, a seasoned world traveler, and a son of the Age of Enlightenment. It was left to the Christian missionaries of a later time to become outraged and to eradicate the traditional island customs. Indeed, one can easily imagine the effect the sexual spectacle would have had on Augustine, had he been able to witness it. One can also assume that it would not have changed his opinion. Instead of admitting that he had been proven wrong by the "shameless" islanders, he would probably have condemned them all as slaves of the devil.

At any rate, we know only too well what would happen to the Tahitian performers if they appeared in the United States today. Any man who performed in a "live sex show" with an eleven-year-old girl would be sent to prison as a statutory rapist. Even worse, as a "child molester" or "pedophile," he could be declared a "sexual psychopath." This means that, before, after, or instead of serving his prison term, he could be committed to a mental hospital for forced psychiatric treatment. If he should ever be released, he would be required to register with the police for the rest of his life. The girl, on the other hand, would be regarded as a juvenile delinquent and could be sent to "reform school." Finally, the entire audience might be arrested for having witnessed, and thereby encouraged, an act of public "lewdness and obscenity."

As this example illustrates, the moral values of modern America differ profoundly from those of precolonial Tahiti. There, people were applauded as valuable members of the community, who are here considered criminal or insane. What Americans now abhor as the moral "corruption of minors," the Tahitians encouraged as practical sex education. What appears sinful to us, often had a religious purpose for them. As a matter of fact, they supported a special order of celebrants (the *Arioi* society) who were trained to give public sexual performances. In short, the Tahitians subscribed to a sexual philosophy that is nearly the opposite of our own.

Should we therefore jump to the conclusion that they were "decadent," "degenerate," "depraved," "morally bankrupt," "animalistic," "sick," or "perverted?" Obviously not. Such denunciations would be entirely inappropriate, because all of their visitors unanimously described the Tahitians as the happiest, healthiest, gentlest, friendliest, and most generous people on earth. Their decline began only after their contact with Western Christians, although even today they retain much of their original free-hearted spirit.

Should we then conclude, to the contrary, that our own standards are wrong, and should we try to adopt the sexual customs of ancient Tahiti? Not necessarily. First of all, a moment's reflection will show that a sudden, radical change of this kind is not feasible. Secondly, even if it could be accomplished, it might well create more social and sexual problems than it solves. Just as the Tahitians were not helped by the imposition of a foreign morality, so we ourselves could come to regret the blind acceptance of values that are foreign to us. In each society the sexual norms are embedded in a large network of other norms, laws, and traditions, all of which have been developed over long periods of time to support each other and to serve a multitude of social purposes. Changes in sexual behavior therefore always affect many other areas of life. It follows that no sexual revolution can do much good, if it makes no allowance for particular historical circumstances and ignores the complexity of cultural traditions.

Indeed, this is exactly what was wrong with the hasty Christianization of the Pacific islanders. A sexual morality that had worked well for them was abruptly replaced with another which hampered the education of their children, disturbed the traditional courtship and marriage patterns, and undermined the institution of the family as they knew it. Worst of all, none of these changes carried any demonstrable benefit. Therefore, the new morality at first demoralized large parts of the population. It loosened the whole social fabric and produced a lengthy period of confusion.

We could, of course, carry our comparative study of moralities still further, in depth as well as in breadth, but by now at least one fundamental insight should already have become clear: There is nothing universal or permanent about sexual norms. On the contrary, when compared cross-culturally, they appear rather capricious and variable. They may seem objective and wholesome to the specific societies which subscribe to them, but outsiders may find them absurd or corrupt. In sum, what, in sexual matters, people call "nature" is usually nothing more than convention.

Sensible men and women have always recognized this truth and acted accordingly. We have seen, for example, that Captain Cook in Tahiti calmly observed a sexual performance which would have provoked a riot and perhaps a lynching in his home country. As an enlightened explorer, he simply honored the sound adage: "When in Rome, do as the Romans do," i.e., respect local customs and do not offend your hosts! In return, this prescription was also followed by a handsome, young Tahitian, whom Cook later brought with him to England. This "noble savage" by the name of Omai conducted himself with great decorum, moved successfully in the highest social circles, and was much praised by the ladies. We can only guess at his sexual behavior, but we know that he did not give any cause for scandal, although this could perhaps be explained by the tolerant attitude of his aristocratic English admirers.

Actually, in this case, a major reason for the mutual respect between "heathen" and Christian was simply the timing of their encounter. Eighteenth-century England was no longer as prudish as it had once been under Puritan rule. (The Victorian 19th century is another matter.) The study of the Greek and Roman classics, various secular modern philosophies, and contact with distant foreign cultures had taught Europeans some religious and sexual tolerance. Indeed, reading reports like that by Captain Cook and meeting people like Omai led many of them to question their traditional moral assumptions and put them into a more liberal frame of mind. In France, Capitain Bougainville published his own account of a voyage to the Pacific, and the great encyclopedist Denis Diderot acclaimed the Polynesian sexual morality in his *Supplement to Bougainville's Voyage* (1796). Thus, gradually, the old rigid sexual attitudes softened in some Western countries. Moral values that had been accepted as absolute, began to be recognized as relative, and people began to criticize their inherited way of life. More and more of them decided to think for themselves and to pursue their own happiness in their own way. Resenting both church interference and government regulation, they demanded freedom from moral tutelage. The ideals of privacy and individual liberty won increasing support and, in the American and French revolutions, finally led to political and social reforms.

This is not to say that Western prudery was dead. Indeed, it was still very much alive in the middle and lower classes, and, as we have briefly mentioned, it regained a great deal of strength in the following century. Nevertheless, among the educated there remained an awareness of uninhibited non-Western sexual customs and, for that matter, of a certain pro-sexual Western tradition. After all, Augustine had never spoken for every one of his fellow Christians. Behind the official moral facade, there had also always been an older, native European sensuality. With the arrival of Christian asceticism, this sensuality had been disparaged, denied, and driven underground, but it had repeatedly surfaced in the Middle Ages at popular festivals, in Renaissance art and literature, in Baroque pomp and pageantry, in rural customs and urban fashions, in earthy folklore and aristocratic splendor, in theater, music, and dance. By the same token, in actual fact the sexual behavior of Westerners was never as joylessly disciplined as their official religious dogmas and secular laws might have suggested. Especially farmers and feudal lords had lived largely by their own, less repressive sexual standards. It was mostly the clergy, and in modern times the bourgeoisie, which insisted on temperance and austerity.

However, after the successful industrialization of the Western world, even the formerly straitlaced middle classes became more tolerant in sexual matters. As their material comfort increased, they realized that the political and economic freedom they had won was incomplete without sexual freedom. Thus, in this century, we have seen a growing trend of sexual liberalization. Drawing on the experiences of non-Western cultures and on Western libertarian traditions, a great many scholars, moralists, and ordinary citizens are today working for a new, humane world without sexual oppression.

For more than a century now, an important part of this work has been the scientific study of human sexual behavior and its social implications. By definition, sex research tends to promote a rational approach to sexual problems and thus combats sexual prejudice, ignorance, and fear. It is in this spirit that the following pages attempt to describe the current state of knowledge in various fields of study. Needless to say, it is not really possible, within the scope of the present book, to deal with all social issues related to sex, but one can gain at least some understanding of their complexity by making a few historical and cross-cultural observations. Therefore, this last part of the text offers a brief analysis of the modern fight for sexual equality, the problem of sexual deviance, recent changes in marriage and family patterns, the fate of the sexually oppressed, and the impact of the present so-called sexual revolution.

9. THE SOCIAL ROLES OF MEN AND WOMEN

In all societies the obvious biological difference between men and women is used as a justification for forcing them into different social roles which limit and shape their attitudes and behavior. That is to say, no society is content with the natural difference of sex, but each insists on adding to it a cultural difference of gender. The simple physical facts therefore always become associated with complex psychological qualities. It is not enough for a man to be male; he also has to appear masculine. A woman, in addition to being female, must also be feminine.

However, once the contrast between men and women has been increased and accentuated in this fashion, it is usually taken as a further manifestation of biological differences which confirm the need for different social roles. Or, to put it another way, sex differences are used to create gender differences which are then explained as sex differences which, in turn, require gender differences, and so on. This may be no more than circular reasoning, but it is socially very effective. For example, in our own patriarchal society males enjoy a socially dominant position. Thus, from an early age, boys are helped to acquire a masculinity that allows them to assume and maintain that position. By the same token, girls are taught to cultivate a submissive femininity. The resulting difference in the male and female character is then described as inborn and used to defend the existing power arrangement. Only those who accept it are normal, and only they can expect to succeed. The male social role is designed to reward masculine men, while the female social role offers its relative advantages only to feminine women. (The aggressive man will run the bigger business; the pretty, agreeable woman will find the richer husband.) In other words, masculinity and femininity are gender qualities which are developed in response to social discrimination. However, once they have been developed, they justify and cement it. The masculine and feminine gender roles mutually reinforce each other and thereby perpetuate the inequality on which they are based.

Obviously, this psychological mechanism can operate only as long as the behavior of men and women does not transgress the generally accepted limits. Every society tries therefore to prevent such transgressions by calling the socially defined gender roles "natural," eternal, and unchangeable. Any person who refuses to accept them is persecuted as a deviant and punished as an offender not only against society, but against "nature" itself. An historical example of such deviance is the case of Joan of Arc who, as a young girl, not only led the French army to victory over the English, but also wore male clothing. In her later trial she was promptly accused of having thus violated the laws of nature.

Over the centuries, many people have, of course, wondered why allegedly "natural" roles should need such rigorous social enforcement. After all, if they were truly natural, they would "come naturally" to both men and women. However, it is noteworthy that the advocates of the so-called natural inequality of the sexes resent nothing more than letting "nature" take its course. Yet, if their arguments were true, there would be no need to deny women equal opportunities, since they would be unable to compete with men. If women were "naturally" inferior, men would have nothing to fear. Therefore, the fact that many men do fear such competition raises sufficient doubt as to the validity of their claim.

The truth is that human desires and capacities have a tendency to go beyond the narrow limits of our traditional gender roles. Indeed, it takes a constant, combined effort by all social authorities to keep this tendency under control. Such social control appears not only externally, in the form of parental guidance, peer-group pressure, and law enforcement, but also internally in the form of concepts and values which determine the self-image of every individual, and it is in the individual mind where the confusion of sex and gender can create the most serious problems.

For instance, men and women who feel that they do not fit the masculine and feminine stereotypes, or who resent them as too restrictive, may also develop ambiguous feelings about their biological sex. They may begin to wish for different bodies which would allow them to play a role more to their liking. Or, to take another example, since men have been told that women are socially and sexually passive, they are usually gravely disturbed by encountering a woman who is socially aggressive and who takes the initiative in sexual intercourse. Confronted with this "lack of femininity" in a woman, a man may feel tempted to dispute her womanhood. If this contention does not hold up in face of the evidence, he may instead begin to doubt his own masculinity and become sexually dysfunctional. Conversely, a handsome, gentle, and passive male may invite ridicule and may be denounced as a "pervert" or "queer." "Real women" may regard him as less than a "real man" and therefore reject him as a sexual partner.

However, the confusion goes still further. The notion that in every sexual encounter there has to be one active (masculine) and one passive (feminine) partner is so persistent that it not only ruins many heterosexual relationships, but also influences the behavior of certain homosexuals who feel compelled to model themselves after these stereotypes. By doing so, they give support to the curious belief that even in sexual relationships between members of the same sex, there always has to be one to play the "man," while the other must assume the role of the "woman." There is, in fact, a general impression that every homosexual couple (whether male or female) consists of one active, masculine and one passive, feminine partner. People who hold this belief are, of course, at a total loss to explain phenomena like the famous homosexual élite troops of ancient Greece, which consisted entirely of male lovers.

All of these views are based on a wrong conclusion drawn from a false assumption. The false assumption states that women are naturally passive, while men are naturally active. The wrong conclusion asserts that every passive person is playing a feminine role and that every active person is playing a masculine role. However, in actual fact neither sex nor gender need be characterized in this fashion. After all, in some human societies the role assignment for men and women is the reverse of our own. In short, there is nothing "natural" or definite about our sexual stereotypes. By the same token, full human equality will not be achieved until it becomes conceivable to both sexes that active and passive attitudes can be appropriate for either of them, and that even two "active" or two "passive" partners can have a rewarding relationship.

This does not mean that, in an ideal future, all human differences will disappear. Indeed, once the old stereotypes have been discarded, the differences between individuals within each sex are likely to increase. Furthermore, under conditions of social equality, these individuals may also happily continue to play different gender roles. There should be no need to point out that there is nothing wrong with gender differences as such. They can greatly enrich our lives, as long as we understand that, in human beings, "different" does not have to mean superior or inferior. In other words, those who demand equal rights for men and women are not asking for drab uniformity, but for a social climate in which variety can flourish without being exploited.

The following pages first elaborate further on the basic concepts of sex and gender and then offer a brief discussion of the different moral standards for men and women. A final section deals with the women's movement and its struggle for sexual equality.

SEX AND GENDER

Earlier in this book, when discussing the development of human sexual behavior, we have distinguished between a person's

- **biological sex** (the male or female characteristics of the body),
- **gender role** (the social role as male or female), and
- **sexual orientation** (the preference for male or female sexual partners).

At the same time, we have also explained that the term "biological sex" refers to people's maleness or femaleness, that "gender role" refers to their masculinity or femininity, and that "sexual orientation" refers to their heterosexuality or homosexuality. In the present context, we will concentrate on the first two of these concepts as they apply to women. (For a detailed discussion of all three concepts see the introduction to "The Development of Sexual Behavior.")

In our initial discussion we have found that biological sex and gender role are not always in perfect agreement: A person can very well be male and feminine or female and masculine. Furthermore, we have seen that both biological sex and gender role are matters of degree: people are male or female to the degree that they meet certain physical criteria; people are masculine or feminine to the degree that their character and behavior fit certain cultural stereotypes. In determining people's biological sex, i.e., their maleness or femaleness, we examine their bodies; in determining people's gender role, i.e., their masculinity or femininity, we examine their attitudes and the way they express them.

Once we have understood the basic difference between the two concepts of biological sex and gender role, we have taken the first step towards understanding the complexity of being a man or a woman. However, this first step is by no means enough. If we really want to get a grip on the subject, we have to introduce still another distinction: that between "gender role" and "gender identity."

So far, we have defined "gender role" rather loosely as the male or female social role, i.e., as the way in which people show their masculinity or femininity. Now we have to admit that this is an oversimplification, because one can look at any social role from at least two different points of view: Role players can be judged according to how they appear to others and how they appear to themselves. After all, people can perform with or without conviction; they can identify or not identify with their roles.

This is also true of gender roles. For example, children with male bodies are expected to play the masculine role, and most often they will readily do so. However, it is entirely possible that, in some cases, this role playing remains a half-hearted, superficial performance and that, in spite of outward appearances, a male child secretly identifies with the feminine role. Indeed, in the long run this feminine self-identification may prove so strong that both the masculine behavior and the physical male characteristics are gladly abandoned in a so-called sex change. It may then become obvious that, from the beginning, the "boy" would have been better brought up as a girl. (See "Transsexualism".) Fortunately, such cases are rare, but they prove that the ultimate criterion for people's gender is neither their physical condition, nor their overt behavior, but only their self-identification. Therefore, when we talk about "gender," we should distinguish between two different aspects:

- **gender role** (the social role as male or female), and

- **gender identity** (the self-identification as male or female).

In most individuals, of course, gender role and gender identity coincide. Thus, for example, most women not only play a feminine role, but truly make it their own. They not only develop and display feminine qualities, but also consider them to be genuine expressions of their "real selves." Many of them may, of course, experience their femininity as crippling and confining, and they may try to broaden its definition, but that does not mean that they do not accept it in principle. They do identify with their roles and only want to see them expanded. Women with genuine gender identity problems are rare. Therefore, when we talk about social issues as they affect women in general, we can usually neglect the correlation between role and identity and simply concentrate on the broader concepts of sex and gender.

As we have seen, "sex" is a biological term, "gender" a psychological and cultural one. Sex is the basis on which gender is built. When babies are born, their sex is quickly determined by a look at their external sex organs, and immediately thereafter the development of their gender begins. At first, the assignment of gender may be demonstrated by nothing more than a male or female first name and a blue or pink blanket. However, soon different parental approaches, caresses, punishments, games, toys, clothes, hairstyles, books, furniture, jewelery, etc. begin to increase the gender differences between boys and girls. Relatives, friends, playmates, babysitters, nurses, and teachers then show that they take these differences for granted and, through their own example, reinforce them whenever they can. Thus, within the first few years of life, children learn not only to identify themselves as male or female, but also to adopt the "proper" masculine or feminine behavior. In short, well before human beings can exercise any rational choice or control in the matter, their gender (i.e. both gender identity and gender role) is "matched" to their sex and becomes permanently established. (For details see "The Development of Sexual Behavior, Infancy and Childhood.")

In theory, the difference between the two genders, need not create any problems and could even be a source of delight, but, as more and more people are beginning to realize, unfortunately in practice it is very often a reflection of injustice and inequality. Most societies, including our own, give females a lower status than males and have less respect for feminine than masculine qualities. Thus, for women, their gender becomes a mark of inferiority. Men, on the other hand, accurately perceive their masculinity as the guarantee of their dominant position. This means that gender also relates to the question of social power and powerlessness. Indeed, in the final analysis it reveals itself as essentially a political issue.

The modern feminist movement has, therefore, long emphasized the political education of women and their participation in public affairs. It has also fought to obtain the vote for women together with other political and legal rights, thereby hoping to change the prevailing power balance between the sexes. Moreover, feminists have also long argued that, once equal rights have been won, men and women will appear to be equal in many other ways. Certain sex differences will, of course, always remain, but the present gender differences may well become much less pronounced and important. Indeed, it would be interesting to see whether any of them would be left at all.

The basic biological facts are undisputed: Only women can bear and nurse children, and, on the average, men are bigger, stronger, and faster than women. Adult male bodies also contain a higher amount of androgen than adult female bodies. However, people are never content with observing these

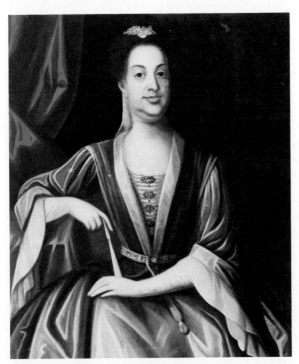
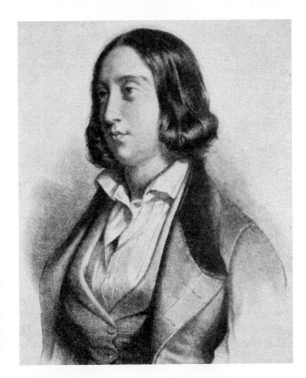

HISTORICAL EXAMPLES OF CROSS-DRESSING

The ancient Greek poet Homer reports that the great hero Achilles was brought up as a girl and wore female clothes until he joined the war against Troy. In addition to this and other legendary figures, however, we also know many historical personalities who wore the clothes of the opposite sex. Such examples of cross-dressing range from the pagan Roman emperor Heliogabalus (3rd century) to the Christian Abbé de Choisy (17th century) and from the peasant girl Joan of Arc (15th century) to Queen Christina of Sweden (17th century). It should not be assumed that all of these men and women had the same motivation for their behavior. It would certainly be an oversimplification to describe them summarily as "transvestites". Actually, some of them were probably transsexuals, and others simply enjoyed shocking their contemporaries or adopted their mode of dress for other, non-sexual reasons. Some also turned to cross-dressing only temporarily and then completely abandoned it.

(Above left) **Edward Hyde, Lord Cornbury** *Colonial Governor of New York and New Jersey. Biologically male, he enjoyed wearing female clothing and even appeared in public dressed as a woman. The official portrait shown here testifies to his lack of embarrassment and to the tolerance of his contemporaries.*

(Above right) **George Sand** *(Lucille Aurore Dupin) 19th-century French writer. Biologically female, she adopted a man's name and mode of dress. For a while she enjoyed the resulting notoriety and freedom, but eventually resumed a more conventional lifestyle.*

(Below) **The Chevalier d'Eon** *18th-century French diplomat and renowned swordfighter. His biological sex was male, but during his long career he switched back and forth several times between masculine and feminine gender roles, living sometimes as a man (left), at other times as a woman (right). However, he continued to display his fencing prowess in both gender roles.*

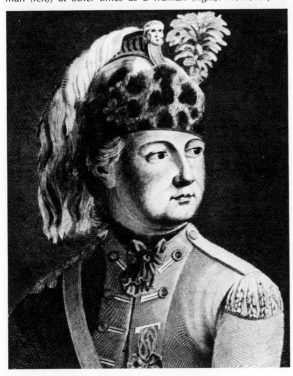
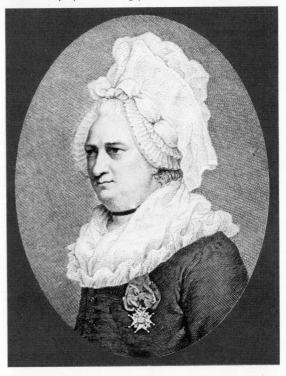

289

simple facts; they always jump to conclusions about their psychological meaning. Thus, in our society, the feminine character stands for passivity, submission, weakness, impulsiveness, and sentimentality, while the masculine character represents activity, aggression, strength, self-control, and rationality. Therefore, men are considered better at fighting, moving heavy equipment, lifting weights, solving technical problems, and abstract thinking; women are said to excel in raising and educating children, working with small, intricate tools, decorating, and communicating. These are all highly questionable generalizations, but even if we accept them as true, we have to realize that, at the present time, it is virtually impossible to say whether they reflect biological inheritance or social conditioning. In fact, males and females are treated differently from birth, and as long as this discrimination continues, their "unadulterated" character will remain a matter of conjecture.

At any rate, in the meantime anthropologists have found and described some societies where the masculine and feminine roles were nearly the reverse of our own, i.e., where women appeared as aggressive providers and men as docile homemakers. (See, for example, Margaret Mead's study *Sex and Temperament in Three Primitive Societies* [1933].) Furthermore, it has been observed that in many "underdeveloped" countries women function as water bearers and are expected to carry heavy burdens over long distances. Many of them also till the soil or catch fish under the "supervision" of men who reserve the easier tasks for themselves.

Ironically, it is not at all unusual for men to let their wives and daughters do all the hard work while claiming at the same time that women are the "weaker sex." Power relationships do not have to make logical sense, and they do not come to an end merely because they do not stand up to reason. After all, in ancient Rome wealthy citizens entrusted the education of their offspring to slaves whom they despised as inferiors, and in more recent times European absolute monarchs used men of "low birth" to help govern their countries and to demonstrate the superiority of aristocratic rule. From a strictly logical point of view it is difficult to justify the specifics of any gender role division or to explain its widespread acceptance. One can only register the fact that the division exists, and that it often implies the denigration and subjection of women.

Male privilege and female subjection, in turn, distort both the masculine and feminine characters. Many men develop a fanatical, anxious pride in their masculinity which colors and restricts nearly all of their actions. This unhealthy attitude, which to others appears both menacing and ridiculous, is perhaps best described with the Spanish word *machismo* (from *macho*: male). Women, on the other hand, have to live up to an unrealistic ideal of "pure womanhood" which robs them of all initiative and exposes them to the injustice of a sexual double standard.

THE DOUBLE STANDARD

The term "double standard" refers to the fact that we have different norms for the sexual behavior of men and women. That is to say, not only our own, but also most other human societies have long held females to a higher degree of sexual restraint than males. Girls and women have traditionally been severely restricted in their sexual opportunities in order to keep them "pure" and "innocent." Boys and men, on the other hand, have usually been encouraged to "sow their wild oats" as demanded by their "animal nature." By the same token, females have often been punished for the smallest sexual transgression, while males have enjoyed considerable sexual license.

Today the double standard operates largely through indirect social pressure, moral indoctrination, rules of etiquette, customs, manners, and taboos, but in the past it was directly and brutally enforced when men beat or even killed their wives, daughters, or sisters for "improper" sexual behavior. The law, which was made by men, also supported the male view and provided harsh penalties for female adultery and the loss of "virginity" before marriage. Male adulterers and seducers were punished only to the extent that they infringed upon the rights of other men. In other words, women were regarded as male property, i.e., they belonged to their fathers, husbands, or brothers. Thus, if adultery and seduction diminished a woman's value, her master had to be compensated for the damage. For example, in ancient Israel the seducer of a girl had to pay her father "money according to the dowry of virgins" (Exodus 22;17), and even in 19th century England a husband could still legally demand some financial restitution from the seducer of his wife.

Obviously, then, the double standard involves more than questions of sexual morality, but points to a more fundamental issue. This issue has recently been redefined as "sexism", i.e., an attitude or a philosophy that uses a person's sex as the basis for all sorts of social discrimination. More specifically, modern fighters for women's rights have used the term "male chauvinism" (after a French super-patriot named Chauvin) to describe the fanatical and unreasonable insistence on male privilege.

Unfortunately, male privilege has a long history and is still firmly embedded in all our social institutions. As we have seen, the double standard for sexual behavior originally reflected the truth that men exercised nearly total economic, legal, and sexual power over women. Societies were organized in such a way that women depended on men who made all important decisions. Men held all political, religious, and artistic authority, while women were confined to the domestic sphere and had no voice in public affairs. In short, people lived under a social system known as patriarchy (Greek, literally: "father rule").

In the meantime, this patriarchal system has, of course, been somewhat modified. Some of its worst excesses have been corrected, but, as women well realize, in principle it has survived to this very day. Indeed, it is still defended by many men as "natural" and inevitable. As proof, they point to a great deal of historical and anthropological evidence which seems to show patriarchy as a universal institution dating back to the earliest ages. However, within the last hundred years this view has repeatedly been challenged by various scholars who claimed that, in some distant past, all of mankind lived under a more benign and humane system of matriarchy ("mother rule"), and that our patriarchal culture is but a sorry deviation from the healthy order of things. In the present context it is not necessary for us to take sides in this controversy, although fairness commands us to state that, so far, no definite proof for the past or present existence of a matriarchal system has been found. What has been found are a number of matrilinear systems, i.e., systems of tracing the family blood line through the mother. This undoubtedly gives women a special status, but does not necessarily imply a socially dominant position. Societies can be matrilineal and patriarchal at the same time.

Still, the once fairly widespread acceptance of matrilinear systems makes an interesting point that may have some relevance here: It is much easier, more "natural," and more accurate to trace the family line through the mother rather than through the father. A baby's mother is never in doubt, while the father may sometimes be hard to determine. It follows that a patrilinear system can work only if women are so closely controlled that all of their pregnancies can be accounted for. Ideally, therefore, they enter marriage as virgins and remain faithful to their spouses. By the same token, a wife's premarital and extramarital affairs are bound to raise questions in her husband's mind about the paternity of his children. He may only be their legitimate and official, but not their biological father. It is true that in some societies husbands do not worry about biological fatherhood and are content with their official role, but in many others, including our own, men have tra-

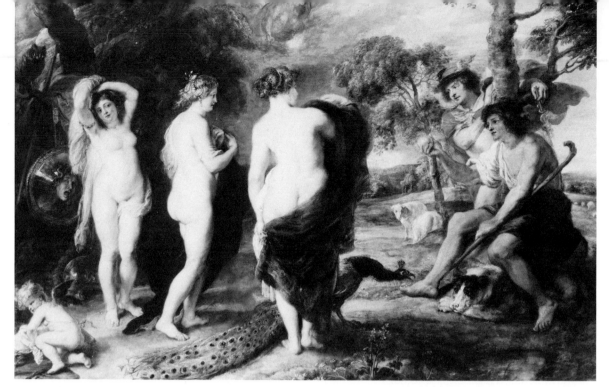

BEAUTY CONTESTS
Both female and male beauty contests have been known among many peoples since ancient times.

The Judgment of Paris *(above)*
The first and most famous female beauty contest in Western civilization was that between the Greek goddesses Hera, Athena, and Aphrodite who chose the Trojan shepherd Paris to be their judge. However, since he found it impossible to judge them by beauty alone, they offered him various bribes. Finally, Paris awarded the prize to Aphrodite who had promised him the love of Helen, wife of the Spartan king Menelaos and the most beautiful woman in the world. Thus, the judgment of Paris led to the Trojan war. Shown here is a painting by Peter Paul Rubens (17th century).

The Island of Women *(below)*
The sexual aspect of beauty contests is stressed in this scroll painting by Hiroshige, a 19th century Japanese artist. The picture illustrates the story of three fishermen who are shipwrecked on an island inhabited only by women. In this particular episode they are being inspected by the ruler of the island who wants to select one of them as her lover.

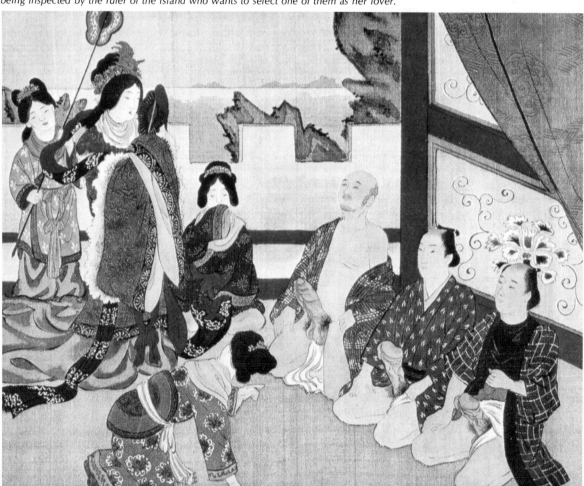

ditionally insisted on raising their "own flesh and blood." However, they could gain this certainty only by restricting female sexual freedom. Consequently, our sexual laws and moral standards have always been stricter for women.

Curiously enough, there have been peoples on this planet (and some of them had survived to the early 20th century) who were unaware of the fact that pregnancies are caused by sexual intercourse. Therefore, for them the whole issue of biological fatherhood could not even arise. Instead, they believed that a woman became pregnant when a spirit entered her body while she was swimming or bathing, or on some other occasion. In other words, for these "primitives" sex and reproduction were unrelated phenomena, although one tribe was found to believe that a man had to feed the growing fetus with his semen through the pregnant woman's vagina.

We do not know at what point in its development the human mind realized the connection between coitus and pregnancy, but we can assume that most societies discovered it a very long time ago. We also know that different societies drew different conclusions from this discovery. Some believed that the female role in reproduction was essential, "because only women can make things grow." The male therefore played merely the role of an assistant who helped matters along. Some societies ascribed equal importance to both sexes, and others regarded the male contribution as decisive. In our Western civilization this latter view eventually became the most widely accepted. The female body came to be regarded as a mere vessel for the male creative fluids. Women were the soil in which men planted their seed (a concept still preserved in our word "semen" which is Latin for "seed").

Thus, women soon found themselves in an inferior, secondary position. Their children did not really belong to them, but to their male "inseminators," just as the grain harvest belonged to the farmer who had sowed it, and not to the field. Indeed, at times it was even believed that a drop of semen contained a fully formed tiny human being, or *homunculus* which, after its deposition in the womb, simply grew there like a flower in a flower bed. At any rate, in the entire reproductive process the female was little more than a passive receptacle. She only nourished life, but did not create it. The true creator was male.

This general shift in perception was, of course, also reflected in religious beliefs. Originally, throughout most of the ancient world, people had worshipped some great "Earth Mother" or life-giving goddess of rebirth and fertility, such as Ishtar (in Babylon), Astarte (in Phoenicia), Cybele (in Phrygia), and Isis (in Egypt). However, the functions of these awesome female deities were gradually taken over by male counterparts. For example, among the nomadic Hebrews there arose a new faith that was later incorporated into Christianity and thus dominated much of Western history: the belief in the male god Yahweh who created the world and Adam, the first man. He also created the woman Eve out of Adam's rib to be his companion, but she allowed herself to be seduced by the serpent and thus was the cause of Adam's fall.

Needless to say, once Woman had been stripped of her creative role and had been burdened with the responsibility for Original Sin, her low social status appeared fully justified. In ancient Israel a wife called her husband "lord" ('adôn) or "Master" (ba'al). While he could repudiate her, she had no such right and, in fact, remained legally a minor throughout her life. The Ten Commandments list wives among a man's possessions. Not surprisingly, therefore, in a traditional Jewish prayer men implored God: ". . . let not my offspring be a girl, for very wretched is the life of woman," and they gladly repeated every day: "Blessed be Thou, o Lord our God, for not making me a woman."

In ancient Greece women fared hardly any better. In early heroic times, Greek women had known some measure of independence, but by the time of Pericles (5th century B.C.) their position had come to resemble that of domestic slaves. An exception was the militaristic state of Sparta, where women enjoyed certain privileges, but, together with men, were subject to lifelong totalitarian regulation. In republican Rome women were also ruled by their fathers or husbands, until they finally became more emancipated in imperial times. The conversion of Europe to Christianity did little for the liberation of women and, indeed, with regard to marriage and divorce, deprived them of rights they had formerly enjoyed. Only in some Northern barbarian countries did the church bring greater sexual equality. However, as a matter of principle, women were still considered inferior. They were respected and welcome in the congregation as long as they remained "modest" and "proper," but had no voice in religious or public affairs. As the Apostle Paul made clear: "But I would have you know that the head of every man is Christ; and the head of the woman is the man. . . . For a man . . . is the image and glory of God: but the woman is the glory of the man. For the man is not of the woman; but the woman of the man" (I Cor. 11; 3–9). Paul then continued: "Let your women keep silence in the churches: for it is not permitted unto them to speak; but they are commanded to be under obedience, as also saith the law. And if they will learn anything, let them ask their husbands at home: for it is a shame for women to speak in the church" (I Cor. 14; 34–35).

Thus, in contrast to many older "pagan" religions, Christianity excluded women from the priesthood and other church offices. At the same time, they were also expected to remain subservient to men at home. The only, and rather belated, religious concession to the female sex was the cult of the Virgin Mary which began to flourish during the Middle Ages. Mary, unsullied by sexual experience, has served as God's vessel by bearing his son. Thus, she had contributed to man's salvation and partly redeemed Eve's guilt. In the eyes of the faithful, this gave women a new dignity. The feminine mystique was further enhanced by the invention of courtly love and the cult of chivalry. In poetry and song the troubadours and other sensitive men extolled the virtues of their noble, irreproachable, and largely inaccessible ladies. However, both the Virgin Mary and the "noble lady" of medieval poets stood for fidelity, purity and propriety and thus symbolized only the passive aspect of womanhood. The active, assertive, sensuous aspect was represented by the image of Woman as temptress, a sexually insatiable animal who drained her victims of their life-sustaining fluids and led them to eternal damnation. Here again the Bible, and especially the Old Testament, provided the appropriate ideology. Christian women-haters approvingly quoted Ecclesiastes: "And I find more bitter than death the woman whose heart is snares and nets and her hands as bands: whoso pleaseth God shall escape from her, but the sinner shall be taken by her." (Eccl. 7:26).

This fear of women eventually grew to a point where it led to open aggression. Indeed, more and more women were directly accused of being in league with the devil. They were tortured until they confessed and then burned, hanged, or drowned as witches. In 1486, the Dominican monks Jakob Sprenger and Heinrich Krämer explained in their treatise on witchcraft *Malleus Maleficarum* (The Witches' Hammer): "What else is a woman but a foe to friendship, an unescapable punishment, a necessary evil, a natural temptation, . . . an evil of nature, painted with fair colors! . . . Women are intellectually like children . . . the natural reason is that woman is more carnal than man. . . . And it should be noted that there was a defect in the formation of the first woman, since she was formed from a bent rib, that is, rib of the breast, which is bent as it were in a contrary direction to a man. And since through this defect she is an imperfect animal, she always deceives. . . . Women also have weak memories; and it is a natural vice in them not to be disciplined." The witch craze raged on for several centuries in both Catholic and Protestant countries and claimed thousands of women as its victims. It was not until the Age of Enlightenment that the fear of female witchcraft stopped haunting the male Christian mind. (See also "Conformity and Deviance, Healthy–Sick".)

The "enlightened" philosophers and writers of the 18th century tried to reduce the female image to more human dimensions. For them, Woman was

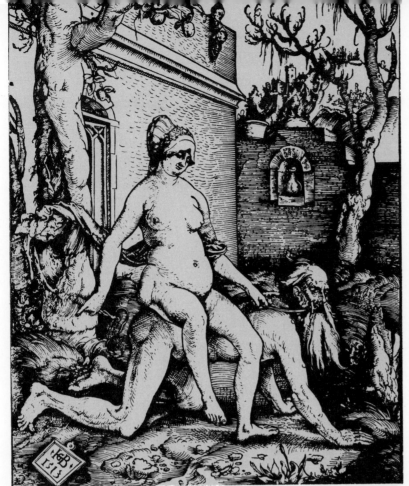

SEXUAL DOMINATION

Although the male sex has in fact dominated the female sex through most of human history, our folklore is rich with powerful images of both male and female domination. The two pictures shown here may serve as examples.

(Top) This 16th-century woodcut by Hans Baldung Grien illustrates the famous anecdote of the philosopher Aristotle playing horse for the prostitute Phyllis. The theme of wisdom being mocked and humbled by beauty recurs in the literatures of many cultures.

(Bottom) 17th-century woodcut satirizing the nearly absolute power of husbands over their wives that was sanctioned by the laws of the time. [The picture is also remarkable for two other reasons: 1. It shows the interior of a 17th-century "big house" with its open, multi-purpose rooms and various activities, such as cooking, card playing, spinning, rocking the baby, and receiving visitors (see also p. 428). 2. The picture further reveals that, in former centuries, "underwear" for women was unknown. Women did not wear "slips", "panties", or "bloomers" under their skirts.]

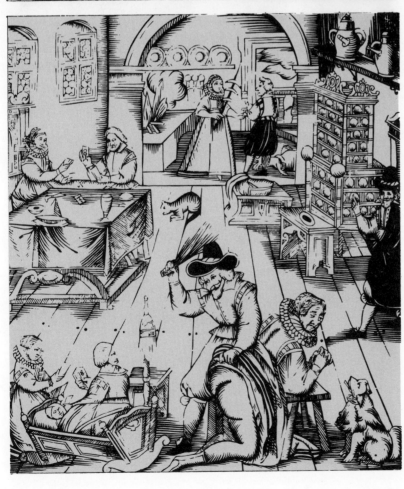

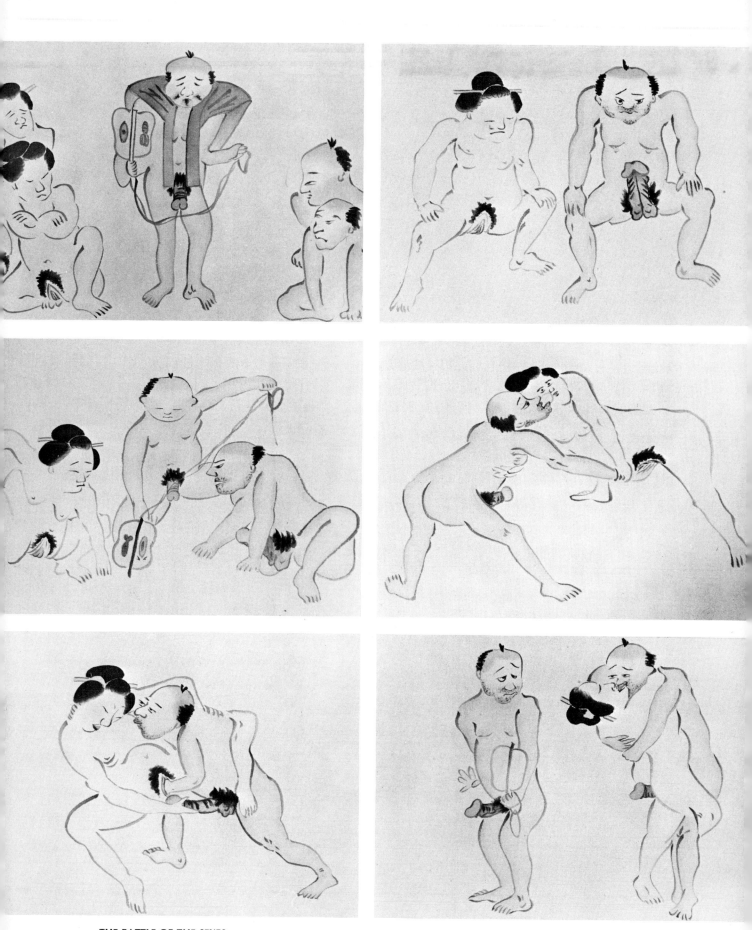

THE BATTLE OF THE SEXES
Pictures from a satirical scroll by Kuroda Seiki (1866-1924) showing a fantastic Sumo wrestling match between men and women.

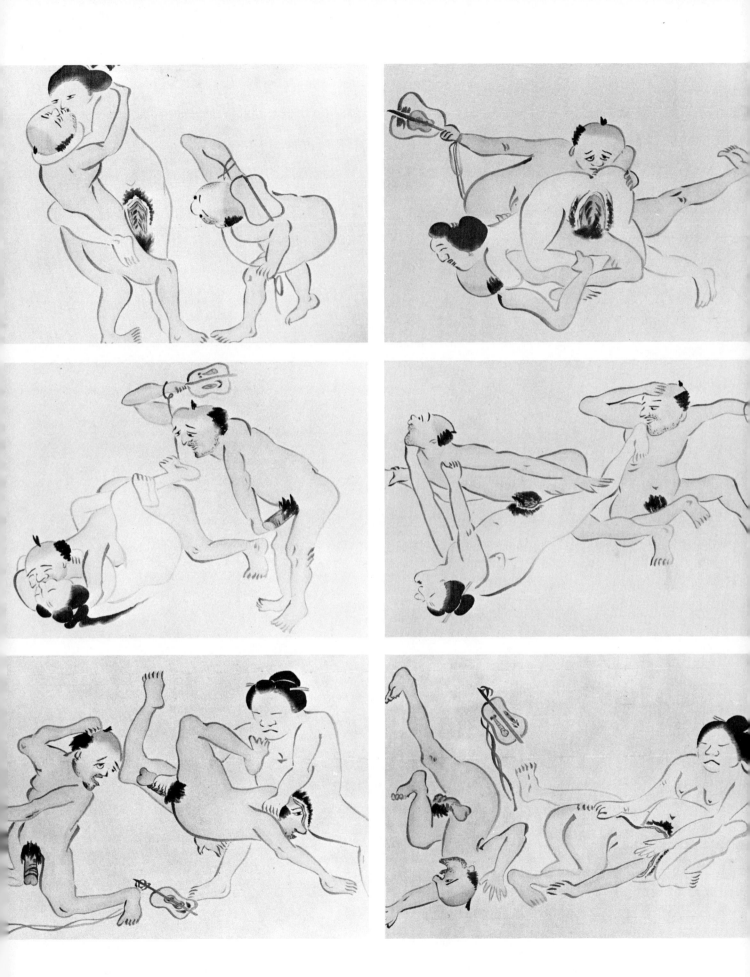

neither the immaculate saint nor the diabolical seductress, but rather a pleasant and useful companion. They treated her with admiration and courtesy, although only very few of them considered her a natural equal. Actually, Jean-Jacques Rousseau spoke for most men of his time when, in *Emile* (1762), he declared: "The man should be strong and active; the woman . . . weak and passive. . . . Nature herself has decreed that woman . . . should be at the mercy of man's judgment. . . . Works of genius are beyond her reach, and she has neither the accuracy nor the attention for success in the exact sciences. . . . The inequality of man-made laws . . . is not of man's making, or at any rate it is not the result of mere prejudice, but of reason." Obviously, in substance this opinion of the female intellect still differed little from that of the earlier witch hunters. Rousseau's "nature" and "reason" were no more natural and reasonable than they had been in the Middle Ages.

Under the circumstances, men saw no logical grounds for giving up the sexual double standard. Thus, as James Boswell recalled in his *Life of Samuel Johnson* (1791), the latter unquestioningly defended the patriarchal and patrilineal system when speaking about adultery: "Confusion of progeny constitutes the essence of the crime; and therefore a woman who breaks her marriage vows is much more criminal than a man who does it." On the other hand, Dr. Johnson also believed that it was easier for women to be faithful, since he considered their sexual needs less pressing. Women had to be more virtuous than men, because, as he once remarked to Boswell: "Women have not the same temptations that we have: they may always live in virtuous company; men must mix in the world indiscriminately."

Dr. Johnson was, of course, the quintessential bourgeois, and his remark about the lack of temptation for women was, to a certain extent, quite true at the time. The rising bourgeoisie increasingly confined its wives inside the house and locked up its daughters in order to shield them from outside influences. Family life became more intimate and exclusive. Outsiders were asked to respect family privacy and the "sanctity of the home." As a result, women became more dependent and domesticated than ever before. Indeed, within the next century, their lives became so restricted that they often gave the impression of being small-minded, incompetent, and devoid of passion. Thus, in a complete reversal of their earlier image, women eventually came to be regarded as less "carnal" than men. Without fear of contradiction, the Victorian English "sex expert" Sir William Acton, in his study *The Function and Disorders of the Reproductive Organs* (1875), therefore reassured his male readers: ". . . the majority of women (happily for society) are not very much troubled with sexual feeling of any kind. . . . The best mothers, wives, and managers of households, know little or nothing of sexual indulgences. Love of home, children, and domestic duties, are the only passions they feel."

Undoubtedly, not only Victorian men, but also many women accepted this "scientific" opinion as accurate. If they themselves did not quite seem to fit the stereotype, they sought the fault in themselves and tried to correct, or at least, conceal it. Still, this sexual oppression and self-oppression also made many of them unhappy and even ill, as became evident in the numerous incidents of female "hysteria" towards the end of the century. However, outside the sexual sphere, some middle-class women had long become more demanding. The French Revolution of 1789 had raised female hopes for full legal equality, and although these hopes were subsequently dashed, a number of feminists had kept battling on for women's right to vote. As a matter of fact, in Acton's time the fight for women's suffrage was already well under way in both Europe and America. Most "suffragettes" were sexually "proper" and "respectable" women, but they were no longer content with their domestic roles. And they were not alone. As more and more women developed a political consciousness, they learned to resent their inferior status. This, in turn, helped them realize that not only social discrimination, but also the sexual double standard had to be abolished, and that both males and females would be the better for it. In short, women began to see that there could be no true political, economic, and sexual morality until they were fully emancipated. The fight against sexual inequality thus became a fight for a more just, more humane society. By freeing themselves, women would also free their oppressors. This basic feminist belief was, over the years, articulated again and again, but it was perhaps best summarized early in the 19th century by the French social utopist Charles Fourier who had said: "The degree of emancipation of women is the natural measure of general emancipation."

THE EMANCIPATION OF WOMEN

The emancipation of women, i.e. their liberation from religious, legal, economic, and sexual oppression, their access to higher education, and their escape from narrow gender roles is not easily achieved. The struggle for sexual equality has a long history and is likely to continue for some time. Even if it should soon be won in the industrial nations, it may well rage on in many "underdeveloped" countries.

In traditionally patriarchal societies any improvement in the status of women has far-reaching consequences and produces fundamental political changes. Therefore it is always resisted by the established powers. However, it seems certain that they will ultimately have to relent, because the emancipation of women is both necessary and desirable. It will provide for a greater degree of social justice and thus benefit everyone. Indeed, from the beginning, the great "feminists" or champions of women's rights have always insisted that they worked in the interest of the whole human race. The feminist movement therefore has always been a humanist movement. Some of its representatives were reformers, others revolutionaries, but virtually all of them worked for a better, more equitable, and more humane world. Much can be learned from their experiences. They often suffered ridicule, persecution, and defeat, but also won admiration, support, and victory. Gradually, they achieved many of their goals. Their opponents, on the other hand, learned that a just cause cannot be suppressed forever. Where needed reforms are consistently blocked, revolution becomes inevitable.

The following pages briefly sketch the history of the modern feminist movement in Europe and America and offer some observations about the position of women in the contemporary world.

The ancient Romans and Celts had granted considerable freedom to women, but with the arrival of Christianity their legal status began to decline. In the Middle Ages single women still enjoyed many rights, but had to surrender them to their husbands upon marriage. Thus, in general, women were second-class citizens. Nevertheless, occasionally individual women were able to break out of conventional patterns and to impress their contemporaries with their accomplishments. The nun Hroswitha of Gandersheim as a playwright, Guillemine of Bohemia as a religious leader, and Joan of Arc as a soldier proved that the female sex was not inferior even in "male" occupations. Medieval queens like Matilda of Scotland (wife of Henry I of England) and Philippa of Hainault (wife of Edward III of England) even exercised a considerable and very beneficial political influence.

The Renaissance saw more women of power, such as Diane de Poitiers, Marguerite of Navarre, Catherine de Medici, and Elizabeth I of England. Some noblewomen also won distinction as writers and scholars, such as Margaret Roper, the daughter of Thomas More. Indeed, the intellectual independence of women grew to a point where it frightened many men who then

THE BEGINNINGS OF FEMINISM IN EUROPE

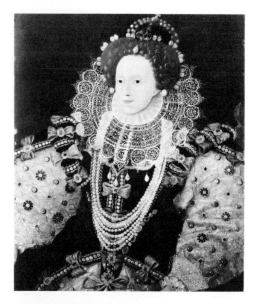

attacked it in vituperative books and pamphlets. The Scottish religious reformer John Knox, for example, in his *First Blast of the Trumpet Against the Monstrous Regiment of Women* (1558), exclaimed: "To promote a Woman to bear rule, superiority, dominion, or empire above any realm, nation, or city is repugnant to Nature; contumely to God. . . . Woman in her greatest perfection was made to serve and obey man, not rule and command him." This Natural-Law argument was to be used many more times in the following centuries not only against female monarchs, but also against any other women with higher aspirations.

However, there were also defenders of women's rights, such as Robert Vaughan, who, in his *Dialogue in Defense of Women, Against Malicious Detractors* (1542) condemned the double standard of morality. Eventually, some women also took the offensive, as for instance in the pamphlet *Haec Vir, Or the Womanish Man* (1620) which declared: "We are as freeborn as Men, have as free election and as free spirit, we are compounded of like parts, and may with like liberty make benefit of our creations." It went on to demand equal treatment for both sexes and to equate the oppression of women with slavery.

In the 17th century a few women, such as the Swedish queen Christina and the French and English writers Mme. de La Fayette and Aphra Behn continued to excel as scholars, novelists and playwrights. In France, learned women began to cultivate "salons," i.e. sexually integrated intellectual circles where good manners, wit, and erudition were esteemed and exercised. That these efforts were not appreciated by everyone can be seen in Molière's comedies *Les Précieuses Ridicules* and *Les Femmes Savantes* which satirize female attempts to enter "high culture." Still, the influence of women on French intellectual life was not diminished and has, in fact, continued to this very day. From Mme. de Sévigné to Mme. de Staël, George Sand, and Simone de Beauvoir, French women have held a position of eminence in French literature.

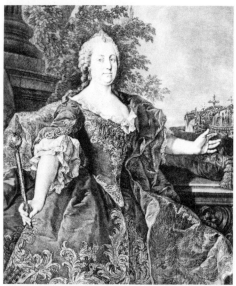

However, while female intellectual brilliance found recognition in exceptional cases, women were not given any political rights. As a matter of fact, with a new growing cult of "nature" even an intellectual education for women came to be seen as inappropriate. Jean-Jacques Rousseau, in his influential *Emile* (1762) flatly stated: "The education of women should always be relative to that of men. To please, to be useful to us, to make us love and esteem them, to educate us when young, to take care of us when grown up; to advise, to console us, to render our lives easy and agreeable. These are the duties of women at all times, and what they should be taught in their infancy." For a very long time this remained the accepted view. When, in 1789, the French Revolution broke out, some attempts were made to secure equal rights and equal education for women, most notably by the Marquis de Condorcet in his essay *The Admission of Women to Full Citizenship* (1790). Unfortunately, Condorcet himself soon became a victim of the revolutionary "reign of terror" and his proposal, along with others, was quickly repudiated. Indeed, in 1793 the National Convention suppressed all women's clubs, societies, and "salons," and denied women all political rights. In the meantime, Talleyrand had formulated the educational policies of the new government which offered girls public education up to the age of eight, after which they were to be kept at home.

WOMEN AS RULERS
The history of Europe has seen several remarkable women as heads of state whose accomplishments compare favorably with those of their male counterparts.

(Top) **Elizabeth I.** *(1533-1603) Queen of England*

(Middle) **Maria Theresa** *(1717-1780) Archduchess of Austria, Queen of Hungary and Bohemia, Empress of the Holy Roman empire*

(Bottom) **Catherine II the Great** *(1729-1796) Empress of Russia*

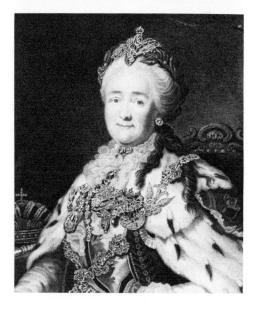

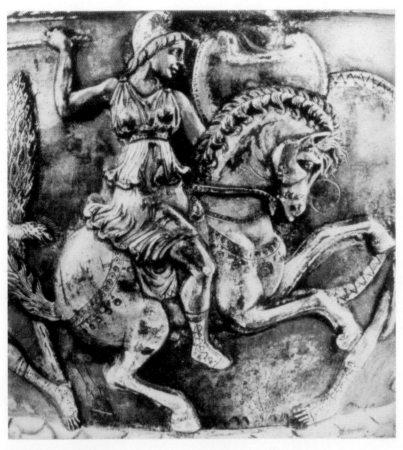

WOMEN AS SOLDIERS

One of the most famous and successful military commanders of all time was a teenage girl: Joan of Arc (1412-31 A.D.) However, for most of human history women have been denied any active role in the military. Curiously enough, the myths and legends of many cultures tell of soldier-like women and even of whole female armies.

(Above) Ancient Roman sculpture of Amazon in combat. The Amazons were a legendary nation of fighting women.

(Below) The Amazon motif is also found in Japanese art, as can be seen in this old anonymous woodcut.

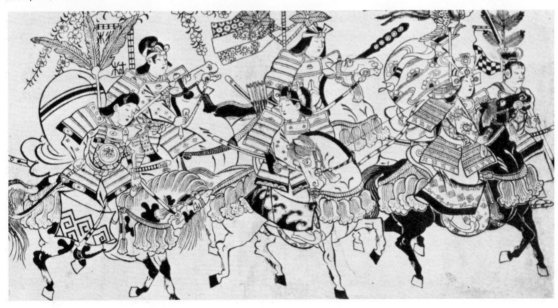

The English writer Mary Wollstonecraft, who had observed the French Revolution at close range, and who admired both Rousseau and Talleyrand, nevertheless felt compelled to protest against this reactionary trend. She therefore challenged both of these male authors in her *Vindication of the Rights of Women* (1792). In direct response to Rousseau she affirmed: "Woman was not created merely to be the solace of man. . . . On this sexual error has all the false system been erected, which robs our whole sex of its dignity." Instead, she demanded full and equal education for all women as a means of escaping sexual oppression. The invocation of "nature" in defense of oppressive policies left her unconvinced. Rousseau had offered this seemingly "objective" observation: "Boys love sports and noise and activity: to whip the top, to beat the drum, to drag about their little carts; girls on the other hand are fond of things of show and ornament—trinkets, mirrors, dolls." Wollstonecraft now replied: "Little girls are *forced* to sit still and play with trinkets. Who can say whether they are fond of them or not?" For her, the different behaviors of males and females arose out of "unnatural" distinctions created by society. In demanding the abolition of these distinctions, she argued for equal opportunity and equal rights. Women should enter all professions and become active in politics. The fight for the "Rights of Man" was more properly broadened to include the "rights of humanity."

Mary Wollstonecraft's book made her famous, or rather notorious, in her time, but after her untimely death was soon forgotten. Instead, the following generations saw the great manifesto of feminism in John Stuart Mill's *On the Subjection of Women* (1869). This brilliant essay by one of the most eminent English thinkers had a deserved influence on the women's movement in Europe and America. Mill wrote it after the death of his wife who had inspired it and who, in a sense, must be considered its co-author. Mill, not content with equal educational opportunities for both sexes, demanded the vote for women and, with others, himself founded the first women's suffrage society. Yet it was not until our century and after an intense struggle by "suffragists" like Lydia Becker and Emmeline Pankhurst and her daughters that English women were finally admitted to the ballot box.

THE FEMINIST MOVEMENT IN THE UNITED STATES

At the time of the American Revolution, American women, just as their European sisters, were clearly an oppressed group. They were generally uneducated and usually had no financial resources of their own. If they earned an income, they rarely had any control over it. Married women were legally dominated by their husbands and completely dependent upon them. Middle- and upper-class women, of course, enjoyed material comfort, but were confined and restricted at every turn by rigid social codes and the sexual double standard. Most important of all, women had no political rights, could not run for office, and were not allowed to vote.

Many women accepted their unequal status without question, but there were also others who took an active interest in political life and who became increasingly dissatisfied with their continued exclusion. The new "enlightened" ideas of liberty, equality, and democracy that were being discussed by men found a strong echo among intelligent women, and when the American colonies prepared for their secession from the English crown, female hopes for sexual equality were naturally high. Thus, one can assume that Abigail Adams spoke not just for herself when, in the spring of 1776, she wrote to her husband John (who later was to become the second president of the United States): "I long to hear that you have declared an independancy—and by the way in the new Code of Laws which I suppose it will be necessary for you to make I desire you would Remember the Ladies, and be more generous and favourable to them than your ancestors. Do not put such unlimited power into the hands of the Husbands. Remember all Men would be tyrants if they could. If perticuliar care and attention is not paid to the Laidies we are determined to foment a Rebelion, and will not hold ourselves bound by any Laws in which we have no voice, or Representation."

However, John Adams promptly rejected her plea in no uncertain terms: "As to your extraordinary Code of Laws, I cannot but laugh.... Depend upon it, We know better than to repeal our Masculine systems. Altho they are in full Force, you know they are little more than Theory.... in Practice you know We are the subjects. We have only the Name of Masters, and rather than give up this, which would compleatly subject Us to the Despotism of the Peticoat, I hope General Washington, and all our brave Heroes would fight."

This answer, although based on firm convictions, was, of course, insincere. Indeed, the claim that men were masters in name only was a clear insult to Abigail's intelligence. Interestingly enough, Adams revealed the real reason for his stance in a letter to a man, James Sullivan, to whom he explained that only property owners should be given the vote. Since few women owned property in those days, they were to be excluded together with all other economically dependent persons. In short, as John Adams well understood, but failed to discuss with his wife, the oppression of women was rooted in economic conditions.

At any rate, the United States of America were founded, and the Constitution was adopted without giving women and slaves their political rights. European women who admired and came to study the new country on visits soon felt their enthusiasm dampened when they encountered the old sexual discrimination and the reality of slavery. For example, the Scottish writer Frances Wright, who published her *Views of Society and Manners in America* in 1820, and who eventually settled in the United States, decided to fight actively for the freedom of slaves, the emancipation of women, and the rights of the urban poor. In the tradition of the Enlightenment, she also opposed the beginning religious revival in America as reactionary and inimical to human progress. Her social experiments and her personal flamboyance made her many enemies, but many of her criticisms were later vindicated. The English writer Harriet Martineau in her *Society in America* (1837) offered a perceptive description of life in the New World, but at times during her visit she had to fear for her own life because she supported the abolition of slavery. Sexual inequality and economic injustice were also attacked by the American writer Margaret Fuller whose study *Woman in the Nineteenth Century* (1845) was one of the most admired books of the time.

In the 1820's and 30's various religious and moral reform movements had attracted a growing number of American women. Education, peace, temperance (i.e., the banning of alcohol), and abolition (i.e., the freeing of the slaves) were the first social concerns to which female American Christians could properly devote themselves. Over the following decades this general reform movement flourished and eventually also came to include a new struggle for women's suffrage. Temperance was, of course, of deep personal interest to women, since alcoholic husbands could spend the entire family income on drinks, and their wives had no legal means to do anything about it. Because of their dependent status, they and their children were left unprotected. The interest in abolition, on the other hand, was entirely altruistic. There were a few great black women in the abolitionist movement, such as Sojourner Truth and Harriet Tubman, but its most prominent representatives belonged to the white middle class.

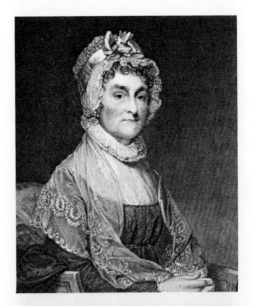

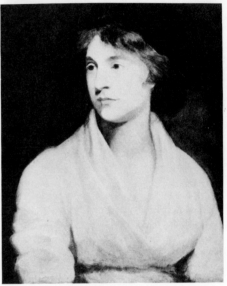

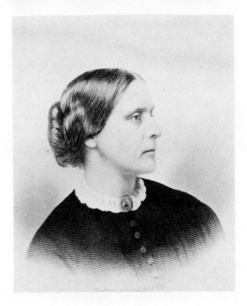

EARLY FEMINISTS
Women have long been struggling for equal rights, a goal that still has not been reached today. Shown here are three famous early feminists.

(Top) **Abigail Adams** *(1744-1818) Wife of John Adams, Second President of the U.S.*

(Middle) **Mary Wollstonecraft** *(1759-1797) English feminist writer*

(Bottom) **Susan B. Anthony** *(1820-1906) The American "Napoleon of the Women's Movement". With her friend Elizabeth Cady Stanton a tireless fighter for women's right to vote.*

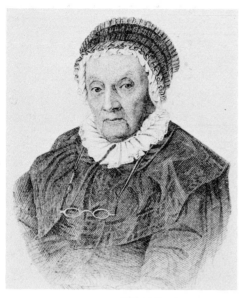

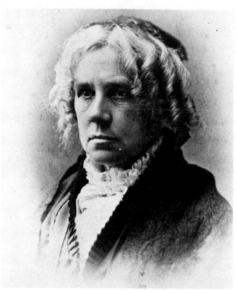

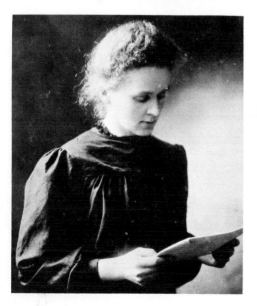

Two of the best known abolitionists were the sisters Angelina and Sarah Grimké. Born in South Carolina, they knew slavery firsthand and, after their move to the North, they wrote and spoke extensively against it. In 1838 Angelina Grimké became the first woman to address an American legislative body when she gave an abolitionist speech before the Massachusetts legislature and took the opportunity to raise women's claim to full citizenship. Two other important abolitionists who turned to feminism were Lucretia Mott and Elizabeth Cady Stanton. They were appalled by some episodes of sexual discrimination within the abolitionist movement and, in 1848, therefore organized history's first "Woman's Rights Convention" in Seneca Falls, N.Y. This convention passed a *Declaration of Sentiments* which echoed the American Declaration of Independence proclaiming: "We hold these truths to be self-evident: that all men and women are created equal; that they are endowed by their Creator with certain inalienable rights; that among these are life, liberty, and the pursuit of happiness." The document then went on to quote the right to change the form of government and stated: "The history of mankind is a history of repeated injuries and usurpations on the part of man toward woman, having in direct object the establishment of an absolute tyranny over her."

The Seneca Falls convention also adopted a set of resolutions, demanding legal and educational reforms and the end of the sexual double standard. Finally, it resolved "that it is the duty of the women of this country to secure to themselves their sacred right to the elective franchise."

These demands were quickly attacked and ridiculed by clergymen and male journalists all over the country. Only a few men had foresight enough to recognize the importance of the women's cause and to support it, among them the great black abolitionist Frederick Douglass, who applauded the feminists in his newspaper and appeared as a guest speaker before subsequent women's rights conventions. The women themselves were undaunted by the hostility they encountered and battled on. Elizabeth Cady Stanton found a close friend and ally in Susan B. Anthony, the "Napoleon of the women's movement," whose tireless work and tactical skill won her national recognition and the respect of her adversaries. The beliefs and experiences of these two courageous women were recorded for posterity in the first three volumes of the massive *History of Woman Suffrage* (1881–86) which they edited together.

The American Civil War (1861–1865) brought the women's movement to a temporary halt, but when the abolitionists' goal was finally achieved and the slaves were freed, women seized the opportunity to raise their demands once more. Indeed, they had reason to hope that, together with black men, they would now be granted the vote. However, this hope was soon disappointed. Over and over again, women were told to wait and not to jeopardize the granting of black voting rights by pressing their own demands at the same time. This well-meaning, but shortsighted argument succeeded in splitting the women's movement and reduced its effectiveness for many years. Even worse, women experienced the most serious setback when, in the Fourteenth Amendment (1868), the Constitution for the first time explicitly defined voters as men.

WOMEN AS SCIENTISTS

For a long time higher education and scientific research were the exclusive province of men. However, once they were given the opportunity, women also began to excel as scientists. Shown here are three women who have made significant contributions to science.

(Top) **Caroline Herschel** *(1750-1848) German-English Astronomer*

(Middle) **Maria Mitchell** *(1818-1889) American Astronomer, Professor at Vassar College*

(Bottom) **Marie Curie** *(1867-1934) French pioneer of modern physics and chemistry. Winner of two Nobel prizes (1903 and 1911)*

Nevertheless, in several other respects progress was being made. Higher education became accessible to females. In the 1830's women's colleges had been founded and, beginning in 1860, some colleges and universities became coeducational. Thus, for example, Elizabeth Blackwell became the first woman to earn a medical degree in the United States. She and her sister Emily, who also became a physician, wrote a book about *Medicine as a Profession for Women* (1860) and inspired many girls to enter this and other formerly "male" fields of study. Feminists also began to concern themselves with dress reform, the fight against prostitution, better working conditions and higher wages, child labor, unionization, and sexual freedom. Some of these issues proved even more explosive than women's suffrage, and many women remained rather cautious and conservative in discussing them. However, some "radical" feminists were less inhibited. Thus, as early as 1871, Victoria Woodhull spoke of an "inalienable, constitutional, and natural right" to "free love," emphatically rejecting the still prevailing double standard. Emma Goldman, and after her Margaret Sanger, campaigned for birth control. Charlotte Perkins Gilman wrote a penetrating analysis of female oppression in her *Women and Economics* (1898). This widely read book demanded economic equality for women as the key to political freedom and criticized the existing family structure.

One thing was obvious to everyone: In the course of the century the United States had undergone a profound transformation. From an agrarian nation of independent settlers it had changed into a largely urban and industrial society with millions of new poor immigrants and vast social problems. The subjection and disenfranchisement of women only added to these problems, because it made their solution more difficult. Other nations which experienced similar pressures finally took corrective action. New Zealand gave women the vote in 1893, Finland in 1906. The First World War produced social upheavals in Europe and secured the vote for women in the Netherlands and the Soviet Union (1917) and, to a limited extent, in Great Britain (1918). Germany followed suit in 1919. Under the circumstances, the lack of women's suffrage in the United States became an embarrassment. Therefore, in 1920, the country finally adopted the Nineteenth Amendment to the Constitution granting the right to vote to women. A struggle of over seventy years had finally been won.

Still, as feminists well knew, this victory was hardly enough, since sexual discrimination continued in many other subtle and not so subtle ways. Unequal pay for equal work, exclusion from influential positions, and innumerable specific legal restrictions denied women equal opportunities in American life. The economic exploitation of women was far from over. The feminist movement therefore supported welfare legislation for maternity and infant care, birth control, stricter labor laws, and government regulation of business. This led to a vicious "red smear" attack by the established powers which denounced feminists as "bolshevik dupes" and "communist conspirators" and accused them of "undermining the family." Primitive and transparent as they were, these smear tactics proved nevertheless to be very successful. Many "respectable" middle-class women were frightened away from the movement and dissuaded from defending their interests.

In 1923 the first "Equal Rights Amendment" was introduced in Congress stating: "Men and women shall have equal rights throughout the United States and every place subject to its jurisdiction." However, this proposed Amendment created dissent even within the feminist movement, because it seemed to eliminate some protective labor legislation advantageous to women. A long and heated debate ensued in political conventions, committees, newspapers, journals, and popular magazines. In the long run, nothing came of it but disunity among women and a decline in their political influence.

It was not until the 1960's that feminism experienced another upsurge. In 1953 Simone de Beauvoir's *The Second Sex* had appeared in English translation, an influential book that analyzed the history and implications of female

Why We Oppose Votes For Men

1.

Because man's place is in the army.

2.

Because no really manly man wants to settle any question otherwise than by fighting about it.

3.

Because if men should adopt peaceable methods women will no longer look up to them.

4.

Because men will lose their charm if they step out of their natural sphere and interest themselves in other matters than feats of arms, uniforms and drums.

5.

Because men are too emotional to vote. Their conduct at baseball games and political conventions shows this, while their innate tendency to appeal to force renders them particularly unfit for the task of government.

Alice Duer Miller,
American novelist and poet, 1915

subjection in Western culture. In 1963 Betty Friedan published *The Feminine Mystique,* openly criticizing the prevailing stereotypical role of the American housewife and mother. Also in 1963 a Presidential Commission issued a report *American Women* which recommended a number of moderate reforms to improve their status. In response to these and other developments, the National Organization for Women (NOW) was founded in 1966 and soon became the largest and best known of various new women's organizations. NOW almost immediately took up the fight for an Equal Rights Amendment and demanded several other drastic reforms, such as the right to abortion. In the meantime, these demands found much wider support than previously, because many middle-class women had become radicalized through the renewed black civil rights struggle, voter registration drives in the South, and the peace movement against the American war in Southeast Asia. Sexual and reproductive liberation could be discussed more openly, as the whole country had become more sensitive to issues of fairness and individual freedom. In the early 1970's the abortion issue was suddenly settled by the U.S. Supreme Court in the feminists' favor. Moreover, Congress finally passed an Equal Rights Amendment stating "Equality of rights under the law shall not be denied or abridged by the United States or by any State on account of sex." This Amendment has now been sent to the states for ratification, and feminists are hopeful that it will ultimately be adopted.

THE STATUS OF WOMEN IN THE WORLD TODAY

Since the early days of the Industrial Revolution women in Europe and North America have made considerable progress towards equality with men, although much remains still to be done. Of course, the industrialization of Western countries at first had not improved the status of women, but had degraded them even further by exploiting them and their children in factories as cheap labor. In the preceding relatively prosperous agrarian culture women had worked on an almost equal footing with men and had been skilled in many occupations. Families were still "producing units," and women received recognition for contributing their substantial share. The factory system changed all that by breaking up the traditional extended family with its large household and by giving people specialized monotonous tasks behind perpetually moving machines. Women and children were, however, paid much less for such work than men, and thus their economic "value" declined. It took many decades of struggle before unionization and legal reform ended the crassest form of this discrimination.

At the same time, middle- and upper-class women were increasingly confined to the home with little to do except to take care of their children. Their husbands no longer worked inside the house, but were absent during most of the day. These idle women often played the role of frail, sensitive creatures who had "the vapours" and fainted in any "indelicate" situation. On the other hand, many of them also became critical of their position in society. They found time to devote themselves to various religious and moral causes and even to become interested in abolition and the women's rights movement. Eventually, both working-class and bourgeois women insisted on change and contributed to the success of feminism. This success still is not total, and, as we all know, even in the industrialized countries women continue to fight for equal rights. Today, however, in addition to economic issues, problems of sexual self-determination have come to the foreground.

It must be remembered, of course, that the relatively liberated and affluent women of Europe and North America are only a small minority of women in the world today. Women in many non-Western countries, and especially in the so-called Third World generally live in a state of subjection and misery. Most of their energy is consumed by a hard and unrelenting struggle for sheer survival. Thus, for them, any talk about "sexual liberation" in the Western sense sounds, at best, irrelevant and, at worst, frivolous. Their concerns are more elementary and more pressing. This became disturbingly obvious, for example, when, in 1975, the United Nations sponsored an "International Women's Conference" in Mexico City. This conference demonstrated a serious communication gap between women from industrial and agrarian societies. It also revealed a stark global picture: More than a billion women (i.e., the majority of the world's female population) live in poor, rural areas. Most of them are illiterate, malnourished, exhausted, or even ill, and are forced to work long hours for little reward. Naturally, men share many of these hardships, but women still bear the greatest burden. In nearly all "underdeveloped" countries boys are favored over girls from the moment of birth, since parents consider sons as a guarantee for their economic security in old age. Girls, on the other hand, marry into some other family. Thus, even under conditions of abject poverty, boys are better fed, clothed, and educated than girls. In emergencies and in case of natural disasters, female needs also take second place. Furthermore, in many poor countries women have few rights and are early given away in marriage with hardly a voice in the matter. Backbreaking work and constant pregnancies then keep them weak and dependent. Attempts by governments and international agencies to raise the general standard of living in poor communities may well have the opposite effect on women by increasing their workload. Under such depressing circumstances, "women's liberation" has a special meaning and, indeed, poses a challenge to the women's movement in the rich and powerful West.

Some of the poor countries have, in the meantime, made great strides toward economic progress and, in some cases, such as in the People's Republic of China, a considerable degree of sexual equality has been achieved. It is also interesting to note that in recent times some "developing" nations, such as India, Sri Lanka, and Israel have chosen women as heads of state, an example that still waits to be emulated in Europe and America. On the whole, one might say that the emancipation of women is no longer a "Western" issue, and that its global implications are increasingly being recognized. There also seems little doubt that the demand for sexual equality will persist until it has fully been granted everywhere.

Reference and Recommended Reading

Beauvoir, Simone de. *The Second Sex.* New York: Knopf, 1953 (cloth); Random Vintage 1974 (paper).

Davis, Elizabeth Gould. *The First Sex.* New York: Penguin, 1972.

Friedan, Betty. *The Feminine Mystique,* 2nd ed. New York: Norton, 1974 (cloth); Dell, 1975 (paper).

Green, Richard. *Sexual Identity Conflict in Children and Adults.* New York: Basic, 1974.

Kanowitz, Leo. *Women and the Law: The Unfinished Revolution.* Albuquerque, N.M.: University of New Mexico Press, 1969 (paper).

Millett, Kate. *Sexual Politics.* New York: Avon, 1973.

Money, John, and Tucker, Patricia. *Sexual Signatures: On Being a Man or a Woman.* Boston: Little, Brown, 1975.

Oakley, Ann. *Sex, Gender, and Society.* New York: Harper & Row, 1972 (paper).

Papachristou, Judith, ed. *Women Together: A History in Documents of the Women's Movement in the United States.* New York: Knopf, 1976.

Ross, Susan C. *The Rights of Women: The Basic ACLU Guide to a Woman's Rights.* New York: Avon, 1973.

Rossi, Alice S., ed. *The Feminist Papers: From Adams to Beauvoir.* New York: Columbia U. Press, 1973 (cloth); Bantam, 1974 (paper).

Russell, Diana E.H., and Van de Ven, Nicole. *Crimes Against Women: Proceedings of the International Tribunal.* Millbrae, Cal.: Les Femmes Press, 1977.

Stoller, Robert J. *Sex and Gender: On the Development of Masculinity and Femininity.* New York: Aronson, 1968.

10. CONFORMITY AND DEVIANCE

Every society develops standards, rules, and norms for the sexual behavior of its members. These norms may differ a great deal from one society and one historical period to another, but in any case they result in dividing people into two groups: those who conform to the norms, i.e., the "normal" persons, and those who deviate from the norms, i.e., the "abnormal" persons or "deviants."

For instance, until early in our century the Siwans in Northern Africa expected all "normal" males to engage in homosexual intercourse, and they regarded those who refused to do so as peculiar or "queer." In contrast, the Rwala Bedouins, who lived on the Arabic peninsula, considered homosexual practices to be so "abnormal" and outrageous, that they put the participants to death.

Turning to our own society, we find that in Victorian times "normal" women were not supposed to have orgasms. Those who did have them or who insisted on them were often branded as loose, immoral, and even sick. Today it is the nonorgasmic woman who is considered "abnormal," "dysfunctional," or "inadequate," and who is offered treatment.

These few examples illustrate not only that sexual norms are relative, but also that deviations from these norms may provoke very different social reactions. In other words, what is sexual conformity in one culture may be sexual deviance in another culture, and those who are considered deviants may suffer very different fates.

As we have seen, sexual deviance can be approached in at least four ways:

- It may be ridiculed as a personal quirk (as in the strictly heterosexual Siwan male),

- it may be condemned as a sign of immorality (as in the orgasmic Victorian woman),

- it may be punished as a crime (as in the homosexual Rwala Bedouin),

- it may be treated as a disease or disorder (as in the nonorgasmic modern woman).

In the first of the above cases the sexual deviance is of no great consequence. The deviant is simply an odd fellow who is easily tolerated. However, the other three cases are much more serious. Once deviance is defined in moral, legal, or medical terms, it becomes a matter of concern for the church, the courts, or the medical profession. As a result, the deviant is no longer regarded as a harmless non-conformist who has a right to be left alone, but as a sinner who needs to be saved, a criminal who needs to be punished, or a patient who needs to be cured.

There are, of course, also some human societies where our particular four examples of sexual behavior would attract no special attention and would, in fact, never be regarded as deviant at all. In such "permissive" societies the sexual standards are broad and flexible enough to accommodate a great many personal peculiarities, and thus both heterosexual *and* homosexual males, orgasmic *and* nonorgasmic females are considered well within the range of normality.

On the other hand, a society with especially rigid sexual norms may put any or all of these different groups of people not just in one, but several deviant categories. We have already mentioned that in Victorian Europe and America, orgasmic, sexually demanding women were often seen as both immoral and sick. Thus, they were subjected not only to pious sermons, but also to psychiatric treatment. Similarly, some countries today regard male homosexuality not only as a sin, but also as a crime and a disease. As a consequence, male homosexuals in these countries face a triple social condemnation—a truly demoralizing experience.

It should be noted, however, that in modern societies the sexual norms can change rather quickly and that triple and double deviance can therefore suddenly be reduced to simple deviance or even complete conformity. An example of such drastic change has recently occurred in the United States where psychiatrists have now removed homosexuality from their list of mental diseases, where several state legislatures have repealed the traditional laws against homosexual behavior, and where a number of Christian churches have ceased to condemn such behavior as sinful. Thus, within a relatively short time, many American homosexuals have been transformed from social outcasts into respectable citizens. Only those who belong to conservative churches, reside in conservative states, or seek treatment from conservative psychiatrists still find themselves defined as deviants in need of "correction."

This leads us to still another important aspect of the problem. In our fast-changing world the moral, legal, and medical standards for sexual behavior may not always remain in agreement and may even become mutually exclusive. That is to say, our very conformity to one standard may come to imply our deviation from another. For example, a modern nonorgasmic woman may be asked by her therapist to masturbate frequently in order to become "fully functional." However, the same woman may be told by her clergyman that masturbation is a sin which will be punished by God. In short, she is given the choice between being either healthy and immoral or moral and sick. No matter how she decides, she ends up violating a sexual norm. By the same token, her therapist who recommends masturbation may thereby break a criminal law. (At least one state in the U.S. makes it a crime to encourage someone to masturbate.) Still, his professional ethics may demand that he give that encouragement. In short, his choice is between being either law-abiding and immoral or moral and criminal. Thus, he, too, is confronted with a dilemma. We could, of course, explore this conflict of norms even further by considering the therapist's possible religious beliefs or the medical views of the clergyman, but the main point of the argument should already be clear: Deviance as well as conformity are relative terms, and their concrete meaning varies with the social context.

Unfortunately, in the past this simple truth has not always been understood. Today it may seem obvious enough to us, but even the most learned and brilliant minds in history often failed to see it. Instead they thought of sexual deviance as an objective quality which arose in the individual and which had to be controlled by society. In accordance with this view, they assumed the existence of a "deviant personality" and devoted most of their efforts to discovering its characteristics and explaining its development. Based on their findings, they then devised various methods for forcing the deviant back into conformity. For many centuries this was the only accepted approach to sexual deviance. Occasionally, there was some variation of emphasis or style, but the results were always strikingly similar:

- During the Middle Ages, when the dominant social force was religion, the problem was defined mainly in religious and moral terms. Thus, the difference between sexual conformity and sexual deviance was seen as the difference between righteousness and sin. Sexual deviants were possessed by the devil or an evil spirit. They could be turned into "normal" human beings only by prayer and repentance. In order to control sexual deviance, society needed more priests and more churches. (By logical implication, sexual conformity could best be preserved in a church state.)

- With the beginning of the Modern Age, the church lost more and more of its power to the secular authorities, and thus the problem began to be defined mainly in legal terms. The difference between sexual conformity and sexual deviance was now seen as the difference between respect for the law and crime. Sexual deviants were "criminal types." They could be turned into "normal" human beings only by punishment and rehabilitation. In order to control sexual deviance, society needed more policemen and more prisons. (By logical implication, sexual conformity could best be preserved in a police state.)

- Finally, the 19th and 20th centuries saw a diminishing trust in political authority and a growing respect for science. As a result, the problem began to be defined mainly in medical terms. The difference between sexual conformity and sexual deviance was seen as that between mental health and mental illness. Sexual deviants were "psychopaths." They could be turned into "normal" human beings only by psychiatric treatment. In order to control sexual deviance, society needed more psychiatrists and more mental hospitals. (By logical implication, sexual conformity could best be preserved in a "therapeutic state.")

In all three of these instances we can observe the same basic ideology at work: The prevailing sexual norms are not to be questioned. Sexual deviance is not to be tolerated. The deviant has no right to his deviant behavior. Special social agents and institutions must be invested with special powers to bring the offenders "back into line" and to impose universal sexual conformity. Human beings in general will achieve and retain their "best" sexual behavior only under some form of totalitarian control.

And a second observation deserves to be made: The social control of sexual behavior may be exercised in the name of "God," "the legal order," or "medical science," but, no matter what the justification, it is always presented as objective, impartial, and "natural." Societies do not like to admit that it is, in fact, nothing more than the control of one group of people by another. The social, indeed, political aspect of the arrangement is rarely discussed, but is hidden behind a smokescreen of religious, legal, or medical jargon.

However, if one really wants to understand the problem of deviance, one has to take a much broader view. It is not enough to focus on the individual deviant and the means of transforming him into some acceptable "normal" person; one also needs to examine those who insist on this transformation and who have defined him as deviant in the first place. Indeed, as such an examination often reveals, the righteousness, respectability, or mental health of the conforming majority is, to a very large extent, sustained and confirmed by the visible presence of sinners, lawbreakers, or mental patients. In other words, deviants perform an important social function. They provide welcome "warning examples" and thereby promote social cohesion and stability among the rest of the population. Their existence also confirms, in a negative way, the dominant values of a society: The existence of godless people confirms the importance of religion, the existence of lawless people confirms the importance of law and order, and the existence of insane people confirms the importance of psychiatry.

Deviance and conformity therefore support each other, and they spring from a common source. It is shortsighted to assume that deviance arises spontaneously in certain individuals and then forces society to take some sort of action. Instead, it is more accurate to say that societies organize themselves in such a way that they create a certain amount of deviance which then helps them to validate the particular norms they have chosen. That is to say, societies produce both their own deviance and their own conformity. Furthermore, it would be an oversimplification to think that deviance exists objectively in some people, and that there is such a thing as an inherently deviant personality or an inherently deviant act. Deviance is not a characteristic of persons or a quality of their behavior. Instead, deviance is the result of human interaction. It is created, maintained, and revoked in social relationships. In short, deviance is best explained as a social role.

Men and women become deviants when they are so labeled either by others or by themselves. For example, someone becomes a heretic when his religious beliefs are found to be false and dangerous by the official religious authorities. As a result, these authorities excommunicate him and, if they have the power to do so, silence him by force. Similarly, someone becomes a criminal when the legal authorities find that his acts have violated the law. As a result, these authorities declare him to be guilty and punish him. Finally, someone becomes a mental patient when his behavior is officially found to indicate a lack of mental health. Psychiatric authorities then pronounce him sick and subject him to treatment.

By the same token, men and women cease to be deviants when they are no longer so labeled either by others or by themselves. For example, they can satisfy the authorities by recanting their heresy and doing penance, by serving their sentences and abandoning their criminal careers, and by being cured of their mental illness. As a result, the labels "heretic," "criminal," and "mental patient" are officially removed, and the former deviants can rejoin the conforming majority. They are received back into the arms of the church, readmitted to respectable society, and restored to the world of the healthy.

This is the basic pattern of conformity and deviance, stripped to its bare essentials. However, in practice the picture is complicated by several additional factors. One of these has already been briefly suggested: It is not at all uncommon for people to label themselves as deviants, i.e., to confess freely to heretical beliefs, to plead guilty to a crime, or to seek treatment for a mental illness. Conversely, in some situations they may also reject the deviant role that is being forced upon them. Instead, they may call it a terrible mistake. Thus, even after their excommunication, they may still claim to be orthodox believers, even in prison they may still protest their innocence, and even in a mental hospital they may still insist on their sanity. Or, as an alternative, people may reject the deviant role on another ground: They may admit having violated official standards, but declare them to be illegitimate and irrelevant. Thus, they may call the traditional catechism ungodly, the criminal code unjust, and the diagnostic manual unscientific.

The authorities, on their part, are sometimes reluctant to affirm the deviance of a certain person. They may refuse to see anything extraordinary in his behavior, even though it is quite unconventional. Or, if he himself insists on being a deviant, they can declare him mistaken, even against his wishes. In addition, they can remove the label of deviant from someone in two other ways: First, they can simply concede an official error by overzealous inquisitors, corrupt judges, or ignorant doctors. Thus, a person burned as a heretic may later be called a saint, a criminal may be exonerated, and a mental patient may be rehabilitated as the unfortunate victim of a false diagnosis. Secondly, the authorities can also decide to reform their dogma, repeal their law, or revise their psychiatric classification system. In none of these cases does the deviant have to change his behavior, yet his conformity is nevertheless restored.

All of this brings up another relevant point: Not everyone who has violated official standards is labeled a deviant, and not everyone who is labeled a deviant has violated official standards. Not all disbelievers come to the attention of the church, not all lawbreakers are caught and convicted, and not all people with bizarre behavior have contact with a psychiatrist. Instead, all of these non-conformists may be accepted as more or less "normal" by their communities. On the other hand, it is very well possible for perfectly "normal" people to be cast in the role of heretics, criminals, or madmen on false evidence. They may then accept or reject that role, but in either case their deviance becomes an undeniable social fact, and they begin to suffer the consequences. They may not really have lost the true faith, but they are still deviants; they may not really have broken the law, but they are still deviants; they may not really have "acted crazy," but they are still deviants.

In view of these and other observations, modern students of deviance have long since broadened their perspective and begun to consider its whole social context. Instead of merely wondering about the origins of deviant behavior in the individual, they now ask: Why and how are certain people set apart from the majority and cast into deviant roles? How do these people react to their role assignment? How does the larger community react to it? Under what conditions can people refuse or leave the deviant role? What are the advantages and disadvantages of the deviant role for the deviant? What are the advantages and disadvantages for everyone else?

Obviously, in this book it is not possible to pursue all of these questions in depth. It is enough if we realize their complexity. For our present limited purposes, we can restrict ourselves to a brief, superficial sketch, and therefore we cut the discussion short with one important final remark: Once people have been successfully labeled deviants either by themselves or by others, i.e., once the label has stuck, they have no choice but to play the deviant role as it is perceived in their particular society. Indeed, very often they enter full-fledged deviant careers and, together with fellow-deviants, develop special deviant subcultures. Thus, for example, a heretic becomes the fulltime leader of a new religious sect, a criminal turns professional and joins a criminal underworld, or a mental patient flaunts his "craziness" and develops a personal following. Eventually, these deviant subcultures may themselves produce their own deviants who then form their own subculture, and so on.

How does any of this apply to the specific case of sexual deviance? Perhaps we find out most quickly if we return to our initial illustrating examples. We had seen that, in Victorian times, orgasmic, sexually demanding females were often regarded as sinful and sick, and that both preachers and psychiatrists tried to save them. They were not just morally condemned as lascivious, but if they were found masturbating, they were medically treated for "masturbatory insanity." If they were not satisfied with the sexual performance of their husbands, they were treated for "nymphomania" or "erotomania." These treatments could go to bizarre lengths and could involve clitoridectomies (cutting out of the clitoris) and even more radical surgery. If the treatment failed to produce a cure, the patients might be forced into regular deviant careers as "loose women" or as inmates in an asylum.

However, by no means all orgasmic females suffered this fate. If they remained undiscovered or if their husbands could keep up with them, they were never labeled deviant and led fairly normal lives. Finally, when religious and psychiatric opinion changed, even highly orgasmic females were declared to be normal, and the problem of excessive female sexual desires vanished altogether. Indeed, in the meantime the situation has nearly reversed itself, and now nonorgasmic women are made to feel guilty. Thus, they may again end up in a psychiatrist's office for treatment and even be given lessons in more "effective" masturbation. If, on the other hand, they truly prefer a life of chastity, or if their husbands prefer them to be nonorgasmic, they are in little danger of being called deviant.

Even more instructive is the example of the homosexual male. As we have seen earlier in this book, there are societies which simply refuse to make an issue out of homosexuality. They may tolerate and even encourage homosexual behavior, but they do not have any "homosexuals." We have also seen that our own society provides for the special social role of homosexual and that people can be assigned to that role more or less arbitrarily. Kinsey's rating scale showed that heterosexuality and homosexuality lie on a continuum, are not mutually exclusive, and need not be permanent. Thus, the question whether any particular person is or is not a homosexual does not have an objective answer, but is decided through social interaction. For example, a soldier caught in a single homosexual act may be forced into a permanent deviant career, while a young male prostitute may regard himself and be generally accepted as heterosexual. Since he performs his homosexual acts only for money, they "do not really count." Thus, if he remains undetected by the police, he may eventually get married and settle into the life of a "normal" family man. (For further details see the introduction to "Homosexual Intercourse.")

However, once a man has been successfully labeled homosexual, i.e., once he has come to regard himself as a "queer," "faggot," or "gay" and is recognized as such, he learns to play his role according to everyone's expectations. Needless to say, these expectations differ in different societies and different situations. Sometimes the role of the homosexual is quite positive: He may be considered a shaman or holy man (as in certain "primitive" cultures), a model citizen (as in pre-Meiji Japan), or a sensitive genius (as in some Western folklore). At other times his role is entirely negative: He may be considered a heretic (as in medieval Europe), a criminal (as in some states of the U.S. today), or a "psychopath" (as in some states of the U.S. today). Furthermore, it must be remembered that, even within the same society, the positive or negative character of the homosexual role can change in the course of time. That is to say, people can cling to the role itself, yet nevertheless reverse its meaning. Thus, a society can maintain that homosexuals are different, yet nevertheless change its moral evaluation of them. This is also true of the homosexuals themselves. For example, in accordance with public opinion, they may think of themselves as "bad" and therefore act irresponsibly. However, after some soul-searching, they may also come to the conclusion that "gay is good" and therefore act like responsible citizens.

Similar observations can be made with regard to the homosexual subculture. Societies which do not make homosexuality a problem neither have "gays" nor a "gay subculture." Our own society has both. Indeed, the American gay subculture contains itself several sub-subcultures, such as that of the "aunties and nellies," the "drag queens," the "hustlers," the "bike and leather crowd," etc. All of these groups cultivate their own social and sexual styles. Still, within recent years, they have also experienced some common changes. In the past, they were usually secretive, suspicious, intolerant, and exclusive; today they have become much more relaxed and open. Moreover, they have now been joined by new, proud, and liberal gay subcultures, such as gay liberation groups, gay students' unions, gay sports clubs, gay churches, gay political caucuses, and gay professional organizations.

As a result of these and other developments, both the self-image and the public image of homosexuals have been greatly improved. More and more people are also beginning to realize that there is nothing intrinsic or permanent in the homosexual role. Apart from their sexual orientation, homosexuals may have very little in common, unless it is slowly acquired under various social pressures. Thus, in America, the old mechanisms of creating homosexual deviance are gradually breaking down. At least some of the more obvious traditional strategies are no longer successful. It is now being recognized, for example, that the psychiatric search for the causes of homosexuality has never been a neutral scientific enterprise. Instead, it was simply an attempt to find new justifications for the control of homosexuals and new methods of doing so. In actual fact, therefore, the psychiatrist looking for the causes of homosexuality rather resembled a Catholic Inquisitor looking for the causes of Protestantism. He was not an objective observer trying to gain some theoretical insight, but a partisan agent of the established order trying to stamp out an aberration. Furthermore, it has now become obvious that, like Protestantism, homosexuality does not have any particular set of causes.

In fact, the two phenomena themselves are virtually impossible to nail down, since both Protestants and homosexuals appear in an endless variety of degrees, shapes, and sizes. In the final analysis, therefore, religious and sexual heresies cannot be usefully studied in isolation. They are the natural product of religious and sexual orthodoxy.

Does this mean that all sexual standards are equal or that they should all equally be abandoned? Is deviance only in the eye of the beholder? Is everything relative? Are there no firm sexual guidelines at all? Should we give up reprimanding people for sexual immorality, punishing them for sexual crimes, or treating them for sexual problems? Obviously not. We have both the right and the duty to do all of these things. After all, nearly every day we see or hear about cases of severe sexual maladjustment leading to conflict and misery. In some of these cases, there are victims who demand protection from various forms of sexual assault, in other cases people suffer from crippling sexual inhibitions, compulsions, or destructive tendencies and ask for professional help. Neither the former nor the latter can long be ignored. No society can survive without a certain minimum of sexual standards or even certain sexual ideals. The enforcement of these standards and the pursuit of these ideals are a direct reflection of a society's moral worth.

By the same token, however, it also well behooves every society to examine and reexamine its sexual values in the light of experience. Furthermore, it should also openly take responsibility for them, instead of hiding behind some alleged "natural order." Historical and cross-cultural studies show all too clearly that sexual violence and misery often spring directly from unrealistic, unreasonable, and unnecessary social regulation. Certainly our own Judeo-Christian civilization has a very dismal record in this regard. The history of sexual deviance in Europe and America is replete with appalling examples of official hypocrisy, cruelty, and fanaticism and thus teaches all of us a very melancholy lesson.

The following pages examine the traditional Western religious, legal, and medical standards for sexual behavior in greater detail. The resulting forms of sexual deviance and the various professional strategies for dealing with them are also discussed at some length. The issue may be further illuminated by a few cross-cultural observations. For the sake of greater clarity, the text has been organized in three separate sections which follow the same basic pattern.

"NATURAL"—"UNNATURAL"

Where the violation of sexual norms is defined as a religious or ethical problem, sexual conformity and sexual deviance are seen as righteousness and sin. Conforming sexual behavior is described as "proper," "moral," and "natural." Deviant behavior is called "improper," "immoral," and "unnatural."

Especially the words "natural" and "unnatural" have always been very popular with moralists, because the invocation of nature is much more effective than an appeal to mere propriety or even morality. Nature does not seem to be subject to human whim and caprice. Therefore it can be presented as an objective, truly impartial authority, an infallible final arbiter in questions of right and wrong. A natural morality can claim to be unchangeable, eternal, and universally valid. By the same token, those who base their moral judgments on nature can imagine themselves to be free of personal bias. In their view, nature itself embodies the rules by which we should live. The intentions of nature can be found with the help of right reason, and once we have found them, we are also obliged to follow them. Only natural actions are moral.

However, this argument rests on a fundamental misunderstanding of both nature and morality. Nature has no intentions, and there is no morality in denying that we are personally responsible for our values. Man is the master of nature and molds it according to his own shifting self-interest. Thus, he encourages or prevents natural occurrences as he sees fit and constantly uses one law of nature to defy another. Indeed, his very life depends on his refusal to let nature take its course. If human beings accepted only that which "comes naturally," they would all end up like a certain eccentric saint, Simeon Stylites, who rejected soap and water and finally had his entire body covered with festering sores. When some of the maggots which fed in these sores fell to the ground, Simeon picked them up and replaced them saying: "Eat what God has given you!"

Fortunately, most people have sense enough not to follow this pious example. They know that human progress has always depended on human disregard for nature "as it is." The history of man is the history of the transformation of nature. In short, insofar as man is a civilized creature, he lives in a world of his own making.

An important part of this man-made world is the system of moral values which determine human behavior. This becomes particularly obvious when we examine the various old and new sexual moralities. As we all know, our Judeo-Christian culture has long believed that the "nature" of sex is reproduction and that any sexual act that does not further this goal is therefore "unnatural." Religious dogmas, popular myths, customs and attitudes, civil and criminal laws, indeed our very language still reflect this belief. For example, when we refer to the human sex organs as "genitals" (Latin: organs of generation) or "the reproductive system" we thereby imply that their "natural" function is that of procreation. However, this is a very selective view, because the sex organs also have many other functions. (See "The Male Sex Organs" and "The Female Sex Organs.") Scientists are, of course, well aware of this fact and do not take the old terms literally. Still, even today nonscientists sometimes persist in trying to derive the "proper" function of these organs from their name. According to this philosophy, God, nature, and logic forbid that the "organs of reproduction" should be used for any other purpose. However, it would make just as much sense to describe the mouth, teeth, tongue, and throat collectively as "nutritionals" or "the feeding system" and then forbid people to speak, sing, whistle, or kiss.

Intellectual honesty requires that we free ourselves from such preconceived, inflexible, and simplistic notions. Instead, we have to recognize that it is never "nature" which decides how the human body is to be used, but always the human will. Man uses his mouth to eat, but also to speak, sing, kiss, smoke, and play the trumpet. He uses his legs to walk and run, but also to jump rope, walk a highwire, play hopscotch, and dance the tango. He uses his sex organs to reproduce, but also to experience pleasure and to give pleasure to his sexual partner.

Any of these uses is as "natural" or "unnatural" as the other. The freedom to modify and improve upon nature is part of the human condition. It is also the very foundation of culture. People today do not simply let their hair and nails grow "naturally," but cut and color them according to fashion. They do not eat their food "naturally" raw, but cook, broil, and bake it. They do not endure "natural" pain, but take pain-killing drugs. They are not content with the "natural" variety of plants and animals, but create new kinds of fruits and breed new kinds of cattle. "Nature" did not intend people to fly and therefore did not provide them with wings. However, very "naturally" they overcame their "natural" handicap and invented the balloon, dirigible, airplane, rocket, and spaceship.

In sum, man alone decides what is "natural" for him, and he alone establishes his moral values. He then projects these moral values into the natural world around him which has no morality of its own. Nature as such is value-free. It has no preferences, no direction, no ultimate goal. Growth as well as decay, health as well as disease, life as well as death are natural. Nature provides both sunshine and rain, heat and cold, edible and inedible plants, fertility drugs and contraceptives. It is the human mind which chooses between them and thus creates the various moralities and ethical systems by which human beings live. Until now these systems have usually been presented as implicit in nature, and therefore they seemed endowed with an objectivity which they did not possess. Today, however, this strategy is no longer acceptable. The time has come to face the sobering truth: We are all responsible for our beliefs and for what we do in their name to our fellow human beings.

SEX AND RELIGION

For thousands of years moral questions were decided on strictly religious grounds. People knew good from bad and right from wrong because they had learned the difference from some superhuman authority. The spirits, the gods, or God commanded the proper course of action and punished any disobedience. In short, morality and religion were virtually identical. Atheistic moral systems did not appear until late in human history. They are the product of civilization.

Still, whether they were religious or not, most moral systems of the past have tried to present themselves as universally valid and therefore have claimed to be free from human influence. Not only the churches, but also authoritarian secular governments have always been strangely reluctant to accept any direct moral responsibility. While they insisted on enforcing very specific moral standards, they usually also refused to recognize them as their own. Religious moralists pointed to "the will of God" or "the intentions of nature"; atheistic moralists invoked "the logic of history," "the laws of dialectic materialism," or some other such fabulous, irresistible forces. By the same token, deviance was defined either in religious terms as "sin," "blasphemy," "idolatry," and "heresy" or in secular terms as "treason," "reactionary behavior," "subjectivism," and "bourgeois decadence." Deviant individuals had to go to confession or engage in public self-criticism. In either case, they were "reeducated" and forced to sacrifice their personal interests to some official dogma.

What we have said about morality in general is, of course, also true of sexual morality. Here again, both religious and atheistic dogmatists have usually judged human actions not by their "subjective" effects, such as pleasure, satisfaction, or happiness, but by their alleged "objective" character. Sexual behavior had to conform to some "higher" transcendental law. In some cases, this law was benevolent, broad, flexible, and sex-positive; in other cases it was oppressive, narrow, rigid, and sex-negative. In the first instance the large majority of people found sexual satisfaction. In the second instance only a small minority was able to do so; all others remained sexually frustrated in various degrees. As a result, their lives were rather nasty, bleak, and brutish. They were unhappy with themselves and intolerant of others.

We do not really know why some societies demand sexual asceticism from their members and others do not. Writers like Friedrich Engels, Sigmund Freud, and Wilhelm Reich have offered different theories about "the origin of the family, private property, and the state," "civilization and its discontents," and "the imposition of sexual morality" which try to find the causes of sexual repression in some distant past when human history somehow "took a wrong turn." However, brilliant as these theories are, they still leave most of the problem unexplained. At the present time we can be sure of only one thing: It is man himself who creates his sexual morality and therefore he also has the right to change it when it begins to threaten his well-being. Indeed, under certain circumstances this right may become his moral duty.

The following pages summarize the teachings of various past and present religions. It should be remembered, however, that modern nonreligious moral systems are just as varied in their sexual attitudes.

Historical Background

The roots of our Western civilization reach far back into antiquity. Indeed, whether we are aware of it or not, many of our present moral convictions reflect events, circumstances, and collective experiences of times that have long since passed. For example, from ancient paganism through Judaism and Christianity, our sexual morality has been influenced by a great variety of religious beliefs. Quite often this influence was not only direct and open, but also indirect, subtle, and concealed. In many instances it persisted even after the beliefs themselves had waned or changed. It therefore appears advisable to cast at least a cursory glance at some of the most important Western religions and especially at their teachings about human sexual behavior.

Ancient Greece and Rome

Generally speaking, the ancient European civilizations had a very positive attitude toward sex. In the present context, however, we can perhaps skip over the civilizations of Northern Europe and concentrate on those in the Mediterranean region, since only the latter had any long-lasting influence on our Western morality.

In ancient Greece, sex was seen as an elementary life force, and thus all sexual impulses were accepted as basically good. Indeed, various gods and goddesses of fertility, beauty, and sexual pleasure were worshipped in special temples or on special occasions, often with orgiastic rites. The Greeks also believed that virtually all of their gods led vigorous and varied sex lives. Therefore they considered it only proper for mortals to follow this divine example.

The Greeks thought so little of sexual abstinence that their language did not even have a special word for chastity. Instead, they devoted themselves to what they called *hedone*, i.e., sensual pleasure in all its manifestations. However, the "hedonism" of ancient Greece was by no means a prescription for sexual license. Rather it was a cheerful enjoyment of life, a grateful appreciation of the human body and especially of its sexual functions. Pleasure was not divorced from reason, but always in harmony with it. The body was never punished or starved for the sake of the soul. Since the Greeks did not believe in a happy life after death, they felt obliged to live every moment on this earth to the fullest.

As youth and physical beauty were greatly admired, youthful bodies were not always covered with clothing, but often proudly exposed. Public nudity was common at many religious festivals, in civic processions, and in beauty contests. Young men exercised at the gymnasium (literally: the place where one is nude). Athletic competitions (including the original Olympic games) were held in the nude, although here women spectators were excluded. In Sparta, on the other hand, there were even nude wrestling matches between boys and girls. Nude male and female dancers entertained guests at parties and other festive gatherings. Temples, theaters, public squares, and private houses were decorated with statues and paintings of nude men and women. The sexual aspect of nudity was openly recognized. Many works of art, in fact, depicted sexual responses and sexual activity. The Greeks felt a constant yearning for beauty, and in their eyes nothing was more beautiful than a young, healthy, nude human body.

Greece was, of course, a male-dominated society, and, during its "golden age," the ideal of beauty was male. Although men usually felt obliged to marry and raise a family, they sought little romantic involvement with their wives. Their most noble sentiments and passionate feelings were reserved for homosexual relationships before and outside of marriage. Here again, they found support in their religion. Gods like Zeus and Apollo and demi-gods like Hercules were believed to have fallen in love with beautiful young men. There can be no doubt that for many Greeks these exalted models were a constant source of inspiration.

In classical Greece love and sexual desire were personified in the youthful, powerful, and unpredictable god Eros. He took possession of human beings

THE EMBRACE OF EROS
(after an ancient Greek vase painting)

The Greeks saw all sexual desire as inspired by the youthful, playful, and powerful god Eros. To resist his embrace would have been not merely futile, but sacrilegious.

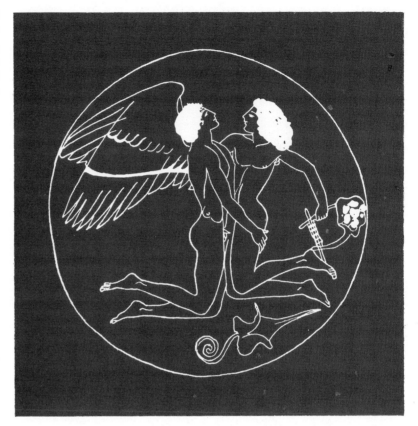

according to his whim, and any resistance would not only have been sacrilegious, but hopeless. All forms of love were of divine origin and had to be respected. This basic belief explains why the Greeks were extremely tolerant in sexual matters and why there was no persecution of sexual "deviants." At any rate, most of our modern, more bizarre manifestations of human sexuality were virtually unknown. For instance, pain and pleasure were never associated, and thus sexual cruelty, "bondage and discipline," and other such practices had no chance to develop.

In this latter respect, Greece stood in sharp contrast to Rome where, especially in imperial days, sexual cruelty and brutality were fairly widespread. Eventually, sex among the Romans became much more crude, coarse, and vulgar than it had been among the Greeks. However, apart from certain eccentricities of the rich, even in Rome the general attitude toward sex was still quite reasonable and realistic.

In Rome, as in Greece, the religious beliefs originally reflected the values of an agrarian society. Farmers prayed mostly for large families, growing cattle herds, and good harvests, and the oldest religious ceremonies were fertility rites. Naturally, in the course of time many of these rites were somewhat changed and refined, but even the urban Rome of the emperors still saw various orgiastic religious celebrations and sexually licentious festivals. Fields and gardens were protected by statues of the fertility god Priapus who displayed an enormous erect penis. Artistic representations of male sex organs were also carried in processions and worn in the form of jewelry as a good luck charm.

However, like the Greeks, the Romans never regarded sex and procreation as inseparable, but accepted all types of sexual activity as divinely inspired and therefore good. Indeed, with the expansion of their empire into areas dominated by Greek culture the Romans directly adopted many Greek customs and beliefs. Thus, the Greek deities Eros and Aphrodite also began to be worshipped in Rome as Amor and Venus. The idealism and nobility of

Greek homosexual love, on the other hand, seem to have been beyond the reach of most Romans. While homosexual relationships were considered normal and natural, they were hardly seen as superior. On the whole, the Roman approach to sex was rather direct, prosaic, and practical.

Summing up, one may say that the religions of both Greece and Rome allowed for the full expression of every human sexual potential. The contrast to our modern religious beliefs is striking. However, perhaps the greatest difference between the ancient and modern attitudes is this: In the ancient world the emphasis was put on the sexual desire itself, not on its object. Thus, men and women were loved not so much because they were desirable in themselves, but because the love felt for them made them appear desirable. Love was a driving force which originated in the lover. It was directed towards others, but its strength or worth never depended on their reactions. This view was well expressed in the Greek saying: "The god of love dwells in the lover, not in the beloved." In short, it was more the god of love himself who was worshipped in every sexual act than the sexual partner.

Because of their religious glorification of physical love, the ancient Greeks and Romans generally had little admiration for people who remained sexually abstinent. It was only in the later Hellenistic period (about the time of Christ) that certain ascetic philosophers found any wider following. These philosophers began to proclaim a conflict between the mortal body and the immortal soul and renounced all material possessions as well as sensual pleasures for the sake of "purity" and "virtue." It is not entirely clear why this new asceticism suddenly became so popular. Quite obviously, however, it had great appeal for the early Christian thinkers.

Ancient Israel

The history, customs, laws, and religious beliefs of ancient Israel are carefully and extensively recorded in the Bible. Thus, in most Western countries where the Bible is still widely read, the general population knows more about the Israelites than about any other ancient people. Under these circumstances, we can restrict ourselves here to a very brief sketch.

In contrast to their polytheistic neighbors, the Israelites believed in only one God, Yahweh, the creator and ruler of the world. He had chosen them as his people and given them his law through Moses. Therefore they felt obliged to live according to his commandments and to reject all other laws and foreign influences.

For the people of Israel the main purpose of sex was procreation. Men and women had the duty to "be fruitful and multiply" (Genesis 1; 28), and there was no greater blessing than a large family. Therefore, when Yahweh decided to reward Abraham, he told him: "I will indeed bless you, and I will multiply your descendants as the stars of the heavens and as the sand which is on the seashore" (Genesis 22; 17). By the same token, sexual abstinence was not only offensive in the eyes of the Lord, but also betrayed an anti-social attitude. As a matter of fact, a person who chose not to have children was regarded as little better than one who shed blood.

Because of their great concern with fertility, the ancient Israelites regarded the male sex organs as inviolate and almost sacred. For example, when Abraham sent his servant out to seek a suitable wife for his son Isaak, he asked him to take a solemn oath. The servant then put his hand under Abraham's "thigh" (euphemism for sex organs) and swore to God that he would not lead his son to marry a Gentile (Genesis 24; 2–4). [This is similar to the ancient Roman practice of touching one's testicles while taking an oath. In fact, the very word "testicle" is the diminutive form of Latin "testis," meaning "witness" for the truth. The same word is, of course, also the root of the English verb "to testify."] The sex organs also warranted special protection. If a woman tried to help her husband in a quarrel with another man by grabbing this man's penis or testicles, she had her hand cut off (Deuteronomy 25; 11–12). Sexually mutilated men were excluded from the congregation.

Various biblical passages (among them the sexually explicit "Song of

**ADAM AND EVE COVERING
THEIR NAKEDNESS**
(14th-century German painting)

*The Bible tells us that, after having disobeyed God,
the first human beings discovered their nakedness
and were ashamed. As a punishment for their sin,
they were then driven from the Garden of Eden.
Thus, among the ancient Israelites, nudity was not
tolerated, and to be stripped naked in public was the
ultimate humiliation.*

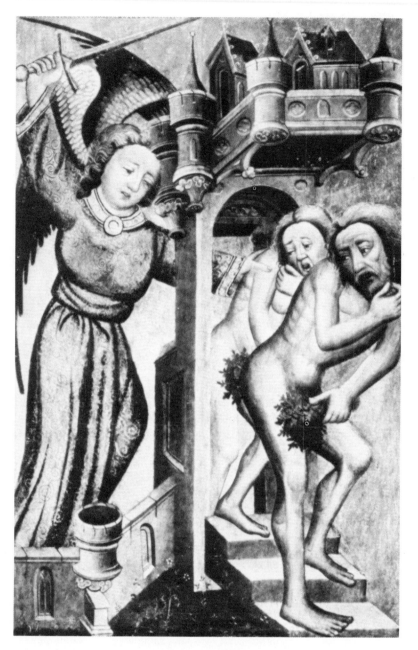

Songs'') make it quite clear that the Israelites thought very highly of sexual
pleasure. Sex was considered a normal part of a healthy life, and it was a virtue to enjoy it. In accordance with this view, newlywed couples were entitled to an extended honeymoon: "When a man is newly married, he shall
not go out with the army or be charged with any business; he shall be free
at home for a year, to be happy with his wife whom he has taken" (Deuteronomy 24; 5).

On the other hand, neither men nor women were encouraged to display
their nude bodies. Nudity was generally regarded as shameful and embarrassing. For instance, an adulterous woman was publicly stripped naked by
her husband as an act of humiliation. Numerous customs and regulations
tried to prevent even the involuntary exposure of sex organs. (In later times
a Jew who exercised in a Greek gymnasium was assumed to have betrayed
his faith.)

Nevertheless, it would be wrong to assume that the ancient Israelites were prudish or puritanical. In most respects their approach to sex was very positive. However, because of their strong emphasis on reproduction, coitus was the only acceptable form of sexual expression. All non-reproductive sex (including sexual self-stimulation) was considered "unnatural" because contrary to the will of God. Homosexual intercourse and sexual contact with animals were even punished by death (Leviticus 20; 13 and 15).

It is important to remember the religious basis of this sexual intolerance. At a time when the Israelites fought for their national and religious survival, they were surrounded by peoples who worshipped numerous gods and idols, and who usually made all types of sexual activity part of that worship. Indeed, we know from the Book of Kings and from the denunciations of the prophets that, at times, even the Israelites themselves had male and female prostitutes attached to the temple in Jerusalem and to various local shrines. However, for the sake of monotheistic purity, this "sacred prostitution," along with all other polytheistic customs, was eventually eliminated from the nation's life. Thus, people began to associate nonreproductive sex with idolatry and to treat it as a major religious offense.

Still, within the relatively narrow framework of marital coitus, sexual pleasure remained well recognized and was actually encouraged. It was only late in Israel's history (about the time of Jesus) that certain peripheral and extremist sects, such as the Essenes, developed strictly ascetic ideals. This sexual asceticism was never representative of Jewish culture as a whole.

The Catholic Church

At the time of Jesus Christ, various ascetic religious movements had begun to flourish in the Roman Empire. There were not only extremist Jewish sects (such as the Essenes) which renounced all sexual pleasure, but also many pagan cults which declared the human body to be "impure" and which demanded that it be neglected, mistreated, or even starved for the sake of the "pure" soul. Jesus himself, however, does not seem to have subscribed to any such notions, but rather followed the more traditional, sexually positive, Jewish teachings. Actually, very little is known about his views on specific sexual issues. He remained a chaste celibate himself, but never praised or condemned the sexual urge as such. In practice, his attitude towards sexual outcasts was compassionate and forgiving (Luke 7; 36–50, John 8; 1–11).

Human sexuality is discussed in more detail by Paul, one of the earliest and most energetic Christian missionaries. Paul, who had not been among Jesus's personal disciples, was apparently influenced by some of the more negative sexual philosophies of his time. His strong condemnation of homosexual behavior can, of course, still be explained as traditionally Jewish (Rom. 1; 26–27, I Cor. 7; 38). However, he goes far beyond this tradition when he sees sexual desire itself as a rather deplorable weakness. Indeed, in clear opposition to Jewish doctrine, he declares celibacy to be superior to marriage (I Cor. 7; 8–9, I Cor. 7; 38).

This ascetic approach to sex was soon developed further by stern and somber Christian scholars, such as Tertullian, Jerome, and Augustine. All of these so-called "Fathers of the Church" had a very low opinion of sensual pleasure. Especially Augustine, a brilliant thinker and writer, proved to be quite influential. He was born and died in Northern Africa, but spent his middle years in Italy where his thinking was shaped by certain then-fashionable ascetic beliefs and philosophies. During his youth and early manhood he had led a relatively active sex life, but after his conversion to Christianity he came to see sex as shameful and degrading. In his opinion, the involuntary bodily responses during sexual intercourse were embarrassing signs of enslavement to the flesh. They proved that human beings were not masters of their own bodies as God had intended them to be. Instead, the sin of Adam and Eve had robbed them and all their descendants of the proper self-control, and thus they were given over to "concupiscence"—lustful desire which seeks self-satisfaction at all cost. A "new" Christian life therefore demanded the strict repression of such lust. Marriage in itself was not evil, because it allowed the spouses to employ their base desires in the noble service of pro-creation. Still, somehow every sexual act, even between husband and wife, remained tainted, and every child born as a result of such an act needed the cleansing power of baptism. Even then the unfortunate disposition towards lust, inherited from Adam and Eve, remained.

Augustine's association of sex with original sin and guilt had a lasting and unfortunate effect on later Christian thinkers. It has to be understood, how-ever, that the entire intellectual and moral climate of the early church was inimical to any cultivation of the senses. The first Christians believed that the end of the world was imminent, and even when it failed to arrive their gen-eral outlook on life remained gloomy and ascetic. Virginity, total abstinence, and the systematic neglect of the body were considered marks of virtue. Monks and hermits were praised and admired for their relentless fasting and their fight against sexual temptation. Even self-castration was considered a moral act. At the same time, intolerance and religious fanaticism scaled new heights. When Christianity finally became the official religion of the Roman empire, the emperors passed strict laws prohibiting certain sexual acts as rel-ics of paganism. Especially homosexuals and other "deviants" from Christian sexual morality were singled out as capital offenders and publicly burned to death. Thus, shortly after the Christians had escaped their own persecution, they began the persecution of others. (See also "Sex and the Law—Historical Background.")

As the Christian church spread and flourished throughout Europe, this early extreme asceticism gave way to a more lenient attitude. Indeed, many members of the clergy themselves married and had families, a custom which prevailed well into the Middle Ages, when it was officially abolished by church leaders. In the course of time, the jurisdiction over sexual offenses shifted away from secular to ecclesiastical courts which now assumed the right to try all matters related to the salvation of souls. (In certain cases, how-ever, the defendant's body was handed over to government authorities for punishment.)

Medieval church policy towards sexual behavior is well documented in so-called penitentials, i.e., books written for the guidance of confessors and providing long lists of sins together with the appropriate penance. In general, these penitentials still show little tolerance of "deviant" sexual behavior or even of a vigorous "normal" marital sex life. It was only later, when Thomas Aquinas and his followers gained a wider influence in the church, that its sexual policies became somewhat more balanced and realistic.

Thomas, the greatest medieval theologian, made a serious effort to ap-proach the subject of sex in a systematic and logical manner. His basic as-sumption was this: It is the "nature" of human sexual intercourse to lead to the procreation of children. Therefore, any sexual activity that does not serve this ultimate end is "unnatural," i.e., contrary to the will of God and sinful.

All the rest of Thomas's sexual philosophy simply follows from this prem-ise. "Natural" sexual activity takes place only for the "right" purpose, with the "right" partner, and in the "right" way (i.e., for the purpose of procrea-tion, with the marriage partner, and by means of coitus). Sexual acts are "un-natural" and sinful to the degree to which they deviate from this triple moral standard. The greatest offense against nature is committed when the wrong purpose (for example mere sexual pleasure) is sought with the wrong partner (for example a partner of the same sex) in the wrong way (for example by means of oral or anal intercourse). Similarly, sexual contact with animals and sexual self-stimulation are very grave sins. Somewhat less sinful is sex with a wrong partner of the opposite sex, such as in rape, adultery, and incest. By the same token, simple "natural" fornication is only a minor transgression as long as it does not lead to pregnancy. In this latter case, however, it becomes a serious "unnatural" act, because the child will be illegitimate and will lack a father's care and attention.

Unlike Augustine before him, Thomas did not see the "right" sexual activ-ity, i.e., marital coitus, as tainted by concupiscence. He merely regretted that

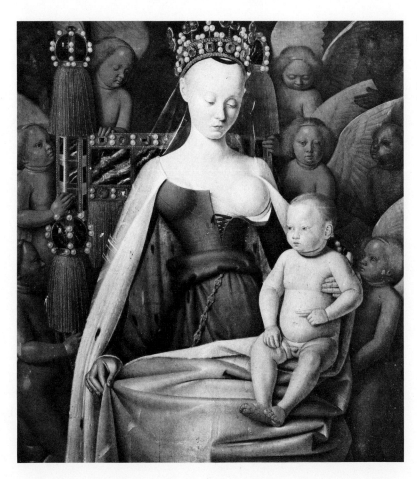

MADONNA AND CHILD
(Painting by Fouquet, 15th century)

The paradoxical image of the virgin mother Mary, which combines the ideals of chastity and procreation, is perhaps the most fitting symbol of the medieval Catholic view of sex.

it involved a loss of rational control. Thus, generally speaking, Thomas had a moderating influence on theological thinking about sex. Nevertheless, even for him sexual abstinence remained morally superior to marriage.

Thomas's insistence on sexual conformity with "nature" or, in other words, his belief in a so-called "natural law" has continued to determine Catholic doctrine to this very day. To be sure, in specific instances the church has modified its medieval views on sex. Especially in our century a certain liberalization has begun to set in. Still, on the whole, Catholics still cling to the same basic assumptions which define most actual human sexual behavior as deviant. Sexual self-stimulation, non-marital heterosexual intercourse, homosexual intercourse, and sexual contact with animals are still considered "unnatural" and sinful in various degrees. Artificial insemination, sterilization, abortion, and most forms of contraception are also rejected. (Only the so-called rhythm method is permissible under certain conditions.) Finally, it remains to be said that the church does not recognize divorces. In sum, with regard to sex the Catholic faith is still one of the most restrictive world religions.

The Protestant Churches

The Protestant Reformation of the 16th century divided the once unified church of Western Europe and gave birth to numerous new Christian churches, sects, and movements, a development which continues to this day.

The first important Protestant leaders, Luther and Calvin, rejected the supremacy of the pope and various other Catholic doctrines, but in regard to sex they retained most of the then traditional attitudes. However, they did attack the custom of clerical celibacy and the glorification of sexual abstinence. Luther, a former monk, himself set an example and married a former

A DIVINE COMMANDMENT FOR HUSBANDS AND WIVES
(17th-century American woodcut)

The first Protestants rejected the traditional celibacy of priests, monks, and nuns, encouraging everyone to get married. Indeed, the English and American Puritans reverted to the sexual laws of the Old Testament confirming reproduction as the main marital duty and the only legitimate purpose of sex.

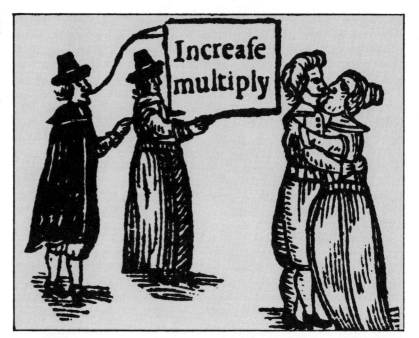

nun, and Calvin also felt obliged to marry in order to lead a more regular and productive life. Both considered women to be necessary, if subservient, companions for men. Calvin in particular saw the role of wife as that of a lifelong close associate of the husband. She was to be more than just a bearer of his children. By the same token, marriage was not simply a means of producing and educating offspring, but a social institution for the mutual benefit of the partners. Sexual pleasure in marriage was therefore moral and proper, provided it did not degenerate into excessive passion or sheer lust.

Calvin's theology had a great influence on the English Puritans for whom the Reformation under Henry VIII had not gone far enough and who eventually emigrated in large numbers to the new English colonies on the American east coast. In view of the harsh conditions under which they had to survive, the Puritans placed a very high value on the integrity of family life. Thus, while they had nothing against sex as such, they were extremely intolerant of any sexual activity outside of marriage. Premarital and extramarital sex was severely punished, as was any form of homosexual behavior or sexual contact with animals. In order to fight temptation, the Puritans also developed strict codes for dress and public behavior. Any seductive appeal to the senses was to be avoided. Under the circumstances, it is hardly surprising that their way of life soon became drab, joyless, and oppressive. Occasional outbursts of mass hysteria, such as in the Salem witch trials, undoubtedly had sexual overtones and prove that the Puritan sexual morality had become unrealistic, fanatical, and destructive. Fortunately, in the following centuries this rigid culture became increasingly diluted by the growing tide of new immigrants with a more liberal heritage. Nevertheless, Puritan attitudes continued to pervade much of American criminal law, especially in the state penal codes. (See "Sex and the Law—Historical Background".)

In the meantime, the various European Protestant churches had, on their part, also come under the influence of new ascetic philosophies. Especially in the second half of the 19th century, during the reign of the English Queen Victoria, an unprecedented prudery swept most Western nations and deeply affected Christian thinking about sex. Originally, this prudery had grown largely outside the church where it was promoted by physicians, psychiatrists, and educators. However, after some initial reluctance most clergymen also rallied to its cause. Indeed, when science finally freed itself from its narrow sexual views, many church leaders remained unable to do likewise. For them, Victorian pseudo-scientific theories had become part of their religious faith. (See also "Sex and Psychiatry—Historical Background".)

Today the many different Protestant churches present a rather varied picture in regard to their teachings on sex. On the one hand, there are fundamentalist churches which retain the strictest possible standards and condemn all sexual activity except marital coitus as sinful. Some of these churches even frown on fashionable clothing, facial make-up, dancing, kissing, embracing, or any other close physical contact between unmarried partners. On the other hand, some modern churches openly advocate complete sexual fulfillment for everyone, regardless of marital status or sexual orientation. Indeed, some churches today not only encourage women to be ministers, but also perform marriage ceremonies between partners of the same sex. Recently some major Protestant denominations, such as the United Church of Christ and the Episcopal Church, have ordained their first openly homosexual clergy.

At present, most of the larger Protestant churches take something of a middle position between these extremes. Many of them recognize the human sexual urge as a gift from God which serves not only the purpose of procreation, but also that of personal enrichment while creating a strong physical and spiritual bond between marriage partners. Noncoital forms of sexual intercourse, contraception, and sterilization can therefore be moral and, under certain conditions, may even be required. Unhappy marriages can be dissolved by divorce. Premarital sex has to be judged according to the circumstances; it is not sinful in itself. In general, people who deviate from traditional sexual norms must be met with compassion and understanding. It is immoral to persecute them in any way as long as they do not harm others. Thus, the governing board of the American National Council of Churches has now officially demanded an end to such persecution. The board also favors full civil rights for all citizens, regardless of their affectional or sexual preference.

Cross-cultural Perspectives

Just as in our own Western, Judeo-Christian civilization, people in other cultures have also found their sexual attitudes influenced by their religious beliefs. These attitudes may range from almost complete sexual freedom to strict asceticism. Indeed, some Eastern religions share certain negative Western approaches to sex. Generally speaking, however, one may say that non-Westerners have always allowed for a greater variety of sexual expression than we have done in the past. Thus, in Africa and Asia the persecution of sexual "deviants" has rarely been as fanatical as in Europe and America. As the scope of the present book does not permit a thorough and detailed discussion, a few selected examples of non-Western religions may serve as illustrations.

Islam

Islam, which dates back to the early 7th century A.D., is the youngest of the great world religions. Its founder, Mohammed, was greatly influenced by Jewish and, to a lesser extent, Christian beliefs, and thus it is not surprising to find that the Koran—the Holy Book of Islam—expresses many moral views that are similar to those of the Judeo-Christian tradition. In addition to the Koran, Moslems recognize the moral authority of the Sharia, a legal code developed after Mohammed's death. (The role of the Sharia is comparable to that of the Talmud in Judaism.)

Islam is not an ascetic faith, permitting as it does temporary marriages (*mut'ah* marriages), some forms of polygamy, and ready divorces. There is no doctrine of original sin or "concupiscence," although certain specific acts are considered sinful. Thus, contraception and abortion have usually been prohibited in Moslem countries which desired a population increase. Furthermore, due to certain historical and cultural traditions (especially in Arabia and Northern Africa), adultery and premarital sex among Moslem women

THE SENSUAL PLEASURES OF PARADISE
(14th-century Turkish miniature)

The religion of Islam never demanded the suppression of sexual interests from its followers. Thus, Islamic literature and art were often highly erotic. The picture shown here depicts the happy afterlife which awaits the righteous after their death when they will sit in shady gardens being served by beautiful heavenly girls (houris).

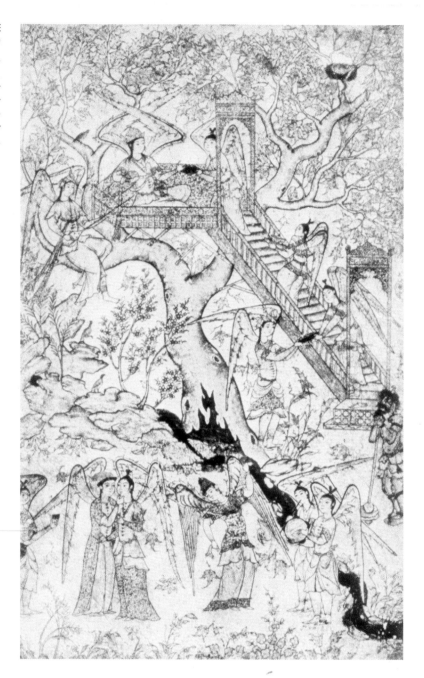

have often been severely punished. Otherwise, however, the Moslem attitude towards sexual "deviance" is comparatively lenient. It is true that the Koran repeats the biblical story of Sodom and Gomorrah and seems to condemn homosexual behavior (Koran XXVI 165–166, XXVII 54–58, XXIX 28–29, LIV 37–38). Indeed, at certain times and in certain places Moslems have demanded that homosexual offenders be put to death. However, in general such persecutions have been quite rare. In actual practice, most Islamic societies have always tolerated homosexual and ambisexual conduct. Where antihomosexual laws were in force, they were of little consequence, since, according to Mohammed, at least two witnesses were required for conviction. It seems, therefore, that consensual sexual behavior suffered few restrictions as long as it remained private. In sum, with regard to sex, the faith of Islam takes a realistic and rather liberal attitude, allowing for a considerable range of human sexual expression.

Hinduism

Hinduism, one of the world's oldest living religions, has no historical founder. Its earliest teachings, which were laid down at about 1000 B.C. in four holy texts called *Vedas,* are believed to have been revealed to wise men who lived along the banks of the Ganges and Indus rivers. (The word Hindu comes from the Persian name for Indus.) Over the centuries, several other holy books were added, among them the *Upanishads,* the *Laws of Manu,* the *Bhagavad Gita,* and epics such as the *Mahabharata* and the *Ramayana.*

These books vary greatly in content, style, and purpose, although in one form or another they support the central assumption of Hinduism—the belief in a Supreme Being, a Highest Spirit or World Soul with which all other souls are ultimately to be united. Since this goal cannot be achieved in one lifetime, reincarnation or transmigrations of the soul are necessary. Man's deeds in one life will determine his state in the next. However, even the lowliest creature has a soul and therefore deserves to be revered.

In practical terms, Hinduism has, on the one hand, given rise to ascetic practices among holy men and other devout persons who rejected all physical pleasure and comfort as an obstacle to the eventual union with the Supreme Perfect Being. On the other hand, there have also been religious movements which celebrated sexual pleasure in all its forms as a path to-

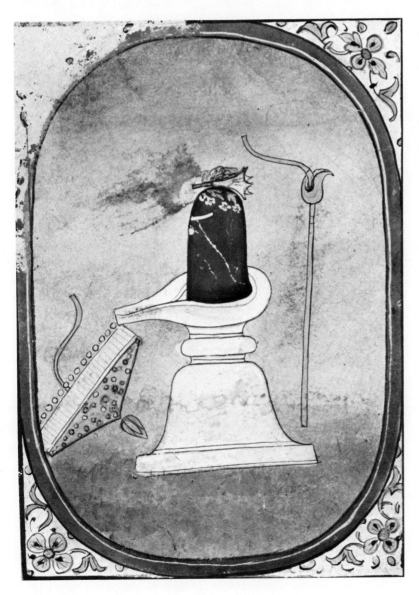

LINGAM AND YONI
(18th-century Indian painting)

For the Hindus, sexual intercourse often had a religious significance, and thus highly erotic images can be found in many Hindu temples. Even more sober temples usually displayed the icon shown here. It is the lingam (male sex organ) set in the yoni (female sex organ), representing the double-sexed deity. As the picture illustrates, offerings are laid on this icon and the honorific umbrella is broken.

wards the Divine. Many famous and sexually explicit works of art and architecture testify to this belief. Indeed, one of the best known early sex manuals, the *Kamasutra* (written in the 2nd century B.C.), treats sexual intercourse as a means of spiritual enrichment and thus is a legitimate expression of Hindu culture. At times, this culture also included polygamy and "sacred prostitution" in temples. Phallic worship, in the form of veneration for the "lingam," an artistic representation of the penis, continues to this day. We know that in India the condemnation and actual persecution of sexual "deviants" has never been long-lasting or severe. Exceptions were adultery and rape. Homosexual acts were usually also abhorred, although in many places groups of homosexual prostitutes called Hijras were allowed to practice openly.

Under the circumstances it is difficult to assess the general influence of Hinduism on sexual attitudes. Over its long history, many different and often contradictory philosophies have dominated different segments of Hindu culture. On the whole, however, Hindus seem to have enjoyed a more positive approach to sex than members of most other world religions.

Buddhism

The principles of Buddhism originated in the 6th century B.C. in Nepal with Siddharta Gautama who was later called Buddha (the Enlightened). Gautama became convinced that human suffering is caused by desire and that man must therefore free himself from his desires (including sexual desires) by a righteous, loving, and spiritual life. A "Noble Eightfold Path" of right belief, right aspiration, right speech, right action, right livelihood, right effort, right thought, and right meditation will lead to "nirvana," i.e., the supreme state of mind, the perfect insight, peace without passion.

As Gautama's moral doctrine spread all over East Asia, his followers divided into two major groups, of which one, the Hinayana (Small Vehicle), maintained his simple and demanding rules of discipline. The other group called Mahayana (Larger Vehicle) greatly expanded on his teachings, absorbing various local religious beliefs, and developing detailed doctrines about heaven, hell, and salvation. Within the two major groups there are numerous subgroups and sects. Gautama's original teachings were not religious in the usual sense of the word, as they said nothing about a Supreme Being or God or even about many minor gods. Instead, he simply pointed the way towards enlightenment through proper living. Self-knowledge, discipline, and kindness led to the gradual liberation from desire and finally to the perfect stillness of nirvana. It was only after Gautama's death that various theologies and mythologies attached themselves to his message. This process, in turn, produced different religious movements and groups which can be compared to churches in the Western sense. However, there was never a specific single sexual dogma. Buddhist attitudes toward sexual behavior varied with local culture and custom. In general, they were positive, practical, and humane. Sexual activity between consenting partners was usually considered a private matter. The persecution of sexual "deviants" was never prevalent in Asian countries. Masturbation, noncoital forms of heterosexual intercourse, and homosexual behavior may, at times, have been ridiculed or discouraged, but did not lead to official harassment. Prostitution often flourished openly. In some cases, it was seen as a useful institution or was even regarded as a respectable profession. Before they were affected by Western sexual attitudes, the Buddhist societies of East Asia were sexually very tolerant. Indeed, a great deal of this tolerance has remained even today.

American Indian Religions

The different native peoples of America held widely different religious beliefs and also differed in their sexual attitudes. It is obvious, for example, that the ancient high civilizations of South and Central America had only little in common with the much simpler cultures in North America, in spite of the fact that their European discoverers mistakenly referred to all of them as "Indian." (America was at first not recognized as a separate continent, but regarded as part of India.) Nevertheless, it is possible to make at least some

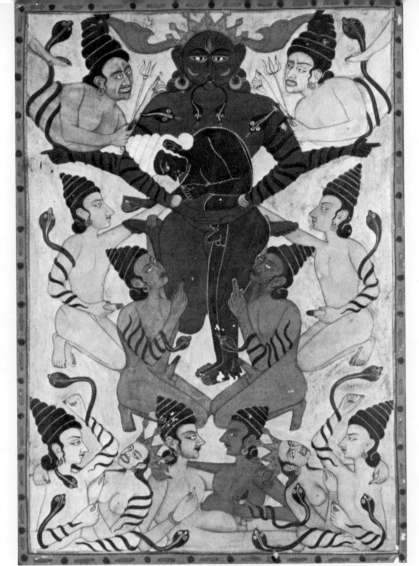

general observations about the American native religions and their view of human sexuality.

Most American Indians believed in various major and minor gods or goddesses and, in some instances, in bisexual or hermaphroditic deities. Some Indian peoples prayed to a Male Supreme Being, others to a Great Earth Mother or other female figure. Among those who lived by farming, fertility rites were common, although these rites rarely had a sexual character. However, sex did play a part in some other ceremonies. Indians in Peru often buried their dead with sexually explicit clay figures and pottery depicting almost every conceivable sexual act. There also seems to have existed some sort of institutionalized "sacred" homosexuality. (On the other hand, in some Central American cultures homosexual behavior seems to have been severely condemned, at least for members of the lower social classes.) While most American Indians observed certain strict sexual taboos against incest and sexual intercourse with a menstruating woman, there was no religious emphasis on chastity. Temporary sexual abstinence was required on special occasions. Childhood sex play was viewed with tolerance. Since marriage took place at an early age, adolescents also encountered little sexual frustration. Single males often enjoyed sexual privileges with the wives of their brothers or those of other male relatives. A married male guest of the family was sometimes granted similar privileges by the host. Sexual "deviance" was usually respected as the manifestation of a person's particular "nature" or "call." For example, a boy who displayed feminine behavior was not "corrected," but allowed to live as a woman and even to become the "wife" of another man. Thus, transsexuals and hermaphrodites encountered few social problems. In

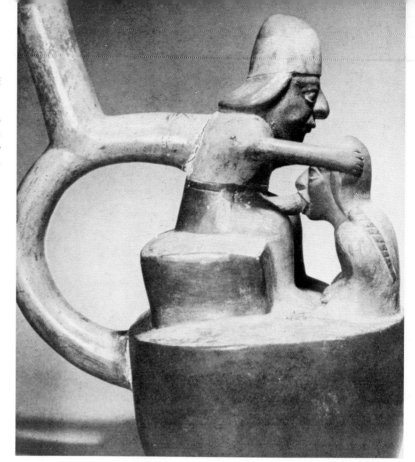

sum, it can be said that virtually all American Indian cultures were extremely
broadminded in sexual matters. Sexual pleasure was considered a necessary
part of life and was therefore everybody's right.

Ancient Polynesian Religions
Before their contact with Western civilization, the Polynesian islanders were
among the sexually least inhibited people on earth. While different Polynesian cultures developed different religious beliefs and social customs, none
of them ever regarded sex as evil, shameful, or dirty. On the contrary, their
gods, goddesses, and priests themselves were models of sexual vigor. Sensual
pleasure and physical beauty were valued very highly. Dancing, singing,
athletic competitions, beauty contests, and sexual exhibitions were regular
features of Polynesian social life. Indeed, in Tahiti there was a special religious order called the *Arioi* society whose members traveled from island to
island as professional celebrants and entertainers giving public sexual performances.

Polynesian children were encouraged from an early age to be sexually active, and they usually also were free to observe adult sexual activity either
at public festivities or in the home. (Sexual contact between young children
and adults was condemned, however, and seems to have been virtually non-
existent.) There were no special puberty rites, but adolescents were allowed
to spend several carefree and sexually active years in youth gangs which
provided their communities with musical, athletic, and sexual entertainment.
Premarital pregnancies were welcomed as signs of fertility and increased a
girl's chances of finding a husband. Furthermore, since the extended Polynesian family system easily absorbed additional children, there was never a
question of "illegitimacy." Marriages were usually monogamous. (Only some
of the highest chiefs had several wives.) However, a marriage was easily dissolved by mutual agreement, and remarriage was just as simple. It also must
be understood that Polynesian monogamy was not entirely exclusive, since
wives were often expected to grant sexual privileges to the male relatives and
house guests of their husbands.

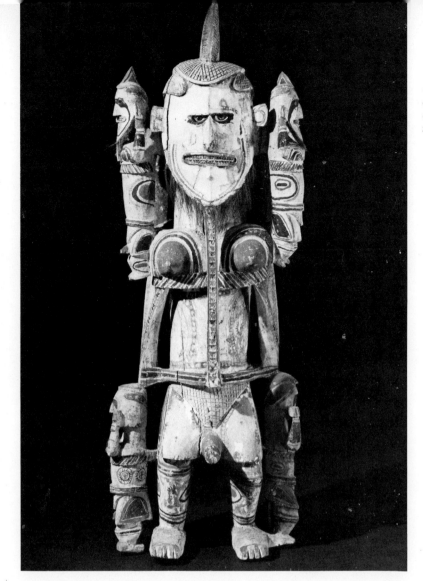

DOUBLE-SEXED ANCESTOR FIGURE
Many of the sexually uninhibited Pacific islanders expressed their worship of the unifying life-force by creating ancestral figures which show both male and female characteristics.

Given the generally tolerant sexual attitude of Polynesians, it is not surprising to find that homosexual and ambisexual activity also flourished openly in their culture and was accepted as natural. Transsexuals were allowed to live according to their preference, and thus certain men simply adopted the role of women. In short, under the circumstances it is questionable whether the term "sexual deviance" has any meaning if applied to ancient Polynesia. To be sure, there were some strong sexual taboos (the very word "taboo" is of Polynesian origin), but they had to do more with class restrictions than with sexual acts as such. There were also firm rules concerning the choice of a marriage partner, but again, they hardly prevented anyone's sexual fulfillment. Various taboos against incest may also be mentioned in this context, although even here exceptions are provided by Hawaii and Rarotonga where brothers and sisters of royal families often married each other. (This practice apparently had no negative effects.) In conclusion one might say that the ancient Polynesian cultures offer perhaps the best proof that a realistic, positive, and humane approach to sex can work and be socially productive.

(**NOTE:** Some of the information in the preceding section has been gathered from various articles in the *Encyclopedia of Sexual Behavior,* edited by Albert Ellis and Maurice Abarbanel, New York: Hawthorn, 1967, which is therefore recommended for further reading. See especially William Graham Cole, "Protestantism and Sex"; Bengt Danielsson, "Sex Life in Polynesia"; Rabbi Samuel Glasner, "Judaism and Sex"; Samuel Z. Klausner, "Sex Life in Islam"; Wu Lien-Teh, "Sex Life in the Orient"; Jelal M. Shah, "Sex Life in India and Pakistan"; Fred W. Voget, "Sex Life of the American Indians"; Robert Wood, "Sex Life in Ancient Civilizations".)

"NATURAL LAW" AND THE LAWS OF NATURE

In the history of human thought few words have created as much confusion as the words "nature" and "law." They can assume very different meanings, and these meanings are not always made sufficiently clear. Indeed, when people use the words in an argument, they often switch from one meaning to another without becoming aware of it and thus trap themselves in logical fallacies.

It seems useful, therefore, to take a brief look at how the concepts of "nature" and "law" originated, how they developed over the ages, and how we can best understand them today.

The Doctrine of Natural Law

In our Western civilization there is an ancient belief that above the imperfect laws written by human legislators one can find a higher, perfectly just, unwritten "natural law" created by God. Human laws are valid only insofar as they correspond to the natural law, and everybody can discover for himself what this natural law demands simply by using his reason.

This belief was well expressed about 2000 years ago by the Roman writer and politician Cicero in his book *Laws* (I, 10): "There is in fact a true law—namely right reason—which is in accordance with nature, applies to all men, and is unchangeable and eternal. . . . It will not lay down one rule at Rome and another at Athens, nor will it be one rule today and another tomorrow. But there will be one law, eternal and unchangeable, binding at all times upon all peoples; and there will be, as it were, one common master and ruler of men, namely God, who is the author of this law, its interpreter and its sponsor. The man who will not obey it will abandon his better self and, in denying the true nature of man, will thereby suffer the severest of penalties, though he has escaped all the other consequences which men call punishment."

In this single, short paragraph Cicero summarizes all the essential features of "natural law": First, it is the direct expression of the Divine Will. Therefore it is universal, eternal and unchangeable. Second, its rules can and must be found with the help of right reason. Third, man has a sacred obligation to obey these rules. Whenever he breaks them, he violates his own "true nature" and therefore automatically punishes himself.

Thus, the concept of a Natural Law implies that moral principles are immanent in nature, and that they tell us exactly how we should behave. As long as we obey them, we fulfill our true destiny. All our actions will not only be natural, but also perfectly moral. In other words, if everybody acted according to his nature, i.e., his "better self," the world could forever live in harmony, justice, and peace.

Cicero was, of course, by no means the first to suggest this appealing idea. Long before him a school of Greek philosophers called Stoics, and before them Aristotle and Plato had made the same basic suggestion. However, even they only updated a much older philosphy. Indeed, as we shall see, the Natural Law doctrine has its roots in some of the earliest religious beliefs of mankind.

The oldest and most primitive form of religion is known as "animism." That is to say, at the lowest stages of civilization man considers natural things —trees, rivers, mountains, the stars in the sky—as "animated" or endowed with feeling and intelligence. He believes that spirits or souls dwell within or behind them, and that these spirits have to be treated with the same consideration as his fellow human beings. In fact, they deserve even greater respect, because they possess superhuman powers with which they can reward or punish him. Thus, all natural phenomena are easily explained: The corn grows because the corn spirit wants to reward man for righteous conduct. The corn fails to grow because its spirit wants to punish man for his transgressions. The river carries the boat because the river spirit is at peace with man. The boat is pulled down into the water and sinks because the spirit has been offended.

This animistic interpretation of nature can, of course, also be described as a social interpretation. Or, to be more precise, man's earliest experience of nature is simply an extension of his social experience. The spirits which surround him everywhere react very much like powerful lords, chiefs, or elders and therefore have to be treated in a similar fashion. In return, they offer protection and help. Thus, the relationship between man and nature is essentially a social relationship governed by the principle of mutual obligation. Man finds himself tolerated and even supported by nature as long as he meets his obligation. However, as soon as he fails, nature becomes angry and punishes him.

As man progresses on his path of civilization, his religious beliefs become more refined and his primitive animism turns into some form of polytheism (Greek: a belief in many gods). The multitude of powerful spirits is gradually reduced to a small number of even more powerful gods, each of whom governs a large segment of nature. Thus, a god or goddess of fertility is responsible not just for a single plant, but for the whole harvest. Boating and seafaring no longer depend on the spirit of each individual river or ocean, but on one great god of all waterways. Needless to say, this more sophisticated religion simplifies life considerably. Still, it does not change man's basic relationship to nature. As a matter of fact, this relationship may remain unchanged even on the next level of sophistication, when polytheism gives way to monotheism (Greek: the belief in one God).

For the purpose of our present argument it does not make very much difference whether the corn grows at the command of a corn spirit, an ancestor spirit, a fertility god, or the Lord God Almighty. The important point is that this growth is caused by a superhuman intelligence in response to human behavior. Sunshine and rain, good and bad harvests, are reward or punishment for man's conduct. Indeed, everything that occurs in nature has some personal meaning for man and is somehow related to his fate. All natural phenomena have the same cause and serve the same end. The law of nature is divine will. There is no differentiation between causal and normative laws. Explanation and justification are one and the same.

Moreover, in these early phases of religious evolution, the divine will manifests itself not only in the laws of nature, but also in the laws of society. Indeed, as we have already mentioned, society and nature are not yet clearly distinguished in man's mind. Both follow the same rules and are experienced the same way. Everything in this world (of which man is an integral part) is governed by powerful, superhuman beings who demand personal, strict obedience. These superhuman beings—the spirits, the gods, or God—are therefore the source of all law, declared and implied, general and specific, known and unknown, written and unwritten. In short, the contrast between an imperfect "artificial" human law and a perfect "natural" law does not yet exist. Even the most trivial social customs, rules, and regulations are of divine origin.

This is the reason why many primitive human societies believe that their political and legal institutions owe their existence to some national deity or a divinely inspired leader. In some societies the rulers themselves claim to be divine or at least of divine ancestry. It is only at higher stages of civilization, when the old customs and laws have to be changed, when people develop some sense of history, and when they learn to show some tolerance for foreign ideas, that they begin to perceive their social order as an arbitrary creation of fallible men. This is the point at which the distinction between a written, imperfect positive law and an unwritten, perfect natural law appears. From now on, perfect justice is restricted to the natural order.

To be sure, for the great monotheistic religions there remain some written laws which are directly inspired by God. They are preserved for all time in the sacred books containing His revelations—the Old and New Testaments and the Koran. However, these laws are rather general in character, cover only a few selected areas of life, and thus have to be augmented by a host of secular human laws. These human laws may, under certain conditions, very well turn out to be unwise and unjust. It is therefore always necessary

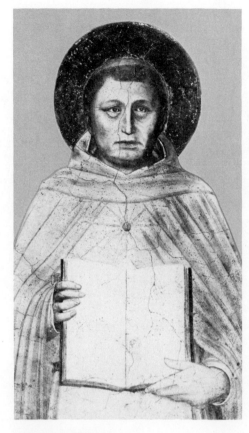

THOMAS AQUINAS
Thomas Aquinas (1224-1274 A.D.) was the greatest medieval theologian and one of the most brilliant proponents of the Natural Law doctrine.

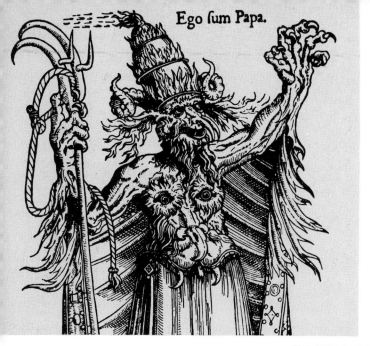

Ego ſum Papa.

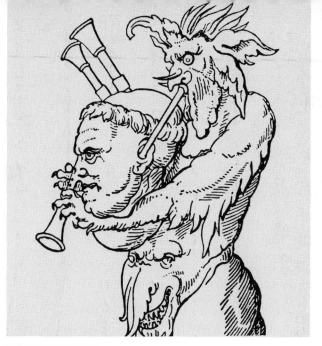

THE IMPACT OF THE REFORMATION

The Protestant Reformation of the 16th century divided the formerly unified Western church, giving rise to new, and often conflicting, religious and moral doctrines. As a result, Christians found it more and more difficult to agree on the "true" will of God or the intentions of nature.

(Left) 16th-century Protestant caricature portraying Pope Alexander VI as the devil.

(Right) 16th-century Catholic caricature portraying Martin Luther as a bagpipe played by the devil.

to measure them against the divine law which is revealed in the Scriptures and the natural law which is implied in nature itself.

In our Western culture, this philosophy was, of course, eventually tied to the doctrines of the Christian faith. (The Jewish and Islamic legal traditions developed along different lines of their own.) Thus, from the end of antiquity well through the Middle Ages, the Catholic church was considered the proper guardian and interpreter of all "higher" law. In his *Summa Theologica,* Thomas Aquinas, the greatest medieval theologian, distinguished four basic types of law:

1. Eternal Law (the justice of God, which is almost identical with His reason),
2. Natural Law (the Eternal Law implanted by God in nature and in the human mind),
3. Divine Law (God's overt revelation of His will), and
4. Human Law (derived from Natural Law).

The first three types of law express the will of a heavenly legislator and therefore clearly fall into the province of theology. Only the fourth type, human law, can be said to have some secular basis. However, since it is derived from natural law (and in specific instances superseded by divine law), its ultimate validity still has to be decided on religious grounds.

The Thomistic view of the law dominated European thinking for many centuries and is, in fact, still held by Catholic theologians today. Obviously, these theologians also believe, as Thomas did, that there can be only one correct interpretation of nature and the Scriptures—the Catholic interpretation. This latter belief, however, is no longer shared by all Christians.

The Protestant Reformation of the early 16th century has, in the meantime, given rise to a great number of new, independent Christian churches which offer a variety of different and even conflicting scriptural interpretations. Furthermore, many of these churches refuse to formulate any detailed official dogma and encourage their members to study the Bible according to their

THE AMERICAN DECLARATION OF INDEPENDENCE
The American Declaration of Independence of 1776 still owes many concepts and phrases to the doctrine of Natural Law. However, the document also reveals a certain ambivalence towards this doctrine. Shown here is the introduction. The key expressions relating to the Natural Law doctrine have been underlined for easy identification.

own lights. As a result, the exact meaning of specific divine revelations has become a matter of opinion.

Not surprisingly, modern Christians also differ in their interpretations of the Natural Law. Instead of a unified church speaking with one voice, we now hear many churches and countless individuals expressing their own diverse beliefs about the meaning of God's creation. Indeed, in the last few centuries this diversity has grown almost to the point of chaos. Thus, the "true nature" of man, which had seemed so obvious in the past, has turned into an ever more elusive phantom.

Because of these developments, the doctrine of Natural Law itself has lost much of its former influence and gone into a gradual decline. Today, legislatures no longer pay much attention to it, but pass their laws simply as an expression of the popular will without invoking any "higher" authority.

The increasing neglect of "nature" as the source of the law has been especially noticeable in England and America, which share a legal heritage quite different from that of other Western countries. English kings gave up some of their "natural" rights as early as 1215 with the signing of the Magna Carta, and in the following centuries their power was limited even further by Parliament. Moreover, a common law founded on practical experience and guided by precedents bound both the King's ministers and his subjects. Thus, unlike the law of continental Europe, English law soon acquired a rather pragmatic character. Legal disputes were more easily recognized as disputes between people, and the key to justice was sought not so much in the Bible as in the Statute Book.

This does not mean, of course, that England and America completely discarded the natural-law philosophy. Indeed, when, in the late 18th century, the American colonies took up arms against the English crown, they used this very philosophy to justify their rebellion. Thus, the Declaration of Independence of 1776 refers specifically to "self-evident truths" and to "the laws of nature and of nature's God." Still, upon closer study, this same document also reveals that its authors were somewhat ambivalent in their attitude or even had second thoughts about the basis of the natural law. For example, in contrast to older traditions they also state that governments derive their just powers not from God in heaven, but from the "consent of the governed" here on earth. It follows that, if necessary, the people have a right to institute a new government, "organizing its powers in such form, as to them shall seem most likely to effect their safety and happiness." In other words, government and law are seen mainly in secular terms as the work of man. The people alone, therefore, bear the ultimate political and legal responsibility.

In contemporary America, the Natural Law doctrine has ceased to play any important practical role. All that is left of it today are a few bizarre vestiges, most notably in the unrevised, older state criminal codes. For example, a number of states still prohibit so-called "crimes against nature," i.e., acts that do not involve actual victims, but run counter to what Jews and Christians once considered to be the will of God. (See "Legal—Illegal, Current Sex Laws in the U.S.") However, the validity of these laws is now being challenged not only by some theologians, but also by modern scientists. As a matter of fact, in the meantime, the whole notion of a normative natural order has been made obsolete by the advance of the natural sciences.

The Natural Sciences and the Laws of Nature

As we have pointed out earlier, primitive man experiences nature as part of society and thus interprets all natural occurrences in social terms, i.e., first and foremost, according to the principle of retribution. Sunshine and rain, good and bad harvests, health and sickness, life and death, are caused by powerful spirits, the gods, or God in response to human conduct. Righteous conduct is promptly rewarded, sinful conduct is automatically punished. There is no differentiation between causal and normative laws. Everything that happens in nature is the direct expression of a superhuman personal will. In short, explanation and justification are one and the same.

This prescientific view of nature could, of course, easily be illustrated with ancient myths and religious beliefs from all over the world. In the present context, however, we can perhaps restrict ourselves to our own Judeo-Christian culture and just mention a few examples from the earliest part of the Bible—the Five Books of Moses in the Old Testament.

In the Book of Leviticus, for instance, Yahweh tells the people of Israel that certain sexual relationships displease him and therefore will not go unpunished. Thus, he declares, among other things: "If a man marries his brother's widow, it is impurity; . . . they shall be childless" (Leviticus 20;21). In other words, religious offense and physical disorder are described simply in terms of cause and effect. An "impure" marriage produces infertility. Even if both the man and the woman were fertile before, their sin immediately and inevitably blocks their normal bodily functions and thus makes procreation impossible. [It will be noted that Yahweh's attitude here is quite different from that expressed earlier in the Book of Genesis (38; 8–10), when he commanded Onan to impregnate his brother's widow and punished him for refusing to do so. (See also "Types of Sexual Activity—Sexual Self-Stimulation.") This apparent contradiction must remain unresolved here. It is a problem for biblical scholars.]

Yahweh also punishes sexual intercourse between the "right" partners which occurs at the "wrong" time: "If a man has sexual intercourse with a woman during her menstrual period, . . . they shall be cut off from among their people" (Leviticus 20; 18). Today, the latter phrase is often interpreted to mean exile or banishment. However, many biblical scholars assert that this interpretation is false, and that the phrase "cut off from among their people" refers instead to sickness and early death sent by the all-knowing Yahweh himself. Thus, again, the crime invariably produces its own punishment.

In the Book of Deuteronomy, Yahweh is even more explicit. His people can receive nothing from nature but what they deserve. If they are righteous and obey the commandments, they will be blessed with prosperity, fertility, gentle rain, and good harvests (Deuteronomy 28; 8 ff.). However, if they should prove to be disobedient, they will be cursed with pestilence, consumption, fever, inflammation, fiery heat, boils, ulcers, scurvy, the itch, madness, blindness, confusion of mind, drought, locusts, worms, and the spoilage of food (Deuteronomy 28; 20 ff.).

To be sure, in many cases Yahweh also relies on human help in carrying out his punishment. Thus, he commands the people of Israel: "If a man has sexual contact with an animal, he shall be put to death; and you shall kill the animal" (Leviticus 20;15). Still, in this as in all other cases, the human executioners are mere instruments of the Divine Will. If they fail in their duty, they will be punished themselves. If, on the other hand, they do as they have been told, they will be promptly rewarded. (For an example see the rewarding of Phinehas who executed a sinful couple [Numbers 25;6 ff.].) At any rate, in the cause of divine justice, human beings never play more than a minor, auxiliary role. Yahweh may use them, but he never depends on them. With or without their assistance, His will is done—as in nature, so in society.

As we can see, for the ancient Israelites the laws of morality and the laws of nature followed the same pattern. Indeed, strictly speaking, there was only one type of law, and it was prescriptive and descriptive at the same time, i.e., it stated not only what ought to happen, but also what would happen in any given case. Retribution could be delayed, but it could not be prevented. In the end, all innocence and all guilt would be revealed, and everybody would be given his due.

We have to remember, of course, that this legal philosophy was by no means restricted to Israel. Similar views were held by many other ancient peoples. The earliest Greek philosophers, for example, saw both the physical and the social world ruled by the twin forces of fate (Moira) and necessity (Ananke). The Greeks also personalized the concept of unfailing justice in the awesome figure of Dike, the goddess of retribution, the ultimate judge of all those who act against the divine order of things. Thus, we can read in a famous fragment written by the philosopher Heraclitus: "The Sun will not overstep his path; if he does, the Erinyes, the handmaids of Dike, will find him out." In other words, even the heavenly bodies follow the commandments of justice. If they deviate from their prescribed course, their offense will be discovered and punished. The laws of nature are essentially moral norms which must be fulfilled by an obedient universe.

The tendency to equate natural with moral laws is characteristic of all pre-scientific thinking, and this thinking changed only with the gradual progress of civilization. It took mankind a very long time to discover that the course of the stars, sunshine and rain, storms and earthquakes, birth defects, epidemic diseases, and the behavior of locusts and worms have nothing to do with human sin or righteousness. In ancient Greece, some philosophers (the so-called Atomists) fairly early developed the notion of an objective causality, but with the rise of the Christian church, their work was increasingly neglected and finally forgotten. It was not until the beginning of the Modern Age, when men like Copernicus, Bacon, Brahe, Kepler, and Galilei started the "scientific revolution" that nature was again studied objectively, i.e., without reference to any divine or human concerns.

When scientists examine a natural phenomenon, they deliberately ignore its alleged religious or moral meaning. Instead, they try to understand it strictly on its own terms. Goodness and badness, justice and injustice do not concern them. They do not make value judgments, but judgments of fact. In short, they do not prescribe what should be, but only describe what is.

A scientist acts on the assumption that the natural and the social order are governed by different principles, and that he can therefore very well explain natural events without having to justify them at the same time. He no longer ascribes any "higher purpose" to nature, but regards it merely as a system of elements which are connected with one another as cause and effect. This connection is independent of any human or superhuman will.

Those familiar with the history of science know, of course, that it did not attain full "objectivity" overnight. Indeed, for many centuries the new, morally neutral principle of causality and the older principle of retribution remained linked in several indirect ways. For example, the first modern scientists assumed that, just like human sin and divine punishment, cause and effect must follow an automatic sequence, and that they must always be in direct proportion to each other. Stronger causes were thought to produce stronger effects. It was further believed that a cause could have only one effect, and that an effect could have only one cause.

In the meantime, these and other vestiges of retributive thinking have been completely eliminated from the scientific concept of causality. Today scientists recognize that cause and effect are only elements in a continuum, and that, as such, they signify nothing more than a regular succession of events. Each cause is the effect of another cause, and each effect is the cause of another effect. Therefore, it seems rather arbitrary to single out any particular cause for any particular effect. Moreover, the connection between cause and effect is no longer considered to be one of absolute necessity, but of mere probability. Under these circumstances, some scientists have, in fact, abandoned the terms "cause" and "effect" altogether, and now speak instead more generally of "conditions" or "components" and "resultants" of an event.

Fortunately, in the present book, we do not have to concern ourselves with all the intricacies of modern scientific theory. For our purposes, it is sufficient to emphasize its basic premise: The natural and the social order are not identical. Nature, i.e., the physical reality surrounding us, can and must be explained without any reference to social norms. The laws of nature are fundamentally different from the religious, moral, criminal, and civil laws of society.

The entire issue can also be summarized in another way: With the advance of the natural sciences, the word "law" has acquired two very different meanings. Where once there was only one law—the will of God—which ruled everything both in nature and in society, we now insist on a sharp distinction between normative and causal laws, and, in formulating the latter, we avoid any reference to possible divine intentions.

The following two laws may illustrate the point:

1. If a woman commits adultery, she will be punished.
2. If water is cooled below a certain temperature, it will turn into ice.

For the prescientific mind, both of these laws simply describe the workings of a divine will. God punishes adultery, God freezes the lakes and rivers, and he does the one as unfailingly as the other. (Still, if he wants, he can also make an exception in both cases. Thus, he can show mercy and let an adulteress go unpunished, or he can perform a miracle and keep a particular river flowing when all other rivers are frozen.)

For the modern, scientific mind, on the other hand, the two laws share only a very superficial resemblance. It is, of course, true that both have the same grammatical structure. Indeed, in the most general and abstract sense, they express the same basic thought, i.e., they connect something as a condition with something else as a consequence. However, it is now widely recognized that the character of this connection is quite different in each case. The first law connects the condition (adultery) with its consequence (punishment) in a prescriptive way, stating that the condition *ought to* be followed by the consequence. The second law connects the condition (a certain low temperature) with its consequence (conversion of water into ice) in a descriptive way, stating that the condition *is* followed by the consequence. The first law designates a *compulsory rule* laid down by some legislative authority. The second law designates nothing more than an *observed pattern*. The first law must be enforced by some superhuman or human agent (the spirits, the gods, God, or the police). The second law "enforces itself," as it were. It takes its course regardless of anybody's opinion or action. A woman who commits adultery may not always be punished. Water which is cooled below a certain temperature always turns into ice.

The difference between normative and causal laws becomes perhaps even more apparent when we consider the ways in which they may change in the course of time. Normative laws are easily amended or even repealed by legislative fiat. The amendment or the repeal then simply replaces the old norm with a new one. Causal laws, on the other hand, change in a very different way, and this change has a different meaning. Indeed, in a certain sense, one might say that causal laws are unchangeable, and that it is only our perception of them which changes. For example, scientists may formulate a certain causal law and then be forced to revise it in the light of new observations. Any such revision, however, produces a greater degree of accuracy in describing the observed phenomenon and therefore does not invalidate the original purpose of the law itself.

Finally, it has to be understood that there are many normative systems in the world, but only one causal system. In the course of its history, the human race has established a great variety of social orders with vastly different and even conflicting norms. Thus, actions that were required at the time were prohibited at another time, and qualities that were praised in one society, were condemned in another. In contrast, there has never been more than one natural order, and it is still the same everywhere today. The reason for this is plain: The natural order has never been and will never be subject to human influence. Human beings can study it and even use it to their advantage, but they cannot change it.

"Nature" as Ideology

When we today look back at the history of human civilization, we see that the strict distinction between normative and causal laws was one of its greatest achievements. Without this distinction the advance of the natural sciences with all of its benefits would have been impossible. Science began only when man finally decided to disregard the divine and human aspects of everything he studied, i.e., when he separated the explanation of natural events from their justification. As a result, he became able to look at nature in a detached, disinterested manner. He no longer assumed that it had any obvious or hidden personal meaning for him, but instead tried to understand it on its own terms. Paradoxically, it was this very detachment, this neutral, "objective" attitude, which enabled man to learn more and more about nature and thus to use it for his own ends.

The objectivity of science is based on the recognition that natural events have no "higher purpose" and do not express or establish any moral values. Scientists know that there is no logical inference from factual reality to ethical norm, from the "is" to the "ought." It does not follow from the fact that an event occurs, that it ought to occur or that it ought not to occur. The fact that in nature water turns into ice if it is cooled below a certain temperature, does not imply that cold temperatures are good or bad, or that water is better or worse than ice. By the same token, the fact that in nature big fish swallow little fish does not imply that their behavior is right, nor yet that it is wrong. The fact that some plants overgrow and destroy other plants says nothing about the moral value of plant life.

However, while nature as such is value-free, human beings cannot live without values and therefore always prefer certain natural phenomena over certain others. Thus, men aboard a ship prefer the lakes, rivers, and oceans unfrozen while men on a sled prefer them covered with ice. Some fishermen like to catch big fish, others prefer to catch little fish. Farmers and gardeners spend their lives cultivating some plants and weeding out others, knowing full well that their weeds may be another man's crop. In short, man constantly selects certain natural things or events as useful and dismisses others as useless. In each case, his selection is guided by his own shifting self-interest, not by some value or norm embedded in nature itself.

Nevertheless, there are still some people today who maintain that nature is built on moral principles or, what amounts to the same thing, that all natural phenomena serve some ultimate end. Furthermore, this ultimate end can supposedly be deduced from nature with the help of "right reason." Thus, everybody who carefully examines nature can discover the law by which he himself should live. This "natural law" guarantees him a way of life which follows the intentions of nature and is therefore perfectly moral and just.

The belief that nature can have intentions clearly implies that it is a superhuman being endowed with will and intelligence, or at least that it is governed by such a being. It follows that the laws of nature do not merely describe observed patterns, but are, in fact, compulsory rules laid down by some legislator. This supreme legislator is either nature itself or God who created nature as an expression of his will. Man's self-interest, properly understood, is therefore best served by obeying God's or nature's commands. As summarized by Sir William Blackstone, the great 18th century legal scholar, in his *Commentaries on the Laws of England:* "As man depends absolutely upon his Maker for everything, it is necessary that he should in all points conform to his Maker's will. This will of his Maker is called the law of nature."

As we have shown earlier, the natural-law doctrine is not and cannot be based on scientific insight, but is essentially religious in character. It reflects a prescientific, mythical view of the world. This fact is, indeed, freely admitted by most Christian proponents of the Natural Law, and even among the adherents of non-Christian faiths it is usually considered quite obvious. Nevertheless, in modern times there have also been repeated attempts to derive "objective" norms from nature without the benefit of religious guidance. As a matter of fact, even some atheistic philosophers have tried to find the foundation of their moral values in "nature."

These modern, non-religious believers in a "natural law" contend, for example, that "finite existence is always unfinished," or that all living things have a "tendency toward completion or fulfillment." Thus, human beings also have certain tendencies toward a particular "natural" way of life which ensures their existential completion or the realization of their inherent potential. Any action which furthers this goal is good, any action which hinders or prevents it is bad. The state or the social order therefore has an obligation to encourage everyone to behave "naturally."

The idea that everything in nature strives towards some sort of completion or fulfillment is, of course, a very old one. For example, in Aristotle's *Metaphysics* (1015a, 13–15) we find the following definition: "Nature in the primary and strict sense is the essence of things which have in themselves, as such, a source of movement." The "essence of things," according to Aristotle, is that singular quality which truly defines them, which makes them what they really are. The essence of an acorn is to become an oak tree, the essence of a tadpole is to become a frog, and the essence of a fetus is to become a human being. The "movement" which "things have in themselves" is their tendency to grow and develop, to realize their potential. It is this movement which produces oak trees from acorns, frogs from tadpoles, and human beings from fetuses. In other words, acorns, tadpoles, and fetuses will always become what they were meant to be unless some outside force prevents it. In that case, their "natural" tendencies would be blocked, and their development would come to an "unnatural" halt. Their "nature" would be deprived of its completion or fulfillment.

However, this view of nature, time-honored and appealing as it may be, is quite incompatible with the demands of scientific objectivity. For a scientist, the growth of oak trees, frogs, and human beings represents only a regular pattern of changes, a probable and, to a certain extent, predictable development. It does not fulfill any inherent needs or express any special tendency towards "completion." Indeed, for someone who merely wants to describe nature without passing judgment on it, all things are always complete as they are.

On the other hand, if any stage of natural development is ever regarded as a stage of incompleteness, then all things are always incomplete. For example, a fetus is incomplete because he is not yet born, a baby boy is incomplete because he is not yet an adult, an adult is incomplete because he is not yet old, and an old man is incomplete because he is not yet dead. If any of these possible changes are described as the realization of a "tendency," then all of them can be described this way. Then there exists not only a tendency towards life, but also a tendency towards death, and both must be equally "natural" and good. Obviously, such a conclusion leaves nobody any wiser.

The truth is that no unprejudiced observation can tell us whether or when a particular living thing is "complete" or "incomplete." In the course of its existence, everything undergoes many different changes, and to say that some of these changes are for the better (i.e., serve its completion) and others for the worse (i.e., deprive it of its completion) is to state a subjective opinion, not a scientific fact. Indeed, the very concept of "completeness" already implies a positive value judgment, just as that of "incompleteness" implies a negative one. The assertion that something is incomplete can only mean that it is imperfect, that something is missing from it which ought to be added. People who argue that the completion of natural things is good and that the lack of completion is bad simply trap themselves in tautologies.

Under the circumstances, an objective observer has no choice but to admit that nature in itself has no tendencies, intentions, meanings, or ultimate goals. Therefore it cannot be taken as a moral guide. Regrettable as this may seem to many people, there simply is no honest way of building a "just" moral or legal system on it. So far, all attempts to find universal values in nature have failed. At worst, they have led to narrow, capricious, and oppressive dogmas; at best, they have produced empty slogans and meaningless maxims which can serve every possible purpose or justify every possible action.

For example, "nature" has been said to require that everybody receive his due. Thus, the ancient Roman moralists thought they had discovered a true natural moral law when they demanded "*Suum cuique!,*" i.e., "To each his own!" However, this law can never create concrete justice, because it fails to answer the crucial question: "What is everybody's own?" This question, the only one that really matters, must already have been decided by some other, positive law or political system. Therefore, the phrase "To each his own!" can be used to justify any such system, the slave state, feudalism, capitalism, or socialism.

Another equally unreliable precept is the so-called Golden Rule or, in other words, the admonition "Do unto others as you want them to do unto you!" At first hearing this, too, may sound like a universally valid "natural" law. However, it would allow any person who enjoys pain to inflict pain on others, even if they do not care for such treatment. Similarly, any alcoholic may, in good conscience, force a hard drink on his neighbor. Finally, if somebody violates the Golden Rule, should it also be violated against him? After all, nobody wants to be punished, even if he has done wrong. Hence, according to the Golden Rule, nobody should punish a wrongdoer. In short, taken literally, the Golden Rule results in the abolition of law and morality.

Still another example is the so-called Categorical Imperative formulated by the German philosopher Kant: "Act only on that maxim whereby you can at the same time will that it should become a universal law!" In other words, a man should act only on thoes principles that he shall wish to be binding on all other men. But what are these principles? They can be the principles of liberal democracy as well as those of fascism, communism, or any other conceivable social order.

The fact of the matter is that, in the course of history, the so-called Natural Law has been used to justify any imaginable moral or political position. Thus, Aristotle declared that some people were destined "by nature" to be slaves. (Nor did the Bible find anything wrong with slavery.) Interestingly enough, when the institution of slavery finally came under attack in modern times, abolitionists also used the Natural Law as an argument. Rejecting the positive, written laws of their time, they appealed to a "higher" unwritten law which declared all men to be created equal and which guaranteed them their inalienable "natural" human rights. The slaveholders remained unimpressed, however, and simply turned the argument around. According to them, God had created nature, and nature had shaped the fate of mankind. History proved that human progress was possible only because superior men gained the freedom to develop their faculties by ruling over their inferiors. Therefore, nature itself demanded slavery as the price of civilization.

Through the centuries, similar inconclusive arguments have been made about the true "natural" form of government. Monarchists, for example, used to point to the hierarchical order of the sky where moons revolved around planets which, in turn, circled the sun. Thus, it was only natural for common citizens to live in the service of noblemen who, in turn, served a king or emperor. Democrats, on the other hand, protested that all heavenly bodies were equally subject to the same law of gravity and that nature therefore also prescribed equal justice under the law for all men. This view did not suit the anarchists, however, who saw the universe as a place of continuous, unrestrained struggle between elementary forces. Therefore, any human legal restraint, even under the pretext of equality, only interfered with the proper workings of nature.

The problem with all of these disputes is not that the ultimate or "true" intention of nature was misunderstood by one or the other side. Nor can it be assumed that an additional dosage of "right reason" would finally have revealed it to all sides. The truth is that no such intention exists and that the quarreling parties simply projected their own value system into nature from where they then retrieved it through circular logic. This is possible precisely because nature has no definite moral content. When used in moral disputes, the word "nature" can mean anything anybody wants it to mean. Thus, it represents the classic example of an "empty formula," a semantic vessel into which each society or group of society pours its own notions about the "right" order of things. In short, it is essentially an ideological term.

This is nowhere more obvious than in the area of sexual morality. We have already described earlier how the ancient Greeks saw the "nature" of sex in pleasure and personal fulfillment. The sexual urge was due to a divine inspiration which drove the lover to unite with the beloved. Any act that approached or accomplished this goal was "natural." In contrast, the ancient Israelites and early Christians believed that the "nature" of sex was procreation and that therefore only one very specific sexual act—coitus—was "natural." Any other sexual activity was "unnatural," and a just society was obliged to prevent it from taking place. The American Indians and ancient Polynesians, on the other hand, felt that even homosexuality, transvestism, and transsexualism expressed the "nature" of particular individuals and therefore had to be respected. Any social interference would have been the greatest injustice and, indeed, a crime against nature itself.

Still no matter how a "crime against nature" is defined—as a specific noncoital sexual act or as its suppression—the definition is always arbitrary and subjective. Objectively speaking, nature can never be violated, because even the violation itself would be entirely natural. Or, as a famous sex researcher once put it: "The only unnatural act is one that cannot be performed."

Therefore, the assertion that certain acts are "unnatural" is never a statement of fact, but always a value judgment. Obviously, it cannot mean that nature prevents these acts from occurring (since actually they occur all the time). It rather means that nature somehow disapproves of their occurrence, or that they are not in nature's best interest. In actual fact, however, nature has no opinion about them one way or the other. The opinion is entirely human. The disapproval does not come from nature, but from very specific men and women who find their personal moral values rejected.

The words "natural" and "unnatural" are expressions of praise and condemnation. They do not provide us with objective descriptions of anything. People who merely want to describe reality without judging it do not use these words. In the neutral view of a scientist, for example, everything is natural, since everything is part of nature. For him, pain is just as natural as pleasure, disease just as natural as health, and death just as natural as life. However, it is obvious that, if used in this neutral fashion, the word "natural" is practically meaningless. Scientists therefore have removed it from their vocabulary and relegated it to the sphere of morals.

When we study the instances in which the words "natural" and "unnatural" are actually used, we always find that they are meant to support definite moral judgments. Needless to say, these value judgments vary with the bias of the speaker. Historical and anthropological research has shown that, in different periods of history and in different parts of the globe, societies have lived by very different moral values. In fact, such differences continue to this day. Nevertheless, also to this day, every society has always presented its own particular moral values as universal, eternal, and unchangeable, i.e., as truly and exclusively "natural." The reason for this is simple: The invocation of "nature" lends any subjective value system an aura of objectivity. It allows people to avoid personal responsibility for their moral positions. Thus, if one dislikes the sexual behavior of one's neighbor, it is easier to persecute him in the name of God or "nature" than in one's own name. In short, we are all too easily tempted to claim that our own tastes and predilections correspond to the demands of "universal justice," the "general welfare," the "divine will," or the "natural order."

However, any such claim is either an innocent delusion or a cynical fraud. An objective analysis proves in every case that the alleged "divine will" or "natural order" represents nothing but the interests of certain individuals, groups, or social classes. This is the very reason why the same God and the same nature can be invoked to justify so many different social policies. As we have seen earlier, even the great monotheistic religions—Judaism, Christianity, and Islam—vary considerably in their interpretations. Moreover, within Christianity itself there are countless churches, sects, and movements with widely divergent views of God's will and nature's law. Thus, using the same Bible to bolster their arguments, some churches recognize divorces while others do not, some churches prohibit contraception while others demand it, and some churches condemn homosexuality while others ordain openly homosexual ministers and perform homosexual marriages.

In any case, it is obvious that today there are Christian churches which no longer share the traditional Judeo-Christian belief that the "nature" of sex is reproduction. To many Christians this belief now appears to have been based on an outmoded, narrow, and arbitrary assumption, and therefore they try to develop a new, more open sexual morality. In doing so they realize, however, that it is not enough to replace one arbitrary assumption with another and to seek the solution in some updated doctrine of Natural Law. Instead, they are beginning to understand that they themselves have to take full responsibility for their sexual values.

This does not mean that the entire moral effort of earlier Natural Law advocates should be ignored or discarded. Indeed, as even its severest critics have pointed out, the Natural Law doctrine has often been used to attack oppressive religious and secular authorities, and thus it has also served the cause of human freedom. In short, in the course of history, the belief in a Natural Law has not only served the prevailing order, but also projected a better order to come. The word "nature" may be an empty formula, but it has sometimes been filled with mankind's best hopes and aspirations. Human beings may not have any God-given, natural rights to life, liberty, and the pursuit of happiness, but in some modern societies they have successfully invoked "nature" to fight for these rights and to win them. The notion of a Natural Law therefore has a utopian, humanistic aspect that deserves to be emphasized and appreciated. In this sense, a critical study of the Natural Law tradition can still teach us a great deal about a truly humane sexual morality.

(Note: In the preceding chapter a number of arguments and illustrating examples have been borrowed from various writings of Hans Kelsen, Karl Popper, Ernst Topitsch, and other representatives of Middle-European *Ideologiekritik*. Although these writers have not dealt specifically with the problem of sexual deviance, their general reasoning is obviously applicable here, and their work is therefore recommended for further study. For a sample of Kelsen's critique of the Natural Law, which has been partly summarized above, see his collection of essays *What Is Justice?*, Berkeley, 1957. The utopian aspect of Natural Law has been thoroughly investigated by Ernst Bloch in his *Naturrecht und menschliche Würde* [Natural Law and Human Dignity], Frankfurt, M. 1961).

LEGAL—ILLEGAL

Where the violation of sexual norms is defined as a legal problem, sexual conformity and sexual deviance are seen as respect for the law and crime. Conforming sexual behavior is "correct," "law-abiding," and "legal." Deviant behavior is "offensive," "criminal," and "illegal."

There is, of course, no question that certain kinds of sexual behavior have to be prohibited by law, because they involve force, fraud, violence, or exploitation, or take place in front of unwilling witnesses. The victims of such behavior are clearly justified in demanding legal protection, and virtually all human societies try to fulfill this demand, at least for their "important" members. In short, no society can survive very long without a certain minimum of sex legislation. However, there have been societies in which large numbers of people were deliberately left unprotected even against the most brutal forms of sexual assault. In these societies the law served only the powerful and privileged and was, in fact, nothing more than a tool of class justice. Thus, slaves and serfs often were "fair game" for their masters. Sometimes, members of religious or racial minorities also were denied their full human rights and could be sexually abused by the majority without fear of punishment.

On the other hand, most modern societies which are devoted to "equal protection under the law" take great pains to punish all sexual abuse, no matter who the offender. Indeed, in their zeal to make the world "safe" for everyone, they sometimes overlegislate and create sexual offenses where otherwise none would exist. Thus, they end up protecting not only the righteous from the wicked, or the wicked from each other, but also the righteous from themselves. That is to say, when the sex laws begin to extend to "victimless crime," they take on a totalitarian character and may themselves victimize many good people.

Still, even the most zealous lawmaker must leave many forms of sexual wrongdoing unpunished. For example, husbands and wives who use sex as a means to degrade each other, parents who keep their children sexually ignorant, teachers who frighten their students with lies about masturbation, or clergymen who call for the persecution of sexual nonconformists may do a great deal of harm. Nevertheless, they are not regarded as sex criminals, and it is doubtful whether any specific law could control them.

All of this leaves us with two conclusions:

1. Law and morality are not the same thing. Undoubtedly, the two are somehow related, but the relationship is not a direct one. Some immoral sex acts may be entirely legal, while certain moral sex acts may be illegal.
2. One cannot simply assume that the purpose of sex legislation is to provide physical or emotional protection. After all, as we have seen, some dangerous behavior may be legal, and harmless behavior may be illegal.

How, then, are we going to find the "true" reasons behind our often puzzling sex laws? Or, in other words, what is the real basis on which societies determine the legality or illegality of sexual behavior? Perhaps we can arrive at an answer by taking a brief look at history.

SEX AND THE LAW

At the beginning of human civilization all laws were religious laws, i.e., they expressed the will of some superhuman authority. The spirits, the gods, or God wanted human beings to behave in a certain way and promptly punished any disobedience. The laws, therefore, practically enforced themselves.

The earliest known sex laws were no exception to this rule. Originally, there was no difference between sin and crime. Sexual offenders were both sinners and criminals, and their punishment was certain. Where human law enforcement was necessary at all, it merely carried out divine orders.

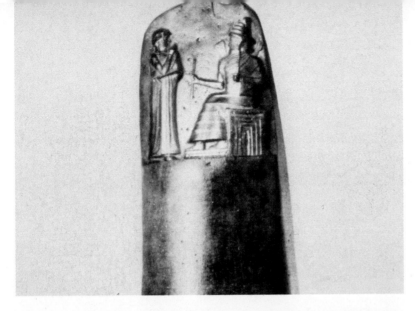

THE DIVINE ORIGIN OF THE LAW

The first great lawgivers of mankind claimed that their laws expressed a divine will.

(Top) Stone in the shape of an erect penis inscribed with the laws of Hammurabi which were inspired by the Sun-god. The relief sculpture at the top of the stone shows the god sitting on his throne instructing Hammurabi who stands before him. (Paris, Louvre)

(Middle) Moses receiving the tablets of the law from Yahweh on mount Sinai. (9th-century Carolingian miniature)

(Bottom) Illustration from a Persian manuscript showing the archangel Gabriel dictating the Koran to Mohammed.

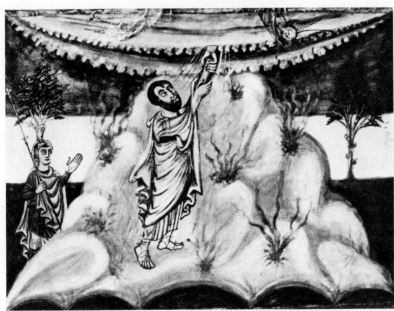

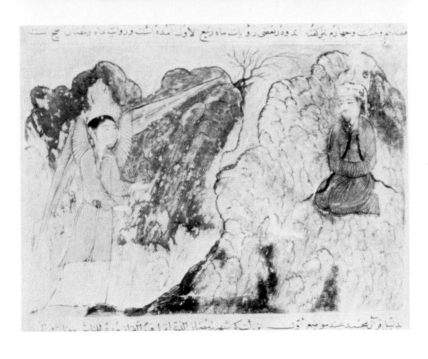

As a matter of fact, this was the prevalent view throughout most of human history. For thousands of years religious belief remained the foundation of all law. The first great lawgivers of the Old World, for example, still openly claimed to be instruments of a "higher" will. Hammurabi received his laws from the Sun-god, Moses was given the Ten Commandments by Yahweh on Mount Sinai, Mohammed had the Koran dictated to him by the archangel Gabriel.

Needless to say, these and various other "divinely inspired" legal codes differed rather widely from each other, especially in regard to sexual behavior. We also know that even some of Yahweh's sexual commandments changed or reversed themselves in the course of time (for example see Genesis 38; 8–10 and Leviticus 20; 21). Still, when we compare the first historical attempts at sex legislation, we also find that they had at least one thing in common: They all covered both social and religious offenses. Sexual behavior was punished not only when it caused harm to other human beings, but also when it merely showed disbelief. Indeed, the latter offense usually carried a harsher penalty than the former. People were much more afraid of divine displeasure than of any personal injury.

Thus, sexual heretics could never claim to be socially harmless. Even if they endangered nobody in particular, they still posed an indirect threat to the community. Their very existence insulted God and invited his retribution. Therefore they could not be tolerated. Their persecution was a religious duty, and any measure taken against them was justified.

This was the basic philosophy of jurists from ancient to medieval times. In their opinion the main function of the law was to restore and preserve God's "natural order." In fact, over the centuries, the control of sexual behavior became the exclusive province of the church. Religion was the most influential moral force, not only in private, but also in public life.

At the beginning of the Modern Age, when the church lost more and more of its power to the secular state, the old prohibitions remained. All over Europe ecclesiastical courts were replaced with secular courts, penitentials with criminal codes, penance with criminal penalties, but the general approach to sexual deviance was the same as before. The state simply adopted the traditional moral standards and enforced them with all its might. Even "harmless," victimless deviants continued to be prosecuted. They just turned from religious heretics into secular "subversives." In the eyes of the law, they somehow still threatened the well-being of the nation.

It was not until after the American and French revolutions in the late 18th century that the state declared its complete separation from the church. This meant, among other things, that the sex laws could no longer directly be copied from the Bible, but had to be based on rational and empirical grounds. As a result, many sexual acts that once had been crimes were now found to be permissible. An "enlightened" citizenry escaped its former moral tutelage and won many new civil liberties. A certain "free sphere" of privacy and personal morality was created, and the law was told to stay out of it. These democratic gains were soon consolidated in the Napoleonic legal reforms which, directly or indirectly, reached most of Western Europe and Latin America. The United States, in their constitution, also proclaimed their independence from religious dogma. Congress was explicitly ordered to "make no law respecting an establishment of religion."

However, the Christian, or rather Puritan, stranglehold on American public life was not so easily broken. For a very long time the state continued to punish not only dangerous crimes, but also mere sins and victimless vices. It simply ignored the growing number of non-Puritans for whom these vices were, in fact, virtues, and who were now prevented from leading a full sexual life in accordance with their beliefs. Indeed, to this very day, when it comes to anything sexual, many American legislators still routinely forget the Constitution.

Fortunately, in recent years the general public has become more sophisticated, and thus it is beginning to understand that sexual freedom is as much a constitutional issue as religious freedom and freedom of speech, for example. A number of states have already liberalized their sex laws, and others are in the process of doing so. It seems, therefore, that, at least in this limited area, the promise of the American Revolution will finally be fulfilled.

These few observations are not meant to imply, however, that religion is the only possible obstacle to rational sex legislation. Even the strictest separation of church and state does not, by itself, guarantee sexual freedom for every citizen. After all, several modern, openly atheistic states, such as the Soviet Union, the People's Republic of China, and Cuba are as intolerant of sexual deviance as any medieval Christian kingdom. Among other things, these countries still prohibit "pornography," prostitution, homosexual acts, and cross-dressing, although none of these offenses involves any victims. Obviously, the prohibitions are now no longer defended on the old religious grounds. Instead, they are based on new ideological dogmas about "Western immorality," "capitalist corruption," or "bourgeois decadence." A closer study of these dogmas could probably discover their long-forgotten religious origin. Or perhaps the desire to create and then persecute heretics is so deeply ingrained in some societies that they use any excuse, religious or secular, to justify it. At any rate, even in our time, there is still much sexual intolerance in many parts of the world. The fight for universal human sexual rights is far from over. (See also "The Sexually Oppressed.")

The following pages briefly summarize the development of European and American sex legislation. In addition, they also offer some cross-cultural comparisons. Because of limited space, sex-related legislation, such as that concerning marriage, divorce, contraception, abortion, illegitimacy, venereal disease, etc. is not mentioned here. The discussion is restricted to laws which directly regulate human sexual behavior in the narrow sense of the term.

Historical Background

In order to understand the present English and American sex laws one has to consider their history. Some of these laws, in fact, are based on the beliefs and customs of primitive ancient peoples and have survived only through a series of historical accidents. Furthermore, unlike the law of continental Europe, for example, Anglo-American law does not yet fully reflect the modern separation of church and state, but continues to enforce a very specific medieval Christian morality. This is particularly surprising in the case of the U.S. which, in its constitution, proclaims complete religious freedom. Nevertheless, in the area of sexual behavior, the constitutional guarantees still wait to be realized. To this day, narrow Christian moral doctrines are legally imposed on the sexual behavior of American Moslems, Hindus, Buddhists, and atheists. Too many American Christians still refuse to accept the fact that, constitutionally, the U.S. is not a "Christian country," but is supposed to be home for all forms of belief and disbelief. Indeed, it can rightly be argued that many current American sex laws are unconstitutional.

The following brief historical survey traces the origin and development of English and American sex legislation. Naturally, in the present context this survey can only be sketchy and incomplete. Even so, it will make the largely religious basis of present legal attitudes indisputably clear.

The Jewish Legal Tradition

The history of ancient Israel is the history of its struggle for national identity and survival. Surrounded and constantly threatened by "infidels," the Israelites made extraordinary efforts to preserve their "true" faith. All of their laws and customs have to be seen in this context.

Early Jewish sex legislation tried to protect "God's chosen people" from four major "evils": a population decrease, the violation of male property rights, the "contamination" with strangers and strange customs, and religious heresy. Thus, the laws encouraged marital coitus at the expense of all other sexual activity and prohibited various forms of nonreproductive sex that were common among neighboring tribes. The refusal to procreate indicated an antisocial attitude and offended the whole nation. Rape, adultery, and illegitimate pregnancies violated the rights of individual men who regarded their wives and daughters as their personal property and who demanded compensation for any "damage." Homosexual behavior and sexual contact with animals were associated with the worship of foreign gods. Thus, they were signs of idolatry or, as the Bible calls them, "abominations," i.e., crimes against Yahweh himself.

Naturally, in the course of time, certain specific sex laws were modified, and others were reinterpreted in the light of changing circumstances. Nevertheless, the general Jewish legal attitude towards sex remained unchanged even at the time of Christ. (See also "Sex and Religion, Historical Background.")

Early Christian Doctrines

The early Christians adopted most of the Jewish legal tradition. Officially, they still lived under the lenient laws of the "pagan" Roman empire, but in their private conduct they followed the stricter biblical standards. Indeed, the first great Christian missionary, Paul, had a very low opinion of man's sexual desires and advocated restraint wherever possible. This attitude was further developed by Augustine and other so-called Fathers of the Church whose views were openly ascetic. Finally, when Christianity became the Roman state religion, this new asceticism found expression in the criminal code. The Christian emperors Theodosius (390 A.D.) and Justinian (538 and 544 A.D.) passed draconic laws condemning certain sexual practices as relics of paganism. Especially the code of Justinian, which survived for nearly 1000 years in the Byzantine (i.e., East Roman) empire, was very intolerant of sexual deviance. For example, Justinian declared that heathen abominations like homosexual intercourse and sexual contact with animals cried out for God's punishment by storm, fire, famine, pestilence, and earthquake, and that the state therefore had the solemn duty to protect the land by executing all offenders. The execution consisted of burning at the stake or live burial, often preceded by torture and mutilation. Justinian's code was a landmark in Western legal history, and it had a great influence on the thinking of medieval jurists.

The Medieval Ecclesiastical Courts

England, Scotland, and Ireland became familiar with Christian legal doctrines through the work of missionaries. Anglo-Saxon law had never been organized into a code. The body of law was customary. Now, together with its new religion, the Christian church introduced a new legal system. English kings also began to enact new secular laws, and, for a long time, both legal systems existed side by side, mutually supporting each other. Eventually, the church acquired jurisdiction over all spiritual matters. Special ecclesiastical courts were set up which dealt with such offenses as heresy, blasphemy, witchcraft, and sexual deviance. These courts did not have the power to impose any secular punishment, however. Instead, they prescribed only a certain penance. By the same token, they were not bound by ordinary rules of evidence, but relied mainly on voluntary confessions. Offenders usually confessed their sins because they feared for their souls. An ecclesiastical court could save them from eternal damnation. The judges, in turn, felt obliged to consider not only concrete actions, but also mere sinful thoughts. The various kinds and degrees of penance were laid down in special books called penitentials, which today give us a fairly accurate picture of medieval ecclesiastical justice.

Generally speaking, the ecclesiastical attitude towards sex was extremely negative. Even coitus between husband and wife was severely restricted. For example, sexual intercourse was forbidden for 3 days after the wedding, during a woman's menstrual period, during her pregnancy, and for several weeks after childbirth. It was also prohibited on Thursdays (Jesus' arrest), Fridays (Jesus' crucifixion), and Sundays (Jesus' resurrection) as well as during official periods of fasting (40 days each before Easter and Christmas). Menstruating women were not allowed to enter the church. Fornication demanded a penance of up to 1 year, adultery for up to 7 years. Masturbation and involuntary orgasms during sleep were treated somewhat more lightly. However, homosexual acts and sexual contact with animals could require a penance of 22 years to life.

To modern minds it may appear strange that there should have been such a great difference between the penance for adultery and that for homosexual acts, for example. However, it must be remembered that, to the medieval mind, these sins belonged to entirely different categories. Nonreproductive types of sexual behavior were offenses against the "natural order" and therefore against God himself. By comparison, sins of "natural" lust, such as seduction, adultery, or even rape, which offended only other human beings, were much less serious.

Penitents usually were expected to dress in a white sheet and to appear barefoot and bareheaded at the church door. They had to carry a heavy candle and were marched down the aisle to the front of the congregation where they made a public confession. Finally, after several weeks or years, when the terms of their penance were fulfilled, they were given a written certificate. Offenders who either refused to confess their sins to the court or failed to do the prescribed penance were excommunicated.

It was perhaps inevitable that, over the centuries, this method of regulating deviance became largely ineffective. First of all, the sexual standards set by the church were utterly unrealistic. Secondly, many clergymen themselves openly flouted these standards. Thirdly, as the system became well entrenched, the act of penance was more and more often replaced with almsgiving and finally with the payment of a fine. This, in turn, set the ecclesiastical courts on a collision course with the secular government. After all, many spiritual offenses also caused real physical harm. Sins against God can, at the same time, also be crimes against people. For example, medieval lords were entitled to a special fee ("merchet") for allowing the daughters of their vassals to marry. If such a daughter ruined her chance for marriage by sexual promiscuity, the lord was cheated out of his fee. In these and similar cases, secular courts had always been entitled to impose fines as a compensation for damage. However, now that the church also collected money through its own courts, the offenders were often unable to make a second payment to the civil authorities or to their victims. As a result, the entire system of ecclesiastical justice began to be questioned.

Finally, when, during the Reformation, King Henry VIII became the head of the English church, he took over some of its jurisdiction and turned various religious offenses into secular crimes. Thus, homosexual acts and sexual contact with animals, for example, which before had required only penance, were declared to be felonies. Offenders were executed and all their possessions confiscated. Queen Elizabeth I even appointed a special Court of High Commission which punished moral and spiritual offenders with fines and imprisonment. This court, however, soon became completely corrupt and turned into a kind of Protestant Inquisition. Therefore it was abolished in 1640.

The Puritan Heritage
When Oliver Cromwell and the Puritans came to power in England, they greatly intensified the persecution of sexual deviants. Cromwell himself never tired of demanding more zeal on the part of prosecutors. In 1650 Parliament passed the so called Puritan Act "for the suppression of the abominable and crying sins of incest, adultery, and fornication, wherewith this land is much defiled, and Almighty God highly displeased." Thus, the religious basis of Puritan sex legislation was made unmistakably clear. The prescribed penalties were the same as those used in biblical times. For example, just as in ancient Israel, adultery was punished by death.

While the Puritan rule soon came to an end in England, it experienced a second flowering in America. The Puritan colonies of New England were, in fact, totalitarian religious states. Most of their sex laws were based on the laws of Moses. The Massachusetts colony, for instance, directly copied the Old Testament when it passed legislation demanding death for adultery, homosexual acts, and sexual contact with animals. Fornication posed a rather difficult problem, because the ancient Israelites had never condemned it as such. Nevertheless, Christians had learned to regard it as a grave sin. The Puritans eventually developed their own approach and specified various forms and degrees of punishment. Fornicators could be enjoined to marry, they could be fined, or they could be pilloried and publicly whipped as a warning example to others. Sometimes all three penalties were combined. In later, more lenient times it also became customary to force fornicators to wear the letter "V" (for Vncleanness) conspicuously displayed on their clothing. Punishment for adultery was then signalled by the letters "AD" or simply by "A." (See also Nathaniel Hawthorne's novel *The Scarlet Letter*.)

In spite of these strict laws and harsh penalties, however, sexual deviance remained quite common among the New England Puritans. Many contemporary reports leave not doubt that illegitimate births were frequent and that homosexual behavior was fairly widespread. This latter fact is, of course, hardly surprising, since the community concentrated its efforts on the prevention of all nonmarital heterosexual contact.

Modern Law

The sex laws in most states of the U.S. today still follow the Puritan model. As the American population moved westward across the continent, the New England penal codes were simply carried along and copied in every new state. Most settlers were content with preserving the legal traditions to which they had been accustomed on the East Coast. Unlike the inhabitants of the Old World, they were not interested in new legal theories or fundamental reforms. Western and Southern Europe had, in the early 19th century, liberalized their sex laws at the command of Napoléon I. The Napoleonic code, which legalized practically all consensual sex between adults in private, had an influence reaching well beyond the French national borders. It was either adopted or used as a model in Italy, Spain, Portugal, Belgium, the Netherlands, and all of Latin America. Thus, most of the world's Catholic countries entered the new Industrial Age with a sensible minimum of modern sex legislation, while the Protestant countries of Central Europe and North America remained tied to the past. Most of their ancient and medieval sex laws were preserved intact. The only real change was a gradual reduction of penalties. For example, while adultery continued to be a crime in Massachusetts, the death penalty was relatively soon replaced with a public whipping, a fine, and imprisonment. Then the whipping was omitted, leaving the fine and the prison term on the books. Finally, even these reduced penalties were considered too severe. However, instead of changing the law, the authorities simply ceased to enforce it.

Another, even more telling example is provided by the case of New York which, unlike Massachusetts, at first did not have a law against adultery. Then, in 1907, a group called "The National Christian League for the Promotion of Purity" pressured the legislature into adopting such a law. From that time on, adulterers could be fined or imprisoned, or both. Nevertheless, almost from the start, there was virtually no attempt at enforcement. The situation was especially grotesque because in the state of New York adultery was the only recognized ground for divorce. Every year the courts routinely granted thousands of divorces on this ground, but also routinely failed to prosecute the guilty parties. It was not until a few years ago that this official exercise in legal hypocrisy finally came to an end when the legislators faced up to their initial mistake and repealed the anti-adultery law that they should never have enacted in the first place.

Unfortunately, to this day, the reform of antiquated sex laws has not made much progress in the U.S. The vast majority of states still insist on legislating and overlegislating morality and thus continue to create for themselves a host of unnecessary social problems. (For a more detailed discussion of some of these problems see below under "Current Sex Laws in the U.S.".)

Cross-Cultural Perspectives

The English and American legal approach to sexual deviance has always been unusually harsh. This becomes quite apparent when one studies the sex laws of other societies. Most of them are much more tolerant. Curiously enough, the experiences of these societies do not seem to be of any interest to Americans. Thus, it is not uncommon to find American legislators quoting the Bible in defense of stricter legal control, but virtually none of them ever considers the available practical record in other countries. Some of these countries have had only minimal sex legislation for more than a hundred years, and by now they know very well what does and does not work. Still most of the discussion in England and America, even among legal scholars, remains parochial, as if nothing could be learned from the experience of others.

Unfortunately, the scope of the present book does not allow for a detailed description of European, African, Asian, and South American sex laws. A very brief selection has to suffice. Nevertheless, the following summaries, inadequate and superficial as they are, may add at least some perspective to the discussion. All criminal codes listed here are those of modern, industrial nations.

The Soviet Union

It is rather difficult to summarize the legal controls of sexual behavior in the Soviet Union. First of all, the various union republics have their own penal codes, and these vary especially in their sex laws. Secondly, deviants of all sorts are often "corrected" without formal arrests and criminal trials. Instead, they may be subject to noncriminal sanctions. Although such sanctions can be quite severe, they do not define the deviant as a "convict" in the regular sense. Persons who are found to lead a "parasitic way of life," for example, may be resettled and forced to work in an assigned job for a certain period of time. Obviously, all of this allows for a great deal of discretion, and thus the criminal law may never be invoked.

Still, one can get a glimpse of the general legal attitude towards sex in the Soviet Union by studying the criminal code of the Russian Soviet Federated Socialist Republic, which is the largest of the 15 union republics. In this code the most serious sexual crime is rape. The law distinguishes between degrees of rape according to the force or violence involved. While simple rape may result in not more than a 3-year prison term, aggravated forms are punished much more harshly (up to 10 years). Gang rape and the rape of a minor can be punished by still longer prison sentences or even death. Child molestation is punishable by imprisonment for up to 3 years. The same offense "in perverted forms" carries a maximum penalty of 6 years. Homosexual acts between men are considered a serious crime. The punishment may range up to 5 years in prison. (The old Czarist law against male homosexual behavior had been abolished in the early days of the revolution, but was reintroduced in 1934. However, now as before, no mention is made of homosexual behavior between females.) There are further strict laws against the making and supplying of pornography (3 years imprisonment). "Pandering for a mercenary purpose" and "keeping dens of debauchery" may be punished with 5 years in prison. In addition, it is a serious offense to "draw minors into criminal activity," such as "begging, gambling, and prostitution."

The Scandinavian Countries

Norway, Denmark, and Sweden have for a long time closely collaborated in the field of administration of justice. Thus, the three countries have developed similar views on what sexual acts should be considered crimes.

Compared to the United States, there is not much legal control of sexual behavior. The most serious offense is rape which, under certain conditions, can be punished with life imprisonment. However, the law recognizes various degrees of rape, and thus in nonviolent and "statutory" cases, such as sexual intercourse with an insane or mentally defective woman, the penalty is much less severe. Sexual contact is punishable as child molestation if one of the participants is under the age of 15 (14 in Norway). Incest is defined narrowly as sexual intercourse between direct ascendents and descendents or brother and sister. It is considered a serious offense, although participants under the age of 18 may escape punishment. There are no laws against "fornication," "sodomy," or "crimes against nature." Adultery and sexual contact with animals are crimes only in Norway, but prosecutions are extremely rare. Homosexual acts are legal as long as they take place between consenting adults in private. (They are punishable only if one of the participants is under the age of 16.) Prostitution as such is also legal, although prostitutes may be arrested under the vagrancy laws and enjoined to find other employment. Lewd and obscene behavior in public is an offense. Obscenity in private, however, does not concern the law. The generally lenient Scandinavian attitude towards "pornography" is well known. Denmark has even lifted the few remaining restrictions and legalized all sexually explicit materials.

The Federal Republic of Germany

The West German sex laws are simple and few in number, comprising only ten paragraphs (§ 174– § 184) of the uniform national German penal code. The code refers to sex crimes collectively as "crimes against (a person's) sexual self-determination" and thus clearly expresses the underlying philosophy of German sex legislation: Sexual behavior is criminal if it interferes with other people's free and healthy sexual development and expression. Accordingly, the code punishes those who have sexual intercourse with partners under their care or authority, such as dependents, apprentices, students, prisoners, mental patients, etc. The seduction of a girl under 16 years of age is also punishable, although the case may be dismissed if the seducer is younger than 21 years. Sexual intercourse with children under 14 years of age is always a crime, and it is illegal to make "adult" pornography available to anyone under 18 years of age. Rape is punished according to the severity of the crime with imprisonment between 6 months and 5 years (more if the victim dies). Sexual intercourse under the threat of force or other threats and impositions carries a penalty of 3 months to 5 years or even up to 10 years imprisonment according to the circumstances. Prostitution as such is not a crime, although operators who provide more than just housing, pimps, and those who encourage prostitution can be punished by several years' imprisonment. There is no law against homosexual behavior between consenting adults. However, homosexual acts are prohibited with partners under 18 years of age, although offenders who are themselves younger than 21 years may go free. (The law here assumes that persons under 18 years are too young and impressionable to make an independent, rational decision for homosexual behavior.) Sexual acts in public can be punished with up to one year imprisonment or a fine. Exhibitionism is prosecuted only in response to a complaint. The sentence can range up to 1 year imprisonment, although it may be suspended if there is reasonable hope that the offender can be rehabilitated by psychiatric treatment.

Japan

In the 19th century the formerly isolated Japan was opened to Western influences and experienced fundamental political and social changes as a result of the so-called Meiji Restoration. In pre-Meiji Japan sex laws were comparatively few and lenient. Homosexual relationships were not considered shameful, but enjoyed a social recognition comparable to that known in ancient Greece. Prostitution also flourished openly in special entertainment districts which were by no means always as sordid as their equivalents in Europe or America. However, as Japan became more westernized, this traditional sexual freedom was more and more restricted. Today the Japanese criminal laws share certain negative Western attitudes towards sex, although on the whole they are still much less oppressive.

There are no laws against homosexual behavior, adultery, fornication, cohabitation, or sexual contact with animals. The encouragement of prostitution, pimping, and pandering are now illegal, however. Prostitutes can be sent to a "women's guidance home" for 6 months in order to be "protected and rehabilitated." Furthermore, there is a law against the public display and sale of "obscene" material. (The Japanese definition of obscenity is rather different from that of Western countries.) The most serious sexual offense is rape, which is punished according to the degree of violence used by the rapist. In simple cases it may carry not more than a 2-year prison term, but if the rape involves a child or results in serious injury or death, the sentence may be life imprisonment. The concept of "statutory rape" is unknown. Sexual molestation, i.e., an "indecent act" with a male or female person which involves force or the threat of force is punishable as "indecency through compulsion." Harmful child molestation (i.e., if the victim is under 13 years of age) can also be prosecuted under this statute. The sentence is usually severe (6 months to 7 years). "Public obscene behavior" carries a maximum prison term of 6 months. On the other hand, several sexual acts which could be considered extremely serious in the U.S. are treated as minor offenses in Japan. For example, a man who "exposes his body in such a way as to cause disgust to the public," or who "secretly peeps into houses, bathrooms, dressing rooms, or toilets" is simply punished with "detention and a minor fine." These acts are listed together with and treated like such offenses as trespassing, starting false fire alarms, and "frightening horses or cows and causing them to run away."

CURRENT SEX LAWS IN THE U.S.

Each state in the U.S. has its own laws regarding the sexual behavior of its citizens. These laws show an astonishing lack of conformity as to the number and character of punishable offenses as well as to the severity of the prescribed punishment. For example, certain sexual acts may be punishable by life imprisonment in one state, yet may not be a crime at all in another state. Furthermore, there is a total confusion as to the terminology used in defining sexual offenses. The various legal terms employed for this purpose are mostly of prescientific origin, and their meaning can differ from state to state.

In addition to their "regular" sex laws, a number of states also have special laws allowing for the commitment and forced psychiatric treatment of offenders. These laws declare certain sex offenders to be "sexual psychopaths" in need of a "cure." Consequently, such offenders, who otherwise would perhaps receive only a suspended sentence or serve a short prison term, can be committed to a mental hospital for an indefinite period or for the rest of their lives. In some states they may even be committed without a trial.

These curious laws were, of course, enacted in the name of science, although there was and is no scientific evidence to support the assumptions on which they are based. Indeed, the very term "sexual psychopath" is unscientific and does not correspond to any particular disease constellation recognized by psychiatrists today. Thus, one and the same person may be considered legally sick in one state and healthy in another. Nevertheless, unsound and unfair as they are, these laws remain on the books because they give an uninformed general public the illusion of preventing sexual violence. However, current diagnostic techniques are incapable of distinguishing between potentially dangerous offenders and those who are not dangerous. At any rate, only very few sex offenders are violent. Furthermore, sex offenders are less likely to repeat their crimes than other types of offenders. Finally, there is little proof that forced psychiatric treatment is an effective tool of rehabilitation. (For further details see "Healthy—Sick.")

The extraordinary diversity and inconsistency of American sex legislation prevent us from describing it accurately within the scope of the present volume. Still, one can recognize certain main areas of behavior that are subject to such legislation. The current legal attitudes towards them are briefly summarized below.

Crimes Involving Victims

Virtually all countries punish sexual acts which involve force, fraud, injury, or exploitation, or which take place in front of unwilling witnesses. In each of these cases there are clearly identifiable victims who complain (or would complain if they could) to the police, and it is obvious that they have a right to be protected. A society that is unwilling or unable to provide such protection cannot survive very long. Thus, quite appropriately, every state in the U.S. has laws against sexual crimes involving victims, and these laws are always vigorously enforced.

However, in many states the laws leave much room for improvement. In some cases they are worded in such archaic and imprecise language that they are no longer effective. In other cases they carry unrealistic and counterproductive penalties, or the manner of their application penalizes the victim along with the offender. A good example are the traditional rape laws, which are now being revised in many states as a result of pressure from women's liberation groups.

The laws may have still another drawback. In their attempt to protect potential victims, they often also prohibit essentially harmless acts and thus, in fact, create crime where otherwise none would exist. On the other hand, legislators may not always be protective enough. As a result, some clearly dangerous sexual behavior may not receive the appropriate punishment.

These and similar problems as well as the laws themselves are discussed in the following paragraphs dealing with specific crimes.

Rape

Ordinary laymen would probably define the crime of rape as "forced sexual intercourse against the partner's will." However, this is not how rape is legally defined in most states of the U.S. First of all, many state penal codes specify that only females can be raped. (Males who rape other males cannot be prosecuted under the rape statutes.) Secondly, these codes usually also recognize cases of rape which involve no force at all and which, in fact, take place with the full consent of the "victim." For example, when a female is "under age," or mentally defective, or drunk, the law simply assumes that she is incapable of consent. It does not matter that she might be quite willing or might even have actively seduced her partner. Any sexual intercourse with her is automatically regarded as rape. Furthermore, this so-called "statutory rape" often is punished just as severely as forcible rape. (Actually, most rape convictions are for the nonviolent statutory type.)

Traditionally, the punishment for rape has always been extremely severe, with prison sentences ranging from one year to life. In many states even the death penalty was common, especially if the offender was black and his victim white. (In recent years there have not been any executions for rape, because the constitutionality of the death penalty itself was being tested in the courts.)

As these few observations already indicate, the American rape laws, although perhaps well intended, may not always be fair. Indeed, in some cases they can lead to patent absurdities. For instance, some criminal codes restrict the act of rape to coitus or attempted coitus. Consequently, forced manual, oral, or anal intercourse, and the apposition of sex organs without penetration must be prosecuted under different statutes. Yet these sexual acts may be even more degrading and injurious to the victim than forced coitus. This applies not only to heterosexual, but also to male and female homosexual rapes as they often occur in prison. There also have been cases where women used guns or other deadly weapons to force men to perform noncoital sexual acts. Such offenses are not considered rape and therefore may not be punished severely enough.

On the other hand, it is obvious that in many cases a "statutory rape" harms no one and is, in fact, a superfluous, artificial, state-manufactured crime which should be stricken from the books. It is neither good sense nor good law to brand male teenagers as felons and send them to prison for years, only because their girlfriends were under the "age of consent." (The age of consent varies from state to state, but it is 18 or 16 in most states.) By the same token, it is highly unreasonable to regard even consensual sexual intercourse with a mentally defective female as rape. Such females should have the same right to sexual fulfillment just as everyone else. By automatically defining any lover of theirs as a rapist, the law does them a grave disservice and, indeed, oppresses them. (See also "The Sexually Oppressed.")

Still another objection to present rape laws can be the manner of their application. Often the female victim is harassed in court by an examination of her sexual history before the alleged rape took place. Her sex life should be irrelevant to the trial, however. After all, even a prostitute has a right not to be raped. Some state codes also require that the victim of rape resist to the utmost. Without such proven resistance, the rapist may go free. Moreover, the prescribed penalties for rape are often so extreme that juries are reluctant to convict. Lighter sentences might produce more certain convictions.

In conclusion, it seems that American legislators could provide greater protection against rape if they treated it as a crime of violence rather than a sex crime. The penalties for rape should differ according to the degree and type of violence used by the rapist. Both males and females of all ages should be protected. The category "statutory rape" should be abolished.

Child Molestation

When persons are sexually molested, threatened, assaulted, or annoyed, they may suffer not only physical injuries, but also psychological damage. This is especially true for very young and helpless persons, i.e., children. Therefore, while everybody should be protected against sexual molestation, children need much stronger protection than adolescents or adults.

Some such protection can perhaps be provided by the threat of harsh criminal penalties. Most state penal codes indeed make this assumption and thus punish child molesters with prison terms ranging from a minimum of 30 days (Wisconsin) to a maximum of life (California). In addition, some states declare such offenders to be "sexual psychopaths" who can be committed to mental hospitals for treatment, and who, even when released, are forced to register with the police. In prison itself, a child molester is usually despised and mistreated by the other inmates who call him "short eyes" or "baby raper" and regard him as the lowest type of criminal.

Unfortunately, a closer examination of American child molestation laws raises serious doubts as to their fairness. First of all, the legal definition of "child" varies considerably from state to state. (In some statutes the term is applied to every person under the age of 18.) Secondly, the age of the offender is not always taken into account. Thus, cases of mutual sex play between adolescents may be treated as "child molestation," with one of the participants being cast into the role of the victim and the other being branded as the molester. Thirdly, the laws often do not distinguish between dangerous molestation and consensual, pleasant encounters which are enjoyed by the child. It is simply assumed that children cannot give consent to a sexual act and that any such act is always harmful. However, this view is irrational and oppressive. (See "The Sexually Oppressed—Children.")

In addition to specific laws against child molestation, there are numerous other laws which try to serve the same purpose. Thus, adults who, in one way or another, have sexual contact with children can also be prosecuted under catch-all statutes such as "Contributing to the Delinquency of a Minor," "Impairing the Morals of a Minor," "Carnal Abuse," "Lascivious Behavior," "Lewdness," "Sodomy," etc. Depending on the circumstances, the laws against "Indecent Exposure" may also apply. If the offender is a close relative, he may be accused of incest.

Studies have shown that by far the greatest majority of convicted child molesters are relatives, neighbors, friends, or acquaintances of their victims. It has also been shown that physical injury occurs only very rarely (in about 2% of the cases). Any potential psychological damage is difficult to assess, and, if it occurs, it may very well be caused more by the reaction of parents and officials than by the sexual act itself. While children understand that coercion, intimidation and physical assault are bad, they may be puzzled and even seriously disturbed by adult hysteria about a gentle and friendly "child molester." It seems, therefore, that it should make a legal difference whether the children are hurt, forced, threatened, or annoyed, or whether they act as willing and satisfied participants. If the latter cases are to be prosecuted at all, they should obviously carry much lighter sentences. Indeed, it may very well be unfair to treat them as crimes in the first place. It also seems only realistic to reduce the age of consent at least to the beginning of puberty. For both sexes the age of 14 seems to be the reasonable maximum. In many cases even lower age limits may be justified. (Actually, the whole notion of age limits for sexual partners deserves to be questioned. Today many people are arguing with good reason that age alone should not be the basis for making otherwise harmless and legal sexual behavior a crime.)

Public Lewdness and Obscenity

Lewdness and obscenity are very difficult to define. They are almost entirely in the eye of the beholder. Nevertheless, it seems possible to describe various instances in which people are annoyed and offended because they are made unwilling witnesses to nudity or sexual behavior.

Such an instance may involve a man who masturbates or exposes his sex organs on a public street, or it may involve several men who have sex in a public toilet and thus shock unsuspecting others who enter upon the scene. Sexual intercourse between men and women may be offensive if it occurs on beaches, in parks, or in other places frequented by the public. Loud and boisterous talk about sex, sexual solicitation, and sexually explicit phone calls can also be quite disturbing to people who have no taste for such things and who want to be left alone. The same goes for sexually explicit billboard signs, window displays, etc., which cannot easily be overlooked by the average person. Finally, men and women may become rightly indignant about being spied upon by a so-called Peeping Tom who watches them in their most intimate moments.

In these and similar cases, society has a clear obligation to protect potential victims by passing appropriate laws and imposing adequate penalties. However, the laws that are now on the books in most states of the U.S. are far from satisfactory. For example, in statutes related to the public exposure of sex organs the punishment is often quite out of proportion to the actual harm done. Sex in public restrooms is often punished not as the public nuisance it is, but as "sodomy" or a "crime against nature" which have entirely different connotations and which may carry excessive penalties. Sexual solicitation, especially among homosexuals, is sometimes punished even in its most polite and unobtrusive forms. Indeed, it is not uncommon for especially discreet individuals to be entrapped by undercover police officers without any further witnesses being aware of the offense. Business advertisements, magazine covers, etc. may be deemed obscene by the law, when, in fact, the vast majority of people find them perfectly acceptable. Occasionally even great works of art have been judged unfit for public view. Laws against "Peeping Toms" may be biased and inconsistent. Thus, as a lawyer once remarked with only slight exaggeration: "If a man is found watching a woman undress in front of an open window, he is arrested as a 'voyeur.' If the situation is reversed, and a woman is found watching a man undress in front of an open window, he is arrested as an 'exhibitionist.' The woman is always simply assumed to be the victim." A further problem with most laws against public lewdness and obscenity is their vagueness which practically invites abuse by overzealous authorities.

Under the circumstances, it seems that the public would be better served if the laws made a clear distinction between those actions that are harmful and those that are merely startling or undignified. The latter should be punished much less severely than the former. Nudity and sexual activity should never be illegal among consenting adults or in front of witnesses who are not personally offended.

Crimes Without Victims

In modern America (just as in many other societies) there is a class of crime that does not involve any victims, but consists of acts committed in private by consenting partners who have no intention of complaining to the police. This so-called victimless crime harms nobody. Indeed, it is perhaps best defined as a transaction or exchange of goods or services between people for their mutual benefit. This transaction concerns only the immediate participants and is not designed to affect anyone else. However, it provides the participants with something they greatly desire and which the law tries to deny them. Therefore, they have no interest in seeing the law enforced. They will neither initiate prosecution nor give evidence to the authorities.

It follows from these observations that, if the government wants to enforce its laws against victimless crimes, it has to adopt extraordinary and often highly questionable methods. Such methods may include systematic spying and snooping, secret surveillance, the use of undercover agents, enticement, and entrapment. However, these elaborate efforts usually produce only very meager results and thus do not justify the expense. The very character of victimless crime leaves most of it undetected. Those few offenders who are caught and convicted are never more than a tiny "unlucky" minority. Since police officials are well aware of this fact, they do not even make an attempt at equal enforcement. Instead, they enforce these laws only periodically or selectively against certain individuals or groups, thus creating a climate of injustice and hypocrisy. These conditions in turn breed new crimes such as blackmail and bribery. Needless to say, eventually all of this leads to widespread contempt for the entire legal system.

In the U.S. the most notorious victimless-crime laws deal with sexual behavior. Because of certain religious and cultural traditions, most American states recognize only two very specific sexual acts as lawful: solitary masturbation and private marital coitus. Any other form of human sexual expression, even between husband and wife, is a crime. Obviously, this makes criminals out of most Americans. As a matter of fact, if the American sex laws were rigorously and equally enforced, the country would have so many sex offenders in prison, that there would not be enough innocent citizens left to guard them.

As we can see, the American laws against victimless sex acts are absurd and dangerous. They create crime where otherwise none would exist. They force harmless behavior underground and produce unhealthy sexual subcultures. They stigmatize untold numbers of respectable people and needlessly force them into criminal careers. They encourage extortion, graft, and police corruption. In short, they are irrational, immoral, and destructive. They themselves victimize many and offer protection to none.

Nevertheless, these laws are sometimes defended on the grounds that they do protect at least some people and that, in a strict sense, there is no such thing as a victimless crime. Thus it is argued, for example, that fornication often leads to unwanted pregnancies or spreads venereal disease. Incest is said to victimize potential offspring by the transmission of genetic defects. Prostitutes are described as the victims of their pimps. Homosexuals are seen as endangered by their lifestyle, because they may be robbed, beaten, or even killed by their casual partners. Sexually explicit books and films are believed to corrupt the minds of those who enjoy them, etc.

However, it is difficult to take such arguments seriously. After all, if any of the above consensual behaviors has undesirable social side effects, they result entirely from the fact that society treats it as a crime. In other words, if the behavior were legal in the first place, the side effects would either not appear at all or be greatly reduced. Unwanted pregnancies are easily prevented by the use of contraceptives. If our sex laws were more reasonable, couples would be better informed, and even the venereal diseases could finally be eliminated. Prostitutes who can ply their trade legally do not need pimps. Homosexuals who have nothing to fear from the law need not seek satisfaction in "one-night stands" with violent strangers. Without laws against "pornography," erotic materials would be of higher quality and might very well diminish in quantity.

It seems, therefore, that the U.S. would do well to follow the example of other Western nations which have abolished most, if not all, laws against consensual sex in private. This policy has also been recommended by various American professional groups and law-revising committees.

The following pages do not cover all private consensual sex acts that are illegal in the U.S. today. The number and diversity of laws is simply too great. Still, a few main areas of legal control are discussed in some detail. Certain problems connected with specific victimless crimes are also mentioned briefly.

Fornication

Fornication may be defined as sexual intercourse between males and females who are not married to each other, and as such it is punishable in many states of the U.S. However, if one of the partners is married to somebody else, he or she may be charged not with fornication, but with adultery.

Curiously enough, some states have traditionally applied different standards to male and female offenders. Thus, a married woman who had sexual intercourse with a single man was punished as an adulteress, while a married man who had intercourse with a single woman was often considered a mere fornicator, and his offense was treated much more leniently. On the other hand, this kind of sexual discrimination usually reversed itself, if the female was under the "age of consent" (18 or 16 years in most states). In this case, she normally went free, while her male partner was prosecuted for "statutory rape," which carries an extremely severe penalty. (See also "Rape.")

The punishment for fornication varies from state to state, but usually consists of a fine (up to $1000) or imprisonment (up to 1 year) or both.

There is no doubt that the laws against fornication are broken millions of times every day, but we can also assume that most offenders are not even aware of the fact that they are committing a crime. The average American remains, perhaps fortunately, ignorant of the extent to which his government may control his private life, and it must be admitted that prosecutions for fornication are quite rare. Nevertheless, as long as the laws are on the books, they can be enforced against anybody who should displease the authorities. Thus, for example, poor, unwed mothers have been tried for fornication on the theory that their imprisonment would prevent them from becoming pregnant again and thereby cut the welfare rolls. The very fact that the women had borne children out of wedlock was taken as sufficient evidence that the crime of fornication had been committed.

Cohabitation

Some states of the U.S. punish fornication only if it is repeated and thus causes the offenders to live in a "state of open and notorious cohabitation." Depending on the state, this crime may be a felony punishable by imprisonment for several years. Needless to say, such a statute has the absurd effect of penalizing couples who live together in an exclusive, stable relationship. Promiscuous individuals, on the other hand, remain untouched by the law.

Seduction

A number of states in the U.S. have laws against "seduction," i.e., a man's coitus with a previously "chaste" woman under promise of marriage. This promise must have been unconditional, however, in order to lead to conviction. For example, if a man promises marriage only in case the woman becomes pregnant or he himself can obtain a divorce, his promise is not unconditional and he cannot be convicted. On the other hand, it does not matter whether the promise of marriage was fraudulent or made in good faith, or whether it was legally binding. The man can be prosecuted even if he is under age or already married. There is sufficient cause for prosecution as long as the promise was unconditional and has not been kept. Indeed, if the man belatedly offers marriage and the woman refuses, he can still be convicted. Nevertheless, if the promised marriage takes place before the man's indictment or before a charge has been filed against him, the prosecution is dropped in most cases. However, if the woman was under the "age of consent" at the time of the seduction, the new husband can still be convicted of earlier "statutory rape."

Some state legislatures have complicated this confusing legal picture still further by various other provisions, exceptions, or requirements relating to the victim's proof of "chastity." Still, in virtually all states which have "seduction" statutes the penalties are quite severe (up to 10 years in prison plus several thousand dollars fine).

There has never been a law punishing women for seducing "chaste" men.

Adultery

Adultery can be defined as voluntary sexual intercourse by a married person with a person other than his or her spouse.

That is to say, adultery can be committed by a married person with an unmarried person, or by two married persons who are not married to each other.

Not all states in the U.S. have laws against adultery, and those that do differ greatly in the degree of punishment. In some states a conviction may result in nothing more than a small fine, in others it may lead to heavy fines and several years imprisonment.

Prosecutions for adultery have become extremely rare in recent decades, although technically this crime may still play a role in divorce cases.

Sodomy and Crimes Against Nature

The U.S. is among the very few modern nations which still have laws against noncoital forms of sexual intercourse. Thus, in most American state penal codes oral and anal intercourse as well as sexual contact with animals are grouped together under such categories as "sodomy" or "crimes against nature," and they are treated as very serious offenses.

It does not matter that these sexual acts may be performed in complete privacy by consenting partners and, indeed, by married couples in their own bedroom. As a rule the law does not make any distinction between the single and the married, men and women, heterosexuals and homosexuals. Noncoital sexual intercourse is punishable under any and all circumstances, and both parties are guilty. Penalties are extremely severe and, depending on the state, may range up to life imprisonment. In addition, offenders may be declared to be "sexual psychopaths" and may be committed for life to a mental institution. If they are released, they may nevertheless be forced to register with the police, so that the government can keep an eye on them.

It can safely be assumed that most Americans are unaware of these laws, and even if they hear about them accidentally, they are likely to misunderstand them. To the average layman, the term "crime against nature" probably suggests some form of environmental pollution or destruction, such as strip mining or an oil spill. The term "sodomy," which is obviously derived from the Old Testament, may suggest some vague religious offense without interest to a modern secular state. In short, the fact that these two curious terms refer to rather common forms of human sexual behavior is by no means obvious, and it is even less clear why these behaviors should be considered crimes. As it turns out, this double mystery can be solved only by a close look at ancient and medieval history.

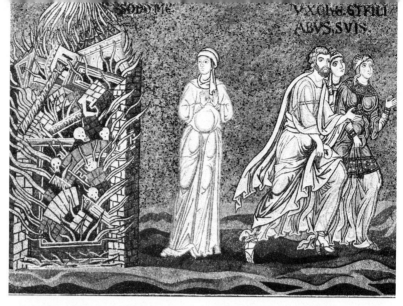

THE CRIME OF SODOMY

Most states of the U.S. today still have laws against "sodomy" or "crimes against nature". These laws severely punish any oral or anal intercourse, even between husband and wife. Originally, however, "sodomy" was a religious offense which could be committed only by men.

(Top) The destruction of Sodom

The early Christians believed that the biblical city of Sodom was destroyed by God, because its male inhabitants had engaged in homosexual intercourse. Modern biblical scholars have challenged this interpretation, but, whether correct or not, it has influenced popular Christian attitudes for more than 1500 years. (Mosaic. Monreale cathedral)

(Middle) The Christian emperor Justinian and his court officials

In order to avert the destruction of their own cities by God, Christian Roman emperors enacted the first European laws against "sodomy" i.e. male homosexual behavior. Offenders were burned at the stake. In the 6th century A.D. the East Roman emperor Justinian (shown here with a halo) confirmed the death penalty for male homosexuals in his famous legal code which greatly influenced subsequent Western legislation. (Mosaic. Church of San Vitale, Ravenna)

(Bottom) Execution of heretics in medieval Spain

In medieval Europe "sodomy" was very often equated with heresy and disbelief. The Spanish Inquisition, for example, persecuted Jews, heretics, and "sodomites" with equal zeal. In 1479 King Ferdinand and Queen Isabella formally decreed that sodomites should be publicly burned alive after the confiscation of their property. The picture by Pedro Berruguete, a painter of the period, shows the method of execution. Modern viewers may be especially intrigued by a curious detail: The stake is equipped with a penis-shaped peg which, placed between the legs of the condemned, holds up the body while it burns. (Madrid. Prado)

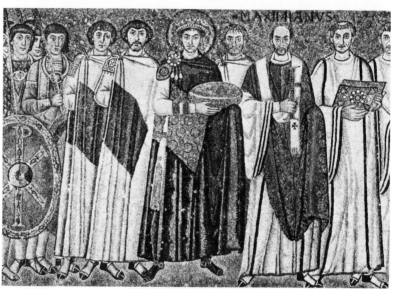

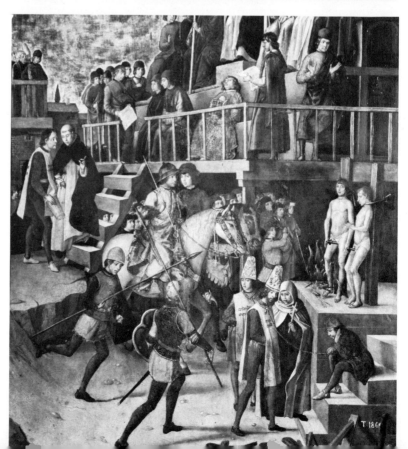

As is well known, in our Judeo-Christian culture the greatest sexual offenses have always been homosexual intercourse and sexual contact with animals. Although these behaviors are quite harmless in themselves, they were, at some early time in Jewish history, associated with the worship of strange gods. Therefore they came to be seen as "abominations," i.e., signs of idolatry. Offenders were punished by death.

The Middle Ages believed that these same sexual behaviors had prompted God to destroy the biblical city of Sodom and therefore referred to them as "sodomy" or "crimes against nature" (i.e. crimes against God's natural order). Anyone who committed these crimes showed disbelief and was automatically considered a heretic. Conversely, heretics were usually also accused of sodomy as a matter of course. For example, when, in the early 14th century, the French king Philippe IV needed an excuse for confiscating the immense wealth of the highly respected Knights Templar, he simply charged them with blasphemy, idolatry, and sodomy. While this charge was utterly false, it nevertheless awakened such deep-seated hostilities among the populace that the entire knightly order was brought to trial and its leadership publicly burned to death. The king, as he had correctly anticipated, was hailed as a defender of the faith and therefore had no trouble pocketing the loot. In the course of time the equation of sodomy and heresy became so well established that every new heretical Christian sect was accused of engaging in "unnatural" sexual practices. Thus, when some of these sects spread to Western Europe from Bulgaria, their members were denounced as "buggers" (from Bulgars), and the word "buggery" became synonymous with sodomy.

In medieval England, sexual heresy, just as any other kind of heresy, was under the jurisdiction of ecclesiastical courts, but in 1533 Henry VIII created the first secular law against "the detestable and abominable vice of Buggery committed with mankind or beast." The crime was declared a felony punishable by death and confiscation of property. Henry's law was repealed under Mary, but revived under Elizabeth I and finally brought to America by the Puritans. For centuries the religious character of the offense was openly admitted. Thus, the original statute of North Carolina, for example, explicitly referred to it as "the abominable and detestable crime against nature, *not to be named among Christians*" and demanded that offenders "shall suffer death *without the benefit of clergy*." Curiously enough, the separation of church and state produced by the American Revolution and codified in the U.S. Constitution did not result in the immediate repeal of the sodomy laws, although their religious origin and character would seem to render them clearly unconstitutional.

Today, the great majority of states in the U.S. still retain their sexual heresy laws, although in some states religious terms like "sodomy," "buggery," and "crime against nature" are now avoided. Other states, however, have seen no need to modernize the language of their statutes. Thus, "sodomy" and "crime against nature" continue to be used, sometimes interchangeably, sometimes side by side. Indeed, in a few states these words have, in the meantime, acquired an ever broader meaning and now cover not only oral and anal intercourse between homosexual or heterosexual partners and sexual contact with animals, but also certain rare and bizarre sexual practices, such as sexual contact with dead bodies (necrophilia).

While the sodomy laws apply to everyone, including married couples, they are now enforced mainly against male homosexuals. After all, heterosexuals can always be presumed to engage only in coitus and to avoid noncoital forms of intercourse. Members of the same sex, on the other hand, cannot engage in coitus with each other and are therefore likely to violate the law when they have sexual contact. Nevertheless, on the whole, prosecutions for sodomy have become quite rare. The main use of the laws today is an indirect one. For example, employers, landlords, bank directors, or insurance executives who want to discriminate against a homosexual routinely point to the sodomy laws which define him as a potential felon. Thus, it seems entirely legal, and even respectable, to fire him from his job and to deny him decent housing, bank loans, and insurance coverage. The sodomy laws have further been used as a basis for denying homosexuals work with certain federal agencies and the military. Indeed, according to a special law passed by Congress in 1952, homosexual foreigners can neither become permanent residents in the U.S. nor obtain U.S. citizenship. (In this context it is interesting to note that there is also still a strong popular tendency to equate sexual heresy with treason and vice versa. Thus, the late Senator Joseph McCarthy and his followers fantasized about subversive "homosexual conspiracies," and the public proved as gullible as in the days of Philippe IV.)

However, it would be a mistake to believe that heterosexuals have nothing to fear from the sodomy laws. As recently as 1965 a man in Indiana was tried for sodomy and sentenced to a prison term of 2–14 years, because, after a domestic quarrel, his own wife had reported him to the authorities. No force had been involved, and after her initial anger subsided, the woman tried to withdraw the charge, but since the crime is an offense against the state, the prosecution could not be halted. Thus, both husband and wife learned to their total surprise how absurd and destructive "justice" can be. Unfortunately, in many states of the U.S. this kind of surprise may still await other married couples, especially as a result of divorce proceedings. For instance, a desperate woman who cannot find any other grounds for divorce may very well accuse her husband of "crimes against nature" in order to prove his "cruelty," and once the charge has been made, the law simply takes its course.

It should be clear from the foregoing that the American sodomy laws are irrational and inherently unjust. They cannot be enforced equally, and no attempt to do so has ever been made. Because of their religious basis, these laws stand out as alien bodies in any modern legal system. The very language in which they are phrased renders them suspect. Even the most serious crimes of violence are never defined in such shrill and emotional terms as the heretical act of sodomy. (For example, no legal code ever spoke of the "abominable and detestable crime of murder, not to be named among Christians.") No other laws carrying comparable penalties are as vague as the sodomy laws. Furthermore, by definition, a "crime against nature" is *the* classic victimless crime. After all, the term itself implies that not any human being, but nature itself is the victim. However, as we have seen, the "nature" which the law endeavors to protect here is not the nature of the natural sciences, but rather an archaic concept of "God's natural order." Modern scientific findings stand in sharp contrast to the philosophy expressed in these laws.

In recent years a number of states have repealed their sodomy laws, although in one state the repeal itself was repealed after intense public pressure. The citizens of that state, perhaps unaware of its true implications, demanded that their sodomy law be reinstated, and the legislature complied with their wish. In view of similar popular sentiments, other state legislatures have proved reluctant to press for reform. It seems, therefore, that the best hope for ridding the nation of these obnoxious and oppressive laws rests with the U.S. Supreme Court.

Unfortunately, this hope was somewhat dimmed in 1976, when the Supreme Court upheld the constitutionality of a Virginia law against sodomy. Since the court made its decision without hearing arguments and without offering an opinion, some lawyers have surmised that it may have rested on a legal technicality and that some future case may yet produce a different outcome. Many thoughtful citizens fervently pray that this interpretation is correct, because otherwise the outlook for the whole nation could be grim. As the deeply distressed president of the American Psychiatric Association pointed out in a letter to the Chief Justice, not only about 20 million American homosexuals, but also about two-thirds of the adult American heterosexual population regularly engage in "sodomy," and thus well over 100 million men and women in this country are summarily branded as criminals. Moreover, psychiatrists and other therapists often feel obliged to recommend the proscribed sexual acts to patients with marital difficulties. Thus, the sodomy laws, which prohibit such acts, undermine the institution of marriage. (The Supreme Court decision was particularly disturbing because it also confirmed the conviction of a Virginia married couple, husband and wife, who were given 5-year prison terms for sodomy with each other.)

One can assume that the idea of "Big Brother" in the marital bedroom is repulsive to most Americans, but it is now high time for them to realize that they still live under a government which denies them the right over their own bodies and feels entitled to interfere in their most intimate relationships. Under such circumstances, any official talk of freedom in America is an insult.

Prostitution

Prostitution is perhaps best defined as "sexual intercourse in exchange for money or some other material reward." However, most existing American laws against prostitution define it rather differently. For example, many states specify that the offense can be committed only by females. As a result, males who sell their sexual services cannot be charged with prostitution, but have to be prosecuted under different statutes, such as the vagrancy or sodomy laws. Moreover, some states have stretched the definition of prostitution to cover even noncommercial sexual behavior that is "promiscuous and indiscriminate." In these states any female who frequently changes her sexual partners can be convicted as a prostitute, even if she never demanded or accepted any pay.

Actually, in the U.S., the most common charge brought against prostitutes is that for "soliciting." That is to say, most states have laws against "soliciting to engage in lewd or dissolute conduct," a misdemeanor which is punishable by a fine or a short prison term, or both. The witnesses against a prostitute are usually undercover police officers who have enticed or entrapped her to commit the offense. At other times, prostitutes are summarily arrested under catch-all statutes such as those against "obstructing the sidewalk" or "disturbing the peace." However, in most cases, they are only briefly detained and then fined, after which they are free to return to their work. The fine thus simply becomes another business expense which is passed on to the consumer. Or, seen in another light, the fine may also be regarded as a crude form of taxation, by which the state tries to share in at least some of a prostitute's illegitimate earnings.

In addition to the prostitute herself, a number of people who may be connected with her business are violating the law. For example, any person, male or female, who encourages or assists prostitutes in their trade (called a panderer or procurer), any person who lives by their earnings (called a pimp), and any person who maintains a house of prostitution (called an operator) is punished more severely than a prostitute. Pimping and pandering are usually felonies punishable by lengthy prison terms. Most states also have laws against a variety of other activities that may be related to prostitution. Indeed, no other sexual offense has prompted so many different and often overlapping statutes as has the single activity of prostitution.

Mention must also be made of a federal law known as the "White Slave Act" or Mann Act which was passed by Congress in 1910. This law defines as a felon any person who transports or aids in the transportation across state lines of any female for the purpose of prostitution, debauchery, or "any other immoral purpose." The penalty is a fine of $5000, five years in prison, or both. This curious law was passed in response to something called "White Slave Traffic," i.e., a vast national or even international conspiracy of procurers and pimps who turned innocent women and girls into prostitutes and then sold them into "shameless, immoral, and involuntary servitude" in various states of the U.S. Whether such a conspiracy has actually ever existed can at least be doubted. It has all the marks of a Puritan paranoid fantasy. At any rate, the "White Slave Act" invited abuse almost from the start.

For example, since the law punishes people for transporting a female (or aiding in her transportation) across state lines for "any immoral purpose," no prostitution need be involved in the crime. It is enough that the female crossed a state line, was somehow "aided" in doing so, and then committed an "immoral act." In other words, an unmarried couple from San Francisco, California going to Reno, Nevada for a weekend and there having sexual intercourse may invite unexpected legal problems, because the man has clearly violated the "White Slave Act." Similarly, a student at Yale (in Connecticut) who picks up his girlfriend at Vassar (in New York) for the Yale-Harvard football game and then celebrates Yale's victory by having sexual intercourse with her before driving her back thereby commits a felony and could spend the next five years in prison.

Unfortunately, these are by no means frivolous examples. On the contrary, over the years many such cases have been prosecuted under the Mann Act. Thus, the perhaps well-intended act became a convenient tool for intolerant zealots with which to harass some hated or envied individual who could not be accused of any other crime. One may wonder, therefore, why the act has not been repealed. After all, if there is still such a thing as "White Slave Traffic," it would better be controlled by laws relating to the deprivation of liberty, kidnapping, assault, tax evasion, etc. An attempt to prohibit "immorality" hardly seems a rational method of liberating oppressed females. Furthermore, the very term "White Slave Traffic" smacks of demagoguery and, to contemporary ears, has embarrassing racist overtones. (Is white slavery worse than black slavery? Or does a black woman also become a white slave if she is helped crossing a state line for an "immoral purpose?")

Prostitution has often been called "the world's oldest profession," and it is true that it has existed at all times among all civilized nations. In certain ancient cultures it had a religious character. Female and male "temple prostitutes" or "sacred prostitutes" offered themselves to the faithful, and their fees went to the temple. However, secular, purely commercial prostitution seems to be nearly as old. Greek and Roman antiquity as well as the Christian Middle Ages were rather tolerant of prostitution. Thomas Aquinas, for example, accepted it as a necessary evil and argued that "even a palace needs sewers." Medieval cities therefore had well-regulated brothels, usually not far from the church. It was only in modern times that certain industrial nations began to close their brothels and to make prostitution illegal. However, since this policy proved unwise in the long run, progressive European countries, such as the Netherlands and West Germany, have again legalized prostitution and tried to improve the prostitute's working conditions. Thus, in these countries, prostitutes no longer need pimps and can count on the police to protect them if they are threatened with violence. They also pay regular income tax on their earnings, like any other citizen.

Before World War I many American cities also had their "red light districts," "cat houses," or bordellos which were more or less tolerated by the authorities. Unfortunately, in the early decades of our century various popular crusades for "purity" or "decency" succeeded in ending this tolerance. By 1925 every state in the Union had enacted antiprostitution statutes. A second wave of repressive legislation arrived with World War II. "In the interest of the war effort" over 650 American communities closed their houses of prostitution. This policy was further encouraged in 1941 by a Federal law, the so-called May Act, which allowed the government to assume police authority in communities which failed to "solve their prostitution problem."

Today it seems rather obvious, however, that making prostitution illegal has not really solved any problems. If, on the whole, there is less prostitution than before, the reason is probably a general relaxation of sexual standards. After all, today young, unmarried people as well as many single adults can easily find "respectable" noncommercial sexual partners. Nevertheless, in many parts of the country, especially in the larger cities, prostitution continues to meet a demand, and so far the law has proved quite incapable of suppressing it. The only certain effect of the law has been a strengthening of the

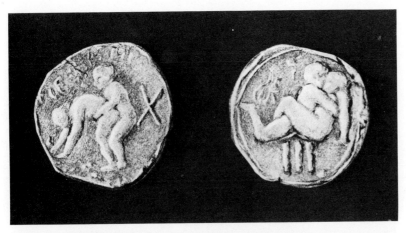

THE CRIME OF PROSTITUTION

Unlike the countries of Western Europe, virtually all states of the U.S. today punish prostitution as a crime. (There are some local exceptions in Nevada). In ancient and medieval times prostitution was widely tolerated and brothels, i.e. houses of prostitution, were common in most cities. In medieval Europe brothels were often located near the church. Brothels also still operated legally in many parts of 19th century America.

(Top) Ancient Roman brothel tokens

(Middle) Medieval brothel

(Bottom) Prostitute awaiting customer in a brothel in New Orleans, ca. 1912.

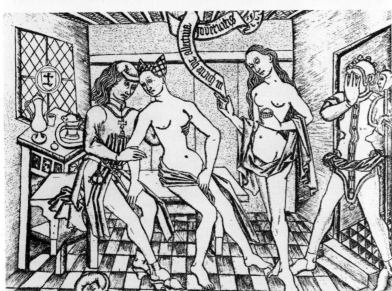

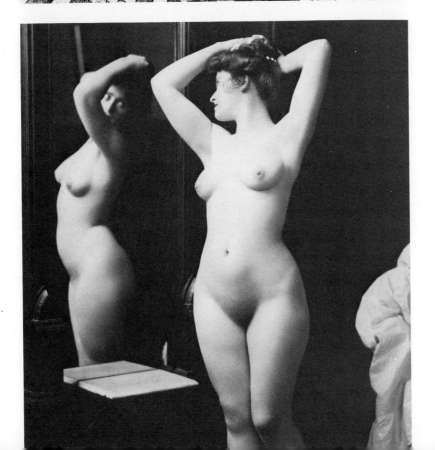

role of the pimp who can now act as the prostitute's quasi-legal advisor and as her protector against the police.

Still, the anti-prostitution laws are usually defended on the grounds that they somehow improve public sexual morality and that they protect at least some women from falling into a life of degradation. It is also pointed out that prostitution is often connected with other crimes, such as robbery of customers, blackmail, and tax evasion. Moreover, there is a fear that legalized prostitution might contribute to the spread of venereal diseases. Finally, it is said that the average citizen does not want a "red light district" or brothel in his neighborhood, and that the legalization and official regulation of prostitution is therefore impractical.

However, critics of the existing laws maintain that they are basically unenforceable and therefore hypocritical, capricious, immoral, and unjust. Far from protecting the reluctant prostitute, they stigmatize her as a criminal and thus make it difficult for her to switch to a more "respectable" career. Furthermore, whenever prostitution breeds associated crimes of violence or theft, they can be prosecuted independently. Indeed, such prosecutions would become much more effective if prostitution itself were legal. In addition, the government could then begin to tax the income of prostitutes. Legalization would also contribute to a better control of venereal diseases, because prostitutes could be given regular checkups. While this would not eliminate the diseases entirely, it would certainly reduce the rate of infection. As for the location of "red light districts," the present European and past American examples should prove that this problem is not insurmountable.

Recent years have revealed still another aspect of the problem. As legitimate sex researchers and sex therapists have provided some of their subjects or patients with paid "surrogate partners" for scientific or therapeutic purposes, they seem to have come close to what the law defines as "procuring," "pandering," or even "pimping." The "surrogate partners" themselves would seem to have engaged in prostitution as defined in many state criminal codes. Nevertheless, no charges seem to have been brought against any of these people, and it is clear enough that they all tried to serve some very "moral" end. However, it is by no means a foregone conclusion that an ordinary prostitute who satisfies an inhibited, handicapped, or dysfunctional customer thereby commits an "immoral act." On the contrary, in some cases she may very well fulfill a truly therapeutic function. (The famous "squeeze technique" now used by many therapists was first taught to a scientist by prostitutes.) At any rate, in the meantime various women charged with prostitution have claimed to be "sex therapists," and, if one wants to be fair about it, this claim is by no means as easily refuted as the police might be inclined to think. It would also seem only reasonable to obtain the opinion of customers. If they really have been helped with their sexual problems by a prostitute, she would have a strong argument in her favor. (Curiously enough, the customers of a prostitute are never asked such questions and are rarely arrested, although, technically, they are also guilty of a sexual offense. Some states have specific laws against using a prostitute, and others can prosecute under different, but related statutes.)

While legalization and regulation or perhaps simple decriminalization seem to be the most rational ways of dealing with prostitution, they cannot remove all of its negative connotations. When all is said and done, there is still something deeply disturbing about the commercialization of human warmth, love, or sexual satisfaction. The thought of human beings treating themselves and each other as commodities remains unpleasant for religious believers and humanists alike. It has therefore often been suggested that society should continue to make every effort to end prostitution. Since we know that punitive measures cannot succeed, a proper sexual and emotional education is advocated as the only way to accomplish that goal. It is believed that if men and women had a healthier attitude towards their own sexuality, they would not use or abuse each other as commercial sex objects.

There is undoubtedly much truth in this argument. However, the real problem seems to lie deeper. The buying and selling of sexual services will not and cannot end as long as any other human services are being bought and sold. In the final analysis, it is the sale of the human body for *any purpose* which creates the problem. Indeed, on the face of it, a sexual purpose seems to be better than most. Over the years, many critical observers have commented upon the strange fact that in our society it is perfectly respectable for people to market their bodies as instruments of labor, but criminal to market them as instruments of pleasure. Thus, a girl is "moral" if she rents her body to a manufacturer at $3 an hour for hard, mindless work in a factory, but she is "immoral" if she rents the same body to the same manufacturer at $30 an hour for sexual pleasure in a hotel room. Obviously, there is something bizarre about such moral values.

One can only hope that our society will soon find a just and workable way of dealing with the problem of prostitution. As indicated above, legalization and regulation have, to a certain extent, been successful in other countries. Some American reformers, however, point out that any form of official registration or control may stigmatize prostitutes for life and make it difficult for them to seek other kinds of employment. Instead, they suggest decriminalization, i.e., the repeal of antiprostitution laws without any further government involvement. This proposal has much to recommend it, although it fails to deal with the tax issue. Some prostitutes have a considerable income, and it would be unfair to leave it untaxed at a time when other workers who make much less money pay increasingly higher taxes.

Incest

Most American state penal codes define incest as coitus between persons related by blood or marriage within the degrees in which marriage is prohibited. This means, among other things, that noncoital forms of sexual intercourse do not constitute incest, and that incest cannot take place between persons of the same sex. (However, such sexual activity may be prosecuted under various other statutes.) It further means that certain sexual relationships may be considered incestuous in one state and not in another, because some states prohibit marriage between first cousins while others allow it. Some states also differentiate between a simple incestuous relationship and an incestuous marriage, treating the latter as a less serious offense. Thus, in one state the maximum penalty for incestuous marriage is 3 years imprisonment and for nonmarital incestuous relationships 20 years. The logic of this, as of so many other sex laws, is mysterious. The maximum penalty in any state for incest is 50 years imprisonment.

Incest prohibitions of one kind or another have existed since prehistoric times and among all peoples. The reason for this is still subject to speculation. It is often assumed by laymen that incest invariably produces genetic defects or somehow leads to "degeneracy," bringing out the worst traits of both the male and the female. However, no professional cattle breeder ever conducts his business according to this belief, and, indeed, there is little scientific evidence to support it. At any rate, the human incest taboo precedes any accurate genetic knowledge by many thousands of years. Another theory proposes that the incest taboo has its roots in the social advantage of marrying outside one's own family or tribe. This allows for the formation of ever larger social groups and thus becomes the basis of progress and civilization. The third, and perhaps most plausible explanation is that the incest taboo contributes to peace and harmony within the family unit which otherwise would be torn by constant sexual rivalries between father and son, mother and daughter, and brother and sister.

Be that as it may, the prohibition of incest is so universal and has been so effective for such a long time that it may almost be said to have become part of "human nature." A sustained sexual attraction between close blood relatives is now rare enough to be considered exceptional. It should be noted, however, that such exceptions do occur, and that, in the past, some societies granted them legal recognition. For example, males of royal descent in an-

THE CRIME OF OBSCENITY

"Pornographic" entertainment is not an invention of our time. In Europe sexually explicit, and even intentionally obscene stage shows date back to Greek and Roman antiquity. About 250 years ago European aristocrats attended such shows in their own private theaters.

(Top) Scene from a classical Greek comedy. Note the large artificial penises (phalloi) worn by the actors. (Ancient Greek pottery painting.)

(Middle) Title page and cast of characters of a comedy written by John Wilmot, Earl of Rochester (17th century). Shown here is a modern reprint.

(Bottom) Private performance in an 18th-century court theater.

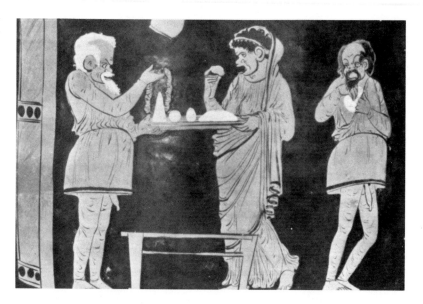

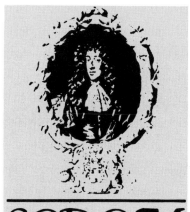

SODOM
or The Quintessence Of Debauchery
by John Wilmot, Earl of Rochester

SODOM

DRAMATIS PERSONAE

BOLLOXINION, *King of Sodom.*
CUNTIGRATIA, *Queen.*
PRICKET, *Prince.*
SWIVIA, *Princess.*
BUGGERANTHOS, *General of the Army.*
POCKENELLO, *Prince, Colonel and Favorite of the King.*
BORASTUS, *Buggermaster-general.*
PINE and TWELY, *Two Pimps of Honour.*
FUCKADILLA,
OFFICINA,   } *Maids of Honour.*
CUNTICULA,
CLYTORIS,
FLUX, *Physician to the King.*
VERTUOSO, *Merkin and Dildoe-maker to the Royal Family.*

With Boys, Rogues, Pimps and other Attendants.

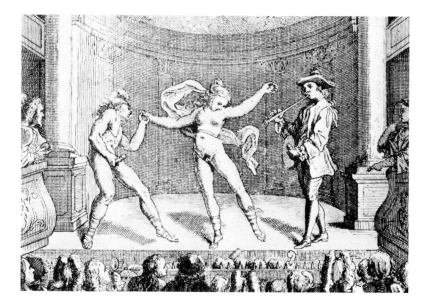

cient Egypt, certain areas of pre-Columbian America, and on certain Polynesian islands were allowed or even compelled to marry their sisters. (These marriages had no apparent negative genetic effect, although the incest continued over many generations.) In some cultures even father-daughter relationships were tolerated under certain circumstances. However, as far as we know, mother-son relationships have never been permitted anywhere.

On the other hand, some cultures have extended the incest prohibition to grandparents, uncles, aunts, first, second, and third cousins, stepfathers, stepmothers, sons-in-law, daughters-in-law, and other relatives. How much such prohibitions can vary is perhaps best illustrated by two passages in the Old Testament which show Yahweh reversing himself on the issue of marriage between a widow and her brother-in-law (Genesis 38; 8–10 and Leviticus 20;21). It will also be recalled that Shakespeare's Hamlet describes the marriage of his widowed mother to his father's brother as incestuous (I,3), although by our present standards it would not be regarded as such. In fact, the modern Scandinavian countries have restricted the definition of incest to coitus between siblings and direct descendents. Moreover, a Swedish government committee has recently proposed the complete elimination of incest from the penal code. After all, it is difficult to see what possible good the laws against incest can still serve today and what damage their repeal could do. The use of contraception could easily allay the fears of those who worry about genetic problems. Children and adolescents could be protected against sexual assault and abuse by their parents or older siblings in the same way they are now protected against any other sexual exploitation.

Private Lewdness and Obscenity

Lewdness, obscenity, pornography, and other such derogatory terms are very difficult to define, because they never refer to anything objective or measurable. All one can say with certainty is that some people use these words to indicate disapproval of nudity and sex or of the manner in which they are presented in stage shows, movies, records, pictures, books, and magazines. Obviously, different observers disapprove of different things, but it seems reasonable to protect all of them from involuntary exposure to anything they might find offensive. In a truly civilized society nobody should be forced to confront sexually explicit behavior or material. The government is therefore well justified in passing strict laws against public "lewdness and obscenity." Indeed, orthodox Jews and Moslems who find pictorial representations of God obscene and objectionable should also be protected. (For further details see "Crimes Involving Victims.")

However, it is quite another matter to have laws against private lewdness and obscenity. People who are not only not offended by sexual activity, but who are positively interested in observing it or even pay for the privilege should not be harassed by the police. It makes no sense to define as criminal anyone who enjoys explicit sexual materials in his own home, who watches "sex films" or live "sex shows" in special private theaters, or who engages in sexual acts in special private "health clubs" or "bath houses." As long as unwilling witnesses are safely excluded, there is no rational ground for official interference. Actually, to some extent, this principle can be applied even to certain "public" places, such as clearly marked "gay bars" or heterosexual "singles bars." When such establishments openly signal their purpose to all potential patrons they acquire a quasi-private character, because no unsuspecting person is ever likely to enter them. A certain general decorum may still have to be required, but, as long as the regular clientele remains undisturbed, there should be no need for undercover police officers to scrutinize every spontaneous gesture for possible signs of "lewdness."

Unfortunately, there have been many cases in the U.S. where men have been arrested for simply holding hands, hugging, or kissing each other in a bar. This harmless behavior appeared "lewd" and obscene" to American policemen, prosecutors, and judges, although in most of the rest of the world it has no sexual connotations and is perfectly acceptable even on the street.

Indeed, American television audiences can regularly observe foreign politicians engaging in such behavior on official occasions. Nevertheless, for some strange reason a show of affection between males is not tolerated in this country. In another display of prudery, some American communities have arrested teenage boys on hot summer days for not wearing a shirt and thus "lewdly" displaying a nude chest. In short, it is clear that the statutes covering "lewd behavior" or "live obscene conduct" are all too easily abused. Moreover, the standards for defining obscenity and the prescribed penalties vary from state to state. In addition, individual cities have passed their own local ordinances, and thus the legal confusion is complete.

However, even more questionable is the legal crusade against "obscene material" or, as it is also often called, "pornography" (literally: writings about prostitutes, from Greek *porne:* prostitute and *graphein:* to write). In 1873 the U.S. Congress passed the first antipornography law in response to intense lobbying efforts by Anthony Comstock, the president of the "New York Society for the Suppression of Vice." This law prohibited the mailing of "obscene" materials. Comstock was appointed a special agent of the Post Office Department and granted the right to open any letter, package, book, or pamphlet passing through the mails. He personally had the power to decide what was lewd or obscene, and since he was a narrow-minded, prudish fanatic, he soon established a dictatorial reign of puritanical terror which lasted over 40 years. Many of his victims were physicians who tried to help their patients with birth control information.

In the meantime, most states have passed "little" Comstock laws of their own. Furthermore, in a 1957 landmark decision (Roth *vs.* U.S.) the Supreme Court held that "obscenity" is not within the area of constitutionally protected freedom of speech or press. The Court also found in 1973 (Miller *vs.* California) that individual states can set their own standards of what should be considered obscene, as long as they observe certain limitations. These limitations allow any work to be declared obscene if (a) the average person, applying contemporary community standards, finds it, taken as a whole, appealing to "prurient interests," and (b) if the work depicts, in a patently offensive way, sexual conduct specifically defined by the applicable state law, and (c) if the work, as a whole, lacks serious literary, artistic, political or scientific value.

From the moment it was handed down, this Supreme Court decision has been criticized by many thoughtful observers as unrealistic, impractical, and worse. After all, terms such as "average person," "community standards," "prurient interest," "offensive," "serious literary, artistic, political, or scientific value" are vague and likely to change their meaning from one time and place to another. It is therefore very difficult, if not impossible, for publishers and producers to know beforehand when and where they might be violating the law. At any rate, the court decision went against the recommendations of a 1970 Presidential Commission which had advocated the repeal of antipornography laws. The carefully documented report of this commission as well as other scholarly studies were simply ignored. Thus, unburdened by any historical knowlege, the Chief Justice even proclaimed that there was "no evidence, empirical or historical," that censorship of sexual subjects in the 19th century "in any way limited or affected expression of serious . . . scientific ideas." Unfortunately, the facts are otherwise. In both the 19th and the 20th centuries censorship effectively prevented the dissemination of scientific knowledge and indeed any rational discussion of sexual matters between scientists as well as between doctor and patient. (For details see "Sex Research" and "Sex Education.")

However, history also shows that sexual censorship tends to strangulate the artistic life of a nation. It is often argued (and was argued by the Chief Justice) that laws against "pornography" are not and will never be directed against genuine works of art. It is further claimed that no serious artist has ever been prevented from realizing his full potential by being forced to observe the limits of "decency" and "good taste." Such arguments sound convincing only to people who are unfamiliar with art history. There are countless historical examples of censors destroying invaluable masterpieces. Indeed, a particularly depressing case concerns one of the greatest works of art of all time, Michelangelo's "Last Judgment." Painted on the wall of the Sistine Chapel in the Vatican during the reign of an enlightened pope, it displeased his prudish successor who ordered a third-rate court artist to paint clothes on all nude bodies, thus ruining Michelangelo's work forever. [Fortunately, in this particular instance the officially appointed vandal had some personal scruples and tried to keep his additions to a minimum. Nevertheless, the damage was done and is now irreparable. There was an outcry of public indignation when, in our own time, another (self-appointed) vandal partly damaged Michelangelo's "Pietà." Even though it proved possible to restore that sculpture to its previous appearance, there was general agreement that it had diminished greatly in value.]

Furthermore, every student of literature can cite dozens of cases in which great novels, plays, poems, and essays have been suppressed as obscene. From the 17th-century English Puritans, who closed all theaters as sinful and thereby abruptly ended one of the most glorious periods of world drama, to modern judges who banned Havelock Ellis's *Studies in the Psychology of Sex*, Joyce's *Ulysses*, Lawrence's *Lady Chatterley's Lover*, and Nabokov's *Lolita*, blue-nosed fanatics have tried to impose their parochial view of scholarship and art on the general public. Even if these fanatics were eventually overruled (sometimes only after decades), the delay robbed the books of much of their deserved impact.

In more recent times, however, prosecutions seem to have switched from books to films and illustrated magazines. The 1973 Supreme Court decision which allowed obscenity to be largely determined by "community standards" is now increasingly being used to punish film makers, actors, publishers, and distributors from all over the United States. Prosecutors can still make use of the old Comstock Act and harass people with federal charges of mailing obscenity. If a narrow-minded small-town jury can be found anywhere, undercover agents can then order the "obscene" material to be sent to that place, and convictions are easily obtained. Thus, the "community standards" of the most backward and bigoted citizens can successfully be imposed on the entire nation. Another possibility of legal harassment is opened up by various crime-conspiracy statutes which allow people to be prosecuted for conspiracy to commit a crime even if it is doubtful that they can be convicted of the crime itself. Or, the crime may carry only a light sentence, while the conspiracy to commit that crime may be punished with years of imprisonment. The penalties in these new obscenity trials are often severe. All of these developments have filled many American artists, actors, directors, writers, and publishers with apprehension. After all, even if some of these absurd convictions in prudish communities are reversed on appeal, the cost in time and money is staggering and may alone be sufficient to put anyone out of business.

Still another problem has been created by recent public concern about "child pornography" or "kiddie porn." Under various public and private pressures, many state legislatures have rather hastily passed draconic laws against the depiction of children or younger teenagers engaging in any sexual activity. Some of these laws make no exception whatsoever and thus apply even to pictures and films that are not legally "obscene." As a result, even scientific or educational works can no longer provide visual research material relating to childhood sexuality or sexual responses during puberty.

In this situation the only hope again lies with the Supreme Court which can modify its decision of 1973 and with the American voter who must realize that ultimately his own freedom of expression is at stake. At present, the American obscenity laws are a disgrace to a "free" country. As George Bernard Shaw observed a long time ago: "Comstockery is the world's standing joke at the expense of the United States."

HEALTHY—SICK

Where the violation of sexual norms is defined as a medical or psychiatric problem, sexual conformity and sexual deviance are seen as mental health and mental illness. Conforming sexual behavior is described as "mature," "productive," and "healthy." Deviant behavior is called "immature," "destructive," and "sick."

Historically speaking, this is a relatively recent view. It originated in the "Age of Enlightenment," and its first proponents were chiefly concerned with obtaining better treatment for deviants. Before that time, sexual deviants had often been regarded as heretics or criminals, and thus they were hated, ostracized, tortured, and even killed with little compunction. After all, nobody doubted that their behavior was prompted by willful malice. On the other hand, the claim that they were, in fact, medical patients suddenly turned their deviance into a disease and relieved them of all responsibility for their actions. Instead of punishment, they now needed medical therapy.

There is no question that the new "enlightened" doctors were more considerate and sympathetic than either the inquisitors or the jailers, at least in the beginning. Instead of the stake or wheel they prescribed special diets, fresh air, cold baths, and moderate exercise. Instead of dark, filthy dungeons they provided clean, bright, and airy hospitals. Even more important, there soon developed a special branch of medicine devoted exclusively to deviant behavior: "mindhealing" or "psychiatry." In short, as compared to their previous fate, the deviants seemed to have made a good bargain.

However, over the years it became rather obvious that the medical interpretation of deviance also had disadvantages. First of all, as the influence of psychiatry grew, many more individuals were said to suffer from sexual "psychopathology" than had ever been accused of sexual heresy or sexual crime. Psychiatrists treated not only cases of "sodomy," "bestiality," rape, and incest, but also many other forms of deviance which had been ignored by the Inquisition and the courts. For example, persons who changed their sexual partners frequently were said to be afflicted with "promiscuity," women who enjoyed sexual intercourse were declared to be victims of "nymphomania," children and adolescents who "abused themselves" had to be saved from "masturbatory insanity," and persons who felt an erotic attraction to members of their own sex, even if they never acted upon these feelings, were described as suffering from a pathological condition called "homosexuality." All of these people and many others who defied sexual convention became candidates for psychiatric treatment, and it was their moral duty to seek such treatment in order to "get well." While they were no longer responsible for their sexual behavior, they had a clear obligation to cooperate with their psychiatrist who tried to "correct" it. If they refused, they had to be treated involuntarily "for their own good."

As the list of sexual diseases expanded, so did the therapeutic arsenal. For instance, in the 18th century masturbators were usually treated with moral exhortations, cool room temperatures, and constant supervision. Later, with the perfection of surgical skills, they were circumcised or infibulated. In the 19th century their sex organs were burned or blistered, the nerves of the penis were severed, or the clitoris was cut out. (This latter operation was also recommended for "excessively" orgasmic women and "nymphomaniacs.") When operating techniques improved still further, the testicles or ovaries were surgically removed. In sum, eventually "medical treatments" of masturbation became so drastic that they began to resemble the medieval tortures which they once had been supposed to replace. The formerly progressive doctors had turned into agents of sexual oppression. (For details see "Types of Sexual Activity—Sexual Self-Stimulation".)

Today we may shudder at these barbarities and dismiss them as unfortunate aberrations or as horror stories from the dark ages of medicine. After all,

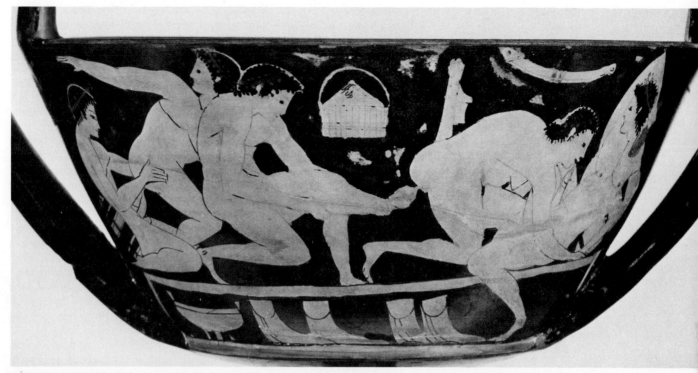

NORMAL–ABNORMAL?
This ancient Greek pottery painting dates from the 6th century B.C., a period when Greece began to enter its "golden age". The picture shows five people engaging in those forms of sexual intercourse that, in later ages, were denounced as "unnatural" and "perverse" by Christian theologians and psychiatrists. The two men on the left are just beginning anal intercourse, the woman and man on the right are beginning oral intercourse, and the man in the middle is about to insert a double "olisbos" (i.e. dildo or artificial penis) into the woman's vagina. Whatever later observers might think of this scene, it is clear from the historical context that it does not represent signs of "decadence" or "moral decay".

we no longer believe in masturbatory insanity, and we know that even "excessive" masturbation is no threat to health. Indeed, there are some psychiatrists today who prescribe it as a means of overcoming sexual inadequacy. However, when we look back a little bit further into the past, we find that the problem has wider implications. Thus, we learn, for example, that masturbation had already been recommended as therapeutic in ancient Rome, and that this view was still held by medieval Islamic doctors. In other words, the medical crusade against masturbation turns out to have been a thoroughly modern phenomenon, restricted entirely to the Western world.

A similar observation can be made in regard to homosexual behavior. We know, of course, that in ancient Greece and Rome such behavior was considered healthy and moral, and that its later condemnation was due mostly to Judeo-Christian religious doctrines. Still, it is perhaps less commonly realized that even in Christian Europe it was, on occasion, used as medical treatment. For example, when, in the 17th century, William of Orange (later King William III of England) fell ill with the smallpox, his physicians suggested that he sleep with one of his pages in order to absorb some "animal spirits" from a young, healthy body. Since the patient was known to enjoy sleeping with his pages, the prescription was easily followed. Naturally, the young man caught the disease from his master, but eventually both of them recovered. (William did not fail to show his appreciation and, in due time, made his page Duke of Portland.) Less than two hundred years later, homosexuality was declared to be a mental disease, and homosexuals began to be treated for it by psychiatrists. Needless to say, in order to be "cured," the patients had to forswear any further homosexual activity. However, in our own century some "radical"psychiatrists again rejected the "sickness theory" and told homosexuals to seek the liberation from their emotional problems in "gay activism" and satisfying sexual relationships. Thus, homosexual intercourse, far from indicating any illness, once more turned into a therapeutic measure. (According to the most recent official position of the American Psychiatric Association, homosexuality as such is not a disease.)

As these examples illustrate, over the years the concepts of sexual health and illness have undergone some extraordinary changes. Behavior which was seen as healthy at one time was regarded as sick at another time, and those who engaged in it found themselves alternately praised and condemned by medical authorities. Indeed, one can almost gain the impression that the "pathology" of sexual acts has never been more than a matter of fashion, and that, throughout history, doctors have promoted or discouraged such acts on no other basis than popular prejudice.

Nevertheless, this cynical view would be wrong. It is, of course, obvious that the medical profession cannot operate outside the general framework of popular moral standards, but in many specific instances it can set its own standards and have them accepted by the public at large. In other words, there are times when the physician can lead and public opinion will follow. The annals of medicine record many such cases, and the "enlightened" conversion of sexual heretics and criminals into medical patients is itself perhaps the most striking example.

Still, even the most progressive physician or psychiatrist who approaches sexual deviance cannot proceed without making some value judgments about the "proper" role of sex in human life. His values may very well differ from those of the official sexual morality, but they will certainly influence every one of his actions. This remains true even if he decides not to take any action at all. Furthermore, any medical or psychiatric "treatment" involves certain fundamental, if sometimes unrecognized, professional assumptions. These have to do with the criteria for health and disease, with the choice between various disease models, the choice of therapy, and with the possibility and urgency of a cure.

It is this whole set of assumptions which has to be examined if one wants to evaluate the medical or psychiatric approach to sexual deviance. As a matter of fact, such a critical examination is essential for doctor and patient alike. If both of them keep an open mind, they may, in many cases, discover that they are not dealing with a medical problem and that any medical intervention would therefore be inappropriate. On the other hand, they may also find that in certain difficult life situations medicine and psychiatry offer the best hope.

In the following pages we will try to describe how some medical and psychiatric assumptions about sexual deviance originated, how they developed in Europe and the U.S., and how widely they are accepted today in other countries.

SEX AND PSYCHIATRY

The word "psychiatry" (Greek: healing of the mind or soul) is only about a hundred years old, although the notion of a disturbed or disordered mind dates back a great deal further. However, previous ages did not speak so much of "mental illness" as of possession, alienation, lunacy, folly, or madness. Originally, these were not medical terms, but merely described any kind of "abnormal" human behavior which puzzled or frightened its observers. People who were "possessed" or who had "gone mad" were therefore treated not by medically trained "mind doctors," but by exorcists, inquisitors, judges, jailers, and sometimes executioners. It was not before the beginning of the Modern Age that the old dungeons, fools' towers, asylums, or madhouses turned into "mental hospitals." The inmates became "mental patients," and special "medical psychologists," "alienists," or "psychiatrists" took charge of them.

This is not to say that in ancient and medieval times physicians paid no attention to madmen. On the contrary, they often tried very hard to find physical causes and cures for madness, because they suspected it to be the result of some bodily disease. Thus, they believed that in many cases a cure of the body would also restore the mind. Still, where treatment proved unsuccessful, they usually agreed with the clergy that some devil, demon, or evil spirit was responsible for the failure, and that a religious response was required.

In pagan Europe the religious response to demonic possession was usually prayer, but sometimes magic incantations and even the shouting of obscenities were considered useful. Some of the possessed were also forced to drink foul smelling potions, or they were beaten, tortured, or starved. These and other drastic measures were supposed to drive the demons out of their victim's body.

Unfortunately, the arrival of Christianity did not bring an end to these cruel and useless treatments. Quite the opposite. Beginning in the late Middle Ages, the belief in demonic possession was strengthened by theologians, and more victims of such possession were found than ever before. An ever growing number of old, young, sick, crippled, simpleminded, or otherwise helpless people were declared to be "sorcerers" or "witches" possessed by the devil. They were hunted down by professional witchfinders, officially diagnosed, and then killed. However, over the years, some physicians began to oppose this systematic holy slaughter, demanding instead new forms of medical treatment. In their view, a witch was simply a person with a sick mind, and, with increasing medical knowledge, this mind could perhaps be cured. Finally, after several centuries of ideological struggle, the new opinion prevailed. The church lost its power to the state, and the old-fashioned belief in witchcraft was replaced with the modern belief in mental illness.

Today we can see that, for a very long time, this victory of science over religion was more apparent than real. Psychiatrists no longer believed in the devil, but their standards for "correct" human behavior were not very different from those of the church. This was nowhere more obvious than in the area of sexual behavior. Virtually all former sins were redefined in medical terms and declared to be mental diseases. Thus, the various forms of noncoital sexual activity turned from religious "abominations" into medical "perversions." Indeed, psychiatric textbooks often showed a strange resemblance to medieval penitentials, with therapy substituted for penance. The only real difference was this: Where sexual deviants were once believed to have lost their souls, they were now merely said to have lost their minds.

Before the beginning of our own century few psychiatrists bothered to question the religious assumptions behind their approach to sex. However, when the First World War produced a "sexual revolution" in Europe and America, the psychiatric profession as a whole was forced to become more critical. As a result, some of the former sexual "perversions" and "deviations" were reclassified as normal "variations" of human sexual behavior, and the psychiatric list of permissible sexual activities began to grow longer. In short, many of those who before had been called mentally ill were suddenly found to have been quite healthy after all.

On the other hand, the number and influence of psychiatrists increased dramatically, because, even with their reduced catalogue of sexual "perversions," they found more than enough patients. After all, in our sex-negative culture there were still millions of men and women with sexual problems, and for them psychiatric treatment seemed to offer the best hope. In addition, the government remained greatly concerned about sexual deviance and hired psychiatrists to detect and cure it wherever possible. Thus, more and more frequently they appeared as "experts" in courtrooms, prisons, schools, and in the military. Most state legislatures also passed special laws against "sexual psychopaths" which, although basically unsound and unfair, created the need for even more official psychiatric expertise. Indeed, over the years the governmental use of psychiatry became so well established that critical observers began to fear the end of individual liberty and the advent of a totalitarian "therapeutic state."

In view of these developments, various contemporary psychiatrists have demanded another radical reexamination of psychiatric assumptions. Some even reject the whole concept of mental illness as a "myth" and search for new ways of understanding abnormal behavior. (For details see "The Medical Model of Sexual Deviance.")

The following pages may help to illuminate this and several other controversial issues by placing them in some historical and cross-cultural perspective.

Historical Background

Present psychiatric attitudes toward sexual deviance cannot be understood without some knowledge of history. Unfortunately, many psychiatrists themselves lack such knowledge and therefore fail to see the true implications of their professional activity. Thus, it does not occur to them that some of their "therapeutic" interventions may be harmful not only to their patients, but to society at large. By the same token, possible beneficial uses of psychiatric knowledge may sometimes remain unexplored. It might therefore be very useful if psychiatrists were trained to look beyond their own immediate place and time.

Needless to say, within the scope of the present book we cannot discuss the entire history of psychiatry. Instead, we have to restrict ourselves to a single limited aspect of it. A few selected examples may show what, through the ages, "regular" physicians and psychiatrists have thought and done about sexual deviance.

Ancient Times

In ancient times people did not distinguish between physical and mental illness or between doctors for the body and doctors for the mind. Indeed, there was no distinction between medicine, magic, and religion. All forms of human suffering were ascribed to spirits, gods, or God, and no treatment could be successful unless it somehow dealt with these superhuman forces. When someone became sick or started to behave in strange ways, he was brought to a priest, shaman, witch doctor, wizard, or magician who performed some sacred ritual. Very often this ritual also included the administration of "medicine," but it was always clear that human actions alone could not effect a cure. Both sickness and health depended on the divine will. Thus, for example, the ancient Israelites were told by Yahweh: "I am the Lord that heals you" (Exodus 15; 26) and "I kill and I make alive; I wound and I heal" (Deuteronomy 32; 39).

In support of this view, the Bible describes how Yahweh sends plagues over Egypt and causes various illnesses in those Israelites who disobey his commandments. He also despatches an "evil spirit" to torment King Saul who therefore becomes subject to recurring black moods and finally ends up committing suicide (I Samuel). A similar fate can befall anyone else who displeases Yahweh, as the Bible warns: "The Lord will smite you with madness" (Deuteronomy 6; 5) and "The Lord shall smite you with madness, blindness, and astonishment of heart" (Deuteronomy 28; 28). Curiously enough, in the biblical view, deviant sexual behavior as such is not symptomatic of madness. However, it may be punished by a loss of certain physical or mental faculties. For some forms of sexual deviance the proper treatment is execution. (For details see "Natural—Unnatural.")

The Greeks of preclassical times also believed in the supernatural cause of human illness and therefore went to their temples for treatment. Their most important early "health cult" was that of Aesculapius, the god of medicine. However, with Greece's "golden age," a critical spirit began to arise, and the old religious beliefs were gradually amended or supplanted by systematic observation. The greatest of the new Greek physicians, Hippocrates (460–377 B.C.) set out to find natural causes for every physical and mental affliction.

For example, he declared that epilepsy, which before him had been known as the "sacred" or "divine malady" was, in fact, produced by a diseased brain. Therefore, magical incantations were useless in treating it. Hippocrates and his followers assumed that the normal functioning of the brain depended on the perfect balance among four essential bodily humors: blood, black bile, yellow bile, and phlegm. (These were related to the "four elements" [air, earth, fire, and water] as well as to the "four temperaments" [sanguinic, melancholic, choleric, and phlegmatic]). Any imbalance of the four humors could produce various diseases and abnormal behaviors. The cure required a proper diet, rest, and, in some cases, sexual abstinence. On the other hand, sexual activity was recommended for females suffering from "hysteria," a condition allegedly caused by a "wandering uterus." (Ancient Greek anatomical teachings were still more fanciful than factual.)

The second great ancient physician was Claudius Galenus, today better known simply as Galen (131–200 A.D.). Galen was born in Pergamum, but spent much of his life in Rome where he had a successful practice and won fame as a writer on medical matters. His teachings followed closely those of Hippocrates, although he also made new discoveries of his own. While he believed in a divine creator, he was nevertheless convinced that physical and mental disorders could be explained rationally. Thus, he reemphasized the importance of the brain and the balance of the essential bodily humors. Galen also developed several striking theories about reproduction and sexual health. For example, he assumed that both sexes produce seminal fluid, and that both men and women can ejaculate this fluid during their sleep. He considered such spontaneous responses natural and necessary, because unreleased semen could become poisonous. Prolonged sexual abstinence could therefore produce serious disorders, such as hysteria, hydrophobia, trembling, convulsions and madness. In view of this danger, Galen recommended moderate, but regular sexual activity. Where coitus was impossible, masturbation was just as useful. Indeed, Galen explicitly praised the example of Diogenes (that famous Greek philosopher with the lamp) who had been known to masturbate frequently for the sake of his health.

Needless to say, neither Hippocrates nor Galen ever regarded noncoital forms of sexual intercourse as signs of mental illness. The ancient Greeks and Romans were sexually very tolerant, and this tolerance was reflected in their medical beliefs. Interestingly enough, many of these beliefs survived well into the Middle Ages and beyond. As a matter of fact, in the Western world Galen remained the supreme medical authority for more than 1500 years. However, given the Christian condemnation of "lust," his sexual theories were largely neglected, then dismissed, and finally forgotten.

The Middle Ages

With the fall of the Roman empire and the arrival of the so-called Dark Ages much ancient medical knowledge was lost. Instead, Europe came again under the influence of magical and demonological beliefs. The Christian church preached the old biblical concepts of health and disease. Abnormal behavior was explained as diabolical possession, and exorcism, prayer, confession, and repentance were the only effective remedies. Sexual behavior was normal only when it could lead to reproduction. However, "deviant" types of sexual activity, such as self-stimulation, homosexual intercourse, and sexual contact with animals were seen not in medical, but religious terms. They were declared to be grave sins.

Beginning in the 7th century, the faith of Islam spread throughout the Middle East and Northern Africa and eventually also reached Spain. The Muslims had great respect for learning and therefore preserved and studied the works of their Greek and Roman predecessors. Since they were especially interested in medicine, they surveyed the entire body of ancient medical writings and soon produced many great physicians of their own. Perhaps the two most important of these are Rhazes (860–930), the "Persian Galen," who created the first "mental ward" at the Baghdad hospital, and Abu Ali Al-Hussein Ben Abdallah Ibn Sina, today better known under his Latinized name Avicenna (980–1037). Avicenna believed with Galen that moderate sexual activity was necessary for the preservation of health and that unreleased semen could turn into poison. He further declared that a man's penis would shrink unless it was strengthened by regular use. On the other hand, excessive sexual intercourse could weaken the eyes and lead to a loss of hearing. It could also produce trembling, insomnia, baldness, and epilepsy. The exact definition of "excess" was different for different people, because some were much stronger than others. Avicenna also provided a first short list of diseases which could impair normal sexual functioning. Among these were hermaphroditism, priapism (a painful, permanent erection), and male homosexuality. This latter disease was caused by a certain physical weakness, either inherited or acquired, which made normal coitus impossible. Homosexuals were spiteful, ill-tempered, effeminate and incapable of gaining or regaining a healthy masculine strength. Any attempt to cure them was therefore doomed to failure.

Condemnatory theories such as this reveal that Islamic medical research was not entirely free of religious bias. After all, for Islamic physicians the Koran was the final authority on every important question. They were further handicapped by a prohibition to cut or dissect human bodies, and they were forbidden to look at a naked woman. Under the circumstances, their scientific advances had to remain limited. Nevertheless, on the whole and compared to their Christian colleagues, they were remarkably objective and open-minded. Certainly their treatment of "madmen" was more humane, because they believed that madness was inspired by Allah rather than by some evil demon or devil.

The high quality of Islamic scholarship and medical practice came to be recognized even in Christian Europe, especially when, in the 13th century, the intellectual emperor Frederick II of Hohenstaufen assembled scholars from various countries at his court and became interested in the writings of the Arabs. He actively supported the University of Salerno and granted it the sole right, in the bounds of the Holy Roman Empire, to grant medical degrees. The physicians trained in Salerno profited from the Arabian preservation of Hippocratic principles and thus had no use for magic or religious ritual. The rediscovery of ancient writers and a growing respect for knowledge soon led to the founding of new European universities. Within the next two centuries, the universities of Padua, Paris, Vienna, Oxford, Cambridge, Prague, and Heidelberg (among others) were established. In short, a rational attitude towards human problems seemed to be gaining ground.

In actual fact, however, progress was difficult and slow. Several eminent Christian physicians who tried to challenge the prevailing demonological beliefs with Greek, Roman, or Arabian clinical observations were accused of heresy or even condemned to death by the Inquisition. Most members of the clergy as well as the laity remained superstitious and ignorant. During the same period there also appeared various bizarre mass movements, such as tarantism and flagellantism, in which great numbers of people all over Europe danced wildly through the streets or whipped themselves bloody in public orgies of self-humiliation. A sense of guilt and sinfulness began to pervade all spheres of life and occasionally led to violent outbursts against Jews, Gypsies, heretics, and other social scapegoats. It also seems that the late Middle Ages developed a strange fear and hatred of women who were increasingly condemned as the vile, wanton, wicked, and lustful sex, a constant temptation for men and their eventual ruin. Females were often seen as instruments of the devil, and, in the course of time, this, together with other frightful fantasies, developed into a new, universal witch craze.

The Modern Age

Today, the witch craze is often seen as a medieval phenomenon. However, the most intense and systematic European witchhunts began at the height of the Renaissance and continued well into the 18th century. It is true that the belief in witches dates back to medieval and even ancient times, but it was

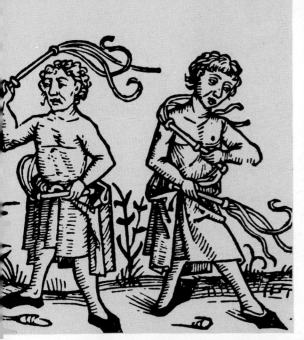
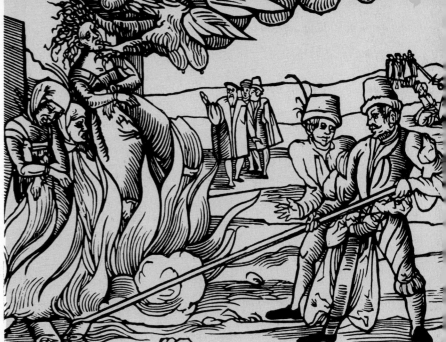

BIZZARE MASS MOVEMENTS IN MEDIEVAL EUROPE

In the Middle Ages Europe saw several mass movements which in later times have often been described as symptomatic of mental illness.

(Left) Flagellants

Flagellants were bands of people who wandered from place to place whipping themselves bloody in public orgies of self-humiliation. It can be assumed that for many of them the practice had sexual connotations. Indeed, flagellation had a second flowering in 18th- and 19th-century English brothels where customers paid handsome fees for being whipped by prostitutes. Thus, a preference for sexual whippings also became known as "the English vice". (Woodcut from the Nuremberg Chronicle.)

(Right) The Burning of Witches

The belief in witchcraft and the persecution of witches reached their height towards the end of the Middle Ages and persisted well into the 18th century. Women who were suspected of being witches were tortured until they confessed and then burned. A closer study of the trial records reveals that the witch craze had strong sexual undertones. (16th-century woodcut.)

not until the end of the 15th century that this belief was shaped into a comprehensive, coherent doctrine. In 1486, just a few years before Columbus discovered America, two German Dominicans, Jakob Sprenger and Heinrich Krämer, published the definitive handbook on witches under the title *Malleus Maleficarum* (The Witches' Hammer). This work soon found the official backing of the church, the state, and the community of scholars. It was read and accepted in every European country and, over the next 250 years, went through more than 30 editions.

The book cannot be discussed in detail here. Suffice it to say that it is one of the most depressing documents of bigotry, cruelty, ignorance, and fanaticism in human history. The text first "proves" that witches exist (those who reject the proof are witches themselves), then describes how they can be discovered, and finally lays down the rules for their trial and execution. Apart from a morbid interest in sexual matters, the authors also reveal an obsessive hatred of women. Thus, they emphasize that a woman is more likely to be a witch than a man. They further declare that "all witchcraft comes from carnal lust which in women is insatiable" and that "those among ambitious women are more deeply infected who are more hot to satisfy their filthy lusts."

Witches were possessed by the devil and often had sexual intercourse with him. They could cause crop failure, disease in cattle, death in small children, infertility in women, impotence in men, and many other disorders, disasters and calamities. The unmasking and extermination of witches was therefore essential for the safety and health of society. Furthermore, the Bible itself was unmistakably clear on the subject: "Thou shalt not suffer a witch to live" (Exodus 22;18). Within a few years, professional witchhunters, sometimes aided by physicians who were trained to search for a special "devil's mark" on the

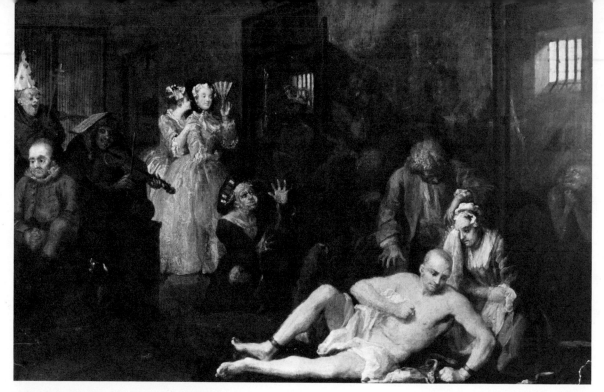

FROM "MADMAN" TO "MENTAL PATIENT"

For centuries in Europe "madmen" were locked up in dungeons, and often they were made to wear chains and fetters. Even the first "hospitals" for the insane were little more than prisons, since they did not offer serious medical treatment. It was only towards the end of the 18th century that certain doctors introduced reforms and thus laid the foundations of modern psychiatry.

(Top) **"Bedlam"**

The Hospital of St. Mary of Bethlehem in London, popularly known as "Bedlam", was the first English insane asylum. Just like a modern zoo, it was a favorite visiting place for curious citizens who came to be shocked and amused by the "antics" of those kept inside. Indeed, the inmates of Bedlam and similar "madhouses" were often treated worse than animals. (Painting by William Hogarth, early 18th century.)

(Bottom) **Pinel frees the insane**

The Frenchman Philippe Pinel was one of the first "modern" psychiatrists. During the French Revolution he was put in charge of the Bicêtre, a large asylum in Paris, and promptly proceeded to free the inmates from their shackles. He also emphasized the need for methodical psychiatric observation and a strictly medical approach to insanity. (19th century painting.)

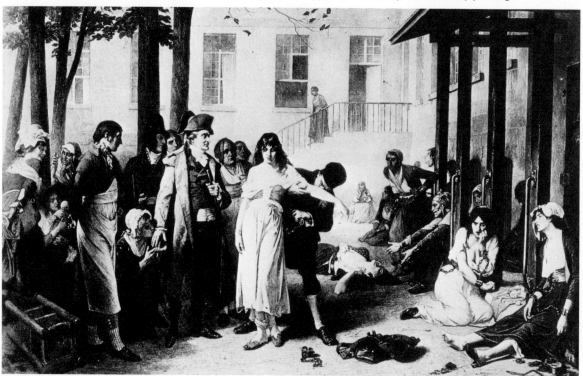

witch's body, began to roam the land and to arrest dozens, hundreds, and eventually thousands of innocent men, women, and children as witches. These unfortunates were tortured until they confessed and then publicly burned to death. The confessions usually implicated relatives, neighbors, and friends, and thus the whole horrible movement fed on itself.

It is important to remember that this movement was equally strong in both Catholic and Protestant countries. The witch craze became truly ecumenical and international, and there was hardly a voice of doubt or protest to be heard anywhere. Still, a few courageous individuals tried to stem this new tide of barbarism, mostly with medical arguments. For example, in 1563 the German physician Johann Weyer published a treatise *De Praestigiis Daemonum* (On the Deceptions of Demons) in which he argued that the diseases attributed to witchcraft were, in fact, due to natural causes and that many of the "poor, perplexed women" called witches were instead mentally ill. Therefore, they should be cured rather than killed. However, this view was rejected by most of Weyer's contemporaries, and the church put his work on the index of prohibited books. Only the Spanish Inquisition, which was busy enough persecuting heretics, Jews, and sodomites remained reluctant to try and execute witches. In Spain the Islamic heritage of caring for the insane was still alive, and thus people accused of witchcraft were often simply declared to be mad and committed to a monastery or asylum.

This latter approach gained wider acceptance in the 18th century and was finally endorsed by the emerging psychiatric profession. The new "mind doctors" took their cue from Weyer and saw the witch craze simply in medical terms. After all, in their confessions the "witches" usually claimed to have performed impossible feats, such as flying through the air, assuming the shape of animals, and causing death by means of a curse or "evil eye." This, together with the openly sexual character of much of their testimony, seemed proof enough that they were, in fact, unrecognized "mental cases" and that "witchcraft" was nothing more than a misunderstood and mishandled "mental health" problem.

Still, nonpsychiatrists pointed out that all confessions were obtained under torture or the threat of torture, and that the court records were kept by the inquisitors, not by their victims. The bizarre sexual fantasies or "hallucinations" ascribed to witches therefore said less about them than about their accusers. However, this argument was quickly seized upon by some writers of medical history who then declared that all participants in the witch trials—witchfinders, witches, and executioners—had been mentally ill.

There is no doubt that the early "alienists" or "psychiatrists" were motivated by a genuine compassion for society's misfits. They not only rescued many of the "possessed" from the clutches of the Inquisition and claimed them as patients for medical science, but also treated these patients more kindly than had been the custom before. Enlightened men like Pinel in France, Chiarugi in Italy, Langermann in Germany, and Rush in America reformed the asylums, freed the inmates from their chains and fetters, and advocated more humane forms of therapy. Unfortunately, however, with regard to deviant sexual behavior the new psychiatric "enlightenment" proved somewhat less beneficial. In the course of the 18th century physicians discovered the alleged health hazards of masturbation, and by the time of the American and French revolutions these hazards came to be seen as extremely serious. Where Galen once had recommended the periodic release of semen as a matter of hygiene, it was now denounced as the cause of nearly all physical and mental disorders. Masturbation weakened the body, softened the brain, and led to impotence, general lethargy, madness, and finally death. Within the next few decades, "masturbatory insanity" became a major threat to humanity's mental health and therefore another compelling reason for preventive psychiatric care. As a result, the psychiatrists became more important and more influential than they had ever been in the past. (For details on the antimasturbation crusade see "Types of Sexual Activity—Sexual Self-Stimulation.")

The prudish 19th century gave rise to various new psychiatric theories about the dangers of masturbation and other forms of sexual deviance. For example, it began to be believed that the weakening habit of "self-abuse" was itself the result of some inherited psychological weakness. In other words, masturbators were already born sick and then could hardly help aggravating their sorry condition. In 1843 a Russian physician named Kaan published a book under the title *Psychopathia Sexualis* (Sexual Sickness of the Mind) in which he explained this double jeopardy of masturbation. (This book, although written in Moscow and dedicated to the personal physician of the Czar, was printed in Germany where it greatly influenced psychiatric thinking. Indeed, more than 40 years later the Austrian psychiatrist von Krafft-Ebing used Kaan's book title for a new, even more famous study of deviant sexual behavior.)

According to Kaan, nearly all human beings were afflicted with a certain "phantasia morbosa" (sick imagination) which predisposed them towards sensual excess. It took only the accident of a faulty diet, a soft mattress, tight clothing, or even mere idleness to trigger the inevitable chain of events. In addition to this dismal theory, Kaan also offered a first list of other, comparatively minor sexual "aberrations," such as the love of boys, homosexual mutual masturbation, the violation of corpses, coitus with animals, and sexual contact with statues. This short list of sexual "psychopathologies" was, of course, soon expanded by other psychiatrists. Furthermore, the ever growing number of new aberrations eventually reduced the once all-important disease of masturbation to second rank. Nevertheless, Kaan's belief in the possible heredity of sexual deviance retained its appeal and was, in fact, strengthened in subsequent years.

Before we turn to these further "scientific" developments, however, it may be useful to comment briefly on the concept of "sexual psychopathology" itself. Quite obviously, in the beginning it was nothing more than the secular version of an old religious dogma. It is hardly a coincidence that Kaan's sexual "aberrations" are virtually identical with the "abominations" of the Bible. Moreover, the parallel of his inherited *phantasia morbosa* to Augustine's "concupiscence" is striking. In short, as Kaan's efforts made clear, science, as the "new religion," was still preoccupied with protecting the old sexual taboos. (For further details compare "Sex and Religion—Historical Background.")

The unacknowledged religious bias of psychiatry became even more evident when, in 1857, the French psychiatrist Morel turned to the concept of *dégénérescence* for the explanation of madness. Morel, who earlier in his life had pursued theological studies, came to the conclusion that progressive "degeneracy" was the cause of most physical and mental illness. The first man (whom the Bible had called Adam) had been of a healthy "primitive type." However, after his nature had become corrupted at some early date, man found himself subjected to weakening external and internal influences. As a result, today we no longer see the original perfect "primitive type," but various imperfect human races as well as a great number of "degenerates." These degenerates usually suffer from hereditary sexual "perversion" and are destined to die out.

Not surprisingly, in the course of time Morel's theory came to be seen as too openly biblical by many of his colleagues, and thus they recast it in more fashionable "objective" terms. It began to be assumed that degeneracy could appear in the course of an otherwise progressive evolutionary process. Still, degenerates retained their basic characteristics, and they, together with their offspring, were inevitably doomed. These ideas were further popularized by great 19th century dramatists like Ibsen and Hauptmann, who described the effects of degeneracy in their most depressing details. Indeed, the novelist Emile Zola presented the "natural and social history" of a whole family, the Rougon-Macquarts, as a case of hereditary progressive decay. The notion of an inborn pathological disposition towards madness and sexual deviance continued to dominate psychiatric thinking up to the time of Sigmund Freud, who finally replaced it with the concept of a traumatic (and largely unconscious) individual life history.

In this context it should be remembered that the 19th century also laid the "scientific" foundations of modern racism. The term "degeneracy" was all too easily applied to whole social or ethnic groups which were unpopular for some reason, and which could now be labeled biologically inferior. Needless to say, such labeling also always implied the charge of sexual "perversion." The logical implications of racism, in turn, led to "eugenic" policies, i.e., official attempts to improve the biological health of the population by preventing the breeding of degenerates. On the other hand, it was felt that the superior races did not breed enough. There was a widespread fear that, sooner or later, the whole of mankind might become degenerate and die out. (This fear seems especially grotesque today when one looks at the population curve between 1800 and 1900.) At any rate, growing racial pride, nationalism, and a rapidly expanding industry prompted many governments to demand a population increase. Procreation was again confirmed as the only "correct" goal of sexual intercourse.

Psychiatry took another important step forward when, in 1883, the German psychiatrist Kraepelin published a textbook offering the first systematic classification of mental diseases. While he remained convinced that all of them had physical causes, he was careful to describe each disease as a distinct entity with its own set of symptoms and prospects of cure. Kraepelin's work became the basis for all later psychiatric categorizations. Inspired by this example, other psychiatrists soon felt encouraged to be ever more specific. Thus, among other things, they drew up new, detailed lists of sexual "abnormalities" or "perversions." These lists sometimes went to extraordinary lengths and, in fact, breathed a medieval spirit of casuistic scholasticism. At any rate, they shared the basic assumptions of traditional Christian moralists: Only coitus between "approved" partners is right; all other forms of sexual expression are wrong. However, as a concession to the modern, secular world, these value judgments were now expressed in medical rather than religious terms. (For details see introduction to "Sexual Maladjustment.")

Curiously enough, towards the end of the 19th century the psychiatric crusade against masturbators began to lose its momentum. Instead, the attention turned to a new group of sexual deviants—persons attracted to members of their own sex. Same-sex behavior had, of course, long been condemned by both Jews and Christians, but it had never before been regarded as a symptom of mental illness. (The medieval Muslim Avicenna had ascribed it to a physical disorder.) However, now this behavior was discovered to result from a specific psychological "condition" which afflicted a certain number of people, and for this condition the new term "homosexuality" was invented. For some time there was a debate whether homosexuality was an outright "perversion," a sign of "degeneracy," or merely a mild "personality disorder" without wider implications. Sigmund Freud did not consider it an "illness," but still saw it as a symptom of "arrested development." Some of his followers became again more severe and called it an indication of "immaturity" or a neurotic fear of the opposite sex. At any rate, in America the "condition" continued to be listed in the "Diagnostic and Statistical Manual of Psychiatric Disorders" (DSM) until 1973 when the American Psychiatric Association finally decided to remove it. Since then, American homosexuals have been officially healthy again. Now only those who are disturbed by their homosexuality (or heterosexuality?) are said to need psychiatric treatment for a "sexual orientation disturbance." (See also "Homosexual Intercourse" and "The Sexually Oppressed—Homosexuals.")

(**Note:** The preceding section is based not only on the standard American histories of psychiatry by Alexander/Selesnick and Zilboorg/Henry [see "Reference and Recommended Reading"], but also includes some historical information from the untranslated German study *Formen des Eros* [2 vols] by Annemarie and Werner Leibbrand, Freiburg Br., München 1972).

Cross-cultural Perspectives

Psychiatrists in other countries do not necessarily share all the professional assumptions of their American colleagues. Especially with regard to sexual deviance psychiatric opinion and practice differ widely from one culture to another. Not surprisingly, the fewest such differences are found in the Western so-called capitalist countries which share a common cultural heritage and political philosophy with the United States. In the so-called communist countries, on the other hand, psychiatry is often assigned functions which would be rejected by most of its Western practitioners. Again, the treatment of sexual deviants offers the most striking example. To a Western observer it is obvious that the present communist societies, whatever their economic or political claims, cling to the sexual standards of the capitalist Victorian bourgeoisie.

Unfortunately, the scope of the present book does not permit a detailed discussion of this phenomenon. Nevertheless, the following few brief notes may help to outline its dimensions.

Western Europe

In Western Europe the practice of psychiatry is quite similar to that in the U.S., although there are fewer psychiatrists, and thus their overall social influence is not as great. After all, it must be remembered that in the 1930's and 1940's many leading European psychiatrists were driven into exile by the rise of fascism. Especially those of the psychoanalytic school found themselves persecuted in every country that came under Nazi domination. The psychoanalytic theory itself was officially condemned as "Jewish science," and all psychoanalytic writings were banned or even publicly burned. In addition, the various European movements for sexual reform were ruthlessly destroyed.

It was not until after the end of the Second World War that European psychiatrists could try to regain their former position of leadership. However, first they had to rediscover their own past, and thus the 1950's and 1960's produced a renaissance of psychoanalysis which, at least with regard to sexual deviance, still dominates European psychiatric thinking at the present time. This becomes manifest especially in official and semiofficial European sex education books and programs which, to this day, are conceived from a strictly Freudian viewpoint. It is interesting to note, however, that most contemporary European psychoanalysts honor the older Freud's critical intentions and are comparatively reluctant to apply the "sickness" label to deviant sexual behavior. (On the whole, they see Freud more as a philosopher and social critic than a clinician.) At the same time, they also feel obliged to question the prevailing "normal" sexual standards.

Naturally, to a certain extent this broadmindedness reflects the more tolerant European legal approach to sex. Generally speaking, there is very little prosecution of victimless sex crimes, and therefore the psychiatric involvement in the legal system is kept to a minimum. Still, where sex crimes do have victims, psychiatric treatment of the offender may be encouraged by the courts. Such treatment is rarely based on psychoanalytic concepts, but normally involves various drug therapies, so-called behavior modification techniques, and even castration and new types of brain surgery (so-called psychosurgery). In the meantime some of these treatments have aroused widespread skepticism as the theories of "radical" American psychiatrists have begun to gain some influence. A further challenge of traditional psychiatric assumptions has come from the Europeans themselves. Perhaps the best known of these recent critics is the British psychiatrist Ronald D. Laing. (For further details see "Critique of the Medical Model.")

The Soviet Union

We know that today in the Soviet Union psychiatry is often used as a means of suppressing political dissent, and that Soviet mental hospitals house all kinds of nonconformists, many of whom would not be considered ill in Western countries. We also know that the present Soviet government espouses a very restrictive sexual morality.

This has not always been the case. On the contrary, in the first years after the revolution the Soviet Union pursued the most liberal and progressive sexual policies in the world. Thus, among other things, it replaced the repressive Czarist sex and marriage laws with a whole body of modern legislation based on the then available findings of Western sex research. Moreover, the Communist Party worked hard to overcome sexual prejudice. For example, the articles on sexual deviance in the Great Soviet Encyclopedia were based on the work of Freud and Hirschfeld. At the same time, Soviet scientists also engaged in new research of their own and conducted experiments in nonrepressive education. The best known of these experiments is perhaps that of the psychoanalyst Vera Schmidt who founded a special children's home in Moscow. In this home the children were left free to satisfy their natural sexual curiosity or to masturbate whenever they felt like it. As a result, they grew up without any sexual guilt feelings and developed friendly and responsible attitudes towards each other.

Naturally, in the early years the Soviet example was a source of pride and inspiration for Western sex reformers who held it up as a model to their own governments. Unfortunately, soon all of this came to an end. In the early 1930s the odious Czarist law against male homosexual behavior was revived and the old bourgeois sexual values were officially reinstated. Premarital chastity was praised and the nuclear family with its traditional sexual roles was again set up as the ideal. At the same time, Stalin started a new wave of general political repression whose effects continue to be felt to this day.

At the present time the Soviet Union still does not permit its citizens much sexual freedom. Soviet psychiatry also explicitly rejects Freud and denies the existence of sexual interests in "normal" children. Childhood masturbation and sex play are considered signs of "premature development" and as a deviation from the norm. The masturbation of adolescents and adults is still called "onanism." It is regarded as a "vice" which demands correction, because it has a pernicious influence on the mind and weakens the body. Male homosexual behavior is considered to be both criminal and sick. However, now as before, little attention is paid to female homosexual behavior. (See also "Sex and the Law—Cross-Cultural Perspectives.")

Cuba

Among the declared goals of the Cuban socialist revolution are the full equality of men and women and a rational and humane approach to sexual problems. However, in practice the Spanish cultural heritage of a sexual double standard and excessive masculine pride (*machismo*) have greatly hampered progress in these areas. Furthermore, there is little official tolerance even of harmless sexual deviance. Special targets of governmental repression are prostitution, "pornography," cross-dressing, and homosexual behavior. Indeed, at times large numbers of homosexuals have been sent to special prison farms or forced labor camps where they have been brutally treated in order to be "reformed." When American and European visitors to Cuba became aware of these policies and denounced them in their home countries, the Cuban government became embarrassed enough to soften its approach. Nevertheless, in principle this approach has not changed even today. Homosexuality is still seen as an infectious "aberration" which has to be corrected. Thus, according to the Cuban National Congress on Education and Culture, "homosexual deviations" are "socially pathological" and must be "prevented from spreading." Homosexuals display an "antisocial character" and therefore must be denied any influence on young people through artistic and cultural activities. Instead, they must be "controlled," "transferred," and "relocated" according to their "degree of deterioration." In short, Cuban officials today still use quasi-medical or pseudo-medical arguments to reduce Cuban homosexuals to the status of second-class citizens and to deny them the most elementary civil rights.

The People's Republic of China

The treatment of "mental patients" in the People's Republic of China combines elements of traditional Chinese medicine, Western medicine, and new political techniques. Mental hospitals are not run exclusively by doctors and their staff, but by so-called Revolutionary Committees which include members of the military and various political workers. By the same token, the patients receive not only drugs and acupuncture therapy, but also ideological counseling. They are expected to engage in "productive labor" and to study the thought of Mao Tse-tung. In addition, there is great emphasis on participation in group activities and on "collective help." Indeed, the social and political aspect of mental illness is considered more important than the medical aspect, and therefore psychiatrists do not hesitate to "put politics in command."

The extent to which the Chinese equate sexual deviance with mental illness is, at the present time, difficult to determine. We know, however, that Freud and his psychoanalytical theory are not accepted in China. We also know, for example, that homosexual behavior is not tolerated, although it is seen as a moral rather than a medical problem. (The last Chinese emperor, who later became an ordinary citizen in the People's Republic, was a homosexual. It is therefore possible that in the public mind homosexuality is now associated with feudalism.) Moreover, there is an official Chinese campaign to stamp out masturbation. From all indications, this campaign seems to be quite similar to that in Western countries about a hundred years ago. Thus, just as in bourgeois Victorian Europe, the public is told that masturbation results in an "overstimulation of the brain, dizziness, insomnia, and general weakness." However, in a new twist of the old yarn, it is now also said to "erode the revolutionary will." In order to avoid these dangers, Chinese teenagers are advised to get sufficient physical exercise, to wear loose-fitting underclothes, and to study the works of Marx, Lenin, and Chairman Mao. In the same puritanical spirit young married couples are warned against having too much sexual intercourse. For instance, a recent advice column in an official Chinese newspaper explains to a young woman that intercourse with her husband must not take place more than one to three times a week, because "indulgence will undermine your health."

(**Note:** Comprehensive and systematic studies of Soviet, Cuban, and Chinese psychiatric practices are difficult to obtain. Most of what can be learned about them in the West is scattered in numerous books and articles written for professional journals. However, some official Soviet and Chinese pronouncements on sexual questions can be found in Steward E. Fraser, ed., *Sex, Schools, & Society, International Perspectives*, Nashville, Tenn., 1972. The Soviet return to bourgeois sexual values is discussed in Wilhelm Reich, *The Sexual Revolution*, New York, 1969. Present Chinese psychiatric treatments are also described by Ruth Sidel in Thomas J. Scheff, ed., *Labeling Mental Illness*, Englewood Cliffs, N.J., 1975. A discussion of homosexual civil rights in Cuba can be found in K. Jay and A. Young, eds., *Out of the Closets, Voices of Gay Liberation*, New York, 1974.)

THE MEDICAL MODEL OF SEXUAL DEVIANCE

As we have mentioned before, whenever a society becomes seriously concerned with achieving or maintaining sexual conformity, it ceases to treat its sexual deviants as harmless individualists, but instead regards them as sinful, criminal, or sick. In other words, where deviant sexual behavior appears as a social issue, it tends to be discussed in either religious, legal, or medical terms.

We have already described in two earlier chapters how the religious and legal frames of reference shape the perceptions of those who use them. (See "Natural—Unnatural" and "Legal—Illegal.") We have also seen that in modern times these traditional approaches to the problem have increasingly been amended or even replaced by a medical or psychiatric approach. The following pages may further clarify this development and point out some of its implications.

The Function of Models

When people are confronted with the unknown or unexpected, they usually try to gain at least some understanding of it by likening it to something familiar. For example, a man who is puzzled by the workings of the brain may liken it to a computer in order to explain them. Needless to say, by making this analogy, the man does not imply that the brain is, in fact, a computer consisting of electronic circuitry, tapedeck, typewriter, etc. Instead, he merely uses the computer as a model or means of comparison. He decides to regard the brain *as if* it were a computer and thereby comes a little closer to finding out how it works.

Similarly, a man who encounters some bizarre human behavior may try to understand it by constructing for himself a certain conceptual model or frame of reference in which his bewildering observations somehow "fall into place." For example, he may ascribe "mad" behavior to demonic possession or see it as God's punishment for a life of sin. That is to say, he decides to regard madness as if it had a supernatural cause. He then finds that, in view of this assumption, the hitherto incomprehensible actions of madmen suddenly begin to make sense and can be explained. In short, he arrives at his otherwise unobtainable insight by using a **religious model** of madness.

However, another observer may not believe in God or demons and thus may choose to assume that madmen are simply victims of unfortunate personal experiences and that they were "driven mad" by what happened to them in the course of their lives. Such an observer decides to regard madness as if it were learned behavior. He uses a **learning model** of madness.

A third observer may reject both of these models and prefer to believe that mad behavior is caused by a lack or loss of health. Thus, he decides to regard madness as if it were a disease. This means that he uses a **medical model** of madness.

There are, of course, many other possible models of madness, and we will discuss some of them later on. Even the three models listed here can be divided into various submodels according to differences in detail. For instance, Christians, Hindus, Buddhists and polytheistic "primitives" may subscribe to different religious models of madness, even if they agree on its supernatural origin. By the same token, different modern scientists may use very different learning models of madness, from psychoanalytic theory to operant conditioning. Finally, in the course of history doctors have used at least two major medical models of madness, depending on whether they traced it to physical or psychological causes. Accordingly, at times they ascribed madness to a diseased body, at other times to a diseased mind.

People choose a particular model to fit their own preconceptions, needs, and purposes, and they usually stick to it as long as it helps to provide them with workable explanations. However, it is not unusual that, upon closer study, a certain phenomenon raises so many new questions that a formerly useful model becomes inadequate and has to be replaced. Thus, for example, when people ceased to believe in supernatural forces and discovered that some forms of mad behavior were caused by physical damage to the brain, they abandoned the religious model of madness in favor of the medical model.

It should be noted, however, that the replacement of one model by another does not defeat its original purpose, but rather confirms the basic principle of all model-making. Models are indispensable, but, by definition, they are never more than temporary structures. A model is supposed to make the strange look familiar, to "make sense" out of what appears to be senseless. As soon as it fails to fulfill this function, it has outlived its usefulness and thereby frees us to look for another, more comprehensive or more precise model which might produce better results. Therefore, it can very well be said that models are made only in order to be tested.

Models are also made in order to be compared to other models. A model always arranges certain concepts, ideas, theories, or points of view in such a way that they invite comparison with other concepts, ideas, theories, and points of view. For example, both the religious and medical models of madness spell out how mad behavior is caused, what should be done about it, and by whom, and to what extent a madman is responsible for his condition:

- According to the religious model, mad behavior is caused by evil spirits, it should be fought with exorcism, and this exorcism should be performed by a priest or other religious authority. The madman is likely to be responsible for his condition by having offended God. However, once he has repented, and the evil spirit has left him, he is saved.

- According to the medical model, mad behavior is caused by a disease, it should be fought with medical treatment, and this treatment should be administered by a doctor. The madman is almost never responsible for his condition, only unlucky. However, once he has successfully responded to drugs, electroshock, psychosurgery, etc., he is cured.

Naturally, if one so desires, one can carry this comparison a great deal further, because both models correspond in many additional details. Thus, where the advocates of the religious model speak of demons, the human soul, divine commandments, temptation, sin, penance, forgiveness, faith, and redemption, the proponents of the medical model speak of germs, viruses, parasites, the human body or the human mind, rules of hygiene, infection, injury, trauma, pathology, therapy, health, and rehabilitation.

The fact that we can make such point-by-point comparisons does not, of course, imply that all models are equal or that we are justified in choosing any model we like as long as we remain consistent. On the contrary, it is precisely when we compare different models with each other that we discover their relative merits. We also have to remember that history records many cases in which a certain model proved to be the only "correct" one and thus rendered all others obsolete. For instance, with regard to certain forms of madness a formerly tentative medical model was later so strongly confirmed by scientific discoveries that it actually lost the character of a model and became the accepted factual truth. (The best known of these cases is perhaps the insanity caused by syphilis.) On the other hand, there have also been cases where a medical model of madness was not only not confirmed, but positively disproved by science. (The best known of these cases is perhaps the alleged insanity caused by masturbation.)

A detailed comparison of models can also help us to recognize each model as a separate entity and to keep it free from adulteration. That is to say, by clarifying the distinctions between different models, we can protect ourselves from conceptual confusion or what some scientists have called a "model muddle." Models must not be mixed. They cannot possibly work if their parts do not fit together logically. A hodgepodge of unrelated assumptions or an amalgamation of heterogenous models can never produce any meaningful insight.

Unfortunately, simple and self-evident as this truth seems to be, it is not always appreciated in practice. Again, the case of "masturbatory insanity" offers perhaps the best illustration: In the 18th and 19th centuries many European and American physicians declared that masturbation softened the brain and led to a mental breakdown. Some also asserted that the harmful habit itself was produced by an inherited abnormal physical or mental constitution. Thus, masturbation was considered to be both the cause and the effect of madness. In any case, masturbators were ill, and their illness required strong therapeutic measures, such as infibulation, clitoridectomy, and castration.

Obviously, those who advanced this view believed that they had thereby created a modern "enlightened" medical model. However, a closer analysis shows that this model still contained a number of traditional "unenlightened" religious elements. For example, the very terms in which doctors spoke of the alleged medical problem ("onanism," "self-abuse," or "solitary vice") were either directly derived from the Bible or otherwise openly judgmental. Furthermore, the useless and cruel "medical treatment" was clearly better designed to punish than to heal. Finally, unlike true medical patients, masturbators were still morally condemned and held responsible for their condition. Therefore, the supposedly medical model of "masturbatory insanity" was, in fact, a religious or moral model in medical disguise.

It should be remembered, however, that such "model muddling" is by no means a thing of the past. It remains a powerful (and usually unrecognized) temptation at all times. This is apparent to any observer of the contemporary psychiatric scene. Today even in one and the same "mental hospital" different psychiatrists may proceed from very different assumptions. Consequently, they may fight the same "disease" with very different types of "treatment" from surgery, drug therapy, and electroshock to behavior modification, group discussion, encounter sessions, and psychoanalysis. Furthermore, it is quite common for psychiatrists to differ in their diagnosis of a particular patient, not only with regard to the kind of illness he may have, but even with regard to the question whether he is ill at all. Naturally, all of this often leads to confusion, not only among the general public, but also within the psychiatric profession itself. As a result, some exasperated psychiatrists have, in the meantime, already begun to demand a radical break with tradition and to proclaim "the death of psychiatry."

Indeed, while the news of its death may be somewhat exaggerated, it seems clear enough that modern psychiatry is in serious trouble. Or, to use an appropriate metaphor, it is suffering from an ever deepening "identity crisis." There is even the possibility that, in the long run, it may not survive as a medical discipline, and the reason for this can again be found in the continued indiscriminate mixing of models. The basic problem is easily stated: Psychiatrists, when dealing with abnormal behavior, are supposedly practicing some form of medicine. However, it is becoming increasingly obvious that many of their professional activities do not really fit into a medical model. Instead, they are much more meaningful in the context of other models. For example, the behavior modification techniques, group encounters, and individual "talking sessions" mentioned above are not medical treatments in the strict sense of the term, and there is no logical reason why people who want them should have to visit a doctor. As a matter of fact, today many such people go to psychologists, lay analysts, and all sorts of family, marriage, sex, drug, or youth counselors. Many of these "experts" have no medical training and do not pursue any medical objectives. By the same token, those who seek their help are not considered sick and therefore are not called patients, but clients. Their difficulties are not defined as symptoms of a disease, but as "adjustment problems," "emotional disturbances," "underdeveloped social skills," "faulty learning," or simply "problems in living."

At the present time the best known and most important nonmedical psychiatric technique is, of course, psychoanalysis. It is true that its founder, Sigmund Freud, was a physician and that he developed his theories in the course of treating his patients. However, over the years he realized that these theories had much wider implications and could not be tied to the practice of medicine. Instead, he saw ever more clearly that he had created a whole new critical education and research system. Therefore, he came to the conclusion that it was unnecessary for psychoanalysts to attend medical school. On the contrary, he hoped that they would take up interdisciplinary studies combining elements of biology, psychology, sociology, the history of civilization, mythology, literature, and other subjects in the humanities. In further recognition of its nonmedical importance, he also recommended psychoanalysis for various people who were not sick, such as artists, writers, and analysts-in-training. Unfortunately, because of certain historical circumstances, Freud's intentions were not carried out by his successors. After his death, psychoanalysis was reconfirmed as a medical specialty, and as such it became part of the vast modern psychiatric enterprise. This development, in turn, could not but add to the growing general confusion. (For a further discussion of the nonmedical character of psychoanalysis see "New Models.")

Naturally, what has been said here about "madness" or "mental illness" in general also applies to sexual deviance when it is defined as a psychiatric problem. Modern psychiatrists may subscribe to very different models of sexual deviance and therefore may also differ greatly in their professional practice. Some may regard every sexual deviant as a sick person and offer him various traditional medical therapies. Others may consider most sexual deviants to be perfectly healthy and refuse to treat them at all. Still others may assume a third position and try to correct even deviants who are not ill using any method that seems to produce results. In short, the apparently medical character of psychiatry is no guarantee that psychiatrists will behave like "regular" doctors and deal with sexual deviants in the same way as with "regular" medical patients.

In view of these circumstances it is perhaps advisable to take a closer look at the medical model and its implications.

Implications of the Medical Model

The medical model of sexual deviance is based on the assumption that it can best be explained as a disease. Or rather, the various forms of deviant sexual behavior are like so many different diseases which have their own causes and symptoms, and which can be medically treated. The assumption further implies that sexual deviants are medical patients, that the classification of their behavior is a medical diagnosis, that this behavior should be corrected by a doctor, and that his attempts to do so constitute therapy. Finally, it is assumed that sexual conformity equals health and that the return to conformity amounts to a cure.

People who make these assumptions do not necessarily mean that a sexual deviant is "mentally ill" or even that there is such a thing as "mental illness." Indeed, they may believe, to the contrary, that all sexual deviants are physically ill and that every illness in the world is physical. In short, the medical model of deviant behavior does not, in itself, suggest a need for "mindhealing" or psychiatry. A few, brief examples may clarify this point:

Physical diseases have traditionally been divided into three major categories according to their causes:

1. **Infectious Diseases,** i.e., diseases caused by some germ or virus, as for instance gonorrhea, syphilis, tuberculosis, or the common cold.
2. **Systemic Diseases,** i.e., diseases caused by some bodily breakdown or malfunction, as for instance a hardening of the arteries, an enlargement of the prostate, or diabetes.
3. **Traumatic Diseases,** i.e., diseases caused by some external agent or influence on the body, as for instance food poisoning, a broken limb, a cut, or a burn.

All three of these categories have, at one time or another, also been used to classify and explain deviant behavior. For example:

- When people discovered that a syphilitic infection can ultimately reach the brain and thus cause bizarre conduct, they began to suspect that perhaps all abnormal behaviors might have similar causes. (In this view, deviance indicated an infectious disease.)

- When people believed in "degeneracy," deviant behavior was ascribed to an inherited weakness, a progressive deterioration of genetic material which manifested itself in "bad nerves" and an overstimulated and misdirected sexual appetite. (In this view, deviance indicated a systemic disease.)

- When people believed in "masturbatory insanity," deviant behavior was traced to the injurious habit of "self-abuse" which overheated the brain and deprived the body of certain essential fluids. (In this view, deviance indicated a traumatic disease.)

It is very important to note that in all three of these examples deviant behavior was ascribed only to physical causes. In other words, a person's behavior was "wrong," because his body was sick. If the body had been healthy, the behavior would have been "right," and it became "right" again as soon as the body was cured. (On the other hand, the behavior remained "wrong," if the body proved incurable.) There was no suggestion of a "mind" or "psyche," "mental illness," or "psychiatry." The entire problem was seen strictly in terms of physical illness and physical treatment. The patient simply needed an ordinary physician.

However, it will be recalled from our earlier historical sketch that in modern times deviant behavior has increasingly been attributed not to physical, but to purely mental diseases. In this view, there is nothing wrong with the deviant's body, but there is something wrong with his mind. It follows that no ordinary physician can cure him, and that he needs instead the help of a "mindhealer" or psychiatrist. Nevertheless, since all psychiatrists are medically trained, they share certain basic assumptions with the physician and thus may also distinguish between infectious, systemic, and traumatic mental diseases.

Unfortunately, in actual practice this approach has not proved to be very useful. Especially with regard to sexual deviance the traditional medical categories have often led to confusing and contradictory propositions. For example, over the years the single mental disease "homosexuality" has been traced to each or all of three different kinds of causes. Specifically, the following theories have been proposed:

- People are homosexual because they were seduced by other, mostly older homosexuals. Therefore, homosexuals must be kept away from young people. (In this view, homosexuality is an infectious disease.)

- People are homosexual because they were born with a certain "weak personality," because they have become senile, or because their "character has disintegrated." (In this view, homosexuality is a systemic disease.)

- People are homosexual because neurotic parents or traumatic early sexual encounters have prevented their normal sexual development. (In this view, homosexuality is a traumatic disease.)

Of course, the psychiatrists who proposed these theories did not always make their underlying assumptions explicit and, in many cases, even remained unaware of them. Indeed, some psychiatrists were clearly embarrassed when these assumptions were spelled out by critical observers. After all, there is something coarse and clumsy about any direct equation of mental and physical diseases. It seems simpleminded to imply that the mind is a thing, a concrete, tangible object or organism which can be infected, break down, or sustain injuries. If such implications are found in psychiatric pronouncements, they are not to be taken literally, but figuratively. The concepts of infection, systemic malfunction, and trauma can be applied to mental diseases only in a poetic or parabolic sense. There are no "mental germs" or vulnerable "mental organs." Therefore, if one wants to classify mental diseases along the same lines as physical diseases one has to take refuge in metaphors.

Actually, as a closer examination reveals, the term "mental disease" itself is metaphoric. That is to say, strictly speaking, a mind cannot be diseased any more than an intellect can be obese or an instinct can be cancerous. One can talk about a "sick mind" only in the sense in which one talks about a "sick joke" or a "sick economy." In fact, just like the words "joke" and "economy," the word "mind" also refers to an abstraction. The mind is a concept, a notion, or an idea which summarizes the activity and function of the human brain. It is obviously not the brain itself. (A brain disease is a physical disease.) Therefore, when we say that somebody's mind is sick, we are actually saying that "the function of his brain" is sick. As a matter of fact, depending on the case, we may be saying that the function of his brain is sick while his brain itself is healthy.

One does not have to be a professor of logic to see that, taken at face value, such a statement is nonsense. It is like saying that the performance of an automobile engine has broken down while the engine itself is in perfect working order—a hopeless contradiction. Yet this kind of contradiction is unavoidable as long as one insists on ascribing a concrete condition to an abstract concept or, in other words, as long as one seriously claims that "the mind can be sick in the same way the body can be sick" and that "mental disease is like any other disease." This claim would make sense only if the mind were indeed a thing and thus could be put in the same logical category as the body. However, as we have seen, no modern scientist makes this assumption.

The situation was different in ancient times when people believed that not only the body, but also the mind was concrete. For example, the ancient Greek word for mind, "psyche," (which forms part of the modern word "psychiatry") originally meant "breath" and then "soul," and this soul was assumed to be located in a certain specific part of the body (the heart, the diaphragm, the liver, or the brain). It was also assumed that the soul was some sort of ethereal creature or spirit and that it could therefore be influenced and even possessed by other spirits. Today no doctor, not even a psychiatrist, believes in spirits or souls. The word "psyche" has now become an abstract, purely technical term and no longer refers to a living and breathing invisible being. In short, when modern psychiatrists talk about a "disease of the mind" they are not talking about an actual disease of an actual organism, but about a metaphorical disease of a theoretical proposition.

It seems necessary to emphasize and reemphasize this simple point because, as experience shows, it is all too easily forgotten. Furthermore, the professional language used by psychiatrists is often "neo-archaic," imprecise, and misleading. For instance, we constantly hear not only about "psychiatry" (healing of the mind), "psychotherapy" (cure of the mind), and "psychopathology" (sickness of the mind), but even about "psychoactive drugs" (drugs that act upon the mind) and "psychosurgery" (surgery performed on the mind). However, these and similar terms do not really mean what they seem to say, and anyone who fails to recognize their metaphorical character is bound to misunderstand them. In other words, since the mind cannot be sick except in a metaphorical sense, it can also only be healed or cured in a metaphorical sense. Psychoactive drugs do not really act upon the mind, but upon the brain and perhaps other parts of the body, and psychosurgery is in fact always brain surgery.

One may, of course, wonder why this kind of loose terminology continues to be employed by professionals who are supposed to know better. Thus, one may well ask: "If a psychosurgeon in fact operates on the brain, why does he not say so? Why does he not refer to his work simply as brain surgery?" The answer is that he is not directly concerned with the brain itself, but operates on it only in order to gain indirect influence on something else. His aim is not so much to alter the brain as the behavior which is determined by the brain. Indeed, he may regard the brain itself as healthy and only the behavior as sick. In a sense, then, it is only the behavior on which he is actually operating. Therefore he thinks of himself more as a "behavior surgeon" than a brain surgeon. Brain surgeons operate only on diseased brains and would never consider operating on a healthy brain. Surgery on a healthy brain must therefore be justified by calling it "psychosurgery," i.e., surgery on the mind. It then becomes, so to speak, surgery by proxy. Once this rationale is accepted, the whole procedure suddenly begins to make sense: A healthy brain may be surgically injured, because this injury results in healing a sick mind.

It is an ironic coincidence that at a time when "psychosurgery" is becoming popular in the Western world there are also reports of Western patients with various bodily diseases traveling to certain backward countries in order to undergo an operation called "psychic surgery." In this type of operation, which is illegal in Europe and America, a "psychic healer" performs imaginary surgery as part of some magic ritual. No surgical instruments are used, no incision is made, and yet in the end the healer claims to have cut out the diseased organ by force of his mental powers alone just as surely as if he had used a knife. In fact, as proof of his accomplishment he usually shows the patient some bloody intestines which supposedly have been left over.

Needless to say, modern Western doctors consider any such magic ritual to be nothing but criminal quackery and an outrageous, cynical fraud. Nevertheless, if only for theoretical reasons, the ideology behind this "fraud" deserves to be taken into consideration when one discusses the concepts of physical and mental disease. It also casts a dramatic and very welcome light on the difference between physical and mental forms of therapy. As a matter of fact, in view of this newly illuminated perspective, we can now clarify our teminological problems in the following manner:

The surgical alteration of behavior which is being advocated in our culture is, in fact, always brain surgery, i.e., ordinary surgery performed on a real organ. The term "psychosurgery" for such an operation is misleading, because it suggests that one can perform surgery on the mind, a wholly imaginary organ or organism. The term "psychic surgery," on the other hand, refers to imaginary surgery on a real organ, such as the brain, the stomach, the liver, or the heart. Finally, as a fourth logical possibility, one can conceive of imaginary surgery being performed on an imaginary organ like the mind. This would perhaps best be described as "psychic psychosurgery."

Perhaps the entire issue can be summarized this way: If one believes in the proposition that both a real organ (like the brain) and an imaginary organ (like the mind) can be subject to operable diseases, one might as well also propose real and imaginary forms of surgery. Thus, one would arrive quite logically at four different possible combinations:

1. *Ordinary surgery,* i.e., real surgery performed on a real organ (like the brain).
2. *Psychosurgery,* i.e., real surgery performed on an imaginary organ (like the mind).
3. *Psychic surgery,* i.e., imaginary surgery performed on a real organ (like the brain).
4. *"Psychic psychosurgery,"* i.e., imaginary surgery performed on an imaginary organ (like the mind).

The first and last of these therapies are "pure," i.e., they are based on matching concepts of theory and practice and thus are logically consistent. "Psychic psychosurgery" is, of course, nothing more than a ceremony, a purely magic ritual, and as such it is out of place in a scientific civilization. It may well have existed in one form or another among ancient or "primitive" peoples, but it is of no practical significance today. Ordinary surgery, which dates back thousands of years, is still recognized and has, in the meantime, been brought up to nearly miraculous standards. It is familiar to everyone and poses no conceptual problems. Truly problematical are only the second and third of the above categories, because they are logically "impure." Fortunately, in our present culture "psychic surgery" is easily dismissed as fraudulent and illegal, but "psychosurgery" is another matter. We know, for example, about the Stone Age custom of trephining, i.e., the practice of cutting holes in someone's skull and thereby allowing evil spirits to escape from the brain. Thus, we know that, as soon as even the most primitive tools (sharpened stones) had become available to man, he used real surgery in the hope of influencing imaginary forces. This ancient hope has persisted and is, in fact, being strengthened today by the continued refinement of surgical tools and techniques. The belief in spirits may have waned, but some modern surgeons remain convinced that the right knife or electrode inserted in the right place inside their patient's skull will control his "psyche."

Indeed, the results of "psychosurgery" are often dramatic enough: Formerly violent patients became docile, sexually aggressive patients lose all interest in sex, etc. However, this is sometimes also true of other forms of physical mutilation, such as castration, which no one has yet dared to call psychosurgery. Many critical observers are therefore unimpressed and demand more "honesty in advertising" and better theoretical justifications. The most serious objections to the practice, however, are based on the fact that it has often been used on unwilling and defenseless patients, such as prisoners and inmates of mental hospitals, some of whom should never have been found guilty or sick in the first place. Especially in the last few years the public outcry against "psychosurgery" has grown so strong that its practitioners have become more cautious, and the number of operations has drastically declined, at least in the United States.

Another important reason for this change has been the development of new "psychoactive" drugs which are now increasingly being used to treat violent, restless, depressed, and schizophrenic patients. People with sexual problems can also be "chemically castrated" by drugs which lower the body's production of testosterone and thus may reduce a person's sexual desire. Unlike a surgical castration, however, this chemical castration is not permanent, but is easily reversed by giving up the drug. In short, today various human behaviors can be provoked, stopped, changed, or revived by pills and injections alone. However, as in the case of "psychosurgery," it is not scientifically correct to say that these interventions act upon the mind, since they clearly act upon the body. The resulting bodily changes then produce a change in behavior. As a matter of fact, both the so-called psychoactive drugs and psychosurgery have led many psychiatrists away from their preoccupation with the "psyche" and refocused their attention on the body. After all, if a disease can be cured by physical treatments, such as surgery and drug ingestion, it may very well be nothing more than a physical disease. Why drag such an elusive concept as "mind" into it? Thus, the old belief in the purely physical causes of all "mental" illness has surfaced again and may well be confirmed in the future. In any case, some of the most critical modern psychiatrists advocate a new emphasis on strictly medical, or rather biological research. At the same time, they have also become very humble about what they can do in regard to moral problems and social issues.

This new-found humility is further reflected in the more recent general concept of illness itself. It is no longer assumed that there is such a thing as a definite, fixed state of health which is sometimes replaced with an equally definite state of illness. Instead, it is now being realized that human beings have to adapt and change throughout their lives and that, by definition, these adaptations and changes give no cause for concern as long as they do not impair normal (i.e., the usual) functioning. By the same token, to the degree that physical and psychological functions do become impaired, i.e., to the degree that the normal continued changes become maladaptive, they might become subject to medical intervention. In this view, health and illness are not clear-cut alternatives or irreconcilable opposites, but rather parts of the life process, and they lie on a continuum.

All of this means that in medicine, just as in any other scientifically based enterprise, there is no room for dogmatism. Especially in the psychological realm the decision of what is or is not maladaptive depends on a great number of individual and social factors which have to be considered in their totality. Furthermore, those who endeavor to offer someone their diagnosis and treatment must not forget to take their own value assumptions into account. Finally, past medical and psychiatric abuses have made it clear even to the average layman that he cannot simply suspend his own judgment when he enters therapy. He also knows that, in spite of certain exaggerated earlier claims, not all of his problems have a medical solution.

Critique of the Medical Model
As we have seen, the development of a concept of "mental illness" enabled medical science to arrive at four different possible kinds of diagnosis: A person could turn out to be

1. healthy in body and healthy in mind,
2. sick in body and healthy in mind
3. sick in body and sick in mind, and
4. healthy in body and sick in mind.

In the first instance no medical treatment was needed. In the second instance a "body doctor" was required. In the third instance this "body doctor" had to be helped by a "mind doctor," and in the last instance only a "mind doctor" could possibly do any good.

This situation was reflected in the increasing specialization of medicine. Psychiatry or "mindhealing" emerged as a separate branch, although its practitioners still received a regular medical training. Thus, they learned to treat not only physical, but also mental illness and became, in fact, "super-doctors" with more skills and more authority than their traditional colleagues. On the other hand, eventually there also appeared various nonmedical "psychotherapists" who were unqualified to treat the body and who treated only the mind. Something of a middle position came to be occupied by the followers of "psychosomatic medicine" (from Greek *psyche:* soul or mind and *soma:* body) which considered illness in both its mental and physical aspects.

A corresponding division also appears in the Diagnostic and Statistical Manual (DSM) of the American Psychiatric Association. Originally based on Kraepelin's system of mental disorders, it has been modernized several times, but it still carries the old implications. The most recent edition of 1968 lists six major categories of abnormal behavior. The first two of these ("Mental Retardation" and "Organic Brain Syndromes") refer to physical problems. The following three categories ("Psychoses Not Attributed to Physical Conditions," "Neuroses," and "Personality Disorders") describe purely mental problems. The final category ("Psychophysiological Disorders") contains "mixed" conditions that have both mental and physical aspects.

It should be pointed out, however, that this classification system has often been criticized even by psychiatrists themselves as arbitrary, heterogenous, unreliable, and invalid. For instance, "psychoses" constitute not only a major category of their own, but also appear as a subcategory of "organic brain syndromes." Disorders such as "neuroses" are defined largely on the basis of psychoanalytic assumptions and thus belong to a different theoretical framework from the other categories. Finally, the category "personality disorders" lists such peculiar subcategories as "sexual deviation," "alcoholism," and "drug dependence." Leaving aside the question of whether alcoholism is not itself a form of drug dependence, one has to ask oneself what scientific information any of these terms really contain. Even if one assumes that sexual deviation and drug dependence indicate some illness (and this is a highly questionable assumption) the classifications themselves do not tell us very much about it. It is rather as if ordinary doctors decided to use diagnoses such as "weakness," "fatigue," "fever," "cough," or "headache." All of these complaints can have a thousand different causes, and so can each of the so-called personality disorders. Furthermore, it is hard to see how they are different from the neuroses.

The most serious criticism of the diagnostic manual, however, asserts that some of its categories are pseudo-scientific, i.e., that they are nothing more than moral prejudices in "objective" disguise. This suspicion is nourished by the history of psychiatry which, in earlier times, had claimed the existence of such diseases as "masturbatory insanity," "pathological mendacity," and "vagabondage." Indeed, until 1973 American psychiatrists officially also regarded homosexuality as a disease. They finally dropped this label only under increasing pressure from gay liberation groups. Thus, as some of them humorously observed, a simple stroke of the pen instantly and miraculously cured hundreds of millions of "patients" all over the world—the greatest mass cure in medical history.

At any rate, experience has shown that a psychiatric diagnosis can be more than a "neutral" medical statement. It often has immediate, and sometimes far-reaching social consequences. People who have been labeled "mentally ill" may be subject to forced commitment to an institution, forced treatment, and all sorts of other drastic interventions. This is particularly true of those who have been so labeled because of their sexual behavior. Their "illness" may well be used as a pretext for isolating, restraining, denigrating, and punishing them. The question of whether they are really ill or not is therefore beside the point. The only important question is what social or moral significance we attach to their "symptoms." A limping, asthmatic, cross-eyed, or near sighted man is certainly abnormal and sick, yet we leave him alone and respect his rights as a person. Even if he should become fatally ill, we would never cure him against his wishes. In contrast, a harmless "sexual deviate" may or may not be sick, yet we insist that he change his behavior and treat him as an inferior human being. It seems, therefore, that sexual deviation as well as some other examples of "mental illness" are essentially moral rather than medical problems.

At least this is the position taken by some recent critics of the medical model of abnormal behavior. In America the most articulate of these critics have been the sociologists Erving Goffman and Thomas J. Scheff and the psychiatrist Thomas S. Szasz.

Goffman, in 1959, wrote an influential essay on "The Moral Career of the Mental Patient" (later reprinted in his book *Asylums*) which examined the human experience of being hospitalized and treated for "mental illness." This experience turned out to be one of humiliation and betrayal. The so-called therapeutic measures revealed themselves as part of a moral ritual by which society stigmatized some of its members.

The same view was elaborated a few years later by Scheff in his book *Being Mentally Ill* (1966). He described chronic mental illness as a social role, the result of scapegoating and victimization. It was, in fact, nothing more than a special label applied to certain deviants and mainly used to ostracize them or to deny them their civil rights. The whole exercise served only the purpose of controlling "residual rule-breakers." The medical jargon and paraphernalia of psychiatry were means of deception which helped to ease the conscience of the community.

However, perhaps the most scathing attack on the medical model of deviance came from inside the psychiatric profession itself. Szasz, in his books *The Myth of Mental Illness* (1961) and *The Manufacture of Madness* (1970), called mental illness a myth and likened the treatment of mental patients by institutional psychiatry to that of witches by the Inquisition. For him, the belief in mental illness is just as false and dangerous as the belief in witchcraft and leads to the same excesses. Psychiatrists do not deal with mental illness and its treatment, but with "personal, social, and ethical problems in living." By mistaking these problems for diseases, and thus assigning the blame for antisocial behavior to some external force, we undermine the principle of personal responsibility and foster the illusion that social conflicts can be solved by medical science.

These and other calls for a critical reassessment have, in the meantime, found a remarkable echo not only among the general public, but also in the therapeutic and helping professions. Even many conservative psychiatrists who rejected the main thrust of the criticism had to admit that it contained enough truth to make them uncomfortable. They were forced to enlarge their field of vision and to recognize, perhaps for the first time, the social dimensions of their professional activity. Instead of concentrating only on the "patient" and his "illness," they had to examine their own role as agents of social control. Consequently, they became more cautious in their pronouncements and more tolerant of deviant behavior.

Especially deviant sexual behavior is now treated much more leniently in psychiatric circles than only a few decades ago. After all, as Kinsey's statistics and numerous other recent surveys have shown, such behavior is far more common than had previously been suspected. Indeed, many forms of alleged sexual deviance have been shown to be "normal" and not deviant at all. If our criminal laws do not yet always reflect this insight it is no longer the fault of psychiatrists who today are often among the most ardent advocates of reform.

Summing up, we can say that those who still use the medical model of deviance now do so with much more sophistication. However, some others (including some certified psychiatrists) have turned to new, nonmedical models in their own practice.

New Models

Earlier in this chapter, we discussed the nonmedical character of psychoanalysis, and we have mentioned Sigmund Freud's hope that it would not be tied exclusively to medical practice. Indeed, any neutral description of the psychoanalytic process reveals that it rests on a learning model of behavior. The analysand (i.e., the person to be analyzed) tries to recall long-forgotten experiences with the help of free association and the recollection of current dreams. His verbal reports are scrutinized by the analyst who looks for certain clues, recurrent themes, or patterns which might give a hint at some repressed early traumatic experience. As soon as this experience or series of experiences have been identified and made conscious, the analysand has regained his chance to deal with them in a rational and appropriate fashion. In short, the psychoanalytic method is essentially a historical or, more specifically, an autobiographical method. The troubled person learns from his own life history that he once learned a "wrong" lesson. This insight then sets him free to profit from future lessons that life might have in store for him.

Psychoanalysis has long been popular in the United States and Europe and has won many prominent followers, some of whom, like Marie Bonaparte and Erik Erikson, for example, have even employed its techniques to study famous historical personalities, such as Edgar Allan Poe and Martin Luther. (Freud himself had written a study of Leonardo da Vinci.) Thus, the nonmedical use of psychoanalysis is well recognized. By the same token, however, many men and women who once might have asked for the services of a psychoanalyst now seek still other nonmedical treatments, such as yoga, meditation, biofeedback, etc. In spite of their differences, all of these treatments have one thing in common: They do not make an assumption of illness and, while they may help some suffering people, they are also applicable to those who merely want to "grow" or increase their personal potential.

Another increasingly popular treatment is known as "behavior modification." It is also based on a learning model of human behavior and employs various techniques of reward and punishment to reinforce behavior which is acceptable while decreasing that which is unacceptable. Again, no assumption of illness is made. Instead, the procedure is entirely pragmatic: "Faulty learning" is corrected without any far-reaching metaphysical speculations. Not surprisingly, however, this uncritical approach has upset many libertarians who have found the techniques of punishment used in the process to be rather repulsive. Moreover, in its early years, "behavior modification" was sometimes used to modify behavior that would better have been left alone. Thus, homosexuals, for example, were subjected to some very bizarre and revolting treatments designed to turn them into heterosexuals. (So far, the reverse has not been tried.) Such abuses have, in the meantime led to justified public outrage and to greater professional caution. There is no doubt, however, that under strict guidelines and in the hands of sensible practitioners, behavior modification can still do a great deal of good.

Still other nonmedical models of deviance have been proposed in recent years. Thomas S. Szasz, for example, who declared mental illness to be a myth, has suggested a "rule-following model" or "game model" of human behavior and misbehavior. According to this suggestion, people slowly learn the rules of the many different games of life, and they also learn to understand which games have priority in which situations. Conflicts arise when people disagree about certain rules, change the rules in the middle of the game, or refuse to learn new rules for new games. Some of these conflicts are external and manifest themselves in social disputes, struggles, or revolutions; others are internal and distort the "normal" individual behavior. These distortions are then often mistaken for "mental illness" when, in fact, they are simply problems in living—a failure to cope successfully with a difficult situation. In other cases, people are called mentally ill in order to remove them from a social game in which they have become obnoxious to others.

Needless to say, Szasz's model is easily reconciled with the "labeling model" used by such writers as Goffman and Scheff. As we have repeatedly mentioned, deviance of any kind is best understood as a label attached to rule breakers by a conforming majority. Any study or treatment of deviance therefore has to take the whole social context into account. Those who mistake deviance (including "mental illness") for an individual problem are shortsighted. Certainly, according to this model, it is not a medical problem.

Fortunately for our discussion, most currently popular models of deviance have been examined in depth by two defenders of psychiatry, Miriam Siegler and Humphry Osmond, in a very illuminating study entitled *Models of Madness, Models of Medicine* (1974). By comparing different models of madness, drug addiction, and alcoholism, they were able to demonstrate the relative advantages, limits, and implications of each model and thus to end some of the present professional confusion. However, the importance of their study does not end there. While they themselves made no attempt in this direction, their method can also easily be applied to the problem of sexual deviance. It seems appropriate, therefore, to include a simplified adaptation of one of their charts in the present text. Since it is self-explanatory, it does not require any additional comment. (See chart on opposite page.)

As already mentioned, however, Siegler and Osmond are far from abandoning the medical model. On the contrary, they believe it to have unique advantages and, indeed, great potential for the future. Of course, they demand a heightened critical consciousness on the part of their colleagues as well as some therapeutic restraint. Psychiatrists must realize that not everyone who seeks their help or is referred to them is mentally ill. Indeed, "screening out" such alleged patients is one of their professional duties. In many such cases, certain nonmedical treatments offer the best hope and should be suggested. Nevertheless, there remains a sufficient number of individual and social problems which can be solved with the help of a medically oriented psychiatry. As a matter of fact, it seems that in the past many psychiatrists have failed because they did not have enough faith in the medical model and did not adhere to it strictly enough. Again, sexual deviance is an interesting case in point.

We had seen earlier that, in Victorian times, alleged mental patients suffering from "masturbatory insanity," "nymphomania," or "homosexuality" had often been treated as both sick and immoral even by their own doctors. However, in the medical model, properly understood, there is no room for moral blame. Quite the opposite: It is the unique authority of a doctor to declare someone sick and thus to absolve him from all responsibility for his condition. In the strict sense, therefore, and by definition, a patient is not a deviant. He may deviate from accepted standards, but he does so with official permission, because as a sick person, he "cannot help it." This means that a psychiatrist, as a doctor, has the power to free sexual nonconformists from their morally negative deviant role and to assign them to the morally neutral sick role. This decision alone can save them from harassment and persecution. By the same token, a psychiatrist who fails to arrive at a clear decision undermines the very foundations of his profession. Any ambivalence, any mixing of medical with moral approaches is detrimental not only to the patients, but also to the practice of psychiatry itself. Indeed, the fact that for so long "mental patients" could be perceived and treated as deviants points to this historical failure of psychiatrists.

On the other hand, it is understandable why people should find it difficult to suspend their moral judgment in the face of "abnormal" sexual behavior.

MODELS OF SEXUAL DEVIANCE*

	RELIGIOUS MODEL	LEGAL MODEL	MEDICAL MODEL	PSYCHOANALYTIC MODEL	LABELING MODEL
CAUSE OF DEVIANCE	Demonic possession or temptation by the devil. Sinfulness	The deviant's "criminal character"	Not always known, but some natural cause (illness) assumed	Individual, largely unconscious life experiences. Arrested or impaired psychosexual development	Labeling by those who cannot tolerate differences
MEANING OF DEVIANT BEHAVIOR	Sin, heresy. Deviant is possessed or evil	Crime	Symptomatic of illness	Symbolic acting-out of unconscious and unresolved childhood conflicts	Determined by those who label the deviant. Today mostly seen as criminal or sick
FORM OF INTERVENTION	Exorcism, repentance, confession	Punishment, sometimes also "rehabilitation"	Medical treatment. Drugs, electroshock, psychosurgery, etc.	Psychoanalysis. Deviant becomes conscious of hidden conflict by means of free association, interpretation of dreams, etc.	Criminal punishment or psychiatric treatment, often involuntary
INTERVENING AUTHORITY	Priest or other religious authority. Sometimes chosen by deviant, sometimes by society	Police, judge, correctional officer. Always chosen by society	Physician or psychiatrist. Sometimes chosen by deviant, usually by society	Analyst. Always chosen by deviant	Today usually a judge or psychiatrist Chosen by those who label the deviant.
RIGHTS AND DUTIES OF DEVIANT	Right to receive exorcism. Duty to atone for sins	Right to be presumed innocent until proven guilty. Duty to accept punishment and to "pay his debt to society"	Right to be considered sick, not evil. Duty to try to get well and to cooperate with doctors	Right to have his behavior interpreted as symbolic, not judged morally. Duty to cooperate with analyst	No rights. No duties
RIGHTS AND DUTIES OF SOCIETY	Right to condemn and isolate sinners. Duty to help them if they repent	Right to protect itself against criminals. Duty to punish them	Right to be protected from sick people who are dangerous. Duty to provide medical treatment for them	No rights. Duty to see deviant behavior as indication of emotional disturbance	Right to control socially harmful deviants. Duty to leave all other deviants alone
GOAL OF MODEL	To save the soul from eternal damnation	To control crime	To cure illness. To help deviant avoid blame by treating him as a medical patient	To resolve deviant's unconscious conflicts	For the intolerant: To maintain the status quo by labeling and "correcting" deviants. For the tolerant: To liberate the oppressed

* This chart is adapted from a similar one used by M. Siegler and H. Osmond in *Models of Madness, Models of Medicine*, N.Y., N.Y., 1974, pp. 16-18.

First of all, in our culture morality and sexual conformity have become nearly synonymous. Furthermore, and most importantly, the general public well realizes that a psychiatric diagnosis is often a "cop-out," i.e., a professional stratagem which helps both doctor and "patient" to avoid facing certain moral issues. Finally, we must remember that many sexual nonconformists are justified in refusing the sick role that is being thrust upon them by well-meaning, but sexually prejudiced doctors. Thus, to return to our examples, masturbators, "nymphomaniacs," and "homosexuals" have successfully fought not only against the pernicious labels of sin and crime, but also against the more benign label of sickness.

Observations such as these tend to support the critics of the medical model who insist on seeing the problem in moral terms, although their morality may well be quite different from the traditional one. Ultimately, therefore, we must hope for the open-minded further study of human sexuality, a continued thorough discussion between all concerned parties, and cooperation on all sides. Difficult as it is, a general commitment to reason still offers the best hope for dealing with nonconformity.

Reference and Recommended Reading

Alexander, Franz G., and Selesnick, Sheldon. *The History of Psychiatry: An Evaluation of Psychiatric Thought and Practice from Prehistoric Times to the Present.* New York: Harper & Row, 1966 (cloth); NAL, 1974 (paper).

Becker, Howard S. *Outsiders: Studies in the Sociology of Deviance.* New York: The Free Press, 1963.

Barnett, Walter. *Sexual Freedom and the Constitution: An Inquiry into the Constitutionality of Repressive Sex Laws.* Albuquerque: University of New Mexico Press, 1973.

Foucault, Michel. *Madness and Civilization: A History of Insanity in the Age of Reason.* New York: Random, 1965 (cloth); Random Vintage, 1973 (paper).

Goffman, Erving. *Asylums: Essays on the Social Situation of Mental Patients and Other Inmates.* Garden City, N.Y.: Doubleday Anchor, 1961.

Kittrie, Nicholas N. *The Right to Be Different: Deviance and Enforced Therapy.* Baltimore, Md.: Penguin, 1973.

Sagarin, Edward. *Deviants and Deviance: An Introduction to the Study of Disvalued People and Behavior.* New York: Praeger, 1975.

Scheff, Thomas J. *Being Mentally Ill: A Sociological Theory.* Chicago: Aldine, 1966.

Schur, Edwin M. *Labeling Deviant Behavior: Its Sociological Functions.* New York: Harper & Row, 1971 (paper).

Schur, Edwin M., and Bedau, Hugo A. *Victimless Crimes: Two Sides of a Controversy.* Englewood Cliffs, N.J.: Prentice-Hall, 1974.

Siegler, Miriam, and Osmond, Humphry. *Models of Madness, Models of Medicine.* New York: Macmillan, 1974 (cloth); Harper & Row, 1976 (paper).

Szasz, Thomas S. *The Manufacture of Madness: A Comparative Study of the Inquisition and the Mental Health Movement.* New York: Harper & Row, 1970.

———. *The Myth of Mental Illness: Foundations of a Theory of Personal Conduct,* rev. ed. New York: Harper & Row, 1974 (paper and cloth).

Zilboorg, Gregory, and Henry, George W. *A History of Medical Psychology.* New York: Norton, 1941.

11. MARRIAGE AND THE FAMILY

Most young Americans today look forward to the time when they can "get married and start a family." In other words, they hope to find a person of the other sex who will make them happy for life and with whom they can share the joys of parenthood in a house or apartment of their own.

All of these expectations seem so natural, simple, and well justified, that it may be hard to believe that young people of other times and other cultures have often felt quite differently. However, as we can learn from historians and anthropologists, our own present forms of marriage and family are relatively new and by no means universal. For example, in some non-Western societies people may marry a person of the same sex or more than one partner of the opposite sex, the marriage may be quite unrelated to happiness, love, sexual intercourse, or procreation, it may not lead to establishing a new household, and it may, from the very beginning, be planned only as a temporary arrangement.

By the same token, in some societies of the past, a family did not consist only of parents and their children, but included a number of other close and distant relatives as well as servants, friends, and permanent guests. On the other hand, sometimes the children's natural father or mother was excluded from the family and remained an unrecognized "outsider." Indeed, in some cases the "official" husbands or wives were themselves children and younger than their legal offspring.

These few observations may suffice to show that it makes little sense to talk about marriage and family in the abstract, as if they had the same meaning for everyone. There are simply too many different forms of marriage and too many different types of family in the world. In short, there are too many exceptions for any rule that we might set up. Marriage and family are actually very difficult to define and even more difficult to explain.

Nevertheless, scholars have often tried to explain marriage and family by pointing to some of their obvious functions. After all, it is a biological fact that sexual intercourse between men and women can produce children, and that these children need adult care and protection for many years before they can fend for themselves. Thus, it has been suggested that, with all of their possible variations, marriage and family are natural and inevitable institutions which provide for the proper raising of children, i.e., ultimately for the survival of the human species. Indeed, the two institutions have been found to serve many additional useful functions, such as providing sexual satisfaction and companionship for the spouses and economic cooperation between all family members. The larger community has also been said to profit from the arrangement, since marriage tends to restrict, regulate, and refine human sexual behavior which might otherwise become promiscuous and barbaric. By the same token, a stable family life has often been seen as the best guarantee of social peace.

Yet, upon closer examination, it becomes clear that all of these worthy goals can also be accomplished without marriages and families. Children do not have to depend on their parents, but can very well be raised by other adults in professional nurseries, daycare centers, schools, and similar institutions. Sexual satisfaction and companionship can be found outside of marriage, and economic cooperation can be achieved in all sorts of ways between all sorts of people. Sexual behavior can be regulated by religious and secular authorities, and social peace can be preserved even in societies which downgrade the family as an institution and subject everyone directly to some totalitarian control.

On the other hand, as already hinted above, in some parts of the globe the institution of marriage has shown such puzzling features that, for a very long time, modern Western observers could not make sense out of them. For example, the theory that marriage always ensures the raising of children by their own parents is contradicted in certain societies by some very strange rules of determining "fatherhood." Thus, among the biblical Israelites who practiced the levirate (i.e., a man's compulsory marriage to his brother's widow), a dead man became the father of children conceived by his widow and his brother. Similarly, among the Nayar in Southern India, a young girl was briefly married to a man who never had a chance to impregnate her, but nevertheless later became the legitimate father of all her children. Even more bizarre: Among the Nuer in Southern Sudan, a woman could marry another woman and be considered the father of that woman's children by some male outsider. Furthermore, the belief that sexual intercourse is the basis or object of marriage loses conviction when one considers the example of the Mojave Indians who allowed adult men to marry baby girls. Or, to give one final illustration, among the Siberian Chukchee, a woman who became pregnant by an authorized lover might marry not him, but a baby husband not older than her own child, and she might, in fact, nurse both of them together at her breast.

Curiously enough, if one looks for an explanation of these customs, one eventually finds that, in spite of their dissimilarities, they have one common denominator, and that it is an economic one. That is to say, in all of the above cases, marriage has little to do with biological parenthood or sexual partnership, but instead is concerned with social legitimacy, official family lines, property rights, and laws of inheritance. In short, it is a method for the orderly transmission and conservation of wealth and status. Its particular form depends on the political organization of each society. This observation, in turn, has prompted some scholars to describe the origin and "true" basis of marriage as economic. Friedrich Engels's study *The Origin of the Family, Private Property and the State*, written in the 1880s, is perhaps the best known example of this approach.

However, while economic factors have undoubtedly played an important role in the development of marriage and family, they cannot explain everything about them. For instance, if only economic considerations were involved, same-sex marriages would long have been common all over the world. Instead, marital partners have nearly always been of different sex. And another point deserves to be made: While marriage usually involves a division of labor between the sexes, one can never predict with certainty how it will work out in practice. What one society calls "men's work," is "women's work" in another and vice versa. It is not true that all wives and mothers everywhere spend their lives as homemakers caring for their children, or that all husbands and fathers work outside the home as providers. Modern anthropologists have found cultures in which these roles were reversed.

Under the circumstances, we are forced to search for still other explanations, and thus some contemporary scholars have suggested that we look beyond the relationships between husband and wife or parents and children. There seems to be more to marriage than that. Indeed, it appears that any such narrow individual concerns are irrelevant to the question. The French anthropologist Claude Lévi-Strauss, for example, cites an interesting clue provided by the natives of New Guinea who state that "the purpose of getting married is not so much to obtain a wife, but to secure brothers-in-law." Accordingly, Lévi-Strauss describes husband and wife as pawns in a larger social game played by their two respective families who use the marriage for the mutual acquisition of in-laws. This means that we are actually dealing with a paradox: Although it is true that marriages produce families, it is also true that families produce marriages as a means of establishing alliances between each other. Such ever-enlarging alliances are the preconditions of civilization. Social progress would have been impossible if people had not found a way of affiliating themselves systematically with other people beyond their immediate blood kin. Fortunately, however, they found it by creating the incest taboo which forced everyone to marry ourside his own family. Thus, families were linked up to form larger groups, and the survival of the human race was assured. (For further details see Lévi-Strauss, "The Family," in the anthology by A.S. and J.H. Skolnick under "Reference and Recommended Reading" below. The essay had appeared earlier in *Man, Culture, and Society,* edited by H.L. Shapiro, New York: 1956.)

It should be pointed out that Lévi-Strauss's explanation of the incest taboo is not considered definitive by everyone. On the other hand, his conclusion about the place of the family in society seems indisputable: The small family of parents and children is not the natural elementary component, cornerstone, or building block of society, as is so often thoughtlessly assumed. In fact, a society does not consist of families any more than it consists of individuals. The old model of a society, state, or nation being made up of people or groups of people is wrong. Societies, states, or nations are not composed of people, but of relationships, and these relationships cannot be understood by simply adding up numbers. With regard to the family, the relationship of those within it to the rest of society is obviously far from static. Families are necessary, but they are not meant to be permanent. On the contrary, society survives precisely because they are continuously being formed, broken up, and formed again by marriages. Adults live with children in a temporary family unit only to give them away in marriage so that they may found their own temporary family units, and so on. Thus, every marriage breaks up the two families of bridegroom and bride while at the same time forging a bond between them and establishing a third, entirely new family. The point of the whole enterprise, however, is the continued transference, realignment, and exchange of social obligations. As Lévi-Strauss summarizes it, quoting the Bible: " 'You will leave your father and mother' provides the iron rule for the establishment and functioning of any society."

It is interesting to note, however, that many past and present thinkers have wanted to see this "iron rule" applied much more strictly than is being suggested by Lévi-Strauss. That is to say, throughout history utopian philosophers from Plato to K'ang Yu-wei have wanted to see marriage and family abolished altogether. Children should therefore be taken away from their fathers and mothers from their day of birth. For example, in Plato's *Republic* wives and children were to be held in common, so that "no parent would know his own child, nor any child his own parent." As a result, all family feelings would be transferred to the whole community. In K'ang Yu-wei's *Book of the Great Equality* (1935), children were to be raised in public institutions, because families were an obstacle to the "perfection of human nature." Similar sentiments have been expressed by certain religious leaders. Indeed, it is striking how many of those who have tried to save or improve mankind have found their efforts obstructed by marital bonds and family loyalties. Thus, as we can learn from the Bible, Jesus himself was quite indifferent to marriage and family as social institutions. He wandered about homeless, remained unmarried, left his own relatives behind, and never showed them any special consideration (Matthew 12; 46–50). When some young men wanted to become his followers, he asked them to ignore their families and to devote themselves entirely to the cause. He even told one of them not to waste time with his father's funeral, but to "go and preach the kingdom of God" (Luke 9; 59–60). Accordingly, the early Christians generally put little emphasis on family relationships and family life. The concept of a close "Christian family" and the idyllic image of the "Holy Family" in Nazareth are products of later historical periods.

There is, of course, little doubt that families can hold an individual down and that they can frustrate ambition, stifle initiative, hamper personal growth, or sabotage noble causes. Occasionally, they can even be downright destructive. It is also clear that entrenched family systems often promote and perpetuate inequality. In short, the family is a very conservative institution, and it usually serves the prevailing social order, whatever it happens to be. By the same token, revolutionaries, reformers, and social visionaries often lose patience with it. Family ties tend to get in the way of sudden social change, even if it is meant to be for the better.

On the other hand, any larger social change sooner or later also affects the family. This fact is illustrated today by the well-publicized "crisis" of marriage and family in our own society. We can now often hear it said that the technological and political changes of our recent history have led to a "breakdown" of the family, and that this, in turn, will eventually lead to the breakdown of society itself. However, these dour predictions do not have to come true and may even rest on false assumptions. As we have mentioned earlier, the family and society do not stand in a static relationship to each other, but exist in a state of dynamic tension, indeed, almost confrontation, in a creative equilibrium subject to constant readjustment. Thus, we may at present simply be going through another phase in which the demands of family and society are being forced to find a new balance.

The following pages are devoted to a more detailed discussion of these and other issues. For the sake of clarity, marriage and family are examined in separate sections. Both of these sections, however, offer some historical and cross-cultural observations and point to future possibilities.

FORMS AND MEANINGS OF MARRIAGE

The English words "marriage" (from Latin *maritus:* husband) and "matrimony" (from Latin *mater:* mother) do not give us any clue as to the origin and meaning of the phenomenon we are trying to discuss here. The same is, of course, also true for similar terms with Latin roots in other European languages. More enlightening is the Germanic word "wedlock" (from Old English *wedlāc:* pledge) which suggests that some sort of promise or contract, i.e., a special relationship between people is involved. Indeed, the best characterization of this relationship is perhaps provided by the German word *Ehe* (from Old High German *êwa:* law).

At any rate, when we compare marriages in different societies and different historical periods, we soon discover that marital partners everywhere have very definite duties toward each other. These duties may not always be spelled out in detail, but they are well understood and readily enforced in each case. Therefore, if we had to look for a common denominator in all the various forms of marriage known to mankind, we might very well find it in the element of mutual obligation. Naturally, this obligation itself can appear in many different forms. It may spring from an informal silent agreement, or it may be loudly proclaimed in a popular celebration. It may extend well beyond the couple to their offspring, to the families on both sides, and even to the entire community. It may be considered permanent, or it may end by mutual agreement or unilateral action. None of this matters here: Some officially recognized mutual obligation exists as long as the partners are married. Where men and women make love and have children without it we do not speak of a marriage, but of an affair, a dalliance, a romance, or a state of cohabitation.

As we can see, marriage is a very special phenomenon which involves more than housekeeping, sexual intercourse, and procreation. These "natural" human activities do not, by themselves, make a marriage. Its real meaning derives instead from social sanctions and expectations. Indeed, as such expectations change from one society to another, marriage is bound to change with them. Therefore, it is not very helpful to talk about marriage in generalities. It seems much more promising to list and describe the possible forms and functions of marriage, and for our present limited purpose it is perhaps best if we begin with a simple classification.

Traditionally, scholars have distinguished between four basic types of marriage:

1. **Monogamy** (i.e., one husband having one wife),
2. **polygyny** (i.e., one husband having several wives),
3. **polyandry** (i.e., several husbands having one wife),   } **polygamy**
4. **group marriage** (i.e., several husbands having several wives).

Monogamy is the prevalent form of marriage today. Polygyny and polyandry (collectively called polygamy) were once practiced in various parts of the world, but now seem to be on the decline. Group marriage has always been rare.

In Victorian times it was often believed that the four basic types of marriage were representative of different stages of human evolution. Thus, the earliest human beings had supposedly lived in a state of indiscriminate promiscuity until they established some form of group marriage. On the next stage of civilization they then entered a matriarchal phase characterized by polyandry. This, in turn, was followed by the patriarchal phase in which polygyny became dominant, and finally monogamy emerged as the crowning achievement of human progress. So far, this beguiling theory has not been confirmed, however. On the contrary, we have learned in the meantime that all four types of marriage have existed since earliest times and under all sorts of technological and economic conditions. Some very "primitive" peoples have always practiced monogamy, while some "civilized" peoples have been and still are polygamous. Moreover, we now understand that each of the four basic types of marriage can appear in several variations. For example, there is quite a difference between monogamy as a lifelong sacramental union and monogamy as a temporary civil contract. Polygyny can mean very different things under different circumstances, such as when a man takes a concubine, or when he marries his brother's widow, or when all his wives are sisters and live under his roof, or when they come from different families and maintain their own separate households. Polyandry can mean that a woman marries several brothers, of whom only the oldest is the official father of her children, or it can mean that she marries several unrelated men who all enjoy equal rights. Group marriage can be the accidental outgrowth of polygamous practices or a conscious "scientific" experiment.

Still, today there is little doubt that monogamy in one variation or another has always been the most common type of marriage. Both group marriage and polyandry have been found only in very few cultures, and polygyny, although permitted in many societies, has almost always been restricted to the wealthier classes. After all, it has never been cheap to purchase and then support more than one wife. Sometimes, of course, wives earned more than their keep as laborers, but even in that case their husband had to be powerful and influential, or he could not have created such an advantage for himself. The other men would have insisted on the same privilege, and this could not have been granted, because "naturally" there is only about one woman for every man. The biological balance between males and females is nearly even, and therefore polygamy can flourish only under exceptional conditions. Such conditions may result from a custom of female infanticide, from frequent wars, in which many men are killed, or from political and religious beliefs that accord a few persons some special prestige. However, where conditions are "normal," and where people are given a fairly equal chance, they tend to favor monogamy.

In view of this fact, one might perhaps call monogamy the "natural" form of marriage, although one should not conclude that everyone will always be happy with it, or that it is practical in every situation. Indeed, even in societies which insist on the strictest monogamy there is often an unofficial toleration of premarital and extramarital intercourse, such as in prostitution, adultery, and homosexual contact. Other societies are still more tolerant and establish monogamy as a flexible or "open" institution from the very start. In addition, they may also permit ready divorces in case of marital failure. At any rate, experience seems to show that one cannot impose a single form of monogamy, or even a single type of marriage on all men and women everywhere. One can, of course, proclaim an ideal, but in real life one has to allow for some improvisation and experimentation.

Nevertheless, even where husbands and wives are given the greatest sexual latitude, marriage is always considered important and is clearly distinguished from nonmarital unions. That is to say, generally speaking, it hardly matters how people arrange, maintain, or modify their marriages, as long as they get married at all. The details may differ from one culture to another, but the principle is nowhere in doubt: Marriage as such is good and must be supported. It also must be proclaimed and made visible to outsiders. For instance, in certain societies married persons are permitted or obliged to dress in a more "dignified" manner than spinsters and bachelors. By the same token, the marital state often carries particular privileges and is celebrated with splendid wedding ceremonies or sumptuous nuptials. These celebrations themselves usually follow some preordained pattern and require their own kind of clothing. In short, there seems to be something special about marriage which makes it different from any other human relationship, and which calls for some public acknowledgment. All of this indicates that marriage serves more than private personal needs, and that it does not exist for the benefit of the spouses alone. Instead, an obvious social interest is involved. It is further obvious that this interest affects not only the form, but also the meaning of marriage, and that the latter can therefore be understood only if one considers both its individual and social aspects.

Of course, in everyday life we normally talk about marriage without worrying much about its precise definition or all of its possible implications. Even professionals are often deliberately vague as they try to illuminate different facets of the phenomenon. Thus, depending on the context, we can find marriage described in very different terms from very different points of view. In American law, for example, marriage may be variously defined as an institution, a status, or a contract. Accordingly, in this country today politicians praise "the institution of marriage," bureaucrats ask other people to declare their "marital status," and lawyers draw up formal "marriage contracts" for their cautious clients, spelling out certain marital rights and duties in advance.

Actually, marriage contracts are neither new nor typically American. Many societies all over the world have known written marriage agreements, if not between bride and bridegroom, then between their respective families. Indeed, in feudal times a marriage contract could seal an alliance between whole tribes or nations. At present, such motives are still formalized on a more modest scale by our own upper classes. Thus, marriage contracts are customary where the possible loss or consolidation of huge family fortunes is involved. After all, in these cases the marriage could well determine the fate not only of two, but perhaps dozens or hundreds of individuals. Still, as a rule, these contracts cover only externals, such as dowry, allowances, financial settlements, inheritance, etc. They rarely say anything about marital conduct in the proper sense and do not concern themselves with questions of intimacy. Therefore, they are in fact mere safeguards or security measures. They accompany and protect, but do not constitute marriage.

This elementary difference has not always been clearly perceived. On the contrary, the fact that marital unions may be protected or guided by contracts and even contain some contractive elements, has led some modern observers to believe that marriage itself is a contract and nothing more. This view also seems to be supported by certain customs and regulations in other cultures. For example, Islamic law explicitly defines marriage (nikāh) as "a contract for the legalization of sexual intercourse and the procreation of children." As such, it is strictly a private matter, requires no religious ceremony, and can be terminated under certain conditions. However, this definition was never meant to be exhaustive and should not be read dogmatically. After all, the custom of mut'ah marriages indicates that the procreation of children need not be essential to the contract. (For details see "Marriage in Islamic Countries.") Furthermore, since it has been possible in Islamic countries for fathers to contract compulsory marriages for their unwilling daughters, it cannot be assumed that the contracting parties are always bridegroom and bride. Similarly, in early medieval Europe, where marriage was a transfer of lordship over a woman from her father to her husband, the bride was not herself party to the contract, but rather its object. Her lot improved only under the influence of the Church, which gave marriage a religious meaning and elevated it to the status of a sacrament.

Needless to say, once marriage had been endowed with a sacramental character, it could no longer be called a contract in any sense of the word. First of all, it was now a vehicle of grace, and thus its essence lay not in any formal stipulations, but in the mutual decision of both partners which made them "one flesh" (Mark 10:8). This reduced both the influence of parents and the importance of economic considerations. As a result, for a while even secret marriages were permitted. Secondly, since the marital relationship mirrored that of Christ with his church, it could not be dissolved: "What God has joined together, let not man put asunder" (Mark 10:9). However, this latter change eventually came to be resented, and therefore the Protestant Reformation returned to the concept of marriage as a civil contract, making it once again possible for Christians to obtain a divorce. In Puritan England, John Milton called marriage a "covenant" which need not bind the parties forever.

The secularization of marriage was, of course, especially welcomed by the emerging bourgeoisie. The bourgeois lived in an increasingly sober world of commodities which were subject to sale, disposal, contract, and regulation, and thus he had less and less sympathy for mythical or supernatural notions. Finally, in the 18th century the German bourgeois philosopher Immanuel Kant felt enlightened enough to put the matter in its baldest terms when he defined marriage as "an association of two persons of different sex for the life-long mutual possession of their sexual qualities" (Rechtslehre, § 24). Much could be said about this definition, but here we can simply point out that it is obviously not universal. The references to "two" persons and a "life-long" mutual possession indicate that only a special form of Western marriage is being considered. Moreover, it should be noted that there is no mention of any contract. After all, irrevocable personal contracts are out of harmony with the modern demands for individual freedom. The lifelong possession of one human being by another is now alien to our whole system of justice. People can no longer legally sell themselves as slaves or buy someone else as a servant for life. Much less are such contracts acceptable in the case of marriage. Indeed, even in ancient Rome marital vows never to separate were invalid before the law. Therefore, the "association" mentioned by Kant must be more than just a legal agreement.

However, it should be apparent that even our contemporary, soluble marriage can never be fully described as a contract. The unique personal relationship that exists between spouses cannot be created, shaped, and maintained by written provisions, clauses, or codicils, or by signatures on some dotted line. This relationship is so intimate that no comprehensive and binding contract could possibly be devised for it, and it goes without saying that nonbinding contracts are worthless. Even simple common sense tells bridegroom and bride not to approach each other in a legalistic spirit, so as not to doom their marriage from the start. On the other hand, they also know that, once a marriage has foundered, it cannot be saved by the law.

These few observations may be sufficient to show that the subject of marriage is too complex for easy generalizations. The precise nature of the marital union itself is elusive, and its role in society varies with changing conditions. Thus, no single definition can capture all conceivable meanings of marriage or fit all of its forms. Still, we may obtain at least some limited insight, if we put the issue in some historical and cross-cultural perspective. The following pages, therefore, briefly sketch the past development and present state of marriage in Western and a few non-Western societies. A concluding section offers some speculations about the future.

HISTORY OF MARRIAGE IN WESTERN CIVILIZATION

Marriage, as we know it in our Western civilization today, has a long history with roots in several very different ancient cultures, of which the Roman, Hebrew, and Germanic are the most important. Western marriage has further been shaped by the doctrines and policies of the medieval Christian church, the demands of the Protestant Reformation, and the social impact of the Industrial Revolution.

When we look at the marriage customs of our ancestors, we discover several striking facts. For example, for the most of Western history, marriage was not a mere personal matter concerning only husband and wife, but rather the business of their two families which brought them together. Most marriages, therefore, were arranged. Moreover, the wife usually had much fewer rights than her husband and was expected to be subservient to him. To a considerable extent, marriage was also an economic arrangement. There was little room for romantic love, and even simple affection was not considered essential. Procreation and cooperation were the main marital duties.

On the other hand, it may surprise many modern couples to learn that in earlier times divorce was often easily granted. Here again, men usually had the advantage when they could simply dismiss their wives, but in many instances women could also sue for divorce. In ancient Rome couples could even divorce each other by mutual agreement, a possibility that has not yet returned to all European countries. Another notable historical fact is the nearly universal stress on the necessity of marriage and the resulting pressure on single persons to get married. This pressure was partially lifted only under the influence of Christianity which, at least for some time, found a special virtue in celibacy. Christian doctrines have, of course, also had their effects on marriage itself, and some of these will be discussed below.

Marriage in Ancient Greece and Rome

In ancient Greece marriage was seen as a fundamental social institution. Indeed, the great lawgiver Solon once contemplated making marriage compulsory, and in Athens under Pericles bachelors were excluded from certain important public positions. Sparta, while encouraging sexual relationships between men, nevertheless insisted on their marrying and producing children. Single and childless men were treated with scorn.

However, while marriage was deemed important, it was usually treated as a practical matter without much romantic significance. A father arranged the most advantageous marriage for his son and then had a contract signed before witnesses. Shortly thereafter a wedding celebration was held and the young couple (who might never have met before) was escorted to bed. All marriages were monogamous. As a rule, the bridegroom was in his thirties and the bride was a teenager. In addition to this disparity in ages there also existed an inequality in education and political rights. Women were considered inferior to men and remained confined to the home. Their main function as wives was to produce children and to manage the household while their husbands tended to public affairs. For their erotic needs, men often turned to prostitutes and concubines. As Demosthenes, the orator, explained it: "We have prostitutes for our pleasure, concubines for our health, and wives to bear us lawful offspring." Many men also cultivated intense emotional and sexual relationships with male adolescents (paiderastia). The legal inequality of the sexes was further reflected in the divorce regulations. It was always easier for a husband to divorce his wife than vice versa. However, since a divorced woman could take her dowry back with her, men normally asked for a divorce only in cases of female adultery and infertility.

The marriage laws and customs of ancient Rome are not easily summarized, because they were rather varied and underwent significant changes in the course of time. Still, without simplifying the issue too much, one may say that marriage and divorce were always personal, civil agreements between the participants and did not need the stamp of governmental or religious approval. Early in Roman history, a husband had considerable power over his wife and children, whom he could punish, sell, or even kill as he saw fit. However, eventually women came to enjoy a better legal position and gained more and more control over their lives and property. Thus, in imperial times husband and wife approached marriage as equals. Yet it seems that there was also a decline in marriage and birth rates, since the emperor Augustus found it necessary to pass drastic laws compelling people to marry and penalizing those who remained single. There were several forms of marriage, the first of which (by usus) involved no ceremony at all. It was established simply by the couple's living together for one year. Divorce was just as informal. A more formal kind of marriage (by coemptio) began with a ceremony in front of witnesses and was also dissolved with a ceremony. Members of the upper classes usually preferred an elaborate ceremony and thus married by confarreatio in front of ten witnesses and a priest. In the case of a divorce, another great ceremony was required. However, all three forms of marriage and divorce were equally valid. All marriages were monogamous. Both men and women usually entered their first marriage in their late teens.

While the Romans tolerated prostitution and concubinage, and had no qualms about homosexual relationships, their marriage laws were remarkably fair to women and thus greatly contributed to their emancipation.

Marriage in Ancient Israel

As we can learn from the Bible, the ancient Israelites had a patriarchal family structure. The status of women was low—they were regarded as the property of their fathers or husbands and could do nothing without their consent. The main purpose of marriage was procreation and the perpetuation of a man's name. Every healthy person was expected to marry. Single men and women were despised. A man could have several wives and concubines. (Jacob married two sisters, Leah and Rachel, and Solomon had 700 wives and 300 concubines.) Divorce was not encouraged, but permitted if a man found some "uncleanness" in his wife. In such a case, he simply wrote her a bill of divorce and sent her out of his house (Deuteronomy 24:1). However, it was virtually impossible for a wife to divorce her husband.

The Bible indicates that the marriage laws and customs of Israel changed somewhat in the course of time. Thus, divorces were increasingly frowned upon, and there was a general trend toward monogamy. Another change concerned the so-called levirate (i.e., the man's obligatory marriage to his brother's widow). This kind of marriage was at times required (Deuteronomy 25:5) and at other times prohibited (Leviticus 20:21). This change was probably related to changing economic conditions.

It was usually the patriarch who selected a bride for his son and who paid a "bride price" to her father. The acceptance of this bride price constituted a legally binding betrothal, which was followed by some wedding celebration when the bride took up residence with her new family. Both males and females married in their early teens, shortly after puberty. Theoretically, therefore, neither sex was subjected to any lengthy period of sexual frustration. Still, because of an unquestioned sexual double standard, men had a far greater opportunity for sexual fulfillment than women.

Marriage in Medieval Europe

The rise of Christianity produced a profound change in European marriage laws and customs, although this change came about only gradually. The first Christian emperors were more or less content with the traditional Roman law. However, under varying political and religious pressures, they alternately broadened and restricted the divorce regulations. They also repealed older laws which had penalized the unmarried and childless, since the new Christian asceticism favored virginity and sexual abstinence over marriage. In most other respects they resisted change. Marriage and divorce continued to be civil and private matters.

In the following centuries, however, marriage came more and more under the influence of the church. Compared to Rome, the newly Christianized countries of Northern Europe had rather barbaric marriage customs and treated women little better than domestic slaves. In Germanic law, for example, marriage was essentially a business deal between the bridegroom and the bride's father ("sale marriage"). The symbol of a successful "bride sale" was the ring (a form of down payment) which was given to the bride herself. Acceptance of the ring constituted betrothal. The full payment of the "bride price" was made on delivery, i.e., when the actual wedding took place. (Since then, the ring has acquired many other symbolic meanings and, indeed, is still used in our modern marriage ceremonies.) The civilizing influence of the church soon refined these primitive customs. According to Roman law and Christian belief, marriage could be built only on the free consent of both partners, and this doctrine was bound to raise the status of women. Furthermore, theologians increasingly found a religious significance in marriage and eventually even included it among the sacraments. This also endowed a formerly rather prosaic arrangement with a new dignity.

Unfortunately, at the same time the church created two new problems: It abolished divorce by declaring marriage to be insoluble (except by death) and greatly increased the number of marriage prohibitions. Now there were three basic impediments to marriage: "consanguinity," "affinity," and "spiritual affinity." Consanguinity (i.e., relationship by blood) was interpreted very broadly up to the 6th or even 7th degree. This meant that nobody could marry anyone more closely related than a third cousin. Affinity referred to a mysterious closeness between the two families of husband and wife. Since the latter were seen as having become "one flesh," all relatives on both sides also became related to each other, a circumstance which made marriage between any of them impossible. Spiritual affinity was said to exist between godparents and godchildren with their families.

As a result of these new regulations, the influence of the church on marriage was greatly strengthened. Very often extensive clerical investigations were necessary to prove or disprove the existence of impediments. For example, marriages that had been entered in ignorance or defiance of such impediments were considered null and void. In these cases the church was therefore willing to pronounce an "annulment." Since divorce was no longer permitted, an annulment was the only way of dissolving a marriage, and thus many married couples who had tired of each other sooner or later conveniently discovered some previously overlooked marriage impediment. The church also began to post so-called banns before each wedding, inviting anyone with knowledge of an impediment to come forward. The growing church involvement in marriage could further be seen in the development of a special religious wedding ceremony. In the first Christian centuries marriage had been a strictly private arrangement. As late as the 10th century, the essential

EARLY MARRIAGE AMONG ARISTOCRATS

Among European aristocrats marriage was often a means of creating political alliances, increasing power, or preserving peace. It was therefore not uncommon for children to be married if this suited the ambitions of their families.

(Top) William II, Prince of Orange (age 14) and his wife Mary Stuart (age 10) daughter of Charles I of England. Painting by van Dyck, 1641.

(Bottom) Wedding of Marie Adélaide of Savoy (age 12) and the Duke of Bourgogne (age 14) at Versailles in 1697. King Louis XIV, the bridegroom's grandfather, can be seen on the right.

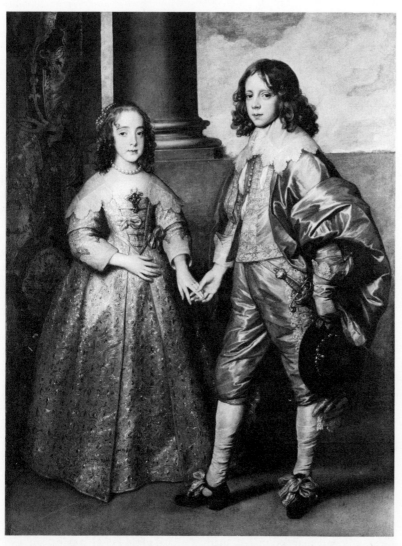

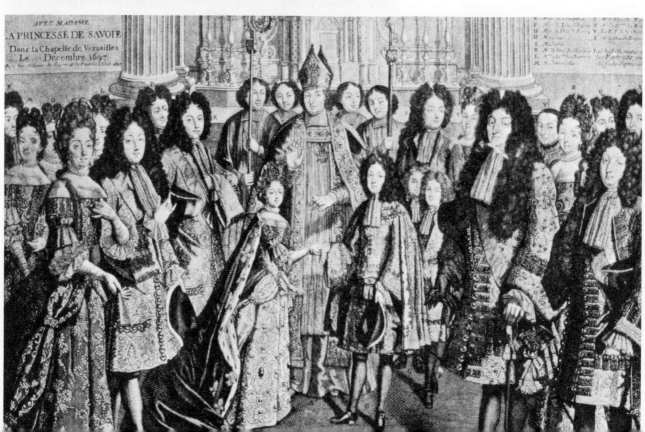

part of the wedding itself took place outside the church door. It was not until the 12th century that a priest became part of the wedding ceremony, and not until the 13th century that he actually took charge of the proceedings. Nevertheless, it remained understood that, even as a sacrament, marriage sprang from the free consent of the two partners, and that therefore neither the parents nor the priest nor the government could affect its validity. It thus became possible for couples to get married secretly if they could not obtain anyone else's approval. It also became possible for very young children to be married, if their parents could coax the necessary consent out of them. Especially aristocratic families often took advantage of this possibility when they found a politically advantageous match for their little sons or daughters. On the average, however, males married in their mid-twenties, and females in their early teens (i.e., soon after their first menstruation).

Today it may be tempting to see medieval marriage in the light of certain lofty religious doctrines and the poetry of the troubadours. However, throughout most of the Middle Ages and for the greater part of the population marriage remained a practical, economic affair. Romantic love hardly had any place in it. Moreover, the social and legal status of women, while somewhat improved in some countries, continued to be very low.

Marriage in Modern Europe and America

The Protestant Reformation of the 16th century rejected the prevailing concept of marriage along with many other Catholic doctrines. Martin Luther declared marriage to be "a worldly thing . . . that belongs to the realm of government," and a similar opinion was expressed by Calvin. The English Puritans in the 17th century even passed an Act of Parliament asserting "marriage to be no sacrament" and soon thereafter made marriage purely secular. It was no longer to be performed by a minister, but by a justice of the peace. The Restoration abolished this law and reverted to the old system, but the Puritans brought their concept of marriage to America where it survived. Luther and other Protestants also reduced the number of marriage impediments. Affinity and spiritual affinity were no longer considered obstacles, and consanguinity was interpreted much more narrowly than before. Thus, even marriages between first cousins became possible.

The Catholic church, in response to the Protestant challenge, took its stand in the Council of Trent and, in 1563, confirmed its previous doctrines. Indeed, it now demanded that all marriages take place before a priest and two witnesses. Among other things, this virtually eliminated not only secret marriages, but also the formerly common informal marriages. These, similar to the old Roman marriages by *usus,* were based simply on mutual consent without formal ceremony. In England they came to be called "common law marriages," and since Henry VIII had broken with Rome, they continued to be permitted until 1753, when the Church of England was put in charge of all marriages (including those of Catholics, but excluding those of Quakers and Jews). This development did not affect the English colonies, however, and thus common law marriages remained possible in America. (As recently as 1970 they were still recognized in several states.)

In most of Europe marriages continued to require a religious ceremony until the French Revolution in 1792 introduced the compulsory civil marriage. Germany followed suit in the 19th century when Bismarck diminished the influence of the Catholic church. Eventually, marriage before some magistrate or government official became the only valid form of marriage in most of the Western world. Religious weddings were still permitted, but only after the civil ceremony had taken place.

Another contested issue was that of divorce. In opposition to Catholic doctrine, the Protestant Reformers did not believe that marriage was insoluble, but favored divorce under special circumstances. The Puritan John Milton in his *Doctrine and Discipline of Divorce* (1643) even advocated self-divorce without the involvement of either church or government. For him, marriage rested entirely on the full compatibility of both partners. Where mutual love

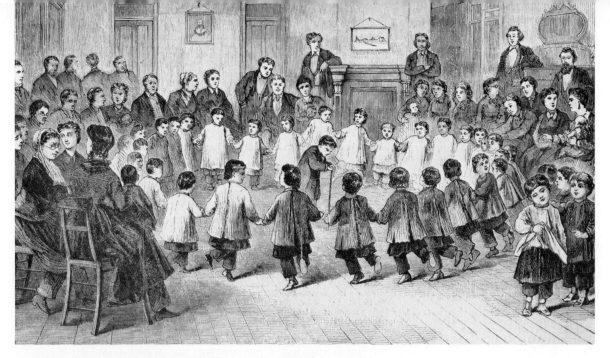

UNCONVENTIONAL FORMS OF MARRIAGE IN 19TH-CENTURY AMERICA

Marital experiments are nothing new. Especially the United States has an interesting history of attempts at marriage reform.

(Above) **The Oneida Community**

Founded by John Noyes in 1848, the Oneida colony in upstate New York cultivated a form of group marriage called "complex marriage" in which theoretically every woman was married to every man. The community also practiced "scientific breeding" in which potential parents were matched by committee for physical and mental health. The picture shows this special breed of children playing in front of their proud parents.

(Below) **Mormon Polygamy**

The members of the Mormon church were relentlessly persecuted, harassed, and ridiculed because of their polygamy. Finally, there were forced to abandon the practice. The picture is a satirical cartoon commenting on the death of Brigham Young in 1877. It shows twelve widows in the same marital bed mourning the death of their husband.

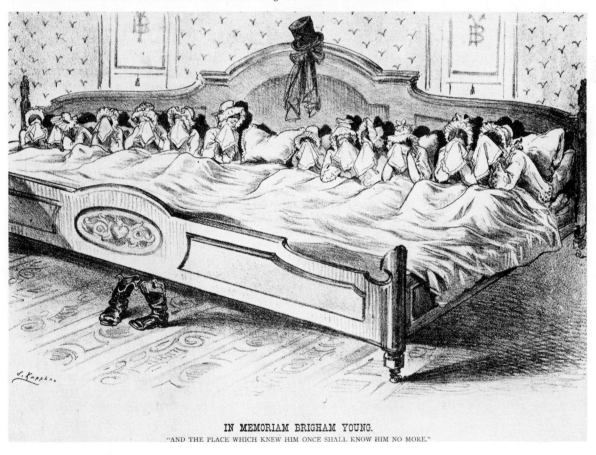

IN MEMORIAM BRIGHAM YOUNG.

"AND THE PLACE WHICH KNEW HIM ONCE SHALL KNOW HIM NO MORE."

was lacking, marriage was a sham and had to be dissolved. However, this philosophy was too far ahead of its time. The English Parliament began to grant some divorces, but the procedure was so cumbersome and expensive that few couples could take advantage of it. A more efficient divorce court was not established until the middle of the 19th century. In colonial America the Puritans permitted divorce in certain specific cases, but it remained prohibited in all Catholic countries until the French Revolution and the Napoleonic code introduced it to France. After Napoleon, divorce was abolished again by the restored monarchy, but it was reinstated by the Second Republic in 1884. Still, divorce remained impossible in Italy, Portugal, and Spain, until Italy finally legalized it in 1970.

Monogamy was and still is the only accepted form of marriage in both Catholic and Protestant countries, although Luther condoned polygyny in exceptional cases. (He "unofficially" permitted Landgrave Philip of Hesse to take two wives.) Nevertheless, such old biblical customs had become repugnant to most modern Christians, and when, in the 19th century, the Mormons revived the practice of polygyny in America, they were so relentlessly persecuted that they abandoned it.

The gradual emancipation of marriage and divorce laws from the control of the church resulted in greater individual freedom and further raised the status of women. The parents began to lose influence over the marital choices of their children, and romantic love became an important factor in marriage. Even so, for most couples until well into the 19th century marriage was still basically an economic arrangement. Moreover, the husband was usually the one who profited most, because he was the "head of the household" and controlled his wife's property. He also had many other rights denied to his wife and was favored by a moral double standard that allowed him considerable sexual license. Under the circumstances, women continued to press for further reforms, a process which even today has not yet fully reached its goal. (See also "The Social Roles of Men and Women.")

MARRIAGE IN NON-WESTERN SOCIETIES

Many Western Christians live under the impression that their own form of marriage is the only "natural" and workable one, and that all other forms are not only sinful, but barbaric. Christians in non-Western countries, however, who are used to observing "exotic" marriage customs at close range, may realize that the matter is not that simple. Human beings are highly adaptable, and they usually develop their particular forms of marriage in response to particular social and economic conditions. When these conditions change, marriage is likely to change with them. The following three examples may illustrate this point. The first form of marriage described here has virtually disappeared under Western influence. The second survives, but is gradually being modernized under increasing pressure. The third represents a radical reform of customs that had become obsolete.

Marriage in Ancient Polynesia

Before their contact with Western civilization, the populations of the many Polynesian islands had their own marriage laws and customs which, however varied, nevertheless had much in common. They were also quite different from those of Europe and America. The Polynesians were sexually quite uninhibited and put a high value on sexual satisfaction. Marriage was considered highly desirable, and very few adults remained single. Widowed and divorced persons also remarried as quickly as possible. Boys and girls usually married as soon as they became adults.

However, the Polynesians were highly conscious of rank, and the marriage customs of the nobility were different from those of the common people. On some islands the nobility practiced polygyny (or polyandry as in the Marquesan Islands). In some cases, noblemen also arranged for child marriages, if this was politically advantageous. At any rate, the upper classes were rather restricted in their choice of marriage partners by complicated social considerations. The lower classes had more freedom in this respect, although most of their marriages were also arranged, or at least required parental consent. Marriage was prohibited between blood relatives to several degrees and outside one's social class. On the other hand, no great formalities were involved in starting a marriage. Bride and bridegroom simply began to live together. Marriages were monogamous, and fidelity was expected. Still, the husband was often allowed sexual relations with his sisters-in-law, and the wife with her brothers-in-law. (In this context, cousins were also regarded as brothers and sisters.) A husband would sometimes also allow his "name brother" (i.e., sworn brother or best friend) and his male guests to sleep with his wife. Under the circumstances, the marital relationship was not a very restrictive one. Still, if a marriage was unsatisfactory, it was easily dissolved by simple private agreement. The property and the children were divided, with the husband usually taking the older boys, and the wife taking the infants and girls. Remarriage was just as easy. Generally speaking, therefore, marriage in ancient Polynesia was a very flexible institution in which prolonged unhappiness of either spouse was unlikely. On the whole, the ancient Polynesians considered marriage a pleasant necessity. This basic attitude reflected their realistic and direct approach to sex and their high regard for physical contentment.

Marriage in Islamic Countries

The faith of Islam has always strongly encouraged marriage and considered celibacy undesirable and exceptional. There is no Islamic tradition of monasteries or vows of lifelong chastity. In many respects the Islamic view of marriage is similar to that expressed in the Old Testament. Thus, for example, the Koran also permits polygyny. Since the time of Mohammed, a man could marry up to four women, provided he could adequately maintain and "do justice" to all of them. In addition, he could have several concubines who did not share the privileges of his wives. Islamic polygyny has survived in many parts of the world to this day. However, even in earlier times it has always been the exception rather than the rule. For most Muslims monogamy was and still is the normal practice.

Islamic culture has, at times, also known a form of temporary marriage known as mut'ah (Arabic:"pleasure"). A man could marry a woman for a predetermined period of time (sometimes only one night), if he paid her an acceptable price or "dower." At the end of the time period the marriage was automatically dissolved. Needless to say, apart from their specific agreement, the woman had no further claim on the man or his property. Mut'ah marriages were usually contracted by men on pilgrimages to Mecca or in other circumstances when they were away from home. However, many devout Muslims opposed and denounced the custom as nothing more than prostitution. It was officially discouraged and eventually became less common.

The Koran does not prohibit divorce, which therefore has always been found in Islamic societies. One form of divorce was that by simple mutual agreement, in which the wife paid her husband a price for her release. Another form was that by repudiation, in which the husband simply told his wife three times that he wanted to divorce her. This was entirely his private business, and he was not required to justify his action to anyone. However, if a wife wanted to divorce her husband, she had to sue for it in court on specific grounds, such as cruelty, desertion, or lack of support.

As this brief summary makes clear, the Islamic marriage laws and customs put men in a clearly privileged position. Women remained legally disadvantaged. More recently, however, industrialization and modernization seem to have made an impact on many Islamic societies that could lead to significant changes.

Marriage in China

In Imperial China marriage was strongly encouraged, as single persons enjoyed little respect. However, marriages were contracted between two families rather than two individuals. Fathers made the best available match for their children, who usually had no opportunity to see each other before the wedding. The purpose of marriage was procreation, i.e., the continuation of the family line. Romantic love between husband and wife was not expected and, indeed, considered irrelevant. The husband enjoyed a privileged status and exercised great power over his family, while the wife had few rights. She owed obedience not only to her husband, but also to her mother-in-law. Husbands could also take concubines for their sexual needs, while wives had no right to take a lover. Divorce was possible, especially if the husband desired it, but the procedure was complicated. Moreover, since a divorce created problems between the families on both sides, it was frowned upon and usually avoided. In actual practice, therefore, even unhappy marriages often remained undissolved.

In the first decades of our century, after the end of imperial rule, the marriage laws began to be reformed, and the founding of the People's Republic finally led to the enactment of a new, modernized code in 1950. The 27 articles of this code are remarkable for their simplicity. They proclaim the free choice of partners and equal rights for both sexes. Older customs, such as concubinage, child betrothal, and the exaction of money or gifts in connection with marriage are prohibited. The code explicitly states that "marriage is based on the complete willingness of the two parties" (Article 3). Consequently, for the contraction of a marriage nothing more is required than registration with the government, which then issues a marriage certificate. Both husband and wife have the right to use his or her own family name. Divorce is easily obtained, if both parties desire it. They simply make arrangements for the care of their children and property, after which they register with the government and obtain a divorce certificate. When only one party insists on divorce, some official attempt at reconciliation is made. If these attempts fail, the divorce is granted. Divorced parents remain responsible for their children and are obliged to make adequate provision for their upbringing. If they cannot agree, an agreement is imposed by a court. Custody of the children may rest with either parent.

At the present time it is difficult for a foreign observer to assess how these laws work in practice, but one has to admit that, at least on paper, they look highly reasonable. They are certainly far ahead of American and most European marriage laws. However, they also contain two rather curious provisions which perhaps need some elucidation. Article 5 prohibits marriage "where one party, because of certain physical defects, is sexually impotent" and where one party suffers from certain specified diseases. In its English translation the language of this article is ambiguous, but it seems to deny the right to marry to many handicapped and chronically ill persons who would enjoy this right in most Western societies. The legal age for marriage in China is now 20 years for males and 18 years for females, although young people are usually encouraged to wait until they are several years older.

MARRIAGE IN CONTEMPORARY AMERICA

Earlier in this book we have discussed the gradual emancipation of women in modern times and its effects on everyday life. While this emancipation is far from complete, it has already produced profound changes in the family structure and in the meaning of marriage. In the past, married women were not allowed to make contracts and were legally prevented from managing any real property that they might have acquired before marriage. Neither could they receive independent income from it. Indeed, all of their premarital property had to be transferred to the husband.

Since that time, women have become legally nearly equal to men. Furthermore, many women now work outside the house, pursue careers of their own and, in some cases, make more money than their husbands. The sexual double standard still exists, especially with regard to laws against sex crimes, but at least some of its worst manifestations have been eliminated. Divorce laws have been broadened, simplified, and made more equitable. Thus,

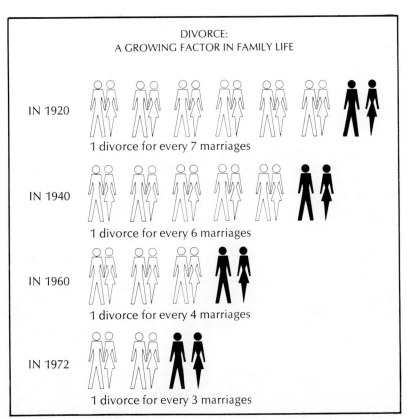

DIVORCE:
A GROWING FACTOR IN FAMILY LIFE

IN 1920
1 divorce for every 7 marriages

IN 1940
1 divorce for every 6 marriages

IN 1960
1 divorce for every 4 marriages

IN 1972
1 divorce for every 3 marriages

women have gained a considerable measure of independence from men, and this has led to some changes in the traditional gender roles.

At the same time, some functions of the family itself have changed. If, in the past, families were mostly producing units in which everyone contributed to some common trade or business, they have now often become mere consuming units. The family members still live, eat, and buy appliances together, but otherwise go their own ways. The children spend several hours every day away from their parents in compulsory school education. After school, they may well be absent for additional hours in youth clubs, on field trips, and at sports events. In many families, both mother and father have outside jobs. Grandparents or sick or disabled relatives live in nursing homes or hospitals, or receive pensions or government assistance at home. Thus, financial and moral family obligations have been greatly reduced.

As a result of these and other developments, marriage today has a quite different meaning than only a century ago. Material considerations have become less important. Instead, it is the sexual attraction between the spouses which prompts them to marry. However, they also know that they can get a divorce if this attraction should wane. In many cases they can further expect that they will be able to care for themselves as divorced individuals, and that, in old age, they will not be a burden to their children. On the other hand, the general improvement of health and the rise in life expectancy now allows husband and wife to look forward to many decades of intimacy, even after the children have grown. The formerly rare silver and golden wedding anniversaries have become realistic possibilities for all young married couples.

Still, not many couples decide to stay together that long. A growing number of them find the demands of strict monogamy for 20, 30, or 50 years too exacting, and, sooner or later, they seek a divorce. Thus, in our century, the divorce rate in the United States has steadily gone up to the point of one divorce for every three marriages, and the trend continues. (See illustration on this page.)

However, the present high divorce rate does not seem to mean that marriage is obsolete, since, in fact, today more people are getting married than ever before. It only means that they no longer conceive of it as a lifelong commitment. Not only in public, but also in private life, men and women have begun to value their personal happiness higher than the maintenance of traditional institutions. Under the circumstances, it is not surprising to find that more and more children live in one-parent families, at least temporarily. Divorced and even unmarried parents often prefer to take care of their children alone, instead of seeking "protection" in some hasty marriage.

American marriage, divorce, and family laws have not yet been brought fully up to date to reflect all of these social changes. This could be one of the reasons why some observers believe modern marriage to be in a "crisis." Actually, this crisis could turn out to be nothing more than a false impression created by the discrepancy between old legal fictions and new practical realities.

THE FUTURE OF MARRIAGE

Many people today are dissatisfied with the institution of marriage as they find it and therefore wonder how they might give it a "new," more agreeable form. Thus, we can now read numerous books and articles which discuss the "crisis of marriage" and which try to offer solutions. For example, some writers propose a "contractual marriage" (i.e., marriage based on an easily terminated private contract), a "permissive marriage" (i.e., marriage permitting extramarital relationships), a "communal marriage" (i.e., group marriage in a commune), or a "quarternary marriage" (i.e., two married couples and their children living together). These and similar arrangements are often felt to be more realistic and durable than our traditional marriage, which is assumed to have "broken down."

However, radical as some of these proposals may seem to some people, they do not really contain anything new. In fact, virtually all "future" forms of marriage that are being advocated today have already existed somewhere at some time in the past. Yet, they have not prevailed. A relatively exclusive monogamy has either long since replaced them or seems in the process of doing so. This means that our present form of marriage is probably based on more solid ground than simple unquestioned tradition. There seems to be something uniquely attractive and appropriate in just two spouses building a life together and, if they are fertile, caring for their own children. Moreover, this seems to be the only marital arrangement in which the partners can be truly equal.

It must be granted, of course, that for thousands of years monogamy has existed without equality, and that women have long been oppressed even where they had only one husband. Nevertheless, as women became more emancipated they have not demanded a return to polygyny. Nor are many emancipated men likely to clamor for polyandry. Group marriage, on the other hand, demands so much discipline that it has never been widely popular. In short, if the future should finally bring full sexual equality, it will also further strengthen the foundations of monogamous marriage.

This is not to say that changes cannot be made. Indeed, our present official ideal of marriage is perhaps justly perceived as too rigid and restrictive. After all, in practice it has never provided complete fulfillment for everyone. Some unofficial "safety valve," "side door," or "escape hatch" always had to be left open. In short, there has always been a need for some marital flexibility. In this respect, the future could bring much progress. Marriage and divorce laws could be made more practical and equitable. Laws against nonmarital sexual relationships could be repealed. The discrimination against unmarried persons could end. Marital status and marital arrangements could become strictly private affairs. There could be more room for individual choices. Some of the possibilities are briefly described below.

Flexible Monogamy

It is easy to imagine a more flexible form of monogamy than that which officially prevails today. Indeed, unofficially there are already many marriages in our society that do not fit the traditional pattern. The following examples may indicate possible future developments.

Open Marriage

The term "open marriage" is now often used for a nonexclusive monogamous relationship. In such a marriage both partners love and cherish each other and do want to live together, but they also permit each other to have other sexual encounters. In fact, they may occasionally even admit a third and fourth partner to their marital bed. This latter practice is today also popularly described as "swinging." Such arrangements are nothing new, of course. They have existed throughout history among many peoples. For example, among certain American Indians and Eskimos it was customary for husbands to offer their wives to their male guests. Many Polynesian men also followed this practice and, in addition, granted their own brothers the same privilege. They themselves, in turn, had sexual access to their sisters-in-law. (In Hawaii such a relationship was known as *punalua*.) But even apart from these socially approved forms of "open marriage," extramarital sex has been silently condoned in many other societies, especially for males. Females were usually more restricted, although in 18th-century Europe upper-class husbands often allowed their wives an "official lover." In one form or another these old customs may well survive into the future.

Temporary Marriage

As mentioned earlier, temporary marriages have, at times, existed in Islamic countries (*mut'ah* marriages). We also know that in old Japan it was possible to contract a marriage for five years or less. In the early 19th century, the great German writer Goethe also entertained a proposal for five-year marriages in his novel *Elective Affinities* (Part 1, Chapter 10). The voluntary continuation of such a marriage could and would follow, if both partners proved compatible. Actually, as divorces have become easier to obtain in most Western countries, marriage has, in fact if not in law, turned into a temporary arrangement for many couples. Today it is no longer unusual for either men or women to marry and divorce two, three, or more partners within a few years. In view of these developments, it has been suggested that the law should officially set a predetermined date for the end of each marriage. At this date the marriage could, of course, be renewed for another agreed-upon period, but without such a renewal, it would automatically be dissolved. Thus, divorce would become unnecessary. However, critics of this proposal point out that fixed time limits of any kind can cast a disturbing pall over a marriage, and that more reasonable "no-fault" divorce laws would serve the same purpose better.

Trial Marriage

Throughout most of European history, farmers have allowed their children premarital sexual experiences in order to insure a compatible match and to test the fecundity of any prospective bride. Thus, well into modern times they practiced a custom variously called bundling, tarrying, sitting up (England), nightrunning (Norway), questing (Holland), and night-courting, trial nights, *Kiltgang, fensterln,* etc. (Germany). According to this custom, a girl could receive a young man in her bed at night, if her parents regarded him as a serious prospect. At first, these nightly visits might not involve any physical intimacy, but if they became more frequent, sexual intercourse was permitted. (Many such relationships lasted for a long time.) However, marriage was always the ultimate goal, especially if the girl became pregnant, and both partners remained well aware of their mutual obligations. Indeed, in some areas the practice became even more formalized as "handfasting," i.e., a regular probationary marriage preceding the "official" marriage by months or even years. All of these customs served the rural populace well for many centuries, until they died out under the influx of strangers who took advantage of them while disregarding their true implications. Still, in our century sexual reformers have repeatedly demanded the reintroduction of similar customs for all citizens. Thus, they proposed a "companionate marriage" (United States), "Ehe auf Zeit" (Germany), or "Probeehe" (Austria). All of these proposals, while differing in details, aimed at avoiding the complications of divorce by replacing it with a simple separation by mutual agreement.

As will be noticed, a trial marriage is very similar to the temporary marriage discussed above. They differ only in that the latter is meant to be transitory, while the former implies a couple's hope for a subsequent permanent union. However, it would seem that none of these reforms are really necessary if our divorce laws are simplified. At any rate, today many young couples already practice some form of trial marriage by simply living together for some time before they get married. Such private, informal agreements are likely to continue and may also become more frequent in the future.

Marriage in Two Steps

A unique variation of the trial marriage has been proposed by the American anthropologist Margaret Mead. According to this proposal, there would be two kinds of marriage: one without and the other with children. Or, to put it another way, marriage would be contracted in two steps, although the second step need never be taken. The first step would bring a young couple together for a so-called "individual marriage." In this marriage the partners would be committed to each other for as long as they wish, but they would not have the right to have children. The next step toward a "parental marriage" could be taken only after both husband and wife have demonstrated their ability to raise and support children. This second-stage marriage would therefore require a special license and ceremony.

Such a reform does not seem practical, because "individual marriages" would always be in danger of producing "illegitimate" children in spite of the ban, and thus the whole two-tiered marriage system would constantly be undermined. Nevertheless, on a theoretical level, Mead's proposal has the great merit of impressing upon young people the responsibilities of parenthood.

Non-Monogamous Marriage

While monogamy in one form or another seems likely to remain predominant in the future, it is not impossible that there may also be a revival of non-monogamous marriages. However, if indeed they should reappear at all, they would now have to be based on complete sexual equality. The following examples may serve as an illustration.

Polygamy

Polygamy in both of its variations (polygyny and polyandry) has, of course, a long and venerable history. Polygyny is condoned in both the Old Testament and the Koran. However, under the influence of Christianity and as a result of growing demands for sexual equality, this form of marriage has long since disappeared in Western civilization and is under attack in other parts of the world. In 19th-century America, the Mormons reintroduced it, but were soon forced to abandon it, at least officially. Nevertheless, polygamy has retained its appeal for some people. It has also repeatedly been pointed out that many Westerners now have begun to practice something like "serial" polygamy by marrying and divorcing several partners in the course of their lives. Thus, it is not inconceivable that in the future some men would again take several wives and some wives would take several husbands if they were legally entitled to do so. Even today a number of people are convicted of bigamy every year, and others, who escape prosecution, live in a so-called ménage à trois with one official and one unofficial spouse. Some day such arrangements might well be officially recognized. Needless to say, every partner in such a marriage would have to be given the same legal rights.

Group Marriage

In a group marriage several husbands are married to several wives or, in other words, all men are married to all women in the group. Such marriages have never been common anywhere, although a few examples have been found among some "primitive" peoples. Still, a famous and rather successful experiment in group marriage was made in 19th-century America by John Humphrey Noyes and his Oneida community. In this community every woman was theoretically married to every man in a system called "complex marriage." Sexual intercourse could take place freely, but procreation was avoided except in special "scientifically" determined couplings. This form of deliberate breeding (a separate issue from the form of marriage) was known as "stirpiculture." After the retirement and death of its charismatic leader, the experiment came to an end. However, in recent years some such experiments have been repeated on a less ambitious scale. In certain contemporary "communes" group marriage has existed and still exists, although in many cases the emotional strain on the partners proved too great and more traditional marriage patterns reasserted themselves. Nevertheless, in the future some attempts at group marriage may continue, and occasionally they may even succeed. Whether they will or should be legally recognized is another question.

Homosexual Marriage

One formerly unmentionable issue which has recently provoked some serious discussion is homosexual marriage. It has, of course, always been possible for two homosexuals to marry each other, if one of them was male and the other female. Indeed, we know that, in the past, some such marriages have turned out rather well. A famous example is the marriage between the British diplomat Harold Nicolson and the novelist Victoria Sackville-West. Both of them sought their sexual fulfillment outside the marital bed, but a deep love and mutual respect kept them together nevertheless.

However, until now our Western civilization has never permitted marriage between partners of the same sex. (The only exceptions are the brief, personal escapades of certain Roman emperors.) A few other civilizations have been more broadminded. Thus, in some American Indian tribes it was possible for a man to assume the role of a woman and to marry another man. Among the Siwans in Northern Africa many men married male adolescents and even paid a higher "bride price" for them than for girls. Still, generally speaking, such customs have always been rare, because marriage was usually associated with procreation. Therefore, even where homosexual relationships were encouraged, they remained pre- or extramarital.

The traditional meanings of marriage have begun to change only recently in some industrial societies. Because of new, reliable contraceptives, procreation has become a matter of choice, and today many men and women marry even though they do not want (or cannot have) any children. Instead, they seek other values in marriage, such as love, companionship, financial security, or professional cooperation, and, as we all know, the law has no objection, but readily obliges. However, it is quite obvious that the same reasons for marriage could also be cited by couples of the same sex. Therefore, if infertile heterosexual couples can get married, it seems unfair to deny this right to homosexual couples.

Many homosexuals, of course, have no desire to be married, but there are also many others who live in stable, sometimes even lifelong relationships, and who suffer disadvantages because these relationships cannot be legalized as marriages. Tax, inheritance, and immigration laws (to name but a few) discriminate against them, and thus they do not find themselves rewarded for their responsible behavior. Indeed, one may say that today our society is still conspiring to keep homosexuals unstable and promiscuous. (For details see "The Sexually Oppressed—Homosexuals.")

However, there are now several Christian churches (especially the Metropolitan Community Church) which perform wedding (or "holy union") ceremonies for homosexual couples. Such a ceremony does not constitute a legal marriage, but at least it gives some recognition to couples who want to make a firm commitment to each other. In some European parliaments (Denmark, the Netherlands) legal proposals have been introduced that would officially allow homosexual marriages. So far, none of these proposals has become law, however. In the United States the chance for the passage of similar laws also appears to be very slim at this time.

THE FAMILY IN HISTORICAL PERSPECTIVE

The word "family" (from Latin *famulus:* servant) originally referred to a group of servants belonging to one man, then, by extension, to all persons ruled by one man or descended from one man, and finally to all persons living together in a man's household, such as servants, wives, children, parents, grandparents, other close and distant relatives, friends, and permanent guests.

These various meanings were still very much alive in medieval English. Indeed, well through the Renaissance the word "family" was used to mean either a body of servants, or the retinue of a nobleman, or a group of people related by blood, or a group of people living together. It was not until the 17th and 18th centuries that the last two of these meanings were combined to describe a new social phenomenon: a small number of close relatives who lived by themselves under the same roof and who were also emotionally close to each other. By the early 19th century this usage had virtually replaced the others, and since then "family" has referred mostly to an intimate domestic group of parents and their children. Thus, we find that today the meaning of the word is both wider and narrower than it had been before. (The same semantic shifts at roughly the same time can be observed in the French *famille* and the German *Familie.*)

This means, among other things, that our present particular concept of family cannot simply be applied to other cultures or even to our own past. If we really want to understand the issue, we have to be more discriminate and, as our philological observations suggest, we should perhaps distinguish between at least three separate phenomena:

1. The **kindred**, i.e., people who are related, whether they live together or not,
2. the **household,** i.e., people who live together, whether they are related or not,
3. the **family** (something now often called "domestic family"), i.e., people who are related and who live together.

In our own present culture it is usually the third of these phenomena, the "domestic family," which dominates the discussion. Kindred systems and household patterns by themselves are now generally neglected as social issues. Instead, the main interest is focused on the one case where they happen to coincide. For example, for the purposes of a recent U.S. Census, "family" was officially defined as "two or more persons related by blood, marriage, or adoption and living together in a household."

Compared to its previous wide range of meanings, this current definition of "family" is, of course, very narrow. Still, upon closer examination, it covers a surprising variety of possible combinations. Even in the simplest case, where a family consists of only two persons, we may find any one of at least a dozen different relationships:

1. A childless married couple,
2. a woman and her natural child,
3. a woman and her adopted child,
4. a man and his natural child,
5. a man and his adopted child,
6. a woman and her natural grandchild,
7. a woman and her adopted grandchild,
8. a man and his natural grandchild,
9. a man and his adopted grandchild,
10. a brother and a sister,
11. two sisters, and
12. two brothers.

Actually, the list could easily be expanded by including great-grandparents, uncles, aunts, cousins, stepparents, stepsisters, stepbrothers, and still other persons "related by blood, marriage, or adoption." According to the U.S. Census, any and all of these social units, even if they comprise only two elements, must be considered families as long as some common living arrangement is involved.

As we can see, the government bureaucrats who use the word "family" in this fashion thereby express a restrictive and modern, but also a "neutral" view. They do not postulate a particular type or ideal of domestic family, but rather look for a practical way of describing present realities. After all, they want simple, descriptive statistics. Thus, for them, all of the above examples represent legitimate families in their own right, not fragments of other, larger families that have "broken up," or become "disorganized."

However, the average citizen may see the matter quite differently. To him, the "two-person family" may not appear as a "real" family at all. Instead, he may regard it as a regrettable exception, a mere vestige or relic of what a family should be. Therefore, he is likely to feel that a husband and his wife or a brother and his sister, for example, do not constitute a family, and that, at the very least, a family should include three persons of two generations: a father, a mother, and a child.

On the other hand, most people today would probably be reluctant to go very far beyond that basic constellation. They would, of course, include any additional number of children, but might begin to wonder whether grandparents, great-grandparents, cousins, uncles, aunts, nephews, and nieces really belong to the family proper. Here again, it will be remembered, the census takers think differently. They say nothing about the size of the family or the degree of relationship between its members. Their decisive criterion is the common household. Thus, the definition of the U.S. Census covers not only the smallest, but also the largest possible domestic family.

Still, in actual fact most modern American families fall somewhat between the extremes. They usually consist of more than two persons, but rarely of more than two generations. Both very large and very small families are now considered atypical. Instead, there seems to be a general trend to reduce or restore the family to a certain "natural" elementary group or "kernel" of a married couple and their offspring. Therefore it seems that the single term "domestic family" is inadequate for a more detailed discussion. If domestic families can come in different shapes and sizes, and if one particular combination is clearly favored today, some further distinction seems to be useful. Such a distinction has been provided by sociologists who commonly list two basic types of domestic family:

1. The **nuclear family** (from Latin *nucleus:* kernel) consisting only of two parents and their children, and
2. the **extended family** consisting of a nuclear family and various other relatives.

(Actually, the extended family, even where it forms a close social unit, is not always "domestic" in the sense that all of its members live under one roof.

THE DEVELOPMENT OF THE MODERN FAMILY

The nuclear family as such is not a new phenomenon, but has long been found in many different cultures. However, its typical modern character and meaning have largely been shaped by the industrial revolution which has transformed it from a producing unit into a consuming unit.

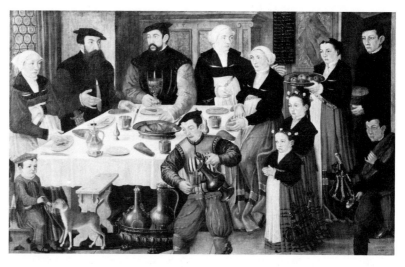

(Top) **Swiss middle-class family in 1559.**
Although painted more than 20 years after the death of Erasmus, the picture still shows the typical family for which he wrote his Colloquia Familiaria. Note the presence of various relatives and several generations under one roof and the demeanor of the children who are portrayed as serious-minded miniature adults, especially the little boy with the dog at bottom left.

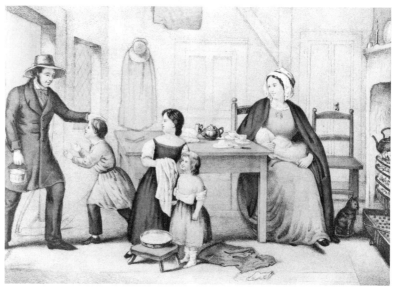

(Middle) **American middle-class family in the 19th century**
The picture shows the "ideal" new nuclear family as it emerged with the Industrial Revolution. The father, a wage earner who works outside the house, is returning home to the warm welcome of his children who have not seen him all day. The mother, who is nursing another baby, is occupied with childcare and other domestic concerns. The household no longer includes grandparents or other relatives.

(Bottom) **"Typical" American Family in the 20th century**
In our own time, the nuclear family with its own suburban home has come to be seen as the only valid model. For several decades now its image has been appearing on countless billboards, in advertisements, commercials, films, radio- and tv-shows as well as in school books. Our picture is taken from a 1972 children's book, Baney's Lake.

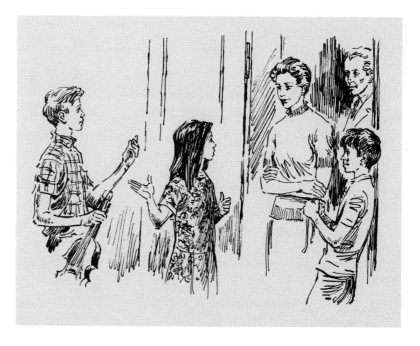

However, they normally live close together and cooperate in many important ways.)

Curiously enough, when this distinction was first proposed, it was often assumed to imply some historical evolution. Indeed, the evolution of the family was believed to have run parallel to that of marriage. Just as monogamy had supposedly evolved out of polygamy, so the nuclear family was said to have evolved out of the extended family. Needless to say, polygamous marriages had always produced extended families, but, according to this theory, even monogamous marriage had once taken place only within a larger context, until it became isolated and independent in the modern industrial world.

This attractive and simple notion went unquestioned for many years, and it must be admitted that it contains a good deal of truth. Nevertheless, like the evolutionary theory of monogamy, it has not stood up as a whole under closer examination. Historians were able to show that the nuclear family had been prevalent in the Western world long before industrialization, and that extended families continued to exist long after it. It was also found that both types of family can easily support the factory system, and that there is no straight evolutionary line leading from one to the other.

However, it is still true that the Modern Age has witnessed some dramatic changes in the European and American family structure, and that the extended family has become increasingly rare. Moreover, the nuclear family has now acquired a different meaning for its members, and thus we seem to be dealing with a new and unique phenomenon.

In this situation it seems appropriate to proceed carefully and to discuss both the traditional extended family and the modern nuclear family in greater detail. The following pages are therefore devoted to this discussion. A concluding section deals with possible future family patterns in our society.

THE TRADITIONAL EXTENDED FAMILY

There are several possible variations of the extended family, and the exact position and function of each of its members can vary accordingly. For example, extended families may result from polygamy or group marriage, and they may be based on sexual equality or on submission to some "head of the household." In the present context we restrict ourselves to the traditional extended family as it existed in the Western world before the Industrial Revolution.

In Christian Europe monogamy was, of course, the only accepted type of marriage, and thus the extended family was usually one in which a married couple, their eldest son and his wife, and perhaps their grandchildren lived and worked together with various other close relatives. In other words, most often it was a family of three or more generations who were engaged in some common enterprise. However, it should be well understood that this kind of family, while common, was by no means universal. Where living conditions were primitive, where people had no land of their own, and where it was difficult to accumulate property, small families were more typical. Indeed, the size and structure of families often fluctuated in response to social changes. Thus, with increased economic opportunity, some nuclear families might expand, become rich, and gain social influence. Or, when faced with some financial threat, they might contract again, consolidating their holdings. By the same token, however, the poor masses in most of medieval Europe could never aspire to the protected life in a big family household. Instead, they lived in very small groups in separate huts or hovels. Obviously, large farm houses, mansions, palazzos, and castles were reserved for the affluent.

Nevertheless, with the beginning of the Modern Age and the growth of commerce, there developed a middle class which could afford to build big, convenient living quarters. Thus, in the cities the modest one- or two-room dwellings of the poor began to be overshadowed by well-made houses, several stories high, in which wealthy officials, merchants, and craftsmen lived with their wives, children, parents, friends, servants, clerks, and apprentices. These "big houses" provided the space for what is now often seen as the ideal extended family or, as it has also been called, "the classical family of Western nostalgia."

Such a family certainly had its advantages. People knew where they belonged and what was expected of them. They ate, drank, slept, learned, worked, and played together under the same roof. From birth to death they were part of an organic whole, growing up and growing old among familiar faces. They all served the common good and shared every joy and every grief with each other. When they were weak, they found ready support, when they were sick or disabled, they found care and protection. In short, they were never lonely, and their lives always "made sense."

It is this feeling of reassurance, this sense of security, which now makes the extended family seem so attractive. However, as historical studies have shown, all that "togetherness" did not really provide much emotional warmth. The main function of the big household was economic. Affection and tenderness were of secondary importance. Not much attention was paid to individual needs and concerns. After all, the parents themselves usually had not married for love, but for material, practical reasons. Furthermore, the wife's status was lower than that of her husband whose wishes always prevailed. Very often there was also a great age difference between the spouses, because many women died in childbirth, and men tended to remarry younger partners. Or, when the master of the house died, his widow married his first assistant in order to keep the business together. A few children were welcome as potential workers, but their parents spent little time with them. Instead, they were brought up by servants and soon sent away as apprentices. Sons of noblemen became pages with other noble families. Many children were simply neglected, and infant mortality was high. For example, in early 18th century London the odds were still 3 to 1 against a child reaching the age of five. Under the circumstances, parents did not become too closely attached to their offspring. Indeed, direct and indirect infanticide was practiced widely. Parents simply let their children suffocate in bed or gave them away to nurses or foster mothers who were known to starve or kill them outright. Even the "enlightened" Jean-Jacques Rousseau, who wrote so sensitively about the innocence of childhood, put his own five children in an orphanage. In these institutions, which provided a welcome supply of domestics and soldiers, the mortality rate was often 80–90%.

We also have to realize that, before the late 17th and early 18th centuries, the "big houses" were, as a rule, noisy and overcrowded. They offered no privacy, but rather were semipublic places. People ran in and out of all rooms at all hours of the day. Visitors appeared unannounced, friends, acquaintances, business partners, clients, solicitors of all kinds walked freely about and sometimes stayed overnight. In addition to its various servants, the household itself usually also contained several permanent guests. There was no formal division between private chamber, workshop, or office. Beds and tables were set up and moved according to need. There were no regular "family dinners," no fixed mealtimes, and many meals were improvised, catered, or bought from the innkeeper next door. A "family life" as such did not exist. Instead, all activities were part of a larger social life. The family was always open to the community and its influences.

It is therefore hardly surprising that, among the middle and upper classes, the relationships between family members were rather formal and cool. In France, husband and wife addressed each other as "Monsieur" and "Madame," in England as "Sir" and "Madam." These official-sounding titles were also used when children spoke to their parents. Noble children called their parents "Milord" and "Milady." Among themselves, the children were no less ceremonious. Instead of using first names, they called each other "brother," "sister," and "cousin." The use of first names, nicknames, and the intimate "Papa" and "Mamma" did not become fashionable until the late 17th century. (After 1800 the English changed their spelling to "Mama," while the Americans used "momma" and later spoke simply of "Mom" and "Dad.")

Obviously, then, for centuries the members of the large European household did not feel much sentimental concern for each other. True intimacy and emotional closeness developed only with the gradual consolidation of the middle class and the growing influence of middle-class values. As the solid citizen prospered, he became ever more industrious, orderly, respectable, disciplined, and domestic; in short, he turned into the now familiar figure of the "bourgeois." This process was well under way by the late 1600's and accelerated through the following century. The "big house" itself began to change. Where once there had been interconnected, open all-purpose rooms, there were now separate, closed chambers for dining, sleeping, reading, and music making. Servants were banned to special quarters "downstairs" or under the roof. Spheres of privacy were established. Business and pleasure were no longer mixed. Workroom and living room became clearly separated. Each house had an "inner sanctum" which was no longer accessible to casual visitors. Indeed, unannounced visits were discouraged. The family "received" only on certain days or *"jours fixes."* At all other times, the family members cultivated each other's company. They gathered around the "family table," played "family games," read "family magazines," and gave "family concerts." Parents took the most tender interest in the welfare and education of their children, who were now regarded as "pure," helpless creatures in need of protection. This protection was found in the family circle. The new ideal was the sheltered, warm, sweet, and idyllic "happy home."

Needless to say, this ideal, which emerged only slowly, was by no means realized everywhere. Both the upper and lower social classes lived very differently. The aristocrats continued much as before in open castles or palaces, surrounded by a tumultuous host of relatives, supplicants, servants, and guests. The poor farmers and common laborers, on the other hand, still lived alone with their wives and children in small, cramped houses, huts, or cabins. As a matter of fact, the bourgeoisie itself often deviated from its own standards as it became more mobile and adventurous. Many men did not care very much for all those quiet evenings with their loved ones. Therefore, they turned the house into a "woman's world" and developed a regular social life of their own in cafés, pubs, guilds, lodges, associations, fraternities, and clubs. As a result, the function and form of the family changed again. It also became clear that the tendency toward family "closeness" was, in effect, a tendency toward reduction in family size. The continued presence of the older generation and of distant relatives was increasingly seen as intrusive. Thus, with the beginning industrialization, the traditional extended family itself gave way to the modern nuclear family.

The "nuclear," "isolated," or "restricted" family is not a recent phenomenon, but has existed in many cultures throughout human history. Indeed, the extended family of several generations is found mostly in relatively advanced, stable, and affluent, but not yet industrialized societies. Very primitive and very sophisticated societies seem to prefer the nuclear family model.

However, nuclear families can vary in the degree of their isolation and restrictedness. For example, before the Industrial Revolution the Western nuclear family was often embedded in a larger social unit, such as a farm or estate, an aristocratic court, or a village populated by relatives. Many older city neighborhoods also kept kinship ties strong, and thus even very small families remained open to the community. Family visits might be frequent and extended; children might freely circulate and feel at home in several households.

On the other hand, we have seen that, beginning in the late 17th century, a trend toward "closeness" reduced the size of many larger households and changed the relationships between the remaining family members. They became more concerned about each other. They needed each other more. The idyllic home of the "bourgeois" became an island of serenity in the gathering

THE MODERN NUCLEAR FAMILY

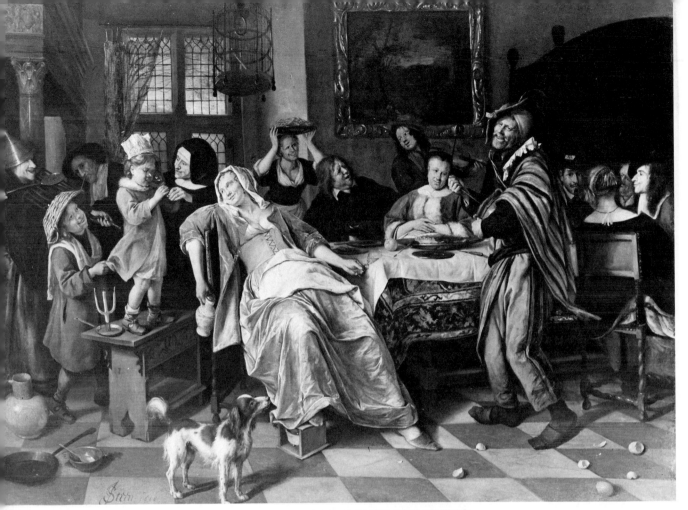

FAMILY LIFE IN THE 17TH CENTURY

The "big house" of the 17th century offered no isolation from the community at large, but allowed family members to mix freely with friends, neighbors, and casual visitors of all ages. Throughout the church year, exuberant celebrations were common. (Painting by Jan Steen 1626-1679)

storm of modernization, a haven secure from the world "out there," from aggressiveness, competition, and class warfare. We have also seen how this home sheltered women and protected the children from sexual and other temptations. Other nasty social realities were also kept safely at bay. The family income was no longer earned inside, but rather outside the house. The division of labor between the sexes became more pronounced as men spent more and more time away from their families as wage earners in factories, shops, and offices. Their wives became almost the only companions of their small children whose care and education was now their main responsibility. (Formerly, these tasks had been divided between mothers, grandmothers, nurses, and servants.) Virtually the only middle-class men who still worked at home were doctors and lawyers in private practice. As a rule, however, the bourgeois family saw its "head" and "breadwinner" only when he returned from his work at night. This work itself remained an abstraction to both his wife and his children.

The removal of productive work from the home into the factories had, of course, important consequences for all family members. It was no longer necessary for any of them to develop strong roots in any particular community or to become attached to a particular house. Instead, they became free to move about, to follow industrial development into new settlements, to "go after the jobs" wherever they might be. Moreover, family connections became less important, as factory work became ever more rationalized and efficient. Nepotism gave way to hiring and promotion on merit alone. By the same token, the new worker, business man, or bureaucrat no longer had to

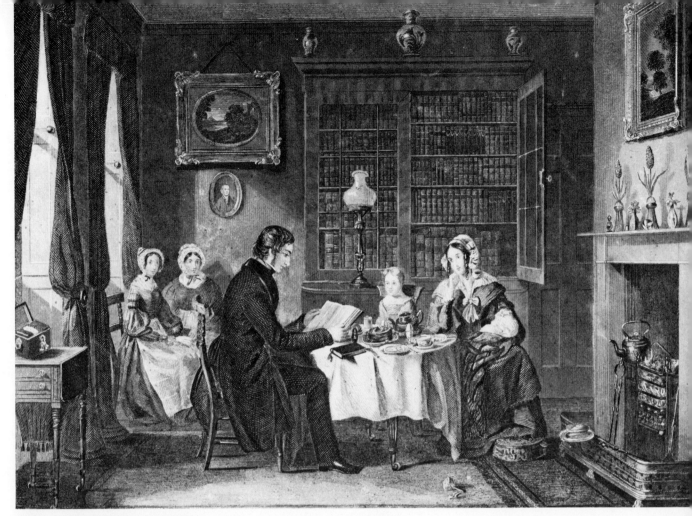

FAMILY LIFE IN THE 19TH CENTURY
By the 19th century, the middle-class home had become a sanctuary, a sheltered place of intimacy and peace. Our picture shows a father reading the Bible to his wife and child. Two female figures (servants?) are listening in the background. (Anonymous etching, early 19th century)

take care of distant relatives. He now worked exclusively for his own small family and this made him more industrious. He could advance faster, since his income had to support only very few people. Thus, the individual husband and father was no longer weighed down by traditions or extensive social obligations. In addition, the education of his children and the care of his aged or sick parents began to be taken over by the state.

In view of these developments, many observers have noted a "fit" between the nuclear family and industrialism. In other words, small, intimate, and mobile families seem best suited to advance the cause of industrialization and, conversely, industrialization seems to encourage the formation of small families. After all, in modern industrial societies there is a general trend toward equality and personal independence. This, in turn, allows for the free choice of a marriage partner, place of residence, and occupation. In an extended family these freedoms are always restricted, because a "wrong" choice would affect too many relatives. Thus, people who want to take full advantage of the new possibilities normally marry late and keep their families small. However, this rule also has its exceptions. Sometimes large families are more useful, because they can serve as a "back-up unit" by providing shelter and aid at crucial moments. This may be especially important for lower-class individuals who try to "move up," although the higher classes often also maintain extensive family ties. Thus, even in fully industrialized societies one can find many men and women who appreciate the traditional extended family or at least a large network of relatives.

Still, by and large, the closely-knit nuclear family has been dominant in

Western societies for the last several generations, and thus it has shaped the general perception of what a family should be: A man and a woman marry for love, have two or three children, live alone by themselves in a "family home" or apartment, and spend all their free time together. The man leaves for work in the morning, while the woman takes care of the children and the house. She also cooks dinner and ministers to her exhausted husband when he returns at night. Once or twice a year, at Thanksgiving or Christmas, there is a brief, ceremonial get-together with other relatives at "Grandma's house," but otherwise everyone keeps his distance and minds his own business.

Obviously, according to this "ideal" model, the family members are relatively isolated from the larger kindred and, indeed, from the rest of the community. However, they are to be compensated for this isolation by a greater emotional warmth inside the nuclear circle. Father, mother, and children are to be the world for each other. A deep mutual love is supposed to keep them together and boost their morale as they compete economically with other small family units. Unfortunately, as many families have discovered, things do not always work out that way. The lack of wider contacts is often perceived as crippling, too much closeness becomes oppressive, and inescapable familiarity breeds contempt. Therefore, almost from the beginning, the modern nuclear family has also been subject to criticism.

In Victorian times, when the "cult of the home" was at its height, this criticism was expressed mainly by great bourgeois writers, such as Flaubert, Ibsen and Strindberg, who denounced the hypocrisy, shallowness, and dullness of middle-class life, and who exposed the suffering and vicious psychological infighting behind the façade of respectability. The family was further criticised on philosophical and political grounds by Friedrich Engels who tied it to the origin and maintenance of private property. Finally, Sigmund Freud provided perhaps the most serious, if indirect, accusation when he described the "happy" nuclear household as the breeding ground of neurosis and sexual perversion.

At any rate, by the late 19th century the disadvantages of the bourgeois family model had also become evident to many average men and women. The emotional hothouse atmosphere of the home began to seem stifling, and what once had been praised as a sanctuary was more and more often condemned as a prison. In the traditional extended family, children had been able to choose between several male and female adult role models; now they had only their parents. Formerly, their early education had been shaped by a number of different people and a variety of influences; now they depended entirely on their own mother and father. Actually, the latter was not even always available. Since he no longer worked inside the house, his children had no clear conception of his social role. Instead, he became simply an abstract "provider" and disciplinarian, a mysterious and distant authority figure. He was occasionally loved, frequently feared, but rarely understood. At the same time, the wife and mother found herself more restricted than ever before. Her greatly increased maternal duties kept her confined inside her "four walls." She could venture outside only for a visit to church or to go shopping. Her world had shrunk, and her functions were narrowly circumscribed. She had to be feminine, motherly, sensitive, "proper," and in all matters of importance she had to defer to her husband.

It is understandable, therefore, that many Victorian women began to resent the nuclear family and their position in it. Thus, it was a signal of things to come when, in Ibsen's *A Doll's House*, the heroine Nora simply walked out on her husband and children. As time went by, more and more women demanded complete legal equality with men and the freedom to develop their full potential as human beings. They began to struggle for the right to vote and the reform of marriage and divorce laws. They also entered the work force in ever increasing numbers. Finally, during World War I, they proved their capabilities in many formerly inaccessible jobs and thereby further emancipated themselves from the home. (See also "The Emancipation of Women.")

Recent decades have seen a continuation of this trend. In many families today both husband wife work outside the house, while the children spend much of their time in a nursery, daycare center, kindergarten, or school. As a result, the emotional ties between family members have become somewhat less constrictive, and a greater tolerance prevails. The influence of peer groups has grown, not only for the children, but also for their mothers. The traditional male and female roles are being reevaluated. The mass media keep everyone in touch with the larger community and its continued transformation. Still, the family circle as such has not widened. Grandparents are rarely part of the household, but live on their own in "retirement villages," "senior citizen centers," or nursing homes. Unmarried relatives move to a "singles' hotel" or apartment building. Thus, the average American family remains fairly small. Indeed, there are now many "fatherless" families consisting only of a woman and her children.

The one-parent family or "core family" is usually described as an "incomplete" nuclear family, and there is a general assumption that it is socially undesirable. The lack of a "father figure" is seen as detrimental to child development, and hasty generalizations are made about "undue" female influence. In the U.S. these comments sometimes even have racist overtones, as mother-child families are frequently found in the poor black population. However, with the rising divorce rate, this family type has also become increasingly common in the white middle class. Indeed, at the present time about 1 out of 6 children in America lives with only one parent, and the number of such households may well increase in the future. After all, our welfare regulations and other government policies often have the effect of breaking up families that would otherwise stay together. Our legislatures have not yet learned how to test new laws through "family impact studies" which would reveal such unintended consequences in advance. Still, in the meantime it should be remembered that the one-parent family is not necessarily bad. In the years following the two World Wars, millions of women have successfully brought up their children alone, and this impressive example should caution us against superficial judgments. Moreover, upon closer examination, many "core families" are discovered to maintain close connections to wider kinship groups and thus turn out to be more open and viable than might have been supposed. Finally, we know that there are also many father-child families which have not received sufficient critical attention.

It is another question whether the nuclear family itself, even when "complete," is still the best available option. Many people today are convinced that small, single households are uneconomical and wasteful, that they are still emotionally unhealthy, that they perpetuate outmoded sterotypical sex roles, and that they produce competitive, egotistical children in an age when universal cooperation seems the only hope of mankind. It is also argued that the modern family no longer has any other function than to provide love and intimacy, and that this is by no means enough to justify its existence. Indeed, since families have been largely relieved of their economic, educational, and protective functions by the state, sexual attachment has become the nearly exclusive basis of marriage, and this basis is notoriously weak. Frequent divorce and remarriage, however, while perhaps practical for the adults, hardly seem in the best interest of the children. Under the circumstances, it is only fitting that a number of thoughtful men and women should continue to search for more stable, "new and improved" family models.

NEW FAMILY MODELS

The disadvantages of the modern nuclear family have prompted many of its critics to look for alternatives. Some reformers want a return to the traditional extended family as it existed before the Industrial Revolution. However, it is unclear how this family type could be reconstituted under present conditions. Furthermore, as we have seen, it also had some very serious shortcomings. It certainly could not accommodate the demands for privacy and individual freedom to which we now feel entitled. On the other hand, slightly extended nuclear families can still be created individually without any drastic social reforms. Yet hardly anyone is convinced that such sporadic minor improvements would make much difference. The real problem seems to lie deeper. Many people feel that their best potential will never be realized unless there is a radical transformation of society as a whole. They believe that a "new man" and a "new woman" have to be created before a better family system can be devised. In their view, the prevailing social order preconditions everyone against achieving true happiness. They find human nature itself deformed by our present unhealthy civilization and therefore demand a "fresh start" and a complete break with tradition. This willingness to experiment is not entirely new, but in the upheavals of recent human history it has become much more widespread than it was before. Thus, today a number of alternative family models are being tried in various parts of the country and the world. The following two examples may hint at the possibilities.

The Kibbutz

The *kibbutz* (Hebrew: "group"; plural: *kibbutzim*) is a form of agricultural collective settlement now common in Israel. The members work for the collective and own everything in common. Married couples have their own living quarters, but take their meals in the common dining room. All children live together in a common "children's house." They are supervised and educated by trained personnel, but may visit their parents for a few hours in the evening. Thus, there is some room for a special relationship between them. However, since even the unmarried adults work for the support of the children and thus consider them "their own," there is a new, wider sense of family in a kibbutz than may be found in the outside world. Marriages are monogamous. They are officially recognized by the granting of a separate, shared room to a young couple. Sexual intercourse between unmarried young people is tolerated, but sooner or later tends to lead to permanent unions. Marriage partners are usually brought in from the outside. Women keep their maiden name and remain (or become) individual members of the kibbutz in their own right.

As can be seen, in this social arrangement there are no families in the traditional sense, because parents and children do not live together. Furthermore, the parents neither work for themselves, nor for each other, nor for their own offspring or other relatives. Instead, work, education, and all social services are shared collectively "from each according to his abilities, to each according to his needs." The kibbutz owes its creation to the idealism of Israeli settlers who wanted to build a more humane society. However, it has sometimes proved difficult to keep this idealism alive with growing prosperity. Moreover, the experiment has not always appealed to everyone, even in Israel. So far, it has not been widely copied in other countries.

The "Commune"

Today the word "commune" is often used for a variety of communal households from "hippie farms" to certain practical arrangements of the urban middle class which tries to reduce the cost of living. After all, it takes nothing more than common sense to see that housing, cooking, washing, sewing, gardening, shopping, child care, etc. are cheaper when provided collectively for several combined nuclear families. Therefore, some such families have begun to pool some of their resources in order to save money. Their "commune" may involve nothing more than a shared house or compound and a more effective use of appliances. However, there are also more radical solutions. Especially in the last decade a number of young, "alienated" people have "dropped out" of society and established an alternative lifestyle living "communally" in the country or in certain city neighborhoods. In America, such movements toward a more "natural" way of living have a long, and sometimes impressive history. At the present time, American "radical" communes still appear in a great variety of forms, depending on the particular aims of their founders. Some are based on strict religious beliefs, others are more secular and hedonistic. Some involve formal monogamous marriages, others practice some type of improvised polygamy or group marriage. Some parents send their children to school, others try to educate them themselves. Some communes practice collective ownership and are economically self-sufficient, others depend on outside income, such as welfare, food stamps, or financial support from benefactors. Some communes have survived for years in relative stability, others have broken up or are lingering on miserably as a warning example to the naïve.

In view of this highly varied picture, it is very difficult to come to any firm conclusions about the contemporary commune. Undoubtedly, in many cases it answers a genuine human need that cannot be fulfilled in the "normal" family as we know it today. The failure of many communes says nothing against their often noble intent. In sum, communal experiments should be expected to continue well into the future. It is always possible that one day some such experiments will provide valuable alternatives that can be successfully copied on a larger scale.

Reference and Recommended Reading

Ariès, Philippe. *Centuries of Childhood*. New York: Knopf, 1962 (cloth); Random Vintage, 1965 (paper).

Goode, William J. *The Family* (Foundations of Modern Sociology Series). New York: Prentice-Hall, 1964.

Horkheimer, Max. "Authority and the Family" in *Critical Theory*. New York: Seabury, 1972 (cloth); 1975 (paper).

Murstein, Bernard I. *Love, Sex, and Marriage through the Ages*. New York: Springer, 1974 (cloth); 1976 (paper).

Shorter, Edward. *The Making of the Modern Family*. New York: Basic Books, 1975.

Skolnick, Arlene S. and Jerome H., eds. *Family in Transition: Rethinking Marriage, Sexuality, Childrearing, and Family Organization*. New York: Little, Brown, 1971 (paper).

12. THE SEXUALLY OPPRESSED

In the l8th century a philosopher allegedly told one of his opponents: "I disagree with what you say, but will defend to the death your right to say it." This noble maxim perfectly summarizes the spirit of an enlightened age which struggled to free itself from intellectual and moral bondage, and which, for the first time in human history, proclaimed universal liberty, equality, and brotherhood. This same spirit also guided the American founding fathers when, in the Constitution of the United States, they guaranteed every citizen freedom of speech, of religion, and of the press.

In the meantime these freedoms have found advocates in many other parts of the world. Over the last 200 years the ideals of tolerance, individualism, self-determination, and personal privacy have been incorporated into the laws of most modern nations. Indeed, our own century has seen a *Universal Declaration of Human Rights* in which all member states of the United Nations pledge their support for these ideals. Thus, at least in theory, the liberation of the human race seems almost complete.

Alas, as we all know, in actual practice things are much less encouraging. Officially, governments may very well subscribe to the famous maxim of that enlightened philosopher, but unofficially many of them still treat all dissent as treason. As a matter of fact, in spite of their libertarian rhetoric, some modern states are more oppressive than the worst medieval kingdom.

All of this is, of course, quite obvious and therefore does not warrant any further discussion here. However, it is not often realized that even in the most tolerant Western countries the tolerance does not extend equally to all spheres of human life. Most notably two kinds of behavior continue to suffer irrational and often severe restrictions: the use of drugs and sexual activity. No public official is yet willing to say: "I disapprove of the drugs you take, but will defend to the death your right to take them," or "I disapprove of your sexual interests, but will defend to the death your right to pursue them." Such pronouncements would still be considered scandalous and irresponsible by most citizens. Drugs and sex remain the great taboos of our civilization.

Actually, in recent times drugs and sex have also begun to be feared by many formerly permissive societies which have been subject to Western influence. It is therefore hardly surprising to find that the celebrated *"Universal Declaration of Human Rights"* says nothing about people's right to control their own bodies. The document only cites the "right to marry and to found a family" and to choose one's marriage partner freely (Article 16). There is no mention of a right to sex education or sexual fulfillment, the free choice of a sexual partner or type of sexual activity, a right to contraception or abortion. Nor is this merely an oversight. Unfortunately, there is little doubt that even today the General Assembly of the United Nations would overwhelmingly reject any official declaration which dared to affirm these rights. Too many member states still consider sex legitimate only within marriage and for the purpose of procreation.

However, it should be well understood that societies which make procreation the only permissible function of sex thereby implicitly condemn most actual human sexual behavior as abnormal or deviant. Thus, solitary masturbation, sex play among children, adolescent sexual experiments, premarital and noncoital forms of marital intercourse, homosexual activity, sexual contact with animals, sex after the menopause—all of these and many other harmless forms of sexual behavior come to be seen as heretical practices which have to be suppressed. This suppression, in turn, creates a universal feeling of guilt and anxiety. Furthermore, since the suppression can never be complete, the development of a sexual double standard and widespread hypocrisy are virtually inevitable. In short, narrow sexual dogmatism always leads to social conflict and a great deal of human misery.

As we have seen earlier in this book, our own Western, Judeo-Christian culture has long been extremely rigid in matters of sex, and thus there is also more sexual hypocrisy and more sexual misery in the West than in most other parts of the world. Our pious forefathers have left us a legacy of intolerance that is difficult to ignore, and which continues to poison our lives to this very day. They were never content with extolling the virtues of procreation, but took the most savage and appalling measures to punish the nonprocreative vices. Sexual nonconformists who were easily tolerated or even esteemed in other societies were stoned in biblical Israel and tortured, mutilated, burned, hanged, or buried alive in Christian Europe.

For example, male homosexuals could be regarded as model citizens in pagan Greece, but for the believers in Yahweh and Jesus they have always been the scum of the earth. The Old Testament demanded the death penalty for sex between males, and so did baptized Roman emperors, Spanish inquisitors, English monarchs, and American colonists. Later, when religion lost some of its public influence, psychiatrists declared homosexuals to be sick and proceeded to treat them, often against their will, with shock or aversion therapy, "psychosurgery," and castration. Finally, in Nazi Germany the "healthy sensibility of the people" allowed homosexuals to be sent to concentration camps where they had to wear a pink triangle on their uniforms (just as the Jews were stigmatized by a yellow star). They were killed by the tens of thousands, and only a few survived. However, unlike the other victims of Nazism, they were never compensated for their suffering. On the contrary, they remained ostracized or were even imprisoned all over again. Indeed, at the present time homosexual behavior is still a felony in most states of the United States, and homosexuals are still being sentenced to long prison terms or committed to mental hospitals as "sexual psychopaths." Even if they are never convicted of any crime, they cannot immigrate, become citizens, or join the Armed Forces. Furthermore, there are still Christian churches which oppose any legal reform and which actively work for the defeat of homosexual civil rights legislation.

Needless to say, all of these barbarities have always been and are now being committed in good conscience by "decent" people with the loftiest motives. Sexual oppression, no matter how harsh or unjustified, has never lacked for rationalizations. These may range from simple religious dogmas to sophisticated pseudo-scientific theories, but regardless of their particular form, they all share one fundamental characteristic: They are not open to logical challenge. Even if they do not make sense or are disproved many times over, they are nevertheless repeated. After all, their real function is not so much to convince the skeptical as to ease the conscience of their proponents, and this task they have always performed remarkably well. Thus, to stay with our example, apart from scriptural quotations, one can now often hear claims by professional "experts" that homosexuality somehow "threatens the survival of the species" or that it "undermines the institutions of marriage and fam-

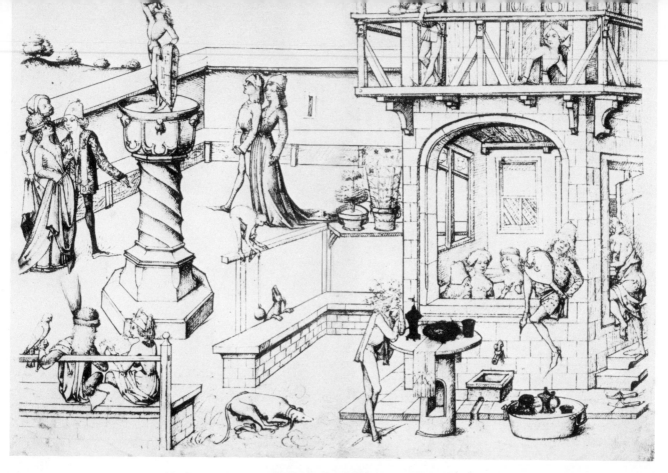

PLEASURES OF THE BATH

Public baths have been popular in many cultures since ancient times. In the past it was not uncommon for men and women to bathe together and to enjoy the mutual erotic stimulation. Indeed, in medieval Europe many bath houses also served as brothels. At any rate, where they did not provide prostitutes directly, they offered ample opportunity for sexual encounters. However, after the end of the Renaissance an increasing prudery and a growing sexual oppression led to the prohibition of public mixed bathing in Europe and America.

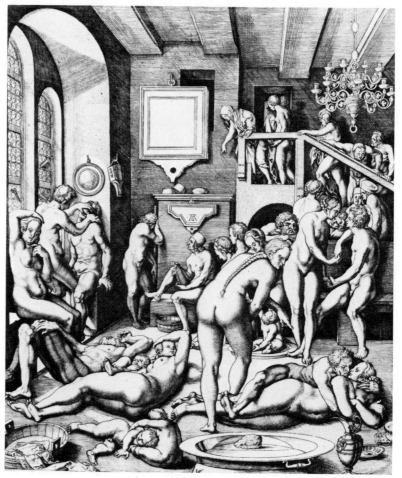

(Top) 14th century drawing showing the pleasures of sexually mixed bathing. Three courting couples are seen in the garden on the left. Behind the open window on the right two men and a woman are soaking in a common tub and are just being joined by another woman. Other guests have already repaired to convenient private rooms upstairs.

(Bottom) 16th century engraving showing a scene in a public bath. The man in the window left is being shaved by a barber, at his feet a family with children is taking a rest, the woman in the center is stepping over an embracing couple, behind them a man is trying to win the favors of a woman, and in the background several men and women are retiring to private rooms upstairs.

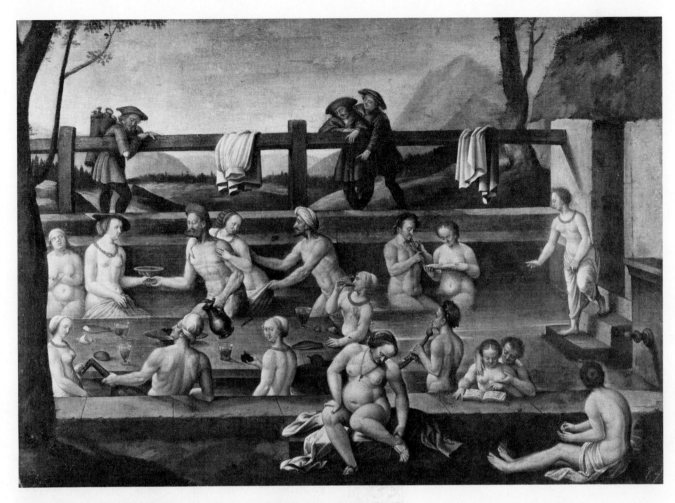

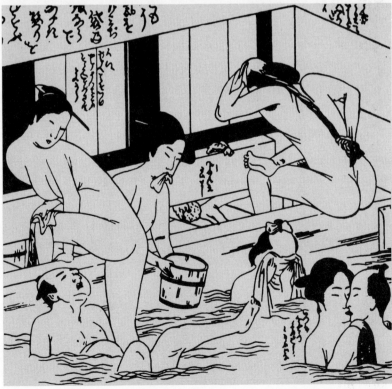

(Top) A 16th century open air bath showing various couples eating, drinking, making music, or engaging in various forms of love play. Note especially the uninhibited couple at bottom right studying a musical score.

(Bottom) 19th century Japanese woodcut showing a public bath. The man at left is admiring the physical charms of an obliging woman. In the foreground right a young couple is shown in an amorous embrace.

ily." The fact that these claims are patently absurd does not in the least prevent them from being put forward. It has often been pointed out that the Islamic and Buddhist societies of Africa and Asia which are well known for their tolerance of homosexuality are also well known for their high birth rates, stable marriages, and strong families. Everyone knows that the world is now threatened with overpopulation. Obviously, the institution of marriage has nothing to gain from being imposed on homosexuals who have no interest in making it work (to say nothing of the injustice perpetrated against their heterosexual partners). On the other hand, there have never been valid grounds why homosexuals should not keep close ties to their relatives and make valuable contributions to family life. However, none of this makes any difference to the intolerant. Since their beliefs are not based on reason, they cannot be shaken by it. In short, when it comes to sexual oppression of this kind, we are dealing not with sober and well-considered judgments, but merely with prejudices.

The oppression of homosexuals is perhaps the most striking and instructive example, but it is, of course, only one among many. The "reproductive bias" of our sexual morality has always produced many other oppressed minorities. Persons with specialized sexual interests, the institutionalized, the infirm, the handicapped and disabled, the aging, children and adolescents, indeed, married couples who practiced contraception or engaged in noncoital intercourse have also been victimized at different times and in various degrees. Moreover, for thousands of years a "double standard" has discriminated against the female sex as a whole. Therefore, if we take them together, we find that the sexually oppressed groups in our society actually constitute an overwhelming majority of the population.

This insight alone should give us serious pause. Indeed, it raises some fundamental and very disturbing questions. For instance: Why would a society first create and then maintain sexual standards that are sure to be violated by most of its members? In other words, why would the majority of any population choose to oppress itself? Or, to give a concrete illustration, why do the American people cling to sex laws that would put virtually everyone behind bars if they were truly enforced? Why would a whole nation want to define itself as a nation of sex criminals? Why do we have this desperate need to feel guilty? What is behind this general urge to be punished?

When these and similar questions are asked, the usual "experts" are, of course, also ready with their prefabricated answers. The religious dogmatists simply talk about "original sin" or "Adam's fall," and since this is strictly a matter of belief, there is no point in arguing about it. However, the same view is sometimes expressed in secularized form by people who speak of an inherently perverse, destructive, or aggressive "human nature." Thus, sexual oppression and self-oppression in America would be nothing more than a manifestation of universal human tendencies, regrettable perhaps, but hardly avoidable. Yet, this hypothesis cannot explain why so many other societies are so much more tolerant. At this point a third explanation is often presented which ascribes all our sexual problems to the evils of our political and economic system. Capitalism, so runs the argument, creates sexual oppression as a drought creates dust; abolish capitalism and you free the sexually oppressed! Unfortunately, this naive assumption is disproved by the continued or even increased sexual intolerance in so-called communist countries, from Albania and Cuba to the Soviet Union and the Peopel's Republic of China. In short, the mere fact that the government takes control of the means of production does not guarantee sexual freedom. The social liberation of the "working class" and its sexual oppression can very well go hand in hand.

The latter example also shows once again that sexual intolerance does not have to be based on divine revelations. To point to religious belief as the cause of sexual oppression therefore explains nothing. It then still has to be explained why some religions are sex-negative and others are not. Even the Bible contains enough material for the support of a tolerant attitude, and, in fact, this material is often quoted by liberal Jews and Christians. Nevertheless,

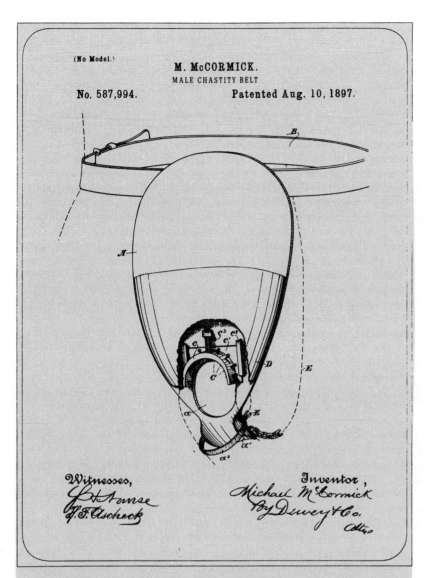

(No Model.)

M. McCORMICK.

MALE CHASTITY BELT

No. 587,994.   Patented Aug. 10, 1897.

Witnesses,   Inventor,
Witnesses   Michael McCormick
                             By Dewey & Co.
                                     Attys

UNITED STATES PATENT OFFICE.

MICHAEL McCORMICK, OF SAN FRANCISCO, CALIFORNIA.

MALE CHASTITY BELT

SPECIFICATION forming part of Letters Patent No. 587,994, dated August 10, 1897.

Application filed November 27, 1896. Serial No. 613,485. (No model.)

To all whom it may concern:

Be it known that I, MICHAEL McCORMICK, of the city and county of San Francisco, State of California, have invented an Improvement in Surgical Appliances; and I hereby declare the following to be a full, clear, and exact description of the same.

My invention relates to the general class of surgical appliances; and it consists in the novel construction and arrangement of the device or appliance which I shall hereinafter fully describe.

The objects of my invention, generally stated, are three, to wit: first, to prevent involuntary nocturnal seminal emissions; second, to control waking thoughts, and, third, to prevent self-abuse.

other cause his thoughts should be running in lascivious channels, these will be diverted. Voluntary self-abuse will be checked, presuming the wearer be desirous of benefit, as he will not take the trouble to relieve himself of the appliance, and he cannot continue his practice without removing it.

If the wearer be irresponsible from any cause, the appliance can be permanently secured to him, as by a protected line E, extending from the lip a' to the back of belt B, and the fastening-strip a² may be of some permanent character, like sticking-plaster, which will prevent the removal of the extremity of the member from lip a'.

Having thus described my invention, what I claim as new, and desire to secure by Letters

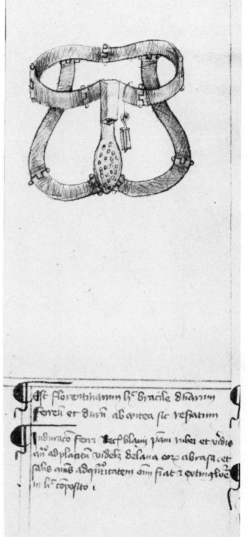

SYMBOLS OF SEXUAL OPPRESSION

(Above) Illustration from a 15th-century manuscript showing a female chastity belt. Such a belt was put on a woman by her husband who kept the key, thereby hoping to prevent her from committing adultery in his absence. The custom illustrates that wives were the property of their husbands who had the right to keep them under lock and key.

(Left) A 19th-century male chastity belt. Such belts or similar contraptions were put on young men by their parents who thereby hoped to prevent them from masturbating. Some worried adult men also put the belts on themselves, because psychiatrists had told them that masturbation would lead to insanity. For a long time this and other absurd psychiatric doctrines were used to justify sexual oppression.

by and large, the sexually positive biblical statements are ignored while the negative ones are stressed. By the same token, the dietary laws of Moses are now widely shrugged off as obsolete, and so are some of his sexual laws, but certain others are fiercely defended, although they are just as archaic. The deeper reasons for this selectivity remain as mysterious as ever.

Under the circumstances, we seem to have little choice but to await further research in this area. In the meantime, however, we do not really have to understand the causes of sexual oppression in order to disapprove of it and to fight against it. Its baneful consequences have been too obvious for too long. Indeed, it is the contemplation of these consequences more than any radical temperament that has always prompted enlightened people to preach greater sexual tolerance. We have, at the beginning of this chapter, quoted a philosopher of the 18th century and mentioned the American founding fathers. They represent a libertarian tradition in our history that can still furnish the means of our emancipation. The authors of the United States Constitution knew the danger of religious and political tyranny and therefore took care to protect the rights of dissenters and nonconformists. Since then, these rights have been further strengthened by numerous decisions of the United States Supreme Court. Indeed, in recent decades the protection of dissent and nonconformity has gradually been extended to the sexual sphere. Thus, Americans now have a constitutional right to marital privacy (Griswold vs. Connecticut, 1965), contraception (Eisenstadt vs. Baird, 1972), and abortion (Roe vs. Wade, 1973). They also may possess and enjoy sexually explicit materials in the privacy of their own homes (Stanley vs. Georgia, 1969). These sexual rights may still be limited, but they provide a basis on which other rights can be built. At any rate, the demand for greater sexual freedom persists and is growing. Even if the Supreme Court, Congress, and the various state legislatures should temporarily try to stall further progress, they will, in the end, have to give in if they want to preserve the principles to which they owe their existence. Democratic government requires autonomous citizens, and if it is an absurdity to deny such citizens the right to their own opinion, it is equally absurd to deny them the right over their own bodies.

Within the last few years, several sexual minorites have formulated their own "bills of rights," thereby challenging the majority to abandon its prejudices. These documents spell out many detailed demands, but, in so doing, they also illustrate the extent of sexual oppression in our society. Finally, and quite appropriately, those who deal with sexual problems in a professional way have felt obliged to summarize the issues in a more general statement. Thus, at the initiative of the sexologist Lester A. Kirkendall, a number of prominent sex researchers have now signed A New Bill of Sexual Rights and Responsibilities (in The Humanist, Jan./Feb. 1976). Among other things, this bill calls for the abandonment of our "reproductive bias" and affirms people's rights to free sexual expression as long as they do not harm others or interfere with their rights. In short, it demands the same freedom with regard to sex that we now take for granted with regard to speech, religion, and the press.

There is, of course, still a great deal of resistance to sexual liberation. Authoritarian politicians, dictatorial judges, orthodox psychiatrists, conservative civic groups, and puritanical churches claim that any loosening of our sexual norms will lead to moral decay and ultimately to the destruction of our society. In support of this claim they usually cite the decline and fall of the Roman empire or some other great nation. However, no competent historian takes this kind of argument seriously, since it cannot be proven. For example, there simply are no statistics about any change in Roman sexual behavior from early to late imperial times. What little we do know does not indicate any significant change between the reigns of Nero (1st century A.D.) and Constantine (4th century A.D.), for example. In any case, Rome fell only under Romulus Augustulus (5th century A.D.), more than a hundred years after it had embraced Christianity and its ascetic sexual doctrines. The conquering heathen barbarians, on the other hand, were sexually much less inhibited. Certainly, classical Greece, Renaissance Italy, and Elizabethan England were quite "permissive" compared to other, less glorious civilizations. Therefore it is rather doubtful that sexual oppression has ever been beneficial to anyone. Indeed, very often it has been the hallmark of sterile and reprehensible cultures like Stalinist Russia and Nazi Germany. Those countries that are dedicated to the ideals of individual liberty will have no difficulty finding their proper course. Sooner or later they will recognize that this liberty is meaningless unless it is extended to the sexual sphere.

The following pages describe the problems of various sexually oppressed groups in our society. One may, of course, with good reason include women as a group among the sexually oppressed. However, since they constitute slightly more than half of the human race, and since their oppression requires a more detailed analysis, they are discussed in a larger special section of this book (see "The Social Roles of Men and Women"). It should also be pointed out that many people belong to more than one group, such as the handicapped teenager, the prisoner with specialized sexual interests, or the aging homosexual who is confined in a mental hospital. Needless to say, in these cases the sexual oppression is all the more severe.

CHILDREN AND ADOLESCENTS

Children are sexual beings from birth. Infants of both sexes are capable of certain elementary sexual responses and can experience some sexual pleasure. At first, their sexuality is rather diffuse, but it becomes more focused as they grow older. Children may begin to masturbate at an early age and learn to enjoy sexual contact with various partners. Where childhood sex play remains uninhibited, it simply continues until puberty brings a dramatic and rather sudden intensification of sexual interests. Adolescents are sexually highly responsive, although in our culture this responsiveness may arrive sooner and be more pronounced in boys than in girls. (See "The Development of Sexual Behavior.")

However, our modern Western civilization does not grant young people the right to sexual satisfaction. In the last few centuries, first childhood and then adolescence have become established as special, protected periods of life in which sexual activity is assumed to be either "unnatural" or dangerous. Thus, most males and females in Europe and America remain sexually frustrated until they are able to marry, i.e., in most cases until they are well over twenty years old. Even worse: They are systematically alienated from their own bodies and indoctrinated with rigid puritanical attitudes which impede their emotional growth. As a result, many of them become insensitive, intolerant, and conformist in sexual matters. Their erotic potential remains underdeveloped and unrefined. This negative conditioning already begins in infancy when mothers deny their babies the most intimate communication by raising them on the bottle, or when they suppress all lustful sensations while breastfeeding them. The deprivation continues when they keep them wrapped up in diapers, clothes, and blankets, instead of allowing them to enjoy complete skin contact and occasional nudity. Finally, the damage is compounded by inflexible daily routines, harsh toilet training, withholding of sexual information, punishment of masturbation, and prevention of exploratory sex play with other children. These and other direct and indirect pressures often succeed in blocking all sexual interests and experiences out of children's minds. This leads to a loss of important primal memories and produces a long period of "latency." (Psychoanalysts ascribe these developments to the "Oedipal conflict.") Puberty then arrives as an unexpected and unpleasant time of trial. The sudden onset of menstruation in girls, more frequent erections and the first ejaculation in boys may be misunderstood as symptoms of a disease. Thus, the lack of sexual knowledge may cause anxiety and confusion. Yet even where adequate knowledge is provided, one basic problem remains: The greatly increased sexual capacity of adolescents cannot be exercised. Modern teenagers may well be told some of the "facts of life," but at the same time they are also informed that for them regular sexual intercourse is out of the question. Therefore, they find themselves restricted to masturbation and various forms of "petting," but even these behaviors are not considered desirable and may actually be denounced as sinful, unhealthy, or immature.

All of this has very serious consequences for the emotional and moral climate in our society. After all, about 40% of the population are sexually mature, but unmarried. Since our official morality makes no allowance for their sexual needs, it creates in our midst a great deal of resentment, hostility, and, indeed, violence. Many young people become openly rebellious or "drop out" of the established system. Those that adapt to it are often emotionally crippled for life. They cannot be happy before they are married and are disappointed thereafter. The reason for this is plain: They are erotically incompetent. Our children and adolescents simply never learn how to be lovers, how to be tender and affectionate, how to give and receive physical pleasure, how to build and maintain mutually rewarding sexual relationships. Instead, they are raised on a steady diet of sexual shame and guilt until some magic wedding ceremony supposedly somehow transforms them into passionate, sensuous, and satisfied husbands and wives. However, in real life such miracles rarely happen. Our sexual rules for the young are therefore not only absurd, but inhumane and destructive.

Many non-Western cultures have shown that this kind of sexual oppression is not necessary. Some American Indian and Polynesian societies, for example, permitted and even encouraged early sexual experimentation in their children. The Muria in Central India even set aside a special building, the *ghotul,* in which children of both sexes spent their nights together. (Similar customs existed among the Trobriand Islanders and the Masai in Africa.) Usually after their sixth or seventh birthday, boys and girls began to sleep in the *ghotul* to which their parents did not have access. Inside, the children practically governed themselves. The older children encouraged the younger ones to become sexually active and instructed them in all sexual techniques. Regular and frequent sexual intercourse was enjoyed as an integral part of childhood and constituted one of the greatest attractions of life in the *ghotul.* Not surprisingly, the Muria children were friendly, graceful, well-behaved, self-reliant, and cooperative. As adults, they lived happily in exclusive and stable marriages. It is only recently with the arrival of compulsory education in government-sponsored schools that this pattern has been disrupted. The "new" Muria children seem to have become just as anxious and inhibited as their counterparts in the rest of the modern world.

Indeed, the "Westernization" of the world has, along with obvious improvements, also brought sexual misery to a great number of formerly satisfied peoples. As we have mentioned earlier, many countries of the so-called Third World are now more puritanical than the old Christian colonialists. Thus, the *Universal Declaration of Human Rights* says nothing about sexual rights. Neither is there any mention of them in the *United Nations Declaration of the Rights of the Child* (passed in 1959). Its ten principles mention the right to a name, a nationality, food, housing, medical care, and compulsory education (!), but are silent about the right to sex education, sexual activity, and the freedom from sexual stereotyping. The document merely states that "the child . . . needs love and understanding" and that he shall, "wherever possible grow up in the care . . . of his parents" (Principle 6). Unfortunately, under present circumstances there is little hope that this declaration will be amended any time soon.

Nevertheless, in those Western countries that are committed to the ideal of individual freedom we can find a growing willingness to extend much of this freedom to children. Thus, in recent years various European and Ameri-

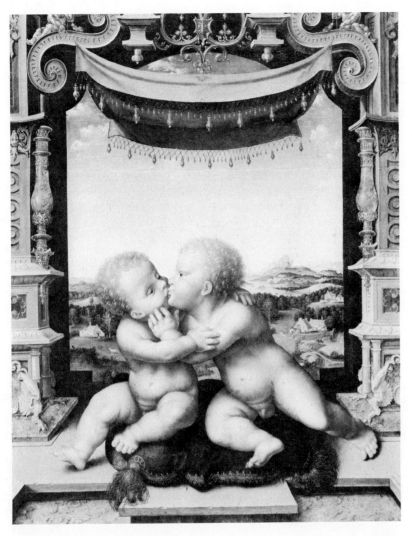

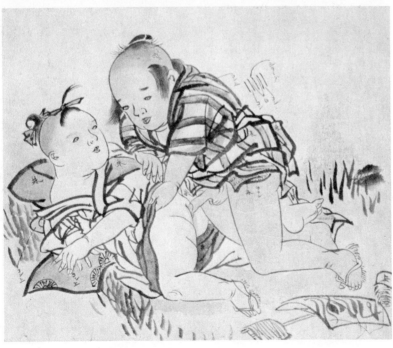

UNINHIBITED CHILDREN

Modern Europeans and Americans often credit Sigmund Freud with having "discovered" the erotic capacities of children. However, in pre-Victorian times and in non-Western cultures these capacities have always been taken for granted.

(Top) European Renaissance artists often painted infants embracing and kissing each other. Shown here are Jesus and St. John the Baptist as children in a painting by Jos van Cleve (1464-1540).

(Bottom) Boy and girl attempting coitus. Scroll painting by Maruyama Okyo, a Japanese artist of the 18th century.

can writers have demanded a more positive sexual education and, indeed, a new "bill of rights" for children that would include sexual rights. These proposals differ in details, but generally agree on these basic points: Children should have the same right to sexual information and sexual activity as adults, and they should not be forced into stereotypical sex roles. This means not only that children would have to be told about contraception, abortion, and venereal disease, but also that they would have to be given access to all "adult" books, magazines, films, and stage shows, including those that are called "pornographic." It further means that children could choose their sexual partners freely (including adult partners), as long as they observed the same decorum as everyone else. "Child molestation" and incest would therefore no longer be crimes unless they involved unwilling children. (Needless to say, at the same time the right and the ability of children to refuse sexual advances would have to be strengthened.) Finally, all sexual discrimination between children would have to cease. Boys and girls would have equal rights to all toys, games, sports, schools, training programs, and occupations.

Undoubtedly, even in the present "permissive" moral climate many parents will find that these suggestions go too far. It is still widely feared that most children would abuse their complete sexual freedom or that they would be exploited by their unscrupulous elders. This fear cannot simply be dismissed, because in our society even many adults are being exploited, and children with their limited strength and experience are all the more vulnerable. However, we should perhaps ask ourselves if it makes sense to condemn sexual activity in children even where no exploitation or any other harm is involved. This also applies to sexual contact between children and adults. By no means all of such contacts are harmful, and it seems irrational to punish them all in a summary fashion.

Less controversy may be created by the sexual liberation of adolescents. It is now commonly agreed that, at least from the age of puberty, boys and girls need accurate information about sexual anatomy and physiology, reproduction, contraception, abortion, and venereal disease. It also seems self-evident that such theoretical knowledge is not enough, and that contraceptives, abortions, and medical treatment of venereal infections must be available to all sexually mature persons regardless of age. (Those teenagers who oppose contraception and abortion should, of course, have the right to refuse them.) It is only fair that girls who can become pregnant and boys who can cause pregnancy should be given the ultimate control over their own bodies. At any rate, their sexual decisions cannot be left up to their parents. Adolescents who are old enough to reproduce are old enough to decide if, when, and how they should become sexually active. It is the duty of society to educate its young in such a way that they can make these decisions responsibly.

If these principles are accepted—and there is a definite trend in this direction—it will be only a matter of time before sex education becomes mandatory in all public schools and safe contraceptives are available from public vending machines everywhere. Moreover, the medical privacy of adolescents will be protected, and parents will not have a veto over their daughter's abortion, no matter how young she might be. All criminal laws against consensual sex acts in private will be abolished, including the notorious laws against "statutory rape." Adolescent boys and girls will be free to choose sexual partners of any age and any sex. They will no longer be declared "delinquents" on account of their sexual habits alone.

Naturally, spelling out these implications of adolescent sexual freedom makes us realize that we still have a long way to go. As a matter of fact, the majority of adults in our society probably prefer to stand pat and resist any further movement. Their concern is genuine, and many of them also have the best interest of their sons and daughters at heart. Therefore it can only help the common cause if their "conservatism" is given a proper hearing. Sexual permissiveness can easily turn into an excuse for emotional neglect. Parents who do not care what their children do, simply do not care for their children.

Sexual freedom means sexual responsibility, not anarchy and license. Boys and girls want, indeed need, firm guidance as they grow up. After all, the development of a human being from self-centered infant to modern citizen repeats, in abbreviated form, the long and arduous civilizing process of the whole human race. This process is not automatic. Spontaneity alone is no longer enough. Some inhibition, coercion, and deprivation will always be necessary.

These may be truisms, but they are sometimes forgotten by overzealous liberationists. Yet, we do not do our young people a favor if we leave them entirely to their own devices. Only if this elementary truth is understood can we begin to grant them sexual freedom. On the other hand, however, we have no right to deny them this freedom, since we know that our present sexual standards are oppressive. It would be a crime to force our children and adolescents into the blind acceptance of a morality that is long overdue for reform.

THE AGING

As we have seen in an earlier chapter, both males and females can remain sexually active into very old age, indeed, as long as they are alive. Of course, serious illnesses or injuries can impair sexual functioning or even kill all interest in sex, but this is true for any age. The fact that in older people the sexual responses are somewhat less vigorous does not mean that they cannot be enjoyed. Under normal conditions, a person's sex life ends only with death. (For details see "The Male Sexual Response" and "The Female Sexual Response.")

However, in the Western world older and even middle-aged persons are often discouraged from sexual activity. They are reprimanded or ridiculed for their sexual interests according to a general assumption that sex in old age is abnormal, indecent, and disgusting. Thus, widows and widowers are scolded by their own adult children for wanting to remarry, residents of nursing homes are sexually segregated and denied any privacy by the staff, aged patients are told by their doctors or nurses to expect and accept a decline of sexual satisfaction, and older homosexuals are refused admission to "gay" bars or bath houses. The common prejudice is particularly strong against sexual relationships between partners of widely different age. A woman who has a much younger husband or lover is frequently viewed with open contempt, and a man with a much younger wife or girl friend is called "dirty." These younger people themselves may be denounced as "neurotic" or suffering from "gerontophilia." Nevertheless, apart from this public harassment, such relationships may be quite satisfying for both partners.

Since all human beings are destined either to die prematurely or to grow old, and since they all need love and affection as long as they are alive, sexual discrimination against the aging is inhumane and barbaric. No one who practices such discrimination or "ageism" can call himself truly civilized. Fortunately, not all societies are prejudiced in this fashion, and even in our own society there are now signs of some change for the better. Young men and women with non-Western backgrounds are often less obsessed with youth and vigor and therefore appreciate the experience and emotional stability of an older sexual partner. They may also be more aware of the fact that age does not have to affect the capacity to provide sexual satisfaction. Since the United States is a country of immigrants and contains a great variety of ethnic groups and subcultures, such open-minded, reasonable, and realistic sexual attitudes can still be found in different parts of the country. By the same token, there are many sociocultural "pockets" in America where an active sex life among the elderly is taken for granted. Furthermore, recent sex research has rediscovered and reconfirmed the sexual interests of the aging, and today there is a growing number of professionals who try to educate the public on this issue. Their efforts are directed primarily toward doctors, nurses, social workers and others who are concerned with the elderly, but they also address a wider audience. There is an obvious need for a general reorientation. Sexual activity can greatly contribute to the maintenance of good health in old age and therefore needs to be encouraged. Nursing homes, rooming houses, "retirement villages," and "senior citizen hotels" must take the sexual needs of their residents into account and allow them to be satisfied. In fact, very often hormone replacement and various physical therapies can be employed to keep sexual interests alive. At the same time, of course, great tact and discretion are necessary in approaching each individual. While it is unfair to ignore an older person's sexual needs, it would also be wrong to exert any pressure to perform or to set up a new sexual achievement standard for the aging. After all, like everyone else, the aging deserve to keep their sexual options and to live according to their own best judgment and ability.

HOMOSEXUALS

Many people enjoy sexual intercourse with members of their own sex, either occasionally or frequently and, in some cases, even exclusively. However, in our particular culture such behavior is generally considered bad and may be severely punished. As a result, all those who feel an erotic attraction to the same sex (and they represent a sizable percentage of the population) find themselves restrained, frustrated, denounced, and persecuted—in short, oppressed.

This oppression already begins with our very language, which today refers to these people as "homosexuals." We have pointed out earlier that it is highly questionable to use this word for any human being, and that, in the present book, we do so only with very specific reservations. (See the introduction to "Homosexual Intercourse.") The fact of the matter is that the term prejudges the issue in the most fundamental way. The ancient and medieval terms for same-sex behavior (pederasty, Greek love, sodomy, buggery, etc.) had always referred to a form of conduct, not a condition. They described acts that might be committed by anybody and did not imply the existence of a particular type of person. In other words, when someone was called a pederast, Greek lover, sodomite, or bugger, he was thereby characterized as a man who did certain things, not as a man who suffered from some inherent peculiarity. Thus, for example, one could not be a "latent pederast" or, in adolescence, go through a "sodomitic phase." Nor was there such a thing as "pseudo-buggery." However, our modern word "homosexual" is different. In its original German form homosexuell it was coined in 1869 by the German-writing Hungarian doctor Benkert. (He wrote under the pseudonym Kertbeny.) Benkert, like many of his medical colleagues, believed that the erotic attraction to the same sex was a mysterious condition typical of a certain small group of people, and that these people were therefore a breed apart from everyone else. In trying to name their condition, he hit upon the awkward, half-Greek and half-Latin "scientific" term Homosexualität. For the "normal" condition of the majority the antonym Heterosexualität then simply suggested itself, and since both words could easily be adapted to other languages, they soon became popular all over Europe.

However, today we know that the basic assumption behind these two categories is false. Homosexual and heterosexual preferences are matters of degree, and they are not mutually exclusive. "Homosexuals" do not suffer from an intrinsic condition, but play a particular social role. Not all societies recognize such a role, and even in our society same-sex behavior is not restricted to "homosexuals." In other words, real life is too varied for these simplistic divisions. There are countless gradations between the extremes, and many people are attracted to both sexes. Those who are singled out as "homosexuals" may have little in common besides this label. Thus, "homosexuality" is not an objective characteristic of certain persons, but rather a deviant status that is conferred upon them by others. By definition, this kind of deviance is possible only in cultures which perceive same-sex behavior as problematic.

Unfortunately, we continue to live in such a culture, and thus the obsolete Victorian medical terms are also still with us. Some contemporary writers try to give them a new meaning or to use them in a modern, less prejudicial fashion, but the misunderstandings persist. In view of this fact, nonprofessional libertarians who want social approval for same-sex behavior now often prefer to speak of "gay people" and "gayness." However, this is a rather dubious improvement. The word "gay" is, of course, older than "homosexual," since it dates back to the Middle Ages when it meant nothing more than "cheerful" or "colorful." Yet, beginning in the 17th century, it also denoted loose morals, and in the 19th century it further referred to a female prostitute (a "gay woman"). In America, the word had still another peculiar connotation. As Bertrand Russell reports in his *Autobiography* (Years 1872-1914), the Quakers in late 19th-century Philadelphia called "gay" any "meaningless" religious custom practiced by non-Quakers. This included all fixed formulas. Thus, for them the Lord's Prayer and the Ten Commandments were "gay." It was not until our own century that the word also became synonymous with "homosexual," but at first this usage was restricted to the "gay" subculture. Its wider acceptance dates only from the last decade. However, short and simple as it may be, the term still draws an artificial dividing line between two sexual camps: "gay" and nongay (now usually called "straight"). Thus, the old pressures toward polarization continue.

Indeed, in recent decades there even has been a polarization between "gay" males and females. Until well into modern times, the same-sex behavior of women never attracted much religious, legal, or medical attention, and there was no special term for such behavior, except the word "tribadism" (from Greek *tribein:* to rub), which referred to mutual bodily friction or manual intercourse (masturbation) between women. Then, in the 19th century, oral intercourse (cunnilingus) between women was described with two new special terms: "sapphism" and "lesbianism" (after the ancient Greek poetess Sappho and the island of Lesbos where she lived). However, gradually all three terms broadened their meaning, and it became customary to call all sexual behavior between women either "tribadic," or "sapphic," or "lesbian." Finally, in our own century, the word "lesbian" replaced the two others, and today it is also used as a noun meaning "female homosexual." Thus, "lesbians" have now emerged as the female subgroup of the general category "homosexuals," i.e., as a special minority within a minority. (In Greek and Roman antiquity the terms "Lesbianist" and "to lesbianize" had already been well known, but had referred exclusively to the sucking of the penis ["active" and "passive" fellatio]. Thus, they had most often been applied to men.)

For several reasons, the modern semantic development was inevitable and even desirable, but before we discuss them, we should once more remind ourselves that all our current terms are based on obsolete, narrow concepts and are therefore essentially oppressive. If it is wrong to speak of "homosexuals" as a distinct and separate group of people, then it is equally wrong to speak of "lesbians" as a distinct and separate group of women. (Fortunately, no one has yet tried to label their male counterparts "Spartans" or "Athenians.") There can be only one justification for any such labels, and that is to identify certain victims of social discrimination. Once this discrimination has ended, the labels will automatically disappear with it.

In the meantime, of course, "homosexual" women do have special problems, because, in addition to being sexual deviants, they are females in a

A HOMOSEXUAL BILL OF RIGHTS

I

BASIC RIGHTS

1. Private consensual sex acts between persons over the age of consent shall not be offenses.

2. Solicitation for any sexual act shall not be an offense except upon the filing of a complaint by the aggrieved party, not a police officer or agent.

3. A person's sexual orientation or practice shall not be a factor in the granting or renewing of Federal security clearance, visas, and the granting of citizenship.

4. Service in and discharge from the armed forces and eligibility to VA benefits shall be without reference to homosexuality.

5. A person's sexual orientation or practice shall not affect his eligibility for employment with federal, state, or local governments.

II

AREAS FOR IMMEDIATE REFORM

1. Police and other government agents shall cease the practice of enticement and entrapment of homosexuals.

2. Police shall desist from notifying the employers of those arrested for homosexual offenses.

3. Neither the police department nor any other government agency shall keep files solely for the purpose of identifying homosexuals.

4. The practice of harassing bars and other establishments and of revoking their licenses because they cater to homosexuals cease.

5. The practice of reviewing less-than-honorable military discharges, granted for homosexual orientation or practice, shall be established, with the goal of upgrading such discharges.

6. The registration of sex offenders shall not be required.

7. City ordinances involving sexual matters shall be rescinded and these matters left to state legislatures.

8. Conviction for homosexual offenses shall not be the basis for prohibiting issuance of professional licenses nor for the revocation of these licenses.

9. No questions regarding sexual orientation or practice shall appear on application forms, personnel data sheets, or in personal interviews.

10. No governmental agency shall use the classification of homosexuality to limit the freedom of any homosexual.

Flyer distributed by a homosexual civil rights organization.
Courtesy: Society for Individual Rights, San Francisco, California

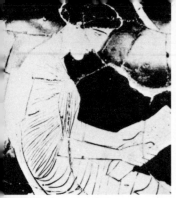
ppho (fl. about 600 B.C.)·
reek poet

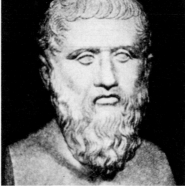
Sophocles (496?–406 B.C.)
Greek dramatist

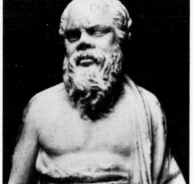
Socrates (470?–399 B.C.)
Greek philosopher

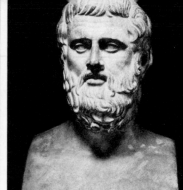
Plato (427?–347 B.C.)
Greek philosopher

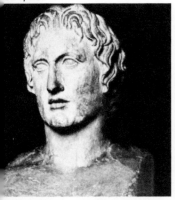
exander the Great (356–323 B.C.)
reek conqueror

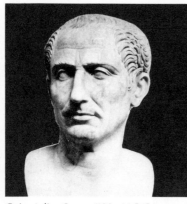
Gaius Julius Caesar (100–44 B.C.)
Roman general and statesman

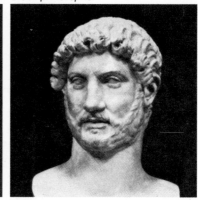
Hadrian (72–138 A.D.)
Roman emperor

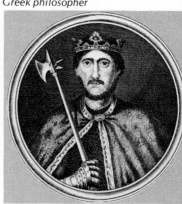
Richard I (the Lion-hearted) (1157–1199)
English king

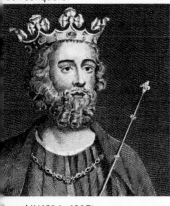
ward II (1284–1327)
glish king

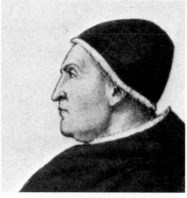
Sixtus IV (Franceso della Rovere)
(1414–1484) Italian Pope

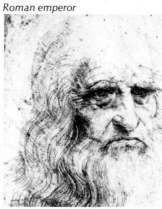
Leonardo da Vinci (1452–1519)
Italian artist and scientist

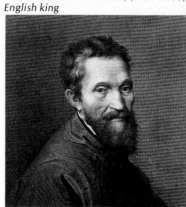
Michelangelo Buonarroti (1475–1564)
Italian artist and poet

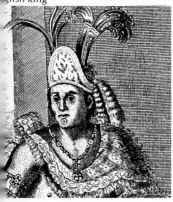
ontezuma II (1480–1520)
tec emperor

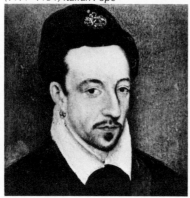
Henry III (1551–1589)
French king

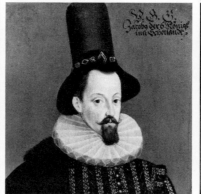
James I (1566–1625)
English king

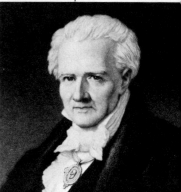
Alexander von Humboldt (1769–1859)
German naturalist and statesman

FAMOUS "HOMOSEXUALS" As Alfred C. Kinsey has pointed out, it is problematical to use the word "homosexual" to describe a person. Such labeling is often arbitrary and over-broad. Especially in the United States today many people have unrealistic ideas about what "homosexuals" are or how they behave. However, throughout history a great number of men and women (many of them quite famous) have felt sexually attracted to members of their own sex either occasionally or frequently, or even exclu-

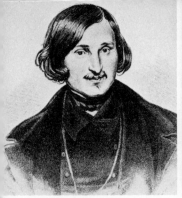
Nikolai Gogol (1809–1852)
Russian writer

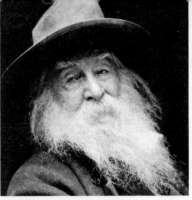
Walt Whitman (1819–1892)
American poet

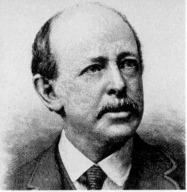
Horatio Alger (1834–1899)
American clergyman and novelist

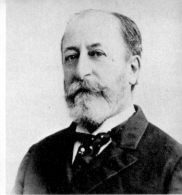
Camille Saint-Saëns (1835–1921)
French composer

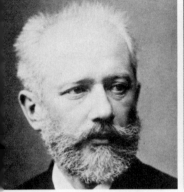
Petr Ilich Tchaikovsky (1840–1893)
Russian composer

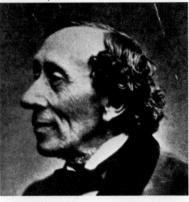
Hans Christian Andersen (1805–1875)
Danish writer

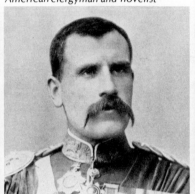
Hector Macdonald (1853–1903)
British soldier

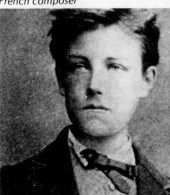
Arthur Rimbaud (1854–1891)
French poet

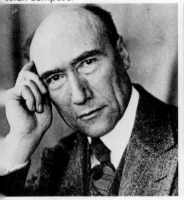
André Gide (1869–1951)
French writer

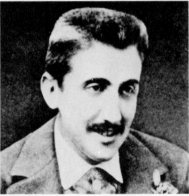
Marcel Proust (1871–1922)
French novelist

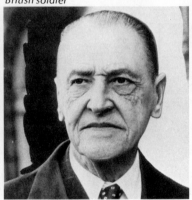
W. Somerset Maugham (1874–1965)
English writer

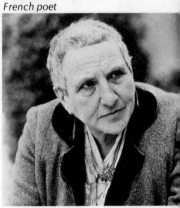
Gertrude Stein (1874–1946)
American writer

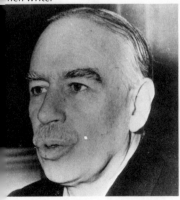
John Maynard Keynes (1883–1946)
English economist

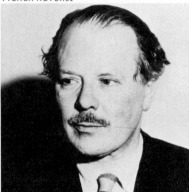
Harold Nicolson (1886–1961)
English writer

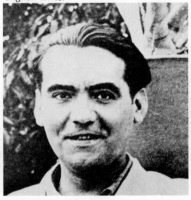
Federico Garcia Lorca (1898–1936)
Spanish poet

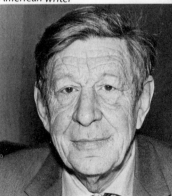
W. H. Auden (1907–1973)
Anglo-American poet

sively. Some acted upon this feeling and were openly proud of it; others suppressed it and led very unhappy lives. Many were even persecuted by their contemporaries and came to a tragic end. The above portrait gallery shows some historical personalities who are known to have had strong homosexual leanings. Obviously, this list is not meant to prove that such leanings make people in any way superior. Still, it can perhaps help to counteract certain false current stereotypes.

x
THE SEXUALLY OPPRESSED   449

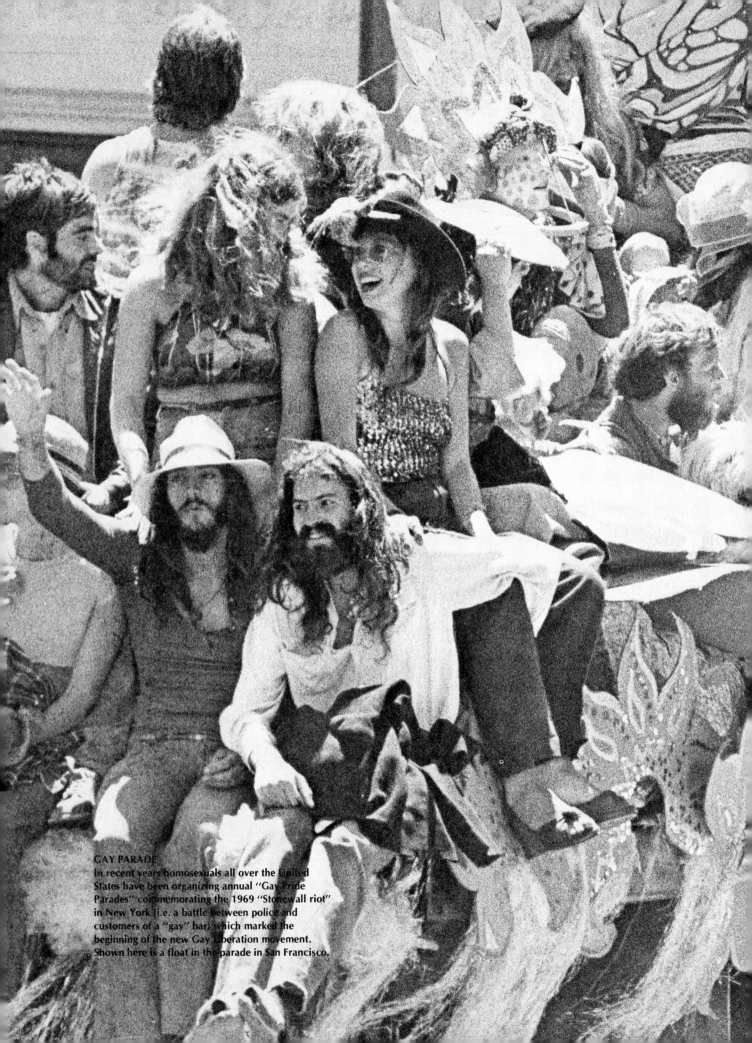

GAY PARADE
In recent years homosexuals all over the United
States have been organizing annual "Gay-Pride
Parades" commemorating the 1969 "Stonewall riot"
in New York (i.e. a battle between police and
customers of a "gay" bar) which marked the
beginning of the new Gay Liberation movement.
Shown here is a float in the parade in San Francisco.

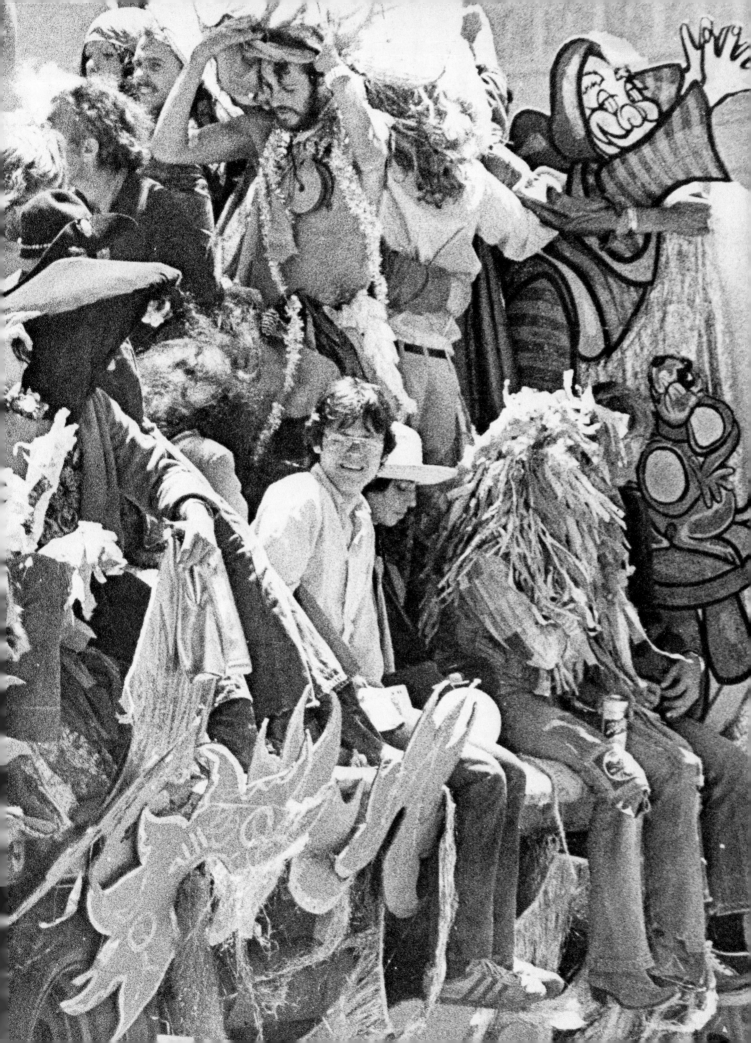

male-dominated culture. If, in general, their sexual behavior is more easily tolerated by the criminal law, it can nevertheless provide a pretext for other forms of official harassment. To cite only one example, in many American courts "lesbianism" is considered sufficient ground to deny mothers the custody of their own children. Needless to say, in housing, employment, military service, etc. they are subject to the same injustices as all "homosexuals." However, in all of these cases their plight is aggravated by the fact that they are female. In short, they suffer a double discrimination, and thus many of them feel that their struggle for sexual liberation is different from that of "gay" males.

We have described in another section how in the Western world religious beliefs, legal doctrines, and psychiatric theories have, for a long time, victimized many harmless sexual deviants and especially homosexuals. (See "Conformity and Deviance.") It is not necessary to repeat the details of this victimization here. May it suffice to say that in the present United States homosexuals are still one of the largest and most oppressed minorities. Since the term "homosexual" for a person is imprecise, misleading, and ultimately inappropriate, it is not possible to total up any meaningful numbers of homosexuals. Still, Kinsey's studies have shown that even by the narrowest and most conservative traditional definition we are talking about many millions of Americans who suffer because of our hatred and fear of same-sex behavior.

Neutral observers have often described this fear as a manifestation of the widespread, irrational fear of physical love in our culture, i.e., as a form of "erotophobia." In fact, recently some writers have used the term "homoerotophobia," or "homophobia" for short, to refer specifically to the irrational fear of love between partners of the same sex. That many people are obsessed with this fear cannot be doubted. Typically, they do not know any homosexuals, do not want to meet them, see them, or hear about them, but would like them to be controlled, contained, put away, locked up, or eliminated. If they discover homosexuals in their own family, they disown them. Very often, however, they live for years very closely with homosexuals at home, at school, or at work without recognizing them. This can happen, because homophobia first creates and then feeds on a stereotype of the dreaded enemy that is completely unrealistic. For instance, in America today the "typical" male homosexual (queer, faggot, sissie, pansy, etc.) is believed to be effeminate, weak, "artistic," and immature. However, in actual fact this type of person is rare among homosexuals. The majority are simply "average", i.e., they look and behave like everyone else, and thus, if they wish, they can remain undetected. Many of them, in fact, make that choice. They either "stay in the closet" or lead an elaborate double life. As a result they are never available to challenge the popular misconceptions.

We should understand, however, that this "straight" masquerade and enforced hypocrisy takes its toll on both the oppressed and the oppressors. The former must waste a great deal of energy on dissembling, and the latter are haunted by foolish fantasies and superfluous apprehensions. This, in turn, forces everyone into a stifling sexual rigidity. Such a state of affairs cannot be considered moral or wholesome by anyone's definition. Many thoughtful observers have therefore long advocated the emancipation of homosexuals. Indeed, in the meantime some vigorous "gay" civil rights organizations and lobbying groups have been formed which try to further this goal. In addition, a growing "gay" press is educating its special audience and the public at large about the realities of "gay" life. In some parts of the country homosexuals have also developed some political power as a voting block that can no longer be ignored. As a result of these and other efforts, much progress has already been made. A significant number of states in the United States have repealed their sodomy laws, the Civil Service no longer bars homosexuals from federal employment, and some local governments have even adopted civil rights ordinances protecting homosexuals against discrimination in housing, jobs, insurance, and other areas. A further boost to the homosexual civil rights struggle has been the 1973 decision of the American Psychiatric Association to remove homosexuality from its list of mental disorders. This decision alone undercut much of the popular rationalization of homophobia.

It is to be hoped that, in the future, all discrimination against homosexuals will end. Sexual orientation, like sex, race, religious belief, and national origin, should not be grounds for denying anyone equal rights. Therefore, the civil rights struggle of homosexuals, like that of other oppressed people, deserves to succeed. However, it would be unfortunate if, in the course of this struggle a "gay" minority became more clearly defined and permanently established as a separate social group. A continued sexual separatism, even on the basis of full equality, would still be oppressive in itself, because it creates artificial lines of division and forces people into false alternatives. The ultimate liberation of both homosexuals and heterosexuals can lie only in the abandonment of all labels and in everyone's freedom to explore his own sexual potential, whatever it may be.

THE HANDICAPPED
AND DISABLED

As we have seen in two previous sections, the human sexual and reproductive functions can be physically and psychologically impaired (see "Some Physical Problems" and "Sexual Maladjustment"). It is also obvious that these functions can be indirectly affected by a great number of nonsexual injuries, disorders, disabilities, and diseases. Indeed, the damage may well be compounded by ignorance and negative social attitudes. Thus, as a rule, physically or mentally handicapped persons find themselves confronted with special sexual problems of their own.

In our society the handicapped and disabled, such as amputees, paraplegics and quadriplegics, and the victims of cerebral palsy, may receive much valuable medical help, but very little support in developing their sexual interests. On the contrary, under the pretext of "protection," their families, friends, doctors, nurses, and teachers often deny them any opportunity to become sexually active or even explicitly discourage them. Many people simply assume that a serious physical or mental handicap precludes any hope for a rewarding sex life. However, this assumption is false. Except for extremely serious cases, in which the sheer need to survive requires all available energy, some form of sexual pleasure is always possible. The fact that this simple truth is not widely recognized only reflects the sensual poverty of our culture.

The situation is especially difficult for those handicapped or disabled persons who live in hospitals, convalescent or nursing homes, or similar institutions. In such places patients usually have very little privacy and little opportunity to meet other people from the outside. Living quarters are sexually segregated. In addition, the staff is often prudish and intolerant. Many doctors, in fact, do not know that their patients are capable of sexual enjoyment and thus never think of discussing the subject. Thus, the men and women in their care remain without guidance, and many possible sexual alternatives are left unexplored. Furthermore, many hospital administrations feel that they cannot permit any sexual activity on their premises, because this would bring them in conflict with the law, and, unfortunately, this concern may be justified. Conservative employees or relatives of patients who disapprove of nonmarital sex might bring suit against the institution. Finally, since many patients are incapable of coitus and therefore practice other forms of sexual intercourse, they may well be guilty of "sodomy" or "crimes against nature" as defined in many state penal codes. This is another reason why doctors may be reluctant to help their patients with necessary sexual experimentations. Needless to say, all of this applies not only to long-term, but also to short-term patients. Many people are hospitalized for only a few months or even weeks and, during that time, are needlessly deprived of sexual intercourse. Not every illness demands sexual abstinence, but virtually no hospital offers its patients an opportunity to become intimate with visiting spouses or lovers. On the other hand, in case of a serious illness, lovers may not even be allowed to visit at all, because they are not officially recognized "family members." Such a regulation is especially insensitive to homosexual patients.

Fortunately, in recent years a more humane and sophisticated approach has been gaining ground. Clinical sex research has shown that a great many of even severely handicapped persons can enjoy sex if they are willing to raise their sexual consciousness and to break out of conventional patterns. As it turns out, very often their partners are happy to go along with them. Indeed, in the meantime special explicit books and films have become available which demonstrate the sexual options open to the handicapped. When these materials are shown in a hospital, they not only help the patients and their families, but also educate the staff. As a result, some institutions have, in fact, changed their policies and now allow their patients to find sexual satisfaction either with other patients or with regular outside visitors.

Unusual problems are faced by the mentally handicapped, especially those who are institutionalized. Still, in principle, everything said above also applies to them. In the past, they were often treated as if they had no sexual interests or sexual rights. As children, the mentally "deficient" or "retarded" were given no sex education of any kind, as adolescents and adults they were forcibly prevented from engaging in any sexual activity and even routinely sterilized against their will. If they wanted to marry, the law would not permit it. However, it is now increasingly being recognized that such unfeeling rigidity is uncalled for. Mentally handicapped children, like all other children, need to learn about conception, contraception, and venereal disease. They also need love and physical affection and therefore should have the right to any sexual activity of their choosing, as long as it is consensual and private. The necessary privacy should be provided by their families or by the institutions to which they are confined. On the other hand, the mentally handicapped also have to be protected against sexual exploitation. This can be done by personal attention, appropriate institutional regulations, and sensible criminal laws. (Laws which define all sexual contact with the mentally handicapped as statutory rape end up victimizing those they are meant to protect.) Where sterilization seems desirable, informed consent should be obtained. Yet, as a matter of policy, the least restrictive alternative should always be preferred. As long as nobody else is harmed, all handicapped and disabled persons are entitled to full sexual fulfillment according to their abilities.

PERSONS WITH SPECIALIZED SEXUAL INTERESTS

Since human sexual behavior is not instinctive, but is shaped by a variety of social influences, different human beings develop different sexual interests and behave sexually in different ways. This fact need not, in itself, create any problems, but most societies set up certain standards or norms for sexual behavior, and if these norms are rigid and narrow, a great number of people may be defined as sexual deviants. (See the introduction to "The Development of Sexual Behavior" and "Conformity and Deviance.")

In our own society the sexual norms have traditionally been extremely restrictive and unrealistic, and thus there have always been many individuals with "sexual problems" or, to be more precise, with social problems which sprang from their need for sexual expression. Their behavior did not fit the prescribed pattern, and thus they found themselves forcibly restrained, frustrated, defamed, and persecuted.

Of course, some social restraint is necessary where sexual acts involve unwilling partners, i.e., where they have clearly identifiable victims. This is the case with rape and all other forms of sexual assault and molestation. However, where sexual behavior is consensual and private, there is no need, and indeed no justification, for social interference. On the contrary, any such interference, whether legal or psychiatric, is intrinsically oppressive, no matter how well intended. It may be that some sexual deviants or eccentrics are maladjusted and could profit from some form of therapy, but this should not be imposed by force. Nor should their sexual abstinence before any "cure" be required. As long as they harm no one else, they deserve to live according to their own values. Even if we perceive them as sexually crippled (and this perception may well be wrong), we have no right to take away their crutches. After all, it would be a double injustice for society first to create such cripples through sex-negative doctrines, emotional neglect, or degrading living conditions and then to punish them once more by denying them the little sexual satisfaction of which they are still capable.

One thing cannot be doubted: Many people in our society have, through no fault of their own, developed sexual interests that lead them far away from our official sexual norm. In the past, such persons were called sinners or heretics, and today they are often denounced as "perverts" or "sexual psychopaths," but regardless of the label, they are, as a rule, deprived of their right to sexual fulfillment, even if it does not interfere with the rights of anyone else. Some, for example, like to be hurt or humiliated during sexual intercourse, others like to dominate their partners, play with urine or excrement, talk "dirty," or watch people masturbate. Still others like to dress in the clothes of the other sex or are sexually dependent on some piece of underwear, a doll, a motorbike, or another inanimate object. The variations are endless, and there is no need to be exhaustive. The main point is that all of these persons with highly specialized sexual interests usually get little support from their communities, have difficulty finding appropriate partners, and most often are left unsatisfied. Many of them are unsuited for marriage and thus live alone and unappreciated in terrible isolation. Not infrequently, they also feel embarrassed and guilty about their desires which they dare not reveal to others. In short, even if they do not come in outright conflict with the law, their lives are likely to be very unhappy.

Yet, with a more tolerant social attitude none of this would be necessary. In fact, we can safely assume that even the most unusual sexual tastes could be satisfied if people were given a chance to look openly for willing partners. In some cases, such partners might have to be paid for their services, but except for totally bizarre or destructive sexual wishes, there should be no lack of gratification. Moreover, society could lend its support by taking suitable action. For example, in 1964 the Swedish physician Lars Ullerstam suggested legal reforms that would permit the establishment of contact bureaus for all erotic minorities. He also proposed specific personal "sex ads" in newspapers and endorsed social clubs in which sexual eccentrics could meet to indulge in their particular fantasies. Certain movie theaters could be set aside to show "sex films" geared to particular audiences, and brothels could be built that would cater to special sexual requests. Indeed, Ullerstam demanded the creation of mobile brothels that could visit suburbs, isolated neighborhoods, hospitals, and nursing homes. The employees of these brothels should be called "erotic Samaritans" and should be highly respected.

Needless to say, when these proposals were first made, they found little public support. In the meantime, however, some of them have been silently adopted in many Western countries. Some European countries have legalized both female and male prostitution along with so-called "pornographic" films, books, and magazines. Even in the United States many cities now have their "adult" theaters, peep shows, bookstores, and "toy shops." There is also a growing number of newspapers and periodicals which publish personal "sex ads." Special "bath houses" offer sexual opportunities to homosexual, and recently even heterosexual, customers. Certain "massage parlors" provide sexual relief for the tired and lonely, and "sex clinics" employ "sexual surrogates" to treat the sexually inadequate. Special clubs organize "swingers' parties" or orgies, sexual "weekend retreats," camping trips, and cruises. Finally, there are hotels and resorts which specialize in sexual recreation.

These developments have undoubtedly helped not only millions of "average" people, but also the sexual minorities, and for this reason alone they ought to be welcomed. Far from proving any "degeneracy" of our civilization, they show, on the contrary, that it has become more enlightened and humane. If some of the new establishments retain an aura of tawdriness and exploitation it is mostly the fault of our outdated laws which force them "underground" or into the arms of unscrupulous hucksters and organized crime. In Europe, elegant, well-appointed, and well-lit "sex shops," "porno theaters," and "sex clubs" are run by respectable people and can be found in the best business districts next to fashion houses and expensive jewelers' stores. Prostitutes can work without pimps in pleasant surroundings. In sum, there is no longer a compulsion to keep sex "smutty" or "filthy." Obviously, if the public were willing, the same improvements could also be made in America.

"SEX ADS"

Both Europe and the United States have recently seen the appearance of newspapers which carry personal "sex ads." Many of these advertisements are directed toward persons with specialized sexual interests, and some are thinly disguised offers by male and female prostitutes. (From a California newspaper 1976.)

PERSONS COMMITTED
TO MENTAL HOSPITALS

In the United States today more than three times as many people are committed to mental hospitals each year than are sent to state or federal prisons. The grounds for such commitment and the commitment procedures vary from state to state, but among the involuntary patients of mental hospitals one may find not only those who are called mentally ill, but also "mental defectives," epileptics, alcoholics, drug addicts, and a variety of other deviants or social nonconformists. Indeed, the term "mental hospital" should not be taken too literally. In actual fact it is often a multipurpose institution: a hospital, a prison, a poorhouse, and an old people's home.

This situation is more easily understood if one considers the history of mental hospitals. Until modern times Western societies usually did not distinguish between the insane, the vagrant, the criminal, and the indigent, but accorded all of them the same treatment. For centuries they were executed, mutilated, banished, or held in bondage, and eventually they were mostly confined. Thus, the first "houses of correction" were built to accommodate many different classes of inmates. The first such institution in Connecticut in 1727, for instance, was meant to house "all rogues, vagabonds, or idle persons going about in town or country begging, common drunkards, common nightwalkers, pilferers, wanton and lascivious persons, . . . and also persons under distraction and unfit to go at large. . . ." Later, when special insane asylums and mental hospitals were established, an attempt was made to keep out the poor (who might enjoy the free room and board), but all sorts of other misfits could be committed simply on the director's assertion that they were mentally ill. As a matter of fact, sometimes no evidence of insanity was required, as for instance in mid-19th century Illinois, where disobedient married women could be committed at the whim of their husbands. These and other blatant abuses subsequently led to more stringent commitment laws, but official relapses have occurred, especially in the 1930s and '40s when a number of state legislatures began to allow the involuntary commitment of "psychopaths," especially "sexual psychopaths." Like the "wanton and lascivious persons" of the 18th century, these "sexual psychopaths" are an ill-defined mixed group of various harmful and harmless sexual deviants who fit no single psychiatric diagnosis. In fact, many of them cannot be called ill in any medical sense. Their "hospitalization" and "treatment" is nothing but an excuse for keeping them locked up somewhere, because if they were treated as criminals they might either not be convicted at all or serve relatively short sentences. (See also "Current Sex Laws in the U.S.")

The commitment to a mental hospital is a civil, not a criminal procedure, and therefore does not offer the procedural safeguards which protect the common criminal. After all, people are committed only "for their own good"; they are to be treated, not punished. As a result, it is extremely difficult for them to assert their rights and, indeed, as "mental patients" they lose virtually all of their rights to the hospital staff. They can be released only if and when this staff declares them to be "cured" or "safe." Moreover, while in the hospital, they may be subjected to various brutal "therapies" from electroshock to "psychosurgery" and "chemical castration." This is particularly disturbing in the case of socially harmless sexual eccentrics and other nonviolent "psychopaths."

Of course, with regard to sexual rights all institutionalized mental patients are equal: They do not have any. Thus, not only the sexually deviant, but also the "normal" inmates find themselves frustrated. Just as in ordinary hospitals, nursing homes, and other such places, there is no privacy and no opportunity for sexual intercourse. Most of what has been said about the aging, handicapped, and disabled therefore also applies here. There is, in principle, no valid reason for such wholesale sexual deprivation. On the contrary, sexual fulfillment could very often contribute to better health and help patients readjust to the world outside. For example, it would surely be beneficial for many of them if they could continue their sexual relationships with visiting spouses and lovers. But even within the institution itself sexual relationships might be feasible as long as pregnancies can be avoided. Certainly, homosexual patients should not have to remain abstinent, if they find willing partners. (Needless to say, sex between patients and hospital staff would have to remain taboo, because the latter enjoy a position of nearly absolute power over the former. This could easily lead to sexual exploitation.) It is clear, however, that significant sexual reforms in mental institutions can be accomplished only if the institutional psychiatrists themselves become more tolerant of human sexual variety and stop labeling every deviant as mentally ill. This would render many of the current "therapies" superfluous and, indeed, often prevent any forced commitment in the first place.

THE IMPRISONED

The inmates of American prisons are, as a rule, deprived of any heterosexual activity. The general public perceives this deprivation as part of their deserved punishment and, so far, has shown little enthusiasm for reform. As a result, the only types of sexual behavior found in prison today are solitary masturbation and homosexual intercourse. This is true for both men's and women's prisons.

Under the circumstances one might suppose that at least homosexuals are sexually satisfied in prison, but this is not actually the case. After all, among prisoners, as in the rest of the population, heterosexuals are in the majority, and their sexual frustration is immense. A great many of them vent this frustration by sexually assaulting younger and weaker inmates, i.e., by engaging in homosexual rape and other forms of vicious and destructive homosexual conduct. Thus, the widespread homosexual activity in prison, far from providing real satisfaction, is basically negative and oppressive. It is usually violent and, in fact, often expresses hate and contempt for its victims. Thus, paradoxically, it reinforces the general homophobia which is so typical of our culture. In short, most prisoners, regardless of their orientation, are likely to lead a degrading and dehumanizing sex life while "inside," and this will certainly leave its mark even after their return to freedom. Furthermore, in many cases it is not only the prisoners who are sexually deprived, but also their spouses or lovers. Wives and husbands may have great difficulty keeping their marriages intact while they wait for the release of their imprisoned partners. However, not all returned prisoners are able to readjust to their previous sexual partners, and thus their marriages or love relationships may break up after all.

All of this seems to suggest that the sexual deprivation and resulting brutalization of prisoners may not be in the best interest of society. Indeed, in the meantime some countries, such as Mexico and Canada, have tried to offer some sexual relief for their prisoners by allowing them "conjugal visits" or holiday furloughs. Such programs have also been tried in Europe and in a few states of the U.S., most notably Mississippi and California. Under a "conjugal visit" program, inmates can be visited overnight in relative privacy by their wives; holiday furloughs or overnight leaves are granted to selected prisoners who can briefly pursue their sexual interests in the community, after which they return to prison. These reforms may not only preserve marriages, but also help to reduce sexual tensions and homosexual attacks among the prisoners themselves.

However, since only a fraction of the prison population is involved, no great overall impact can be expected. Furloughs are exceptional by definition, and "conjugal visits" naturally exclude unmarried and homosexual partners. It should also be pointed out that there have never been conjugal visit programs in female prisons. In view of these facts, the existing modest sexual relief programs are therefore inadequate. At best, they are first steps in the right direction. The general sexual oppression of the imprisoned can be brought to an end only through a comprehensive reform of our entire penal system.

Reference and Recommended Reading

Altman, Dennis. *Homosexual: Oppression and Liberation*. New York: Avon, 1973.

Boggan, Carrington E., M.C. Haft, Ch. Lister and J.P. Rupp. *The Rights of Gay People* (An American Civil Liberties Union Handbook). New York: Avon, 1975.

Brenton, Myron. *Sex and Your Heart,* New York: Coward McCann, 1968.

Butler, Robert N. and Myrna I. Lewis. *Sex After Sixty: A Guide for Men and Women for Their Later Years*. New York: Harper & Row, 1976.

De la Cruz, Felix F. and la Veck, Gerald D., eds. *Human Sexuality and the Mentally Retarded*. Baltimore: Penguin, 1974.

Farson, Richard. *Birthrights: A Bill of Rights for Children*. New York: Macmillan, 1974.

Gochros, Harvey L. and Jean, eds. *The Sexually Oppressed*. New York: Association Press, 1977.

Heslinga, K. *Not Made of Stone: The Sexual Problems of Handicapped People*. Springfield Ill.: Ch.C. Thomas, 1974.

Katz, Jonathan. *Gay American History: Lesbians and Gay Men in the U.S.A.* New York: Crowell, 1976 (paper).

Martin, Del, and Phyllis Lyon. *Lesbian/Woman*. New York: Bantam, 1972.

Mooney, T.O., et al. *Sexual Options for Paraplegics and Quadriplegics*. Boston: Little, Brown, 1975 (paper).

Ullerstam, Lars. *The Erotic Minorities*. New York: Grove Press, 1966.

13. THE "SEXUAL REVOLUTION"

At the end of the Second World War, Wilhelm Reich introduced American readers to some of his earlier writings under the title *The Sexual Revolution* (1945). Explaining that this revolution went to the "roots" of human emotional, social, and economic existence, he presented himself as a radical (from Latin *radix*: root), i.e. as a man who examines these roots and who then fearlessly speaks the truth that sets humanity free.

The truth, according to Reich, was that Western civilization had made people sick by imposing on them an unnatural, destructive sexual morality. However, thanks to various modern social and scientific upheavals, the natural human life functions were finally awakening after a sleep of thousands of years. The future would restore sexual health and, for the first time, bring full human autonomy.

Reich left no doubt that, in the interest of human happiness, he hoped for profound political changes, and thus, when he spoke of "revolution," he meant it quite literally. In this respect he upheld the tradition of many earlier writers. After all, for a long time before him fighters for sexual freedom had defined themselves as rebels and revolutionaries. Notably, the American feminist movement had never been shy about using such terms. During the First World War, for example, Margaret Sanger had published a magazine *The Woman Rebel*, and as early as 1868 Elizabeth Cady Stanton and Susan B. Anthony had edited a suffragist newspaper *The Revolution*. Indeed, even in 1776, at the birth of American independence, Abigail Adams had threatened her husband John with a "Rebelion" of women unless they were given political rights. (For details see "The Social Roles of Men and Women—The Emancipation of Women".)

This brief hint may suffice to remind us that the so-called sexual revolution is not a sudden, isolated phenomenon, but that it is related to the many other revolutions of modern times, most notably the industrial revolution which began in 18th-century England, and the subsequent political revolutions in America and Europe. If the American Revolution was not yet explicitly concerned with sexual liberation and even failed to discuss the emancipation of women, it nevertheless laid the groundwork for later changes by proclaiming a natural human right to the "pursuit of happiness." The French Revolution of 1789 directly addressed many sexual issues, and while the best of its impulses soon came to naught, it succeeded in freeing the criminal sex laws from the influence of the church.

In 19th-century France and Germany several new "small" revolutions tried to speed up the process of modernization and to expand individual rights, but they failed. Repressive marriage and family laws and the denial of suffrage kept women "in their place." Literary censorship hampered the free flow of ideas and kept the public sexually ignorant. Nevertheless, when technological progress made the mass production of condoms possible, many men and women began to plan the size of their families and thus quietly started a "contraceptive revolution." As a result, they gained at least some measure of sexual self-determination, even if it remained unrecognized by the state. Eventually, however, the gap between traditional ideology and practical reality grew so wide that a drastic readjustment was all but inevitable. This readjustment was brought about by the First World War which announced the collapse of the rigid old political order. In 1917, when the revolution came to Russia, it expressly included equal rights for women and universal sexual freedom in its program. Thus, for the first time, a "sexual revolution" became official government policy.

Unfortunately, as Reich described in his book, after a few years the Russian Revolution betrayed its libertarian goals by becoming sexually oppressive. Reactionary laws were reinstated, and soon, together with many other civil rights, the right to free sexual expression vanished. Reich concluded from this observation that the mere transfer of power from one social class to another was not enough, and that a much more profound transformation was required. Indeed, he felt that such a transformation was already well under way in the United States and other enlightened Western democracies. Therefore, it was no longer a question of wealth or poverty, communism or capitalism, but simply a question of individual autonomy, of a "self-governing character structure." This was an ideal that had to be realized in defiance of all existing political systems with the help of natural science.

The self-governing, autonomous individual is, of course, essentially a *bourgeois* ideal. It is a model of human existence that reflects the interests and hopes of the modern Western middle classes, and thus it has always provided the impetus for the middle-class revolutions of the past. However, it seems that the political revolutions of our own century no longer follow this pattern. The Russian, Chinese, and Cuban revolutions, for example, did not serve the ends of the bourgeoisie and had little patience with individualism. Therefore it hardly comes as a surprise to find that they also failed to produce an increase in sexual freedom. Indeed, they even cancelled some freedoms that had already been won. (A good illustration is Cuba which, like most other Catholic countries, had abolished its sodomy laws as a result of the French Revolution and the following Napoleonic reforms. Yet after its recent "socialist revolution," Cuba once more began to harass homosexuals.)

By the same token, in the bourgeois, capitalist societies of the West which are dedicated to individual freedom, the sexual revolution continues. The right to sexual self-determination is considered as important as ever, and, indeed, various sexual liberation groups are working hard to extend it. In the United States, the struggle for an Equal Rights Amendment, legal abortion, the repeal of sodomy, prostitution and obscenity laws, and an end to discrimination against homosexuals are perhaps the best known current examples. At the same time, more and more people also take advantage of those sexual rights that have already been granted. Thus, the movement toward sexual emancipation is still gaining in strength.

However, some contemporary observers do not believe this movement to be part of the bourgeois revolution, or any other revolution, for that matter. Instead, they prefer to speak of a natural evolution, a gradual development without abrupt and dramatic changes. In support of this view, they point to the persistence of courtship and marriage patterns, the survival of many traditional moral values, and the rather conventional behavior of "average" men and women. The "evolutionists" further remind us that pre- and extramarital sex, contraception, abortion, homosexual behavior, prostitution, and "pornography" are nothing new. Actually, these norm violations may well have been just as common among our ancestors as they now seem to be among ourselves. Since reliable statistics for past generations are not available, we simply have no way of knowing whether any revolutionary changes have, in fact, occurred. The prevailing impression of changing sexual mores may not be due to any loss of restraint, but merely to greater candor.

There is clearly some merit in this supposition. Generally speaking, people today are less hypocritical about their sexual needs than they used to be, and thus behaviors that were once concealed or denied are now being discussed quite openly. This, in turn, can create a misleading, idealized picture of the past. Still, even if we assume that in actual fact our ancestors behaved very much as we do, one very important difference remains: When they violated traditional sexual standards, they usually suffered from guilt. They certainly did not advertise their breach of convention or demanded it as a right. They accepted the rules even if they could not help breaking them, while we today feel entitled to setting up "easier" rules of our own.

It is this change in attitude, more than anything else, that amounts to a revolution. Instead of blindly following inherited customs, we now decide for ourselves what sexual activity is proper. Therefore, even if our overt behavior remains the same, it now has a different meaning. We have learned that there are alternatives, that there is nothing eternal or sacred about our sexual morality. We no longer submit to blanket taboos or suspend our judgment. In short, we have become used to questioning the legitimacy of our traditions.

At least in this sense, the talk about a "sexual revolution" is fully justified. We have to remember that significant social changes occur not only when people change what they do. It may be enough that they change the way they think about it. It may be enough that different behaviors become defensible, that moral options develop which did not exist before. The old sexual standards seemed unassailable as long as they were taken for granted. However, today radical changes of all sorts have become conceivable and even plausible to many formerly uncritical men and women. Thus, past and present are no longer reliable guides to the future. Religious dogmas have been replaced by scientific hypotheses, certainties by doubts. At the same time, our choices and responsibilities have increased. There is cause for great joy as well as for great anxiety. In the area of sex, as in so many other areas of life, virtually anything seems to have become possible.

Obviously, an introductory textbook such as this cannot cover the "sexual revolution" in all of its aspects. Therefore, the following pages briefly discuss only three issues which are receiving special attention today—sex research, sex education, and the difficulty of creating new, sensible sexual standards. For further study, the bibliographies at the end of this chapter and at the end of the volume are recommended.

SEX RESEARCH

The study of sexual functioning and behavior has a long history dating back to ancient times. For example, Greek philosophers like Plato and Aristotle discussed the causes and the merits of homosexuality, and physicians like Hippocrates discovered important facts about human reproduction. Further discoveries were made in Rome by physicians such as Soranus, who wrote the first treatise on contraception, and Galen, who developed the first coherent sexual theory. After the fall of the Roman empire, the victorious Northern barbarians lost much of this ancient knowledge, but some of it was preserved by Islamic physicians in the Middle East and Africa, who reintroduced it to medieval Spain and Italy. Finally, the end of the Middle Ages saw the birth of modern experimental science in several European countries. Renaissance scholars and artists showed a new interest in the human body and began to examine it in ever greater detail. To cite only one famous example, the notebooks of Leonardo da Vinci contain various explicit sketches of sexual responses, coitus, fetal development, and other such matters. These sketches, which could have been made only from direct observation, prove that Leonardo was no longer content with relying on ancient authorities, but con-

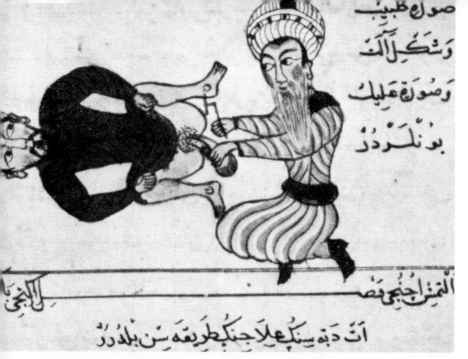

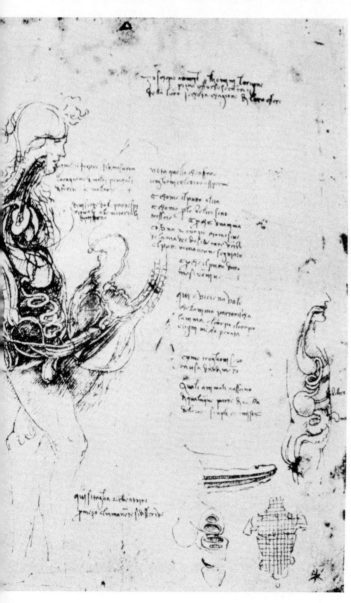

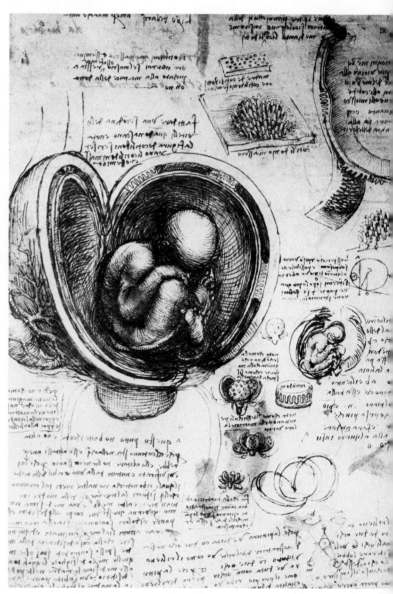

EARLY SEX RESEARCH

During the Middle Ages much of the ancient medical and sexual knowledge was preserved by Islamic physicians, some of whom also offered new theories of their own. Later, during the Renaissance in Europe, artists and scholars began to conduct systematic anatomical research.

(Left) Drawing from the manuscript of a Muslim surgeon showing surgery being performed on a man's sex organs. (15th century.)

(Below) Two pages from the notebooks of Leonardo da Vinci showing anatomical studies of coitus (left) and of fetal development (right).

ducted anatomical studies of his own. The work was then carried even further by famous anatomists like Fallopius, Bartholin, and de Graaf, who dissected human corpses and thus contributed to a better understanding of the internal sex organs. (See "The Female Sex Organs.")

Naturally, the increase in anatomical knowledge in the 16th and 17th centuries was of great medical value, since it enabled doctors to treat their patients much more effectively and even to help them with certain reproductive problems. Unfortunately, in the 18th century, the medical profession also took a giant step backward and created a great deal of new sexual misery by "discovering" the alleged health hazards of masturbation. Ancient physicians like Galen had been convinced that masturbation was sometimes necessary and healthy, because unreleased semen could become poisonous. Now, "enlightened" medicine turned the ancient therapy into a modern disease by declaring that the regular loss of semen weakened the body and could, in fact, be fatal. (See "Sexual Self-Stimulation.")

Ironically, the medical campaign against masturbation was launched at a time when libertarian philosophers had begun to discard the ascetic Christian doctrines about sex, and when various explorers returned home with news of sexually uninhibited "noble savages" in distant parts of the globe. The French Capitain Bougainville and the English Captain Cook found sensuous, happy peoples in Tahiti and on other Pacific islands, and this discovery cast serious doubts on the sexual standards of Europe. Writers like Voltaire and Diderot openly criticized these standards as inhumane, and the French Revolution finally raised the demand for legal reforms and greater sexual freedom. In England, the traditional emphasis on reproduction was questioned by the pious but nevertheless pragmatic Thomas R. Malthus in his *Essay on Population* (1798), which predicted that sooner or later the increase in population would outrun the food supply. In order to avert this disaster, he advocated "self-restraint" and late marriage. However, such measures were soon deemed inadequate by more audacious spirits who therefore proceeded to popularize contraception. Perhaps the most important of these efforts was undertaken by the American physician Charles Knowlton in his book *The Fruits of Philosophy, Or the Private Companion of Young Married People* (1832). This volume, although written in a sober and even moralistic tone, offered the most comprehensive description of contraceptive techniques since the days of Soranus. Still, in spite of its scholarly merits, it displeased the authorities, and Knowlton was fined and imprisoned.

This episode, among others, was a clear signal that the established powers were ready to take their stand. Western churches and governments were not interested in the progress of sex research and, in any case, did not want its results to be known to the general public. The following decades proved that the signal had been understood. Many researchers became themselves highly intolerant and remained content with defending the *status quo*. Psychiatry emerged as a new medical discipline. Its practitioners took up the fight against "self-abuse" and advanced ever more fantastic theories about its causes and consequences. The French psychiatrists Morel, Magnan, and Charcot strengthened the old morality by ascribing unconventional sexual behavior to "degeneracy" which produced sexual "perversions." Russian, German, and Austrian doctors developed the concept of "sexual psychopathology" which was blamed for all deviations from the sexual norm. Finally, in 1886 the Viennese psychiatrist Richard von Krafft-Ebing deplored, listed, and classified these deviations in his influential textbook *Psychopathia Sexualis*. Just as the title itself, large portions of the text were written in Latin, so as to make them unintelligible to ordinary readers. (For details see "Conformity and Deviance—Healthy–Sick.")

It was not until the beginning of our own century that a more critical attitude gained some ground. Sigmund Freud dismissed the concept of degeneracy and explained "abnormal" sexual behavior as the result of traumatic childhood experiences. At the same time, he offered a keen and unflattering analysis of modern civilization. More practical research was done by Havelock Ellis, Iwan Bloch, and Magnus Hirschfeld, who published voluminous studies of sexual behavior, thus laying the groundwork for a new academic discipline: "*Sexualwissenschaft*" (sex science) or "sexology." This kind of work was later continued by American scientists like Kinsey, Masters, and Johnson.

Another important research effort concerned the venereal diseases. In 1906 Wassermann developed his famous test for syphilis, and in 1910 Ehrlich and Hata found the first successful cure. The discovery of penicillin by Fleming in 1928 then prepared the way for our present effective methods of treatment.

The First World War (1914–18) shook the existing moral order and led to greatly increased sexual freedom. Women became more emancipated and rejected their traditional gender roles as too confining. They and other sexually oppressed groups found new arguments in the work of anthropologists who made cross-cultural studies of sex. Once more, the Pacific islands supplied the material for a moral lesson. In the 1920s and '30s Bronislaw Malinowski and Margaret Mead studied the Trobrianders, Samoans, and other "primitives," and confirmed that neither our Western ideals of sexual behavior nor our concepts of masculinity and femininity are universal. These studies also proved that greater sexual tolerance need not lead to moral decay. In 1951 Clellan S. Ford and Frank A. Beach summarized a vast amount of anthropological data in their book *Patterns of Sexual Behavior* and arrived at the same conclusion.

Today, sex research continues on numerous fronts and is increasingly being accepted. Indeed, occasionally it is even taken too seriously or burdened with too many expectations. For instance, some laymen believe that modern sex research has produced entirely new human insights. However, this is only partially true. After all, the most "revolutionary" discoveries of Freud (infant sexuality), Kinsey (the great extent of homosexual behavior and the high sexual responsiveness of adolescents), and Masters and Johnson (the superior orgasmic potential of women) had already been common knowledge in ancient and medieval times. This knowledge had been suppressed only within the last few centuries and only in the industrialized West. Thus, in many cases our modern sex researchers have merely revived some very old truths.

This realization does not take any credit away from recent accomplishments, but it shows that it may be useful to put them in some historical perspective. The following pages make this attempt by briefly describing the work of a few outstanding researchers. A concluding section deals with present concerns and possible future developments.

PIONEERS OF SEX RESEARCH

Specific sex research in the modern, narrow sense originated in the 19th century. This research was begun in several Western countries by men and women of different backgrounds using very different methods. Most of these pioneers had to fight long and hard for public acceptance, and some were even ostracized by their colleagues or persecuted by their governments. Nevertheless, eventually their work proved its usefulness, and today there is a generally recognized body of scientific sexual knowledge which continues to grow.

The scope of the present book does not allow us to list more than a few outstanding scientists. Still, brief and incomplete as it is, this list can perhaps provide some insight into the history and the problems of sex research.

Sigmund Freud (1856–1939)

Sigmund Freud, the Austrian physician and founder of the psychoanalytic theory, began his career as a neurologist in Vienna, where he had to treat many so-called hysterical patients. These were people who suffered from some "impossible" physical dysfunction, i.e., according to all standard tests they were healthy and should have been able to function normally. By inter-

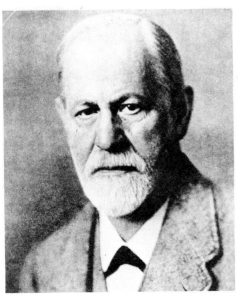

Sigmund Freud

viewing such patients over long periods of time, Freud discovered that their mysterious disabilities were caused by unconscious sexual conflicts. This and other discoveries eventually led him to a special form of therapy called psychoanalysis (Greek. Literally: examination of the soul or mind), in which the patient by means of "free association" gradually revealed the hidden source of his problems to the analyst and, most importantly, to himself. Once the conflict was brought "out into the open," and thus became conscious, it could be handled rationally. In this sense, the patient was then "cured."

The scope of the present text does not allow for a detailed discussion of the psychoanalytic theory which was greatly expanded and repeatedly revised over the years. Freud's writings comprise 24 volumes in their English-language edition, and, to this day, any attempt to popularize his highly sophisticated and complex thinking remains a questionable enterprise. Nevertheless, at least some aspects of Freud's theory are briefly summarized in another part of this book. (See introduction to "The Development of Sexual Behavior".)

Freud was a truly cultivated man of wide-ranging interests, a master prose stylist, and an uncompromising thinker. All of these qualities undoubtedly contributed to his eventual success and international fame. However, at first Freud's theories were not well received at all. The general importance he ascribed to sex and especially his rediscovery of the sexuality of children caused a storm of controversy and made him almost an outcast among his scientific colleagues. At the University of Vienna he became a lecturer and later a professor, but was never given a seat on the faculty. Still, his medical practice, his lectures, and his major books *The Interpretation of Dreams* (1900), *Three Essays on the Theory of Sexuality* (1905), *Totem and Taboo* (1913), and *Beyond the Pleasure Principle* (1919) secured him a wide following. Moreover, he was able to gather around him several young and brilliant disciples. Over the years, Freud had the satisfaction of seeing the psychoanalytic movement spread all over Europe, although some of his former students eventually broke with him and established psychoanalytical schools of their own. Still, towards the end of his life most of his work seemed to have been in vain. In Nazi Germany psychoanalysis was outlawed as "Jewish science," Freud's books were publicly burned and his followers persecuted. Finally, in 1938, when Hitler invaded Austria, Freud had no choice but to go into exile in England where he died of cancer the following year.

Since his death, Freud's influence has continued to grow, especially in America. Even though many of his views have been challenged, and some of his assertions have actually been disproved, his work as a whole stands as a towering achievement in Western intellectual history. In an age of prudery and hypocrisy Freud approached sexual matters in a strictly scientific spirit. By discussing sexual behavior openly and soberly in precise language, he helped to establish it as a proper subject of study. He also broadened the whole concept of sexuality and thus laid the foundation for important later research.

Havelock Ellis (1859–1939)

Henry Havelock Ellis, an English scholar and essayist, early in life became interested in a scientific approach to sexual problems. He studied medicine and obtained a degree, but never practiced regularly. Instead, he turned to writing and, over the years, made many important contributions to a better understanding of human sexuality. His most famous work are the *Studies in the Psychology of Sex* which were published in seven volumes between 1896 and 1928. When the first volume appeared it was denounced as obscene, and the public scandal quickly led to a confrontation with the law. An accused bookdealer pointed to the scientific value of the work, but the judge dismissed this argument as nothing but "a pretense, adopted for the purpose of selling a filthy publication." As a result of this judicial attitude, the entire work remained legally unavailable to the general public until 1935. Only members of the medical profession were allowed to read it.

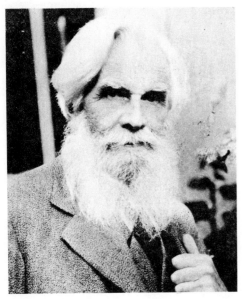

Havelock Ellis

Nevertheless, the author's fame and influence grew steadily in Europe and America. He corresponded with Freud (who adopted several of Ellis' scientific terms and phrases) and was active in the movement for sexual reform. He was one of the most articulate early champions of general sex education and the emancipation of women.

Iwan Bloch (1872–1922)

Iwan Bloch worked as a physician in Berlin, specializing in the study of venereal diseases. His research in this field soon won him wide recognition. However, he also wrote extensively on other sexual matters and was active in the sexual reform movement. In his two major works *Das Sexualleben unserer Zeit* (*The Sexual Life of Our Time*) published in 1907, and the three-volume *Handbuch der gesamten Sexualwissenschaft* (*Handbook of Sex Science in Its Totality*) published from 1912 to 1925, Bloch emerges as one of the pioneers of modern sex research.

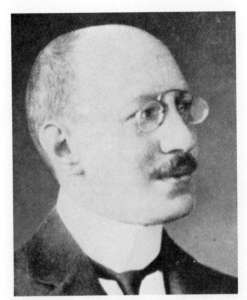

Iwan Bloch

Magnus Hirschfeld (1868–1935)

Magnus Hirschfeld, a German physician, first worked as a general practitioner and then as a specialist for "psychological sexual disorders" in Berlin. Through his medical practice and his own scientific research he became aware of the psychological and social problems of homosexuals and soon reached the conclusion that their legal persecution was unjust, irrational, and inhuman.

In 1897 Hirschfeld founded the *Wissenschaftlich-Humanitäres Komitee* (Scientific-Humanitarian Committee) for the scientific study of homosexuality. The Committee also attempted to provide practical help to individual homosexuals. As part of his scientific and humanitarian work Hirschfeld also began to edit the *Jahrbuch für sexuelle Zwischenstufen* (Yearbook for Sexual Intermediate Stages) which tried to educate the professional community as well as the nation at large about homosexuality and other sexual matters. Over the years, this scientific journal carried articles by many important writers, such as Havelock Ellis, Freud, and Bloch. A recurrent theme throughout all volumes is the fight for repeal of antihomosexual laws in Germany.

With the turn of the century, Hirschfeld's Committee grew into the *Institut für Sexualwissenschaft* (Institute for Sex Science) which, in 1919, was signed over to the new democratic German government. The institute contained laboratories, large collections of sexual materials, and a research library. It also offered counseling and treatment to the general public. Poor patients were helped free of charge.

In 1921 Hirschfeld founded the *International Congress for Sexual Reform* which, seven years later, developed into the *World League for Sexual Reform*. Among the members and supporters of this league were Sigmund Freud, Bertrand Russell, Judge Ben Lindsey, and many other sex reformers.

In 1933, when Hitler came to power in Germany, the Nazis raided Hirschfeld's Institute in Berlin, destroyed the collections and burned the books. Hirschfeld himself, who happened to be absent at the time, found himself exiled and died two years later in France.

In Nazi Germany the persecution of homosexuals and other "deviants" continued and quickly reached unequalled proportions. Many of them died in concentration camps. After Hitler's defeat, the few survivors remained uncompensated for their suffering. It was not until the late 1960s that Hirschfeld's earlier work finally bore fruit. The German anti-homosexual laws were repealed and the full sexual and civil rights of German homosexuals were finally recognized.

Magnus Hirschfeld

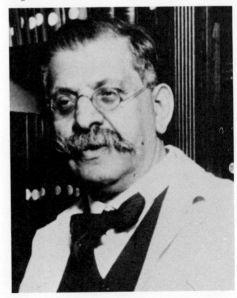

Wilhelm Reich (1897–1957)

Wilhelm Reich studied medicine in Vienna and, under the influence of Freud, became a practicing psychoanalyst. His work at the Viennese free psychoanalytic clinic brought him in contact with many poor patients and, in studying them, he turned his attention to their social and economic condi-

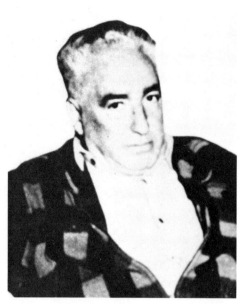

Wilhelm Reich

tions. He soon began to feel that Freud and his followers unduly neglected these problems and that, in order to achieve general sexual health, some political change was needed. Reich therefore studied the works of Karl Marx and, when he moved to Berlin in 1930, he joined the Communist Party. He also helped to organize a communist sexual-political organization (Sexpol) and lectured widely to working-class audiences.

During this period Reich also wrote extensively about sexual and political questions. The most important of his books (which were translated into English and partly rewritten in the 1940s) are *The Function of the Orgasm* (1927), *The Imposition of Sexual Morality* (1932), *Character Analysis* (1933), *The Mass Psychology of Fascism* (1933), and *The Sexual Revolution* (1936). In these studies Reich dealt with sexual and other dysfunctions, the origin of sexual oppression, the psychological mechanisms that cause people to embrace fascism, and the history of the sexual reforms and their subsequent repeal in the Soviet Union.

Because of his radical views, Reich soon became a very controversial figure. The Communists felt increasingly uncomfortable with his ideas of sexual liberation and in 1933 formally expelled him from the party. In the meantime, he had also made many enemies among his professional colleagues and, in 1934, Reich was expelled from the International Psychoanalytic Association. Needless to say, there was also no longer any room for him in Nazi Germany. His books were publicly burned, and he fled to Denmark and later to Sweden and Norway. Finally, in 1939, he settled in the United States.

Towards the end of the 1930s Reich's interest in politics gradually gave way to a preoccupation with biology. Where once he had tried to integrate the theories of Marx and Freud, he now turned away from both. Instead, he claimed to have discovered the "orgone," i.e., a basic life energy which he believed to be necessary for the preservation and restoration of health, and which could be accumulated in specially designed boxes for therapeutic purposes.

Virtually all scientists who heard of his new theory quickly dismissed it as nonsensical. Unfortunately, as Reich's scientific claims became ever more fantastic, he also became increasingly irrational in his daily personal life. It was therefore very difficult to continue to take him seriously. In 1954 the federal Food and Drug Administration in Washington came to the conclusion that Reich's work amounted to nothing more than dangerous quackery and obtained an injunction ordering the destruction of all "orgone accumulators" and virtually all of his writings. The injunction also banned any further discussion of the orgone theory and, in fact, even made the very use of the word "orgone" a crime (at least for Reich and his associates). However, the list of books that were to be destroyed included not only Reich's newest biological writings, but also major earlier works such as *Character Analysis* and *The Mass Psychology of Fascism* which contained no mention of the orgone theory. Reich refused to obey the injunction, claiming that scientific questions could not and should not be settled in court. As a result, he was sentenced to two years in prison for contempt and, just as before in Nazi Germany, his books were officially burned. Reich himself died soon thereafter in the Lewisburg Penitentiary in Pennsylvania.

Today, Reich's work (with the exception of the orgone theory) has regained some general recognition. His therapeutic techniques, which combine verbal communication with special massages, have been found useful by many new therapists. Furthermore, Reich's original insistence on seeing sexual problems in political terms is again beginning to be appreciated. On the whole, he is now considered to have been one of the most important writers on sexual matters.

Alfred C. Kinsey (1894–1956)

Alfred C. Kinsey was a zoology professor at Indiana University in Bloomington when, in 1938, he was asked to give some lectures about the biological aspects of sex and marriage. Turning to the professional publications in this field, his discovered that most of them were highly speculative and based on inadequate statistical samples. He also found that the available literature could not answer some of the simplest questions put to him by his students.

Kinsey therefore realized the need for a major new study of human sexuality and, with the help of some volunteer subjects on campus, began to compile the first of many thousands of individual sex histories. In 1939 he went outside the university and interviewed people in small surrounding towns as well as inmates in the state prison system. It soon became clear, however, that the entire project would take many years to complete and would require considerable funds. These funds were eventually obtained from the university and various public and private foundations. Thus, Kinsey and his associates Wardell B. Pomeroy, Clyde E. Martin, and Paul H. Gebhard, were able to continue their work. In 1947 the Institute for Sex Research was incorporated, and, by 1959, it had accumulated more than 18,000 individual case histories, all taken by personal interview.

Kinsey's abundant material formed the basis for two major books: *Sexual Behavior in the Human Male* (1948) and *Sexual Behavior in the Human Female* (1953). These monumental studies contained detailed statistics about the sexual behavior of ordinary Americans of all ages, all walks of life, and from all parts of the country. The figures revealed an astonishing range of behavior and made it obvious that most American sex laws were completely unrealistic. For example, it came as a great surprise to the public (and to Kinsey himself) that homosexual behavior was not at all exceptional, but fairly widespread, and that many other allegedly deviant acts were quite common among otherwise "normal" men and women. The books also contained many new insights into the physiology of sexual responses and offered a critical review of previous studies.

Naturally, the publication of Kinsey's work created a sensation, and he soon found himself both praised as a courageous scientist and condemned as a mindless and shameless destroyer of intimacy. As happens quite often in such cases, however, not all of his critics really bothered to read the entire text. In fact, even today many of Kinsey's findings have not yet entered the public consciousness. In the meantime, Kinsey's pioneering work still stands out as a model of scholarship and lucid writing. So far, there has been no comparable study anywhere in the world.

After Kinsey's death in 1956, the Institute for Sex Research continued under the directorship of Paul H. Gebhard. Several new books, such as *Pregnancy, Birth, and Abortion* (1958), *Sex Offenders* (1965), and *Male Homosexuals* (1974) have been published and other major studies are under way. The institute is also open to trained researchers who can take advantage of its large library and its vast special collections. All case histories, however, remain confidential and are not available except to the institute staff.

William H. Masters and Virginia E. Johnson
(1915 –   , and 1925 –   )

William H. Masters was still a young man when he decided to devote his life to sex research. He studied medicine, specialized in obstetrics and gynecology, and became a professor at the Washington University School of Medicine in St. Louis, Missouri. As a medical researcher he first won recognition for his work on hormones. However, in 1954 he turned to the direct observation of human sexual responses. In 1957 he was joined in this project by psychologist Virginia E. Johnson, who eventually became his wife.

Since research of this kind had rarely been attempted before, Masters first encountered many difficulties. At the beginning he had to rely mainly on prostitutes as subjects of study and only later was able to find a sufficient number of "average" men and women as volunteers. These volunteers were observed in the laboratory during various sexual activities and their responses were measured and recorded by sophisticated instruments. In many cases they were also filmed.

For about ten years this research was carried out under university auspices

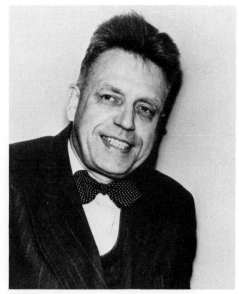

Alfred C. Kinsey

Masters and Johnson

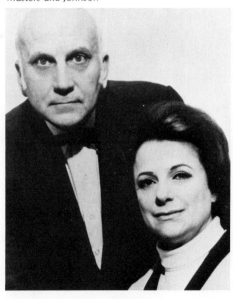

until, in 1964, Masters established his own Reproductive Biology Research Foundation near the campus, financed by individual donors and several philanthropic foundations. Two years later, Masters and Johnson published their first major study, *Human Sexual Response* (1966).

The authors disproved many popular myths and fallacies about sex and also challenged some traditional professional beliefs. Especially certain psychoanalytic assumptions about female sexuality turned out to be in direct conflict with the physiological facts. Since Masters' and Johnson's work continues to be of unusual interest, it is reported in greater detail in another part of this book. (See "The Male Sexual Response" and "The Female Sexual Response.")

As a result of their work, Masters and Johnson gained a better understanding of human sexual functioning and, in 1959, they began a program of treating married couples with sexual problems. Eventually, they also treated unmarried individuals together with their partners, and, in some instances "surrogate partners" were provided. The program proved to be surprisingly effective, and the therapists therefore published their findings in a second major study, *Human Sexual Inadequacy* (1970). Because of its importance, this study is also partly summarized in a special section of this book. (See "Sexual Inadequacy.") Masters' and Johnson's treatment program continues to this date. In addition, they are also engaged in several other long-range research projects.

THE FUTURE OF SEX RESEARCH

Modern sex research has contributed greatly to a better understanding not only of sex and reproduction, but also of human behavior in general. Nevertheless, there is much that still has to be learned. In fact, many scientists agree that, so far, we have taken only the first few steps into a vast, new, unexplored territory. Nobody can say where these steps will eventually lead us.

We need to know still more about the physiology and biochemistry of sexual responses. Thus, new research is being conducted on the role of hormones and other glandular secretions (such as those produced by the bulbourethral and greater vestibular glands, for example). There is also some hope that the continued study of the reproductive process may lead to a reduction of infertility, a better control of birth defects, and more effective contraceptives. In addition, scientists are seeking for vaccines or other preventive methods that could finally end the venereal disease epidemic. Some researchers are turning their attention to the sexual capacities of people with various handicaps, or they study the effects of sexual activity on the aging and on persons with a damaged heart. Furthermore, by systematically comparing sexually dysfunctional young people with older people who once had the same problems, but overcame them, sex therapists may learn to become more successful and may even discover how to prevent sexual inadequacy altogether.

The study of sexual behavior in a wider sense is also important. For example, it would be very useful if Kinsey's original work could be repeated today, and if similar large statistical surveys could be made in other countries. This kind of research can greatly illuminate the problems of sexual conformity and sexual deviance. If we want rational public attitudes and workable sex laws, we need to find out a great deal more about the various sexual minorities, including sex offenders. We also need a better understanding of gender identity problems, such as transvestism and transsexualism. Very few studies have been made of female homosexuals. Indeed, the entire subject of homosexuality remains shrouded in mystery and mired in confusion. It seems that, so far, only the wrong questions have been asked. Anthropologists, sociologists, economists, and even political scientists may find new ways of approaching such matters. However, it is not only the sexual minorities that need to be studied and explained. The presumed majority is just as mysterious. We therefore have to start questioning even our most innocent assumptions. Such a critical spirit can not only teach us more about ourselves, but also prevent us from becoming self-righteous and intolerant. We will also have to re-member that, while sex is a fascinating subject, it is never more than a small part in a much larger picture. We are not likely to understand very much about sex until we realize that it is, at most, only one aspect of the whole human personality. In the final analysis, therefore, it is the human race and the human condition that have to be studied. Sex research, properly under-stood, is destined to transcend the narrow confines of any single discipline.

SEX EDUCATION

Sex education, as it is understood today, was unknown until about 200 years ago. In ancient and medieval Europe sex was seen as an integral part of life, not as a separate, problematical issue which needed special study. Sexual knowledge was acquired spontaneously together with all other kinds of knowledge. Children did not live in a "protected" world of their own, but took part in virtually all adult work and leisure activities. Since the majority of the population lived on farms close to nature, boys and girls had ample opportunity to observe the mating of animals. Indeed, it was not uncommon for people to share their house with their cattle. Neither the highest nor the lowest social classes enjoyed much personal privacy, but there was also no squeamishness or embarrassment about the natural bodily functions. Families were used to bathing and sleeping together in the nude. Courtships and preg-nancies were discussed openly, and women gave birth to their babies at home. The "facts of life" were never a secret to anyone, and as soon as they reached puberty, both males and females were considered ready for mar-riage. (See also introduction to "The Human Body.")

Even at the beginning of the Modern Age, when a new urban middle class started to exchange important information in print, sex was not yet treated as an isolated topic. Thus, educational books for children, like the *Colloquia Familiaria* by Erasmus of Rotterdam (1522), approached sex simply and straightforwardly as a normal part of domestic life, giving it no more and no less emphasis than other matters of general interest.

However, in the course of the next few centuries people adopted a very different attitude. First childhood, and then adolescence, began to emerge as special, "innocent" periods of life, in which the individual had to be shielded from the temptations of the adult world. An increasing prudery saw everything sexual as dirty and dangerous. Masturbation was discovered as a universal problem and declared a serious threat to health. By the time Jean-Jacques Rousseau formulated his "enlightened" educational theories in *Emile* (1762), sex had become a highly mysterious and deeply disturbing subject. (See the introductions to "Infancy and Childhood" and "Adoles-cence.")

Rousseau believed that all children were born in a "natural" state of "holy innocence" which had to be preserved as long as possible. For him, sexual ignorance was bliss, at least in childhood. After puberty, sexual information was justified only in answer to direct questions, but even then it was advis-able to stifle further curiosity by making the adolescent disgusted with the subject. Perhaps it was best if the educator used "dirty words" for sex organs and sexual functions and stressed their connection with the most repulsive bodily excretions. On the other hand, one had to be careful not to arouse any premature passions by becoming too explicit. Indeed, the educator always walked a very thin line. A single inappropriate remark could ruin his pupil's life.

In many respects Rousseau expressed the attitude of his age. However, there were other influential educators, especially in Germany, who suggested a different approach. While they shared Rousseau's basic belief that children were innocent, and that sex was dangerous, they saw early "sexual enlightenment" as the only effective way of combating the danger. In their opinion, sexual ignorance was even worse than sexual knowledge, because it led to harmful misconceptions and wild fantasies. Furthermore, it was impossible to fight masturbation without discussing it freely. In short, if sex education had its distasteful side, it was nevertheless a necessary evil.

In accordance with this general view, the first formal sex education classes were instituted in some "progressive" schools. These classes aimed, above all, at creating a sense of modesty and wholesome fear. Everything had to take place in an atmosphere of utter seriousness. Any suggestion of pleasure or joy was to be avoided. As a matter of fact, it was proposed that students should be prepared for a sex education class with a special and very meager diet which would weaken their bodies and thus prevent dangerous desires from being aroused. As an additional safety measure, an indirect approach was recommended. Beginning with a description of plant and animal life, the teachers could gradually lead up to the touchy subject of human reproduction. Still, they must not become too specific. It was enough to hint that women bore their children "under the heart" and gave birth in great pain. Naturally, the danger of death in childbed could always be emphasized. In the same somber spirit, some educators also preferred to demonstrate the anatomical difference between the sexes by inviting their students to the morgue and showing them naked male and female corpses. In addition, children were taken to hospitals and insane asylums to observe syphilitic patients and madmen who were described as victims of masturbation. Some schools used books containing allegedly true reports about adolescents who had died miserably as a result of "self-abuse," in spite of the best medical treatment. Students were also encouraged to read stories about seduction, abandonment, infanticide, and similar gruesome matters. In short, the real purpose behind the whole enterprise was not so much to educate the young about sex as to warn them against temptation.

As already mentioned, these early sex education programs were developed in a few model schools, and they reached only the children of the rising middle classes and the lower aristocracy. Sex education for all segments of society was not considered until after the French Revolution in 1789. Educators appealed to the new democratic French government to make such education mandatory and especially to provide medical instruction for girls about menstruation, pregnancy, birth, and baby care. If these plans had been carried out and followed through to their logical conclusion, they would undoubtedly have accelerated the emancipation of women. Unfortunately, the revolutionary momentum was soon lost. Not only in France, but all over Europe, the middle classes became increasingly powerful and conservative. Even the earlier limited educational experiments were abandoned. Thus, only a short time after its introduction, the subject of sex disappeared again from the curriculum.

Nevertheless, in the early 19th century, adults still had free access to some positive sexual information. Both in Europe and in America a number of serious "marriage manuals" were published, which took a very reasonable attitude towards sex and also described various methods of contraception. These books were not always scientifically correct (some important facts about human reproduction had not yet been discovered), but at least they tried to be helpful. Furthermore, around the middle of the century, new technical processes made the mass production of condoms possible. As a result, more and more people began to plan the size of their families.

The Christian churches were, of course, well aware of these developments, but took no official stand on the matter. Even most Catholic bishops preferred to remain silent and instructed their priests not to upset parishioners who acted in good faith. It was only later, when rapid industrialization and a rising nationalism prompted governments to demand a population increase, that the churches became more outspoken. Finally, the politicians and clergymen were joined by various civic groups which feared for the very survival of civilization, and which called for a "Christian" crusade against contraception and other "immoral" practices.

In the U.S. the most successful of these new crusaders was Anthony Comstock, the secretary of the New York Society for the Suppression of Vice. Comstock had begun his career as a fighter against the "demon alcohol," but later devoted his life to the eradication of "obscenity." With his slogan "Morals, not Art or Literature," he set out to prevent the dissemination of sexual knowledge and to end all public discussion of sexual matters. His intense lobbying efforts persuaded Congress in 1873 to pass the so-called Comstock Act, which made it a felony to mail any "obscene, lewd, or lascivious book, pamphlet, picture, writing, paper, or other publication of an 'indecent character'." Comstock himself was made a special agent of the Post Office. This gave him the right to open other people's mail, and soon he was able to establish a veritable reign of puritanical terror.

In Comstock's opinion, one of the greatest obscenities was contraception. Thus, under the new law, contraceptive devices could no longer be imported or shipped across state lines, and even the mailing of contraceptive information was prohibited. As a result, Comstock could take on even the medical profession, and, like any true fanatic, he had no scruples about using immoral means to achieve his "moral" ends. For example, he or one of his followers would obtain the address of some kindhearted physician and write him a tear-drenched letter, pretending to be a poor, sick mother of many children on the verge of killing herself, and begging for some advice on how to prevent further pregnancies. If the physician responded, he was promptly arrested and sent to prison. Naturally, this also meant the end of his career. When, in 1914, Margaret Sanger started to write about contraception, Comstock had her indicted. However, since she left the country, he could not obtain a conviction and therefore decided to punish her husband instead. Using the standard method of entrapment, one of Comstock's undercover agents succeeded in buying a birth control pamphlet from the unsuspecting Mr. Sanger, who was therefore imprisoned. For the aging Comstock, this turned out to be the last heroic deed in defense of "decency." He died before his victim had served his full sentence.

As we have repeatedly pointed out, in the second half of the 19th century, most Western nations were gripped by an unprecedented prudery. Ignorance and hypocrisy carried the day, and thus many hard-won civil liberties were quickly surrendered. The phenomenon is, of course, also known as Victorianism, after the English Queen Victoria, whose reign fell into this period. Still, we have to realize that the sexual repression was international. England and the United States were neither better nor worse than other countries. The reasons for this historical development are still not entirely clear. Perhaps it was related to the general process of industrialization.

While we do not really know why the Victorians were so afraid of sex, we nevertheless understand how this fear could spread and grow. An important contributing factor was censorship. Once the assumption had been made that children and adolescents were endangered by sexual information, the even-

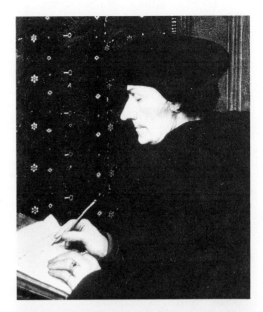

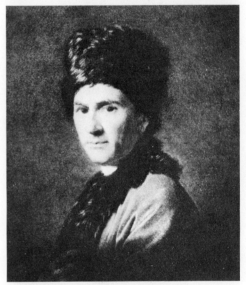

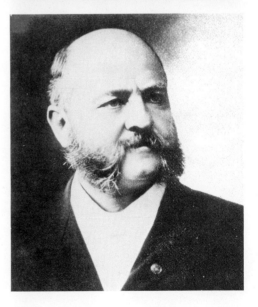

CHANGING ATTITUDES TOWARD SEXUAL KNOWLEDGE
With the rise of middle classes in Europe and America sexual information became increasingly restricted. This trend, which has reversed itself only in our century, is well illustrated by the efforts of the three men shown here.

(Top) **Erasmus of Rotterdam** *(1466?-1536) Wrote very frankly about sex in his "children's book"* Colloquia Familiaria.

(Middle) **Jean-Jacques Rousseau** *(1712-1778) Supported the sexual "innocence" and ignorance of children in* Emile.

(Bottom) **Anthony Comstock** *(1844-1915) Tried to save even adults from "obscenity" and therefore lobbied for censorship through the "Comstock Act."*

tual active suppression of such information even for adults was only a question of time. Over the years, the public simply became more and more sensitive. The 16th and 17th centuries had produced the first examples of a special "children's literature," but even these were later found to be too indelicate. The 18th century created a "purified" Bible for children, but, in the 19th century, a second and more thorough purification was deemed necessary. Even the traditional catechisms were no longer considered chaste enough and therefore had to be rewritten. Soon the procedure was applied to the other "classics" as well. Ancient Greek and Latin authors appeared in new, censored editions. In England, a "Family Shakespeare" was published which omitted all "indecent" words and phrases. Thus, not only children, but also their parents were protected. Needless to say, the new "adult" books had to conform to the same "pure" standards. In short, both the young and the old began to live in an artificial world from which all references to sexual functions had been removed.

On the other hand, people were secretly obsessed with sex. Since it could no longer be openly discussed, it became a dark and threatening force. Unknown dangers lurked everywhere. Even the most innocent words and actions acquired sexual overtones. It became important for any well-bred person to notice such overtones and to ignore them at the same time. Eternal vigilance was the price of chastity. Finally, "good taste" developed to the point where a "decent" citizen was expected to keep books by male and female authors separated on the shelf, thus avoiding the accusation that he favored sexual promiscuity.

The Victorian "conspiracy of silence" created an atmosphere of perpetual panic. It was generally believed that innocence, modesty, decency, and purity were under constant attack, and that any measure taken in their defense was justified. It was also assumed that whatever people did not know about sex could not hurt them. Thus, boys and girls grew up in complete ignorance about the most elementary biological facts. Quite often, they were even deliberately misinformed. They also heard occasional vague talk about various diseases caused by masturbation. Many adolescents were subjected to cruel and useless "treatments" in order to "cure" them of this "solitary vice." Some developed such an overwhelming sense of guilt that they committed suicide. Those who reached adulthood usually remained uninformed and superstitious. Sexual fear continued to permeate their entire lives. However, there was no one who could educate and reassure them. With the acceptance of censorship they had lost the right to understand the functions of their own bodies.

Over the years, this sexual ignorance exacted a horrible price from society in the form of unhappy marriages, unwanted children, and wasted lives. Its full cost in human suffering will, of course, never be known. Still, at the end of the 19th century, at least some of this suffering was so obvious that it simply could no longer be overlooked. An ever growing number of men and women became nervous, depressed, or even physically ill because of their sexual problems, and any treatment remained ineffective until these problems were recognized. Physicians like Freud, Bloch, and Hirschfeld, who tried to help such patients, were therefore forced to conclude that the silence had to be broken and that the time for reform had come. Thus, they began to educate first their professional colleagues, and then a wider adult public about sexual matters. Finally, when the adults had overcome their fears, adolescents and children could also again be included in the discussion. This, in turn, cleared the way for an entirely new and comprehensive approach to sex education.

Note: For a description of sex education in 18th-century Europe the preceding text has largely relied on the hitherto untranslated study *Sexualunterdrückung* by Jos van Ussel, Reinbeck b. Hamburg, 1970. Information from this important study has further been used in other parts of the present book. However, the study contains more material than can or should be summarized in a textbook such as this one. It is to be hoped, therefore, that van Ussel's work as a whole will soon become available in English.

Early in our century the right to sexual knowledge reappeared as a public issue. Especially after World War I, many Western countries began to debate the merits of lifting all sexual censorship for adults and of including some sex education in the normal school curriculum. Sex researchers and physicians wrote new explicit sex manuals or offered public lecture programs (see "Sex Research"). Not surprisingly, in the U.S. as well as in Europe, the first advocates of sex education met with considerable opposition. However, their persistent efforts finally led to more rational public attitudes. Since we can list here only a few examples, we have selected three individuals from different fields and three organizations with different goals and approaches. The individuals belong to America's recent past; the organizations are still active today.

Benjamin B. Lindsey (1869–1943)

Benjamin Barr Lindsey served as a judge on the juvenile court in Denver, Colorado, where he became concerned with the connection between poverty and juvenile delinquency. He drafted numerous legislative proposals and contributed greatly to an improved juvenile justice system in Colorado and other states.

His social concerns also led him to lecture widely to popular audiences all over the country and, in 1925 he and Wainwright Evans, a journalist, wrote a series of articles dealing with the sexual problems of adolescents. Collected in a book under the title *The Revolt of Modern Youth*, these articles created a great deal of controversy, since Lindsey approached unconventional sexual behavior in a rational and nonjudgmental manner. As a result, many conservative political and religious leaders accused him of corrupting the morals of the young. In 1927 his next book *The Companionate Marriage* (also written with Evans) caused an even greater public outcry. In this book Lindsey advocated, among other things, sex education and birth control information in public schools. In view of the continued sexual oppression of the young, he also proposed a new form of marriage called "companionate marriage" which he defined as "a legal marriage, with legalized birth control, and with the right to divorce by mutual consent for childless couples, usually without payment of alimony."

The book made Lindsey internationally famous. However, while his rather moderate and reasonable proposals were widely supported in the U.S. as well as in Europe, he also found himself again accused of immorality by various conservative religious groups. His political opponents quickly seized the opportunity to drive him from the bench in Colorado. Lindsey then moved to California where he served as a judge in Los Angeles until his death.

Today Judge Lindsey is largely forgotten, but in his time he was well known all over the world as one of the most engaging and effective spokesmen for sexual reform.

Margaret Sanger (1883–1966)

Working as a nurse with women in the poorer sections of New York City, Margaret Sanger saw a great deal of sexual misery. She soon came to the conclusion that, in order to give her patients effective help, she had to teach them how to avoid unwanted pregnancies. She promptly set out to do so and also began to write about the subject. (It was she who coined the term "birth control.")

Margaret Sanger felt very strongly that every woman should have the right to control her own body and, in 1914, she began to espouse the view in her magazine *The Woman Rebel*. Of the nine issues that appeared, seven were suppressed by the Federal authorities and Mrs. Sanger was indicted for "sending obscene literature through the mails." However, since she was able to win considerable public support for her work, the case was dismissed in 1916.

During that same year, Margaret Sanger and her sister opened a birth control clinic in the Brownsville section of Brooklyn. This clinic was almost

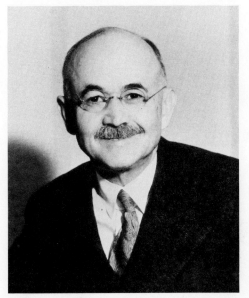

Benjamin B. Lindsey

Margaret Sanger

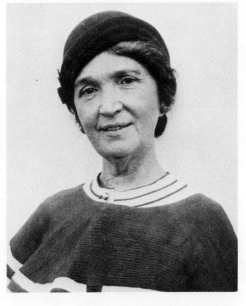

immediately closed by the authorities as a "public nuisance." The sisters were accused of having violated the state obscenity laws and, as a punishment, they were sentenced to 30 days in the workhouse. Still, after having served the sentence, Margaret Sanger continued her work undeterred until, in 1929, the Sanger Clinic was raided and the files were confiscated. Again, public support led to an eventual dismissal of the case. Finally, in 1936, a Federal Appeals Court affirmed the right of physicians to prescribe contraceptives "for the purpose of saving life or promoting the well-being of patients."

In 1921 Mrs. Sanger founded the American Birth Control League, and in 1929 she organized the National Committee on Federal Legislation for Birth Control. Ten years later the League combined with another group to form the Birth Control Federation of America, which in 1942 became the Planned Parenthood Federation of America. In 1953 Margaret Sanger became the first president of the International Planned Parenthood Federation and devoted much of her remaining time and energy to the cause of birth control in Asia.

In spite of Margaret Sanger's great personal success and eventual vindication, there remained legal obstacles to the effective spread of birth control information in many parts of the U.S. even after her death. Federal law still prevented such information from being sent through the mails, and many states retained laws against the use and sale of contraceptives. It was not until 1965 that a Connecticut law prohibiting contraception even within marriage was declared unconstitutional. In view of this Supreme Court decision, Massachusetts in 1966 amended its own law to allow contraception when prescribed by a doctor, but only to married couples. It took another six years to have this amended law also struck down as unconstitutional. Finally, in 1970, the U.S. Congress removed the last Federal restrictions related to contraception.

Bertrand Russell (1872–1970)

In the course of his long life, Bertrand Russell, the English mathematician and philosopher, made substantial contributions in many different fields of human knowledge and championed a great number of humanitarian causes. All of this is well known and therefore need not be repeated here. However, modern sex educators owe him a special gratitude for his courageous fight for sexual rights and a rational approach to sexual problems.

When Russell's own children were growing up he and his wife founded a coeducational school in which the students were given considerable freedom. His experiences with this school (1927–1932) greatly influenced his views on education. In 1929 he published *Marriage and Morals,* a book dealing with human sexual relations both inside and outside of marriage. In this book he argued for more and better sex education of the young, sexual intercourse before marriage, the option of extramarital relations for both husband and wife, and divorce by mutual consent for childless couples. Russell made these proposals because he believed in marriage as a social institution and, in fact, wanted to strengthen it by combating ignorance, hypocrisy, and sexual exploitation. In some respects his position was quite similar to that taken two years earlier by Judge Ben Lindsey. Not surprisingly, just like Lindsey, he was quickly denounced as immoral and when, during the Second World War, he came to the U.S., outraged conservative groups turned on him with a vengeance.

In 1940 Russell was appointed professor of philosophy at the City College of New York. However, certain parents of City College students went to court and filed a taxpayer's suit to have the appointment annulled. The parents' lawyer argued that Russell's books were "lecherous, salacious, libidinous, lustful, venerous, erotomaniac, aphrodisiac, atheistic, irreverent, narrow-minded, untruthful and bereft of moral fibre." Moreover, as an individual, the author had condoned homosexuality and led a nudist colony in England. Russell's philosophical writings were dismissed as "cheap, tawdry, worn out, patched up fetishes and propositions, devices for the purpose of misleading the people."

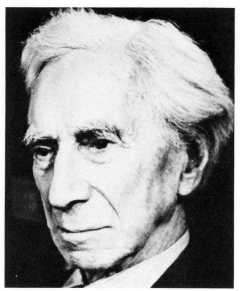

Bertrand Russell

The judge who heard the case agreed that Russell's books contained "filth" and "immoral and salacious doctrines" and promptly denied him the right to teach. In the view of the court, the appointment had been an illegal attempt to establish a "Chair of Indecency" at the college and therefore violated "the public health, safety, and morals of the people." Since Russell himself was not a party to the proceedings, he had no means of reply or redress. The Board of Higher Education in New York did not appeal the decision, because Mayor La Guardia feared the political consequences. Bertrand Russell went on to lecture at Harvard and later at the Barnes Foundation near Philadelphia. Nevertheless, his experience in New York continued to cast a shadow over the rest of his stay in America.

Planned Parenthood

Thanks to the efforts of Margaret Sanger and other champions of birth control, the *Planned Parenthood Federation of America* was established in 1942. The Federation now has its headquarters on 810 Seventh Avenue, New York, N.Y. 10019. There are also several regional offices around the country as well as affiliated committees and councils in every state of the union. The respective offices are listed in the telephone book of almost every large city.

Planned Parenthood, which has grown considerably over the years, provides reproduction information and voluntary birth control services to the general public. It also trains professionals and paraprofessionals for work in the family planning field.

The International Planned Parenthood Federation is a worldwide organization composed of family planning groups from 79 nations which helps provide birth control services in more than 100 countries. Today the activities of Planned Parenthood represent perhaps the most extensive organized effort to bring at least some theoretical and practical sexual knowledge to men and women everywhere.

SIECUS

SIECUS, the *Sex Information and Education Council of the United States,* was formed as a voluntary health organization in 1964. The members come from various professional disciplines, such as medicine, psychiatry, anthropology, sociology, education, and religion. The organization tries to "establish man's sexuality as a health entity, . . . to dignify it by openness of approach, . . . to give leadership to professionals and to society, to the end that human beings may be aided toward responsible use of the sexual faculty and toward assimilation of sex into their individual life patterns as a creative and recreative force."

In conjunction with these efforts, SIECUS has published a number of books, pamphlets, and study guides related to sexual problems and issues a quarterly SIECUS Report. It also provides consultant services to communities and schools and supports a nationwide program of sex education. The SIECUS national headquarters is located at 137–155 N. Franklin, Hempstead, L.I., New York 11550.

The National Sex Forum

In 1968 The National Sex Forum was established in San Francisco under the auspices of a religious foundation and soon became internationally known as a center for innovative methods in sex education, sex therapy, and counseling. The Forum produces its own printed materials, videotapes, and educational films which cover the whole spectrum of human sexual activity. They are used in so-called SAR (Sexual Attitude Restructuring) programs which are attended by professionals from many fields, but which are also open to the general public. The films are further made available to medical schools, colleges, churches, and other institutions.

In addition to such practical projects, however, the Forum has also encouraged advanced and specialized research. Therefore, in 1976, The Institute for Advanced Study of Human Sexuality was founded. It is a graduate school for persons wishing extended professional training in the area of human sexuality. The Institute is qualified under California law to grant four academic degrees: Master of Human Sexuality, Doctor of Arts in Human Sexuality, Doctor of Human Sexuality, and Doctor of Philosophy in Human Sexuality. The Institute's comprehensive academic programs, sophisticated instruction methods, and excellent physical facilities make it one of the most important enterprises in the field of higher sex education today.

Both The National Sex Forum and The Institute for Advanced Study of Human Sexuality are located at 1523 Franklin Street, San Francisco, CA, 94109.

THE FUTURE OF SEX EDUCATION

In 1970 the *Federal Commission on Obscenity and Pornography* made its official report to the President and Congress recommending "that a massive sex education effort be launched. . . . It should be aimed at achieving an acceptance of sex as a normal and natural part of life and of oneself as a sexual being. It should not aim for orthodoxy; rather it should be designed to allow for a pluralism of values. It should be based on facts and encompass not only biological and physiological information, but also social, psychological and religious information. . . . It should be aimed, as appropriate, to all segments of our society, adults as well as children and adolescents."

These few sentences very well describe the goals and methods of modern sex educators and provide sensible guidelines for the future. It is now widely agreed, for example, that sex education has to be positive rather than negative as it so often was in the past. People must learn to accept rather than reject their sexuality. Furthermore, it is clear that in our present secular culture sex education, like any other education, cannot afford to be dogmatic. It is equally obvious that it must involve more than the biological "facts of life" or a description of "genital plumbing." Indeed, sex education today has to go well beyond the narrow subject of reproduction to include a discussion of sexual feelings and fantasies, pleasures, beliefs, superstitions, and dysfunctions. It must further discuss sexual attitudes in different societies and historical periods, erotic art, sex legislation and, indeed, "sexual politics." Finally, it cannot be restricted to children, but must address itself to the whole population.

After all, education, properly understood, is a life-long process. Human beings can learn as long as they are alive. And they learn not only as solitary private citizens—families, communities, professional groups, political parties, and even entire nations can change their sexual attitudes as a result of sex education. They can adopt healthier lifestyles, more sensible moral standards, and a greater sexual tolerance. This, in turn, can contribute to a greater degree of individual and collective happiness.

There is no doubt that much of our present sexual misery springs from simple ignorance. Some sexual and social problems even are the result of outright misinformation. People who misunderstand normal bodily functions and elementary human behavior often fall victim to crippling inhibitions or fears which poison all of their relationships. Great sex educators have always realized this, and even many doctors have acted upon this insight in their clinical practice. Thus, we have seen earlier in this book how in recent years the medical model of sexual deviance has, in many instances, been supplanted or even replaced by a learning model. Physicians and psychiatrists have developed new special kinds of therapy that can best be described as forms of education. Psychoanalysis, for example, can be explained as an autobiographical method, an educational process in which the analysand, under the subtle guidance of the analyst, educates himself about his own life history. (For details see "Conformity and Deviance, Healthy–Sick.")

The various modern, more specific "sex therapies" can also be characterized as forms of education. Masters' and Johnson's treatment of sexual dysfunctions, for instance, combines factual information with practical exercises which help men and women to learn or relearn satisfying sexual behavior. Similarly, the "Sexual Attitude Restructuring" program developed by the Na-

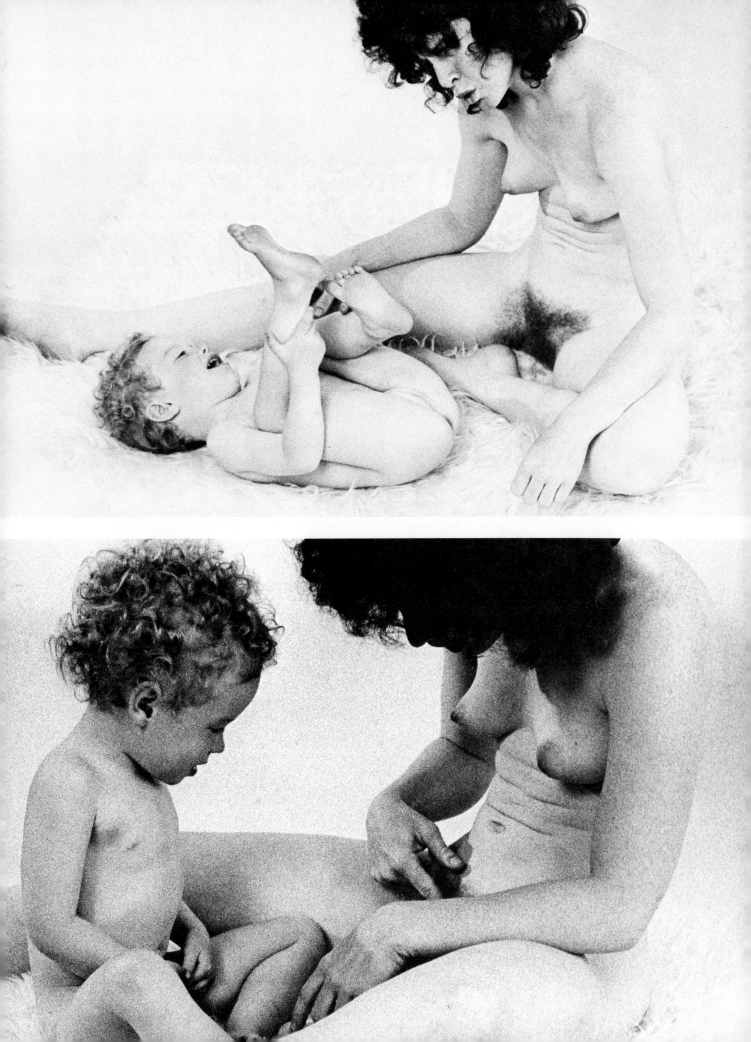

tional Sex Forum educates the participants about their own attitudes and thus shows them the way to greater understanding and personal sexual fulfillment. All of these and many similar developments support our earlier contention: Sex education is more than just theoretical instruction about the sex organs, their function, and their use. Instead, it combines both theory and practice in a never-ending process of developing all mental and physical human capacities. In short, sex education in the full sense of the term is education of the whole person as a sexual being.

It follows from these observations that conscious sex education should begin at the time of birth. Infants have to become familiar with their own bodily responses, they must learn to receive and express affection, and they must be helped to develop the appropriate self-identification as male or female. At the same time, however, care must be taken not to force them into obsolete, narrow gender roles. Sexual stereotyping of this kind is unfair to children and may well prevent them from realizing their full human potential. Needless to say, no information on any subject should be withheld from children if they show interest in it. This also applies to the subject of sex. Private, personal matters should remain private, but otherwise no holds need be barred. Anything covered in the present book, for example, can be discussed with children, if the right tone is found, and if the language is adjusted to their level of comprehension.

Since sex education is necessarily concerned with moral values, it is, of course, the primary privilege and responsibility of parents. Nevertheless, just as in any other field of study, schools can make a very important contribution by imparting some broader biological, psychological, legal, historical, and cultural knowledge. Thus, they may prove to children that a dispassionate, academic approach to sex (as to many other controversial subjects) has its own advantages. This, in turn, might eventually have a wholesome influence on the level of public discussion.

However, the transmission of sexual knowledge need not be confined to the home and the schools. Churches, youth organizations, the Red Cross, Planned Parenthood, public libraries, museums, and zoological gardens can also offer special programs dealing with the various aspects of human and animal sexuality. Publishers could provide more and better books, pamphlets, magazines, comics, and record albums for the sex education of children. Film producers could make entertaining, but nevertheless educational films about sex for the whole family or specifically for youth audiences. Television stations could create special sex education programs for various age groups. The possibilities seem endless and, at this date, have scarcely been perceived, much less exhausted. The daily press, as well as students' newspapers, could devote more space to the sexual problems of the young and even feature regular sex education departments. Certain contraceptives could be made available much more freely in public vending machines, and they could be accompanied by leaflets with detailed information about contraception and venereal disease. Such information could also be routinely included in every package of menstrual napkins or tampons.

Obviously, some elements in this continuous educational campaign would focus on reproduction in all of its aspects, but others would also emphasize the emotional aspect of sex and talk about the pleasure that can be part of sexual activity. Indeed, the capacity for such pleasure should be carefully nourished. Unfortunately, today any attempt to do so still meets with a great deal of public resistance. We have discussed the sexual experiences of young people elsewhere in this book, and we have seen that in our society few adults encourage or even condone such experiences. Under the circumstances, the practical side of early sex education is likely to remain neglected for a long time to come. Still, it should be clear to everyone that the lack of practice is a serious flaw in any educational program. After all, nobody expects students to learn dancing only by listening to lectures or reading books. Neither can they learn to drive an automobile just by studying a description of it. In short, sex education as it exists and is being advocated today is still handicapped by some very fundamental restrictions imposed on no other educational discipline. Even where students are given enough information, they are never permitted to put the content of their lessons to any concrete test. They cannot prove themselves in actual situations with real sexual partners, accumulate and sort out their own impressions, or learn by trial and error. These curious limitations give all official attempts at sex education a peculiar aura of unreality, if not insincerity, and undermine the credibility of even the most competent educator.

Of course, unofficially many young people do engage in sexual intercourse and thus try to gain some practical knowledge. However, because they must do so without adult approval, their experiences are not always as pleasant, rewarding, or instructive as they might otherwise be. Moreover, their partners are often of the same age and equally inexperienced and insecure. Many societies past and present have believed that boys and girls should be sexually initiated at puberty by experienced older partners. Yet, the sex laws in most states of the U.S. still take a very dim view of sexual contact between adolescents and adults. (See "Conformity and Deviance, Legal–Illegal.")

By the time they leave high school, many young Americans have some practical sexual experience, however unsatisfactory, and in college they normally find ample sexual opportunities. A growing number of colleges offer courses on human sexuality and also provide birth control services on campus. Young men and women who do not go to college can take advantage of Planned Parenthood and various other public and private sex information and counseling services. Recent years have seen a proliferation of such services, and they help great numbers of people from all levels of society. To give only one striking example: Some physicians have now produced their own sex education films and videotapes and make them available on private monitors in hospital rooms. This is especially appropriate in maternity hospitals, where many women are grateful for the opportunity to watch special explicit programs on childbirth, childcare, contraception, sexual intercourse after delivery, and similar topics.

Another source of adult sex education are the mass media in every form. In particular certain sexually oriented popular magazines have done much to educate the public about sexual techniques, erotic art, legal and philosophical issues related to sex, and the history of sexual customs. These magazines are often officially condemned as "obscene" or "pornographic," but it is only fair to acknowledge that they sometimes contain valuable sexual information in simple language. In many cases they fill a gap left open by more "respectable" publications. This is also true of certain so-called "pornographic" movies. Undoubtedly, many of them are disgusting, exploitative trash, but some of the most graphic "hardcore" films have also been beneficial and educational for timid or inexperienced audiences.

On the other hand, it is often correctly pointed out that much of our contemporary "pornography" paints a highly unrealistic picture of human sexuality and thus can mislead certain naive readers or viewers. Indeed, some sex educators have considered this danger to be serious enough to censor or prohibit the material in question. However, we must remember that for centuries much more harmful misinformation has been found in medical and psychiatric textbooks, encyclopedias, marital guides, police training manuals, catechisms, pastoral letters, and devotional literature. As a matter of fact, even today dangerous sexual misconceptions continue to be spread in certain religious pamphlets which are sold by the millions at church doors all over the country. Some of these booklets may well have a crippling effect on an unsophisticated young mind. Furthermore, they often also foster prejudice and sexual intolerance. By comparison, most "pornography" seems relatively harmless.

In any case, censorship is hardly the answer. In a pluralistic society such as ours, the "best" sexual knowledge can be found only through unhampered research in all directions, and the "proper" sexual values have to emerge from a vigorous public debate in which all opinions are given a hearing.

By and large, this already describes the situation today and is likely to characterize it in the future. Thus, ultimately, we can hope to arrive at a point where "sex" once more ceases to be a titillating or threatening special problem. Instead, it will again become a natural aspect of human life, attracting neither too much nor too little attention. As in former, less repressive ages, sex education will then simply be part of everyone's general education as a human being.

THE PROBLEM OF SEXUAL ETHICS

Throughout history, men have wrestled with the problem of sexual ethics or, in other words, with the question whether their own or other people's sexual behavior was good or bad. Today this question is as important as ever, although the answer has now become much more difficult than it was in the past.

All ethical standards are, of course, based upon certain fundamental beliefs, convictions, or assumptions, and the sexual ethics of any given society reflect its assumptions about the purpose or "nature" of sex. For example, there have been peoples on this planet who were unaware of the causal connection between sex and procreation. Obviously, these peoples arrived at different standards for sexual behavior than those who believed that procreation was the only purpose of sex.

In our own society this latter belief has long been espoused by religious authorities, and thus it has also determined our traditional sexual morality. However, in modern times the advance of science and technology, the gradual loss of faith, and the increasing communication between different cultures have created a pluralism of values that was formerly unknown. As a result, we now find ourselves in a new historical situation. In the course of our lives, we encounter a great variety of conflicting opinions about the purpose of sex and are forced to choose between a number of competing value systems.

The following pages briefly discuss this development and describe some of our present and future options.

RELIGIOUS TRADITION   Our ethical heritage is often described as "Judeo-Christian." That is to say, our moral values are explained as typical of the Jewish and Christian religions and, to a certain extent, this explanation makes sense. However, the two religions themselves have been subject to various other ancient and modern influences of which we are not always aware. Indeed, directly or indirectly, our attitudes have also been shaped by Near-Eastern mythologies, Greek philosophies, Roman laws, and Germanic customs. Furthermore, even if we concentrate only on the "Christian" tradition, we find that it had different meanings at different times. Historical studies show, for example, that the Christian approach to sex has varied widely over the centuries, and that the meaning of these variations is by no means as obvious as we might think. To give only one illustration: Today we tend to equate piety with sexual modesty, yet Chaucer's England, with all its bawdry, was a much more religious country than the prudish England of Queen Victoria. Nevertheless, on the whole, one can say that Judeo-Christian sexual doctrines have, for a very long time, dominated our lives, and that many of these doctrines have been rather arbitrary and narrow. Most of the time, most Jews and Christians believed that the only justification of sex was the procreation of children.

In ancient Israel, all possible pressure was brought to bear on everyone to "be fruitful and multiply." Coitus between husband and wife was encouraged, but any other form of sexual expression was taboo. Even marital intercourse was considered sinful at the time of the wife's menstruation, i.e. when she was unlikely to conceive. Indeed, the "worst" non-reproductive sins, homosexual intercourse and sexual contact with animals, were declared to be "abominations" or signs of idolatry. Thus, they became religious offenses. They violated God's natural order, and anyone who engaged in them was a sexual heretic. He could not be tolerated among the faithful and therefore was put to death.

The early Christians rejected many Jewish beliefs and traditions, but with regard to sex they more or less followed the law of Moses. Indeed, soon they developed even stricter laws of their own and, for a while, disparaged all sexual pleasure in favor of chastity. The procreation of children within marriage was recognized as legitimate, but complete abstinence was considered superior. This new ascetiscism softened somewhat in the course of time, but the negative basic attitude remained. The medieval church still saw the only "natural" function of sex in reproduction.

The Protestant Reformation did not bring greater sexual tolerance. On the contrary, while they attacked the Catholic cult of celibacy, many Protestants (especially the Puritans) retained the traditional reproductive bias and punished all sexual activity outside of marriage. Indeed, they even revived the laws of the Old Testament against the non-reproductive sexual heresies, and their philosophy then provided the basis of modern sex legislation in England and America. (See "Conformity and Deviance—Legal–Illegal.")

MODERN CHALLENGE

The old Judeo-Christian sexual standards first came under attack at the end of the Middle Ages. The renaissance of Greek and Roman thought, the change from a feudalistic to a capitalistic economy, technological innovations, the beginning exploration of the globe, the growth of commerce, and the birth of modern science encouraged people to become independent and to question many formerly sacred beliefs. Moreover, as a result of the Protestant Reformation, the old religious unity and certainty disappeared. An increasing number of new Christian sects offered their own interpretation of God's will, and while most of them still agreed on questions of sexual ethics, their quarrels in other areas could not but undermine their overall influence. At any rate, eventually they came to differ even in matters of sex and then quoted the same Bible in support of very dissimilar or even mutually exclusive positions. Under the circumstances, many men and women turned away from the churches and sought moral guidance elsewhere. Values that had been considered absolute, slowly became relative in a general process of secularization.

The "Contraceptive Revolution"

As modern research led to a better understanding of the human sexual and reproductive functions, the conscious control of reproduction became much easier than it had been before. Sometime in the late 17th or early 18th century, condoms made of animal intestines became more widely available. (There are still conflicting theories about the exact origin of the condom. For all we know, in one form or another it may already have been used in ancient times.) At first, these condoms were probably used mainly as a protection against venereal disease, but their contraceptive value did not go unappreciated for long. Finally, in the 19th century, the mass production of rubber condoms became possible and encouraged an ever-growing number of people to practice contraception. Gradually, other efficient methods were added, such as the diaphragm in the 1880s, the IUD in the 1930s, and the "pill" in the 1950s, resulting in a wide range of contraceptive choices. At the same time, private and public organizations developed which tried to make these choices available to the public. In most countries today, men and women can easily prevent pregnancies if they so choose.

The "Population Explosion"

The invention of reliable contraceptives and the increasing willingness to use them gave the human race as a whole some reason for hope, as it rather suddenly found itself confronted with a new problem: the threat of overpopulation.

Actually, this problem had already been perceived at the end of the 18th century by Thomas R. Malthus, but when, in the following decades, the population growth of some European countries failed to keep up with the demands of industrialization, religious and political authorities dismissed Malthus' warnings and even actively encouraged higher birth rates. In the meantime, however, the truth has reasserted itself with a vengeance: The population growth on this planet has become explosive and is about to outstrip the available resources.

It is estimated that the human species has existed for at least three million years, yet as recently as three centuries ago it numbered only about 500 million individuals (i.e. a little more than twice the present population of the United States). However, by 1850, only two centuries later, the number had doubled to 1 billion, and by 1930 it had doubled again to 2 billion. Only thirty years later, in 1960, the number had reached 3 billion, and only fifteen years later, in 1975, the world population had grown to 4 billion. This means, among other things, that of all human beings who have ever lived, about 25% or one quarter are alive today. It also means that, if the present trend continues, the number of people will double again in only 35 years and then reach the staggering figure of 8 billion. (See chart on p. 89)

Without going into details about the causes and consequences of this development, there is no doubt that it forces us to reexamine the reproductive bias of our traditional morality. There is no escape: If men and women continue to "increase and multiply" to their fullest capacity, they will soon render life on this earth intolerable or even impossible. If, on the other hand, they want to reduce the present high birth rates to a defensible level, they have to divorce their sexual behavior from the purpose of procreation. The complete sexual abstinence of billions of people cannot be considered a realistic alternative.

The Struggle for Individual Rights

The movement toward human self-determination, which began at the end of the Middle Ages, has, in the meantime, led to profound social and political changes. First religious reformers, then scientists and philosophers, and finally ordinary citizens emancipated themselves from absolutistic rule. Popes and kings were openly defied, as a desire for "enlightenment" prompted everyone to use his own powers of reason and to question all established authority. Individualism, equality, and independence were the new ideals, and in order to accommodate them, democratic forms of government were established in the United States and Europe.

The "enlightened" autonomous individual claimed that he had "natural human rights," and that among these were the right to life, liberty, and the pursuit of happiness. He also demanded freedom of religious belief and the right to speak, read, or print anything he desired. However, it soon became clear that there was nothing "natural" about any of these rights. On the contrary, they could result only from conscious human struggle. They were not really "nature's gift," but mankind's achievement. They had to be fought for, and once they were won, they had to be guarded, because they were easily lost. Furthermore, at first the new freedom was granted only to male members of the white middle and upper classes—women, slaves, the poor, and certain ethnic minorities were excluded to various degrees. It was only when these oppressed groups began their own civil rights struggle that they gained some measure of autonomy.

Today the struggle for individual rights continues and is, in fact, growing both wider and more intense. In the United States, women, blacks, and other ethnic groups still do not feel that all discrimination against them has ended and that some "affirmative action" on their behalf is required. Not only that —their demands are now being echoed by other, formerly silent minorities, such as the aging, the young, single adults, homosexuals, the handicapped, inmates in mental hospitals, and others. Each of these minorities has its own axe to grind, but in the present context we can point to one complaint which they have in common: For a very long time, they have all been victims of sexual oppression. (See "The Sexually Oppressed.")

However, today the sexually oppressed are no longer content with their lot, but demand the same freedom as everyone else. They are no longer apologetic about their desires and refuse to accept the status to which they have so long been assigned. By the same token, those who want to continue the present oppression now find that they must explain and justify their policies, and this is increasingly difficult, since they mostly reflect religious dogmas and do not have a rational basis. Under the circumstances, we can hope that the struggle for sexual liberation will succeed. It is part of the general struggle for the extension of individual rights and thus represents an exciting and constructive movement toward a society that is more open, more just, and more free. After all, by granting more rights to more people, we do not abolish all moral, legal, and political authority; we merely make it more democratic. (See also "The Social Roles of Men and Women—The Emancipation of Women.")

A "NEW MORALITY" FOR THE FUTURE

The modern challenge to religious tradition is deeply disturbing to many people who feel that it signals the end of our civilization. They do not want any change and, especially with regard to sexual ethics, they do not believe in progress. Instead, they believe that any loosening of the old strictures will lead to sexual chaos, and that sexual standards are worthless unless they are absolute. Still, in the meantime even some deeply religious men and women have become aware of the immoral effects of the old dogmatism, and they have searched for a new, more humane morality. Forgetting their ancient fears, they have embraced the modern ideals of individualism and self-determination, and they welcome the strict separation of church and state. Thus, they no longer want religious beliefs to influence our criminal law, for example. Even in the sexual sphere, they now accept the principle which John Stuart Mill had proclaimed in his famous essay *On Liberty* (1859): "The only purpose for which power can be rightfully exercised over any member of the community, against his will, is to prevent harm to others. His own good, either physical or moral, is not sufficient warrant. Each person is the proper guardian of his own health, whether bodily, or mental and spiritual."

We must understand, however, that this principle breaks with a moral tradition of thousands of years. Throughout most of human history, people have not been their own "proper guardians," but have left all decisions about their spiritual health in the hands of religious and political authorities. Only these "higher" authorities could determine what was good or bad in everyone's conduct, and they possessed the right to silence any dissent. It was not until rather recently that some democratic societies dared to subject their moral assumptions to rational scrutiny and public debate.

This development was brought about mainly by two factors: The growing struggle for individual rights and the realization that even the most altruistic motive is no justification for moral despotism. Indeed, as the great Christian writer C.S. Lewis once put it: "Of all tyrannies a tyranny exercised for the good of its victims may be the most oppressive." Selfish, greedy, and lecherous tyrants may sometimes grow weary, but a man who persecutes other people for their own good does so with a clear conscience, never relents, makes no exceptions, and shows no regard for the consequences. A democratic society therefore defends its very foundations when it respects the autonomy of its members and protects them from being tormented by "omnipotent moral busybodies."

Unfortunately, even where democratic values have been accepted in theory, they are not yet always upheld in practice. For example, although the United States Constitution proclaims individual freedom, there is still a great deal of oppression in the sexual sphere. Indeed, every now and then the old puritanical tyranny reappears and tries to put everyone in the same sexual straitjacket. Thus, in the late 19th century, American lawmakers passed the Comstock Act against mailing "obscene" material. In the early 20th century, they criminalized adultery where it had been legal before and closed the traditional brothels. After the First World War, a new drive against "vice" resulted in the general prohibition of alcohol. In the 1930s and '40s public hysteria about "perversion" led to the widespread adoption of laws against "sexual psychopaths." In the 1950s, fantasies about a communist "queer" conspiracy prompted a wave of repressive federal legislation against homosexuals. Now, in the 1970s, still another massive effort is being made to stamp out "pornography" and to end prostitution by arresting the customers.

However, experience shows that these and similar moral crusades rarely have the intended result and may actually make matters worse. Comstock's fanaticism denied generations of women adequate sexual and contraceptive knowledge and thus was directly responsible for much of the misery which Margaret Sanger and others tried to alleviate. The criminal statutes against extra-marital sex resulted in the monumental hypocrisy of the courts granting thousands of divorces on grounds of adultery and never prosecuting the guilty parties. The closing of brothels forced many prostitutes into the streets where they needed the "protection" of pimps. The prohibition of alcohol gave a tremendous boost to organized crime, the "sexual psychopath laws" and the legal discrimination against homosexuals created new oppressed social groups while producing no practical benefits for the general public. The current "war on pornography" is again wasting huge amounts of tax money in questionable legal attempts to harass publishers whose products are eagerly bought by millions of readers. At the same time, these readers are being victimized by ever-increasing violent crimes.

Actually, the problem goes even deeper than that. The old puritanical tyranny oppresses not only a few sexual sinners and heretics, but also a great number of righteous, "average" citizens. Sex researchers and therapists have found that rigid moral beliefs can literally make people sick and cause a variety of sexual and social dysfunctions. Furthermore, such beliefs often needlessly deprive men and women of much potential pleasure, breeding frustration, envy, and even violence. The biological facts, at least, cannot be disputed: In modern times the age of the onset of puberty has been lowering steadily, while the average life expectancy has been rising. As a result, for people in general there has been a significant increase in the number of sexually responsive, but non-reproductive years.

Under the circumstances, the reproductive bias of our traditional sexual ethics has become even less defensible than before. Nothing worthwhile is accomplished by making people feel guilty about desires that could well be a source of happiness, health, and mutual appreciation. Instead, it would seem more "decent" to develop a more humane, more flexible code of ethics. Today, we need to encourage not only procreational, but also recreational sex.

Of course, once we accept recreation as a legitimate purpose of sex, many of our traditional moral standards, criminal laws, and psychiatric assumptions no longer make sense. There is no longer a valid reason, for instance, to restrict sexual intercourse to marriage, and thus the condemnation and criminalization of sex between unmarried partners can only seem arbitrary and unjust. By the same token, the old sexual heresies, abominations, or non-procreative "perversions" have to be judged by their objective social effects, and in some cases these effects may well prove desirable. Moreover, if sex is to be enjoyed for its own sake, contraception will have to be made available to everyone from the age of puberty, and the old taboos against advertising contraceptives on radio, television, or billboards will have to fall. Indeed, in the meantime the "population explosion" has already forced many countries to run large-scale, permanent contraception campaigns, using all public media. Some also distribute free contraceptives to anyone who wants them, including unmarried adolescents.

There is no need here to spell out all possible implications of a future "recreative" sexual morality. In the present context it is enough if we realize that some drastic changes are likely and that, even in the sexual sphere, we may eventually have to "think the unthinkable." For example, a few hard-pressed governments have now begun to fight the increase in population with "disincentives" (i.e. penalties) for large families and are debating the possibility of compulsory sterilizations. Other governments are preaching premarital sexual abstinence while simultaneously raising the age at which people can get married and denouncing all forms of sensuality or "indulgence" within marriage itself. If strictly enforced, such policies can lower the birth rate, but, needless to say, they also promote political totalitarianism. Democratic governments, therefore, may rather decide to pursue the opposite course. Perhaps only total sexual freedom can really succeed in stabilizing the population.

These few hints may suffice to show that the "sexual revolution" is far from over, and that not all sexual and marital experiments of our time are frivolous aberrations. As we may also gather from these hints, by no means all of the experiments will prove to be successful in the end. Some may even turn out to have very destructive results, forcing us to abandon them and to begin our search anew. However, in any case it seems safe to predict that both failure and success will increasingly be judged in practical terms. The final arbiter will be experience, not some unquestioned religious dogma. In short, to a much greater extent than before, our sexual morality will have to stand up to reason.

This is not meant to imply that moral standards can be entirely rational. Certainly, science alone cannot tell us what we should do as sexual beings. At best, it can make us alert and critical, but it cannot by itself establish a code of sexual ethics. Value judgments are essentially unscientific. There is no objective way of making ethical choices. In questions of good and evil, we will always depend on feelings, beliefs, and moral traditions.

Therefore, the great religions, including our own, still have an important role to play in shaping our sexual attitudes. As long as we live our faith humbly and prudently, it will comfort us and teach us how best to serve our fellow human beings. It may no longer be able to offer us instant solutions for every moral dilemma, but at least it can give us some general guidelines. Even the fact that, in the past, religion has often been used as a pretext for cruelty and sexual oppression can today help our moral enlightenment. Understanding the suffering caused by religious zealots can keep us properly modest in our moral claims.

Reference and Recommended Reading

Brecher, Edward. *The Sex Researchers.* rev. ed. New York: New American Library, 1971.

Fromm, Erich. *The Art of Loving.* New York: Harper & Row, 1956 (cloth); 1974 (paper).

Guyon, René, *The Ethics of Sexual Acts.* New York: Knopf, 1958.

Kirkendall, Lester and Whitehurst, Edward, eds. *The New Sexual Revolution.* Buffalo: Prometheus Books, 1971.

Kosnik, Anthony, et al., *Human Sexuality: New Directions in American Catholic Thought.* New York: Paulist Press, 1977.

Lippmann, Walter. *A Preface to Morals.* New York: Macmillan, 1929 (reissued 1964, Time-Life Books).

Pomeroy, Wardell B. *Dr. Kinsey and the Institute for Sex Research.* New York: New American Library, 1973.

Reich, Wilhelm. *The Sexual Revolution: Toward a Self-Governing Character Structure,* 4th ed. New York: Farrar, Straus & Giroux, 1969 (cloth); Simon & Schuster, 1975 (paper).

EPILOGUE

202

NOW THANK WE GOD FOR BODIES STRONG

KINGSFOLD 8 6 8 6 D

traditional melody of England and Ireland
arranged by Ralph Vaughan Williams 1872-1958

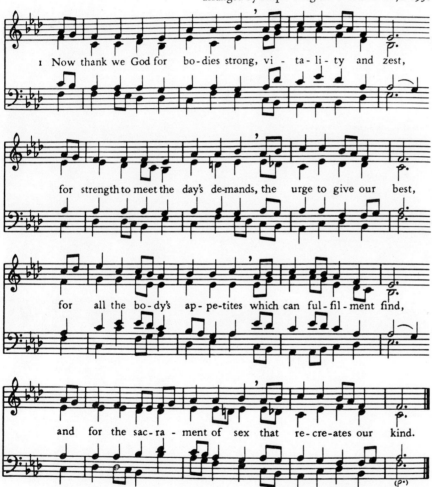

1 Now thank we God for bo-dies strong, vi - ta - li - ty and zest,

for strength to meet the day's de-mands, the urge to give our best,

for all the bo-dy's ap-pe-tites which can ful-fil-ment find,

and for the sac-ra-ment of sex that re-cre-ates our kind.

2 We thank him too that he has given
the gift of human minds,
and for the thrill of piecing out
the pattern that one finds–
to see in science and in art,
in lore of every kind,
that we, in searching out life's ways
do but discern his mind.

3 And most of all we thank him for
the highest gift of all:
that body, mind and all our powers
respond to Spirit's call.
Though kin to beasts and born of flesh,
in mortal bodies dressed,
yet God has linked our souls to his:
they nowhere else can rest.

Derwyn Dixon Jones 1925–

A GLOSSARY OF SEXUAL SLANG

Oh perish the use of the four-letter words
Whose meanings are never obscure!
The Angles and Saxons, those bawdy old birds,
Were vulgar, obscene, and impure

But cherish the use of the weaseling phrase
That never quite says what you mean!
You'd better be known for your hypocrite ways
Than as vulgar, impure, and obscene.

(ANON.)

In our society it is not always easy to talk about sex. As we have seen in this book, the current standard terms for sex organs and sexual behavior are often pretentious, difficult to pronounce, imprecise, and misleading, while the simpler, more graphic slang expressions are considered "dirty" and cannot be used in polite conversation. Furthermore, there is now a growing army of sexologists who are busy coining new words and expressions every day, and who are confusing not only the general public, but also each other with their various cabalistic and neo-archaic professional jargons. At the same time, many formerly silent sexual minorities are speaking out, trying to free themselves from negative semantic labels or to give them a new, positive meaning. As a result of all this, discussions often lead nowhere, misunderstandings abound, and communication breaks down.

This is especially true for the communication between different age groups. The older generation has been trained to speak "properly" about sex, but most young people have an instinctive aversion against "heavy" Greek and Latin terms, and they sense the prudery and cultural snobbery which led to their official adoption. After all, when translated, these terms often say neither more nor less than our suppressed Anglo-Saxon words, and thus, from a purely logical standpoint, there is no reason why they should be considered superior. In-deed, in almost any area except sex, the vernacular is preferred.

Most of our modern "dirty" words were once perfectly clean, and even today many people find nothing wrong with them, but use them regularly in private. At any rate, they are usually the only sexual terms young people know, and it goes without saying that anyone who wants to teach or counsel them must be familiar with their language. The exclusive use of "four-letter words" in the classroom is hardly desirable, but sometimes it can at least break the ice. By the same token, students and confused persons who feel that they are being understood by their teachers or counselors are more likely to ask those questions that really trouble them.

Of course, as any intelligent student will soon discover, our sexual slang also has serious shortcomings. While it is often forceful, vivid, and even humorous, it can also be biased, narrow, and simpleminded. It does not always help us to understand what it attempts to describe. In this respect, some carefully chosen professional terms may prove much more practical. Under the circumstances, it seems advisable to provide both teachers and students with a double glossary of sexual standard terms and sexual slang. Such a glossary "works both ways" and can therefore help them to bridge the "communication gap." It may also be useful to doctors, social workers, police officers, and other professionals in their work. Finally, it may be welcome to ordinary citizens who want to understand modern "underground" literature or the "sex ads" in certain magazines.

Obviously, the following brief glossary is not complete. New terms and phrases are being invented all the time, and many old ones go out of fashion. Some slang expressions are also confined to particular geographical regions or change their meaning from one region to another. Still, the few words listed here can give the reader a first impression of the "unofficial" sexual language in most of the United States today.

STANDARD TERMS	SLANG TERMS	STANDARD TERMS	SLANG TERMS
I. THE HUMAN BODY			
		rectum	*ass*
anus	*asshole, bung hole, butt hole*	scrotum	*bag, sack*
breasts	*boobs, headlights, knockers, tits*	semen	*come, cream, cum, jism, load, love juice*
buttocks	*ass, behind, buns, butt, fanny, rear*		
clitoris	*button, clit*	syphilis	*bad blood, haircut, Old Joe, pox, siff, syph*
gonorrhea	*the clap, a dose, the drip, gleet, morning drop, a strain, the whites*	testicles	*balls, family jewels, gonads, gones, nuts*
hymen	*cherry, maidenhead*		
menstruation	*the curse, wearing the rag*	venereal disease	*social disease, VD*
penis	*cock, dick, dong, joy stick, meat, organ, pecker, peter, poker, prick, rod, tool, wang, weenie*	vagina (or vulva)	*bearded clam, bearded lady, beaver, box, cunt, honey pot, manhole, muff, pussy, quim, snatch, toolbox, twat*

II. HUMAN SEXUAL BEHAVIOR

STANDARD TERMS	SLANG TERMS
ambisexual(ity)	AC/DC
an ambisexual person	switch hitter, trade
anal intercourse	assfucking, cornholing, the Greek way
anilingus (licking of the anus)	reaming, ream job, rimming
condom	French letter, love glove, raincoat, rubber, safe, safety
cunnilingus	cunt lapping, eating out, eating pussy, French art, frenching, muff diving
ejaculation	coming
ejaculation during sleep	wet dream
to ejaculate	to come, to shoot
erection	boner, hard-on
fellatio	blowing somebody, blow job, cocksucking, doing somebody, French art, frenching, going down on somebody, sucking somebody
group sex	daisy chain, gang bang, group grope
homosexual	male: cocksucker, fag, faggot, fruit, gay, homo, nellie, pansy, queen, queer, sister female: dyke, lessie, lez
masturbation	beating off, beating one's meat, hand fuck, hand job, jacking off, jerking off, pocket pool, rubbing off (females), whacking off
prostitute	male: hustler, stud female: B-girl, hooker, lady of the evening, streetwalker, working girl
sexually excited	horny, hot, juicy (females), turned on
to have sexual intercourse	to ball, to bang, to fuck, to get laid, to get into somebody's pants, to get a piece, to get a piece of ass, to get some tail, to have the banana peeled, to hump, to lay somebody, to make somebody, to make out with somebody, to roll in the hay, to rub bellies, to score, to screw

SLANG TERMS	STANDARD TERMS
AC/DC	ambisexual(ity)
ass	buttocks or rectum
asshole	anus (the rectal opening)
B & D	Bondage and Discipline: sadism (see also s/m)
B-girl	a female prostitute
bad blood	syphilis
bag	scrotum
to ball	to have sexual intercourse
to ball somebody	to insert one's penis in either the vagina or rectum of a sexual partner
balls	testicles
to bang somebody	to insert one's penis in either the vagina or rectum of a sexual partner
bearded clam, bearded lady	vulva or vagina
to beat off	to masturbate
to beat one's meat	to masturbate
beaver	vulva or vagina
behind	buttocks
to blow somebody	to fellate somebody (to suck somebody's penis)
blow job	fellatio (sucking the penis)
boner	erection
boobs	breasts
bottom man	a man who has a penis inserted in his rectum
box	vulva or vagina
broad	girl
bull bitch, bull dyke	a masculine looking lesbian
bung hole	anus (the rectal opening)
buns	buttocks
butch	masculine looking
butt	buttocks
butt hole	anus (the rectal opening)

SLANG TERMS	STANDARD TERMS
button	clitoris
cherry	hymen
chick	girl
chicken	a male adolescent
chicken hawk,	a man who prefers male adolescents as sexual partners
circle jerk	group masturbation
clap	gonorrhea
clit	clitoris
closet queen	a male homosexual who does not admit his homosexuality
cock	penis
cocksucker	a male homosexual
come	semen
to come	to have an orgasm
to come out (of the closet)	to admit one's homosexuality
to cornhole somebody	to insert one's penis in the rectum of a sexual partner
cream	semen
cum	semen
cunt	vagina or vulva
cunt lapping	cunnilingus (sucking the vulva)
the curse	menstruation
daisy chain	group sex
dick	penis
discipline	sadism
to do somebody	to suck somebody's sex organs
dong	penis
a dose	gonorrhea
drag	clothing of the opposite sex
drag queen	a male homosexual who sometimes wears female clothes
the drip	gonorrhea

SLANG TERMS	STANDARD TERMS	SLANG TERMS	STANDARD TERMS
dyke	a female homosexual (lesbian)	honeypot	vulva or vagina
to eat somebody	to have oral intercourse	hooker	a female prostitute
to eat somebody out	to engage in cunnilingus (to suck somebody's vulva)	horny	sexually excited
		hot	sexually excited
to eat pussy	to engage in cunnilingus (to suck somebody's vulva)	to be hung	to have a large penis
		to hump somebody	to insert one's penis in either the vagina or the rectum of a sexual partner
fag, faggot	a male homosexual		
fag hag	a woman who prefers the company of male homosexuals		
		hustler	a male prostitute
fairy	a male homosexual	to jack off	to masturbate
family jewels	testicles	to jerk off	to masturbate
fanny	buttocks	jism	semen
FFA	"Fist Fuckers of America" i.e. men who enjoy certain sadistic practices (see also s/m)	John	the customer of a prostitute
		joy stick	penis
		juicy	sexually excited (females)
fistfucking	inserting a hand or fist into the rectum (a dangerous practice that can lead to serious injuries)	to knock up	to make pregnant
		knockers	breasts
		lady of the evening	a female prostitute
flagwaver	exhibitionist	to lay somebody	to have sexual intercourse
French active	a person who sucks somebody's sex organs	les, lessie, lez	a female homosexual (lesbian)
		load	semen
French art	oral intercourse	love glove	condom
French kiss	an open-mouth kiss	love juice	semen
French letter	condom	maidenhead	hymen
French passive	a person who has his or her sex organs sucked	to make out	to have sexual intercourse
		to make somebody	to have sexual intercourse
to french somebody	to suck somebody's sex organs	manhole	vulva or vagina
fruit	a male homosexual	meat	penis
fruit fly	a woman who prefers the company of male homosexuals	morning drop	gonorrhea
		M/S	Master/Slave (A confusing misinterpretation of s/m, since the master is a sadist (s), the slave a masochist (m). See also s/m and B/D)
to fuck	to have sexual intercourse		
to fuck somebody	to insert one's penis in either the vagina or rectum of a sexual partner		
gang bang	group sex or gang rape (several persons raping the same victim)	muff	vulva or vagina
		muff diving	cunnilingus (sucking the vulva)
gay	homosexual	nellie	an effeminate male homosexual
to get into somebody's pants	to have sexual intercourse	nelly	effeminate
		nuts	testicles
to get laid	to have sexual intercourse	Old Joe	syphilis
to get off	to have an orgasm	organ	penis
to get a piece of ass	to have sexual intercourse (not necessarily anal intercourse)	pansy	an effeminate male homosexual
		pecker	penis
to get some tail	to have sexual intercourse	peeping Tom	voyeur (a man who watches people undress or having sexual intercourse)
gleet	gonorrhea		
to go down on somebody	to suck somebody's sex organs	peter	penis
		prick	penis
golden shower	urination on a person's body	pocket pool	masturbation
gonads	testicles	pox	syphilis
gones	testicles	pussy	vulva or vagina
Greek active	a man who inserts his penis in his partner's rectum	queen	an effeminate male homosexual
		queer	homosexual
Greek passive	a person who has a penis inserted in the rectum	quim	vulva or vagina
		raincoat	condom
the Greek way	anal intercourse	to ream somebody	to lick somebody's rectal opening (anus)
group grope	group sex		
haircut	syphilis	ream job	anilingus (licking the rectal opening)
hand fuck	masturbation	rear	buttocks
hand job	masturbation	rice queen	a homosexual who prefers Asian partners
hard-on	erection		
to have the banana peeled	to have sexual intercourse	to rim somebody	to lick somebody's rectal opening (anus)
head lights	breasts	rod	penis
homo	a male homosexual	to roll in the hay	to have sexual intercourse

SLANG TERMS	STANDARD TERMS	SLANG TERMS	STANDARD TERMS
to rub bellies	to have sexual intercourse	to swing both ways	to engage in both heterosexual and homosexual intercourse
to rub off	to masturbate (females)		
rubber	condom	swinger	a sexually promiscuous person
sack	scrotum	swishy	effeminate
safe	condom	switch hitter	an ambisexual person
safety	condom	syph (or siff)	syphilis
to score	to have sexual intercourse	tea room	public toilet
to screw	to have sexual intercourse	tea room queen	a male homosexual who seeks partners in public toilets
to screw somebody	to insert one's penis in either the vagina or rectum of a sexual partner		
		tits	breasts
to shoot	to ejaculate	tool	penis
short eyes	child molester	tool box	vulva or vagina
siff (or syph)	syphilis	top man	a man who inserts his penis in his partner's rectum
sissy	effeminate		
sister	a male homosexual	trade	an ambisexual man
sixty-nine (69)	simultaneous mutual oral intercourse	trick	1. a casual sex partner or
s/m	sadistic/masochistic (See also M/S and B/D)		2. a customer for prostitution
		to trick	to find a casual sex partner
snatch	vulva or vagina	to turn a trick	to find a customer for prostitution
social disease	venereal disease	turned on	sexually excited
soul kiss	an open-mouth kiss	TV	a transvestite
spade queen	a homosexual who prefers black partners	TS	a transsexual
		twat	vulva or vagina
steam queen	a homosexual who frequents bath houses	VD	venereal disease
		versatile	willing to engage in all forms of sexual intercourse
strain	gonorrhea		
streetwalker	a female prostitute	wang	penis
stud	1. a sexually very active man or	water sport	urination on a person's body
	2. a male prostitute	wearing the rag	having a menstruation, to menstruate
to suck somebody	to fellate somebody	weenie	penis
sugar daddy	an older man who pays his sexual partners	wet dream	ejaculation during sleep
		to whack off	to masturbate
to swing	1. to be sexually promiscuous or	the whites	gonorrhea
	2. to engage in partner swapping	working girl	a female prostitute

BIBLIOGRAPHY AND RESOURCE GUIDE

The main references for the present book are given in the body of the text itself, in brief notes following specific sections, and at the end of each chapter. The following select bibliography again lists the most important of these references and also provides an introduction to other educational resources.

I. BASIC RESOURCE GUIDE

1. BIBLIOGRAPHIES

American Library Association, Task Force on Gay Liberation, Social Responsibilities Round Table. *A Gay Bibliography*. Box 2383, Philadelphia, Pa. 19103.

Indiana University, Institute for Sex Research Library. *Catalog of the Social and Behavioral Sciences, Monograph Section of the Library of the Institute for Sex Research, Indiana University, Bloomington, Ind.* 4 vols. Boston: G. K. Hall, 1975.

Reisner, Robert G. *Show Me the Good Parts: The Reader's Guide to Sex in Literature*. New York: Citadel Press, 1964.

Seruya, Flora C. *Sex and Sex Education: A Bibliography*. New York: Bowker, 1972.

Sex Information and Education Council of the United States (SIECUS). *Human Sexuality: A Book List for Professionals*. 137-155 N. Franklin, Hempstead, N.Y. 11550, 1970.

University of Michigan Library, *Sex in Contemporary Society: A Catalogue of Dissertations*. Ann Arbor, Mich.: Xerox University Microfilms, 1973.

Weinberg, Martin S. and Alan P. Bell. *Homosexuality, An Annotated Bibliography*. New York: Harper & Row, 1972.

2. ENCYCLOPEDIAS AND HANDBOOKS

Beigel, Hugo G. *Sex from A to Z: A Modern Approach to All Aspects of Human Sex Life*. New York: Daye, 1961.

Comfort, Alex. *The Joy of Sex: A Gourmet Guide to Lovemaking*. New York: Crown, 1972.

———. *More Joy*. New York: Crown, 1973.

Ellis, Albert and Maurice Abarbanel, eds. *The Encyclopedia of Sexual Behavior*. New York: Hawthorn, 1967.

Goldstein, Martin, Erwin J. Haeberle and Will McBride. *The Sex Book: A Modern Pictorial Encyclopedia*. New York: Herder & Herder, 1971.

Hegeler, Inge and Sten. *An ABZ of Love*. New York: New American Library, 1974.

Money, John and Herman Musaph, eds. *Handbook of Sexology*. New York: Elsevier North-Holland, 1977.

Scott-Morley, A. *Encyclopedia of Sex Worship*. London: Walton, 1967.

3. DICTIONARIES

Dorland's Illustrated Medical Dictionary. 23rd ed. Philadelphia: Saunders, 1957.

Partridge, Eric. *Shakespeare's Bawdy*, rev. ed. New York: Dutton, 1947.

———. *A Dictionary of Slang and Unconventional English*, 2 vols. London: Routledge & Kegan, 1961.

———. *A Classical Dictionary of the Vulgar Tongue*. New York: Barnes & Noble, 1963.

Reissner, Albert. *Dictionary of Sexual Terms*. Bridgeport, Conn.: Assoc. Booksellers, 1967.

Rodgers, Bruce. *The Queen's Vernacular: A Gay Lexicon*. San Francisco: Straight Arrow, 1972.

Schmidt, J. E. *Cyclopedic Lexicon of Sex*. New York: Brussel & Brussel, 1967.

Trimble, John. *5,000 Adult Sex Words and Phrases*. North Hollywood, Calif.: Brandon House, 1966.

Wentworth, Harold and Stuart B. Flexner. *Dictionary of American Slang*. New York: T. Y. Crowell, 1975.

4. PERIODICALS

Archives of Sexual Behavior. Edited by Richard E. Green, M.D. Plenum Publishing Corp., 227 West 17th Street, N.Y. 10011. Quarterly.

AASECT Newsletter. American Association of Sex Educators, Counselors and Therapists, 5010 Wisconsin Ave., Suite 304, Washington D.C. 20016.

Cohabitation Research Newsletter. Compiled and edited by Eleanor D. Macklin, Ph.D. Dept. of Human Development and Family Studies, N.Y.S. College of Human Ecology, Cornell University, Ithaca, N.Y. 14850.

EMKO Newsletter. 7912 Manchester Ave., St. Louis, Mo. 63143. A monthly digest of sex information. Free.

Erickson Educational Foundation Newsletter. Erickson Educational Foundation, 1627 Moreland Avenue, Baton Rouge, La. 70808.

Family Planning Digest. The Bureau of Community Health Services, Health Services Administration, Department of Health, Education and Welfare, 5600 Fishers Lane, Room 12A-33, Rockville, Md. 20852. Free.

Family Planning Perspectives. Center for Family Planning Program Development, 515 Madison Avenue, N.Y., N.Y. 10022. Free.

Forum: The International Journal of Human Relations. 909 Third Avenue, New York, N.Y. 10022.

Information, Education, Communication in Population. East-West Center, 1777 East-West Road, Honolulu, Hi. 96822. Free.

Journal of Homosexuality. Hawarth Press, 130 West 72nd Street, N.Y., N.Y. 10023.

Journal of Marriage and the Family. The National Council on Family Relations, 1219 University Ave., S.E., Minneapolis, Minn. 55414.

Journal of Sex and Marital Therapy. Behavioral Publications, 72 Fifth Avenue, N.Y., N.Y. 10011.

Journal of Sex Education and Therapy. American Association of Sex Educators, Counselors and Therapists, 5010 Wisconsin Ave., Suite 304, Washington, D.C. 20016.

Journal of Sex Research. Society for the Scientific Study of Sex, Inc., 12 E. 41st St., N.Y. 10017. Quarterly.

Journal of Sex Role Research. Dr. Phyllis A. Katx, Graduate Center, CUNY, 33 West 42nd Street, N.Y., N.Y. 10036.

Medical Aspects of Human Sexuality. Clinical Communications, Inc., 18 East 48th Street, N.Y., N.Y. 10017.

Ms Magazine. 370 Lexington Avenue, N.Y., N.Y. 10017.

Newsletter of Division 34. American Psychological Association, 1200-17th Street, N.W., Washington, D.C. 20036.

News Service. International Planned Parenthood Federation, Western Hemisphere Region, 111 Fourth Avenue, N.Y., N.Y. 10003. Free.

Options. Newsletter of the Association for Sexual Adjustment in Disability, P.O. Box 3579. Downey, Ca. 90242.

Sex News. P. K. Houdek, 7140 Oak, Kansas City, Mo. 64114. Monthly digest of resources.

Sexual Law Reporter, 3701 Wilshire Boulevard, Suite 700, Los Angeles, Cal. 90010. Bi-monthly.

SIECUS Report. Sex Information and Education Council of the U.S. All SIECUS publications available from Behavioral Publications, 72 Fifth Avenue, N.Y., N.Y. 10011.

Successful Marriage: A Newsletter Offering Practical Information to Help Make Your Marriage Work. DJT Publications, 115 East Armour Blvd., Box 1042, Kansas City, Mo. 64141.

5. FILM PRODUCERS AND DISTRIBUTORS

Center for Marital and Sexual Studies, 5199 East Pacific Coast Highway, Long Beach, Ca. 90804 [Sexual Dysfunctions].

EDCOA Productions Inc., 12555 East 37th Avenue, Denver, Col. 80239 [Sex Education].

Focus International, Inc., 505 West End Avenue, New York, N.Y. 10024 [Sex Education and Therapy].

Hallmark Films and Recordings, Hallmark Educational Division, 1511 E. North Avenue, Baltimore, Md. 21213 [Sex and the Mentally Retarded].

John Wiley & Sons, 605 Third Avenue, New York, N.Y. 10016 [Sex Education for Adolescents].

Medical Film Library, 18740 Ventura Boulevard, Suite 302, Tarzana, Cal. 91356 [Sex Therapy].

Multi Media Resource Center, 1525 Franklin Street, San Francisco, Ca. 94109, publishes the "Multi Media Resource Guide" [All Aspects of Human Sexuality].

New Day Films, P. O. Box 315, Franklin Lakes, N.J. 07417 [Male and Female Roles].

Perennial Education, 1825 Willow Road, P.O. Box 236, Northfield, Ill. 60093 [Family Planning].

Serious Business Company, 1609 Jaynes Street, Berkeley, Ca. 94703 [Women].

SIECUS Film Sources for Sex Education, 137-155 N. Franklin, Hempstead, N.Y. 11550 [Sex Education].

Singer, Laura J. *Sex Education on Film: A Guide to Visual Aids and Programs.* New York: Teachers College Press, 1971.

Stanfield House, 900 Euclid Avenue, P.O. Box 3208, Santa Monica, Cal. 90403 [Mentally Handicapped].

6. SEX RESEARCH AND EDUCATION PROGRAMS

Human Sexuality Program, University of California, San Francisco, School of Medicine, 350 Parnassus Avenue, San Francisco, Ca. 94143 [Course for Health Professionals].

The Institute for Advanced Study of Human Sexuality, 1523 Franklin Street, San Francisco, Ca. 94109 [A graduate school for professionals, offering Master's and Doctor's degrees in Human Sexuality].

The Institute for Sex Research (Kinsey Institute), Indiana University, Bloomington, Ind. 47401 [Research Library and Summer Study Program in Human Sexuality].

S.A.R. (Sexual Attitude Restructuring), The National Sex Forum, 1523 Franklin Street, San Francisco, Ca. 94109 [Intensive Course for Professionals].

Social Work Institute for the Study of Sex (SWISS), University of Hawaii, School of Social Work, Hawaii Hall, Honolulu, Hi. 96822 [Summer Training Institute for Social Workers].

7. ORGANIZATIONS AND INSTITUTIONS

American Association of Marriage and Family Counselors, 225 Yale Avenue, Claremont, Calif. 91711.

American Association of Sex Educators, Counselors and Therapists, 5010 Wisconsin Ave., N.W., Suite 304, Washington, D.C. 20016.

The American Institute of Family Relations, 5287 Sunset Blvd., Los Angeles, Cal. 90027.

American Medical Association, Department of Community Health and Health Education, 535 North Dearborn Street, Chicago, Ill. 60610.

American Psychological Association, Task Force on Psychology, Family Planning and Population Policy, 1200 Seventeenth Street, N.W., Washington, D.C. 20036.

American Public Health Association, 1015 Eighteenth Street, N.W., Washington, D.C. 20036.

American School Health Association, 107 South Depeyster Street, Kent, Oh. 44240.

American Social Health Association, 1740 Broadway, New York, N.Y. 10019.

Association for Voluntary Sterilization, 14 West 40th Street, New York, N.Y. 10019.

Bureau of Community Health Services, Health Services Administration, Department of Health, Education and Welfare, 5600 Fishers Lane, Room 12A-33, Rockville, Md. 20852.

California Institute for Human Sexuality, P.O. Box 77671, Los Angeles, Ca. 90007.

Carolina Population Center, University of North Carolina, University Square, Chapel Hill, N.C. 27514.

Center for Family Planning Program Development, Division of Planned Parenthood-World Population, 1666 K Street, N.W., Washington, D.C. 20006.

Center for the Study of Sex Education in Medicine, 4025 Chestnut Street, Philadelphia, Pa. 19104.

Child Study Association of America, 9 East 89th Street, New York, N.Y. 10028.

Center for Population Research, National Institute for Child Health and Human Development, National Institutes of Health, Room A-721, Landow Building, Bethesda, Md. 20014.

Community Sex Information, Inc., 888 7th Avenue, N.Y., N.Y. 10019.

East-West Center, 1777 East-West Road, Honolulu, Hi. 96822.

E. C. Brown Center for Family Studies, 1802 Moss Street, Eugene, Or. 97463.

Educational Foundation for Human Sexuality, Montclair State College, Upper Montclair, N.J. 07043.

Erickson Education Foundation, 1627 Moreland Avenue, Baton Rouge, La. 70808.

Institute for Advanced Study of Human Sexuality, 1523 Franklin Street, San Francisco, Ca. 94109.

Institute for Family Research and Education, 760 Ostrom Avenue, Syracuse, N.Y. 13210.

Institute for Sex Research, Inc., Indiana University, Room 416, Morrison Hall, Bloomington, In. 47401.

International Academy of Sex Research, State University of New York Medical School, Health Sciences, Department of Psychiatry, Stony Brook, N.Y. 11790.

International Family Planning Research Associates, Inc., 2960 West 8th Street, Los Angeles, Ca. 90005.

International Planned Parenthood Federation, 18-20 Lower Regent Street, London, SW1, England.

National Alliance Concerned with School-Age Parents (NACSAP), 3746 Cumberland Street, N.W., Washington, D.C. 20016.

National Council of Churches, Commission on Marriage and the Family, 475 Riverside Drive, N.Y., N.Y. 10027.

National Council on Family Relations, 1219 University Avenue, S.E., Minneapolis, Minn. 55414.

National Gay Task Force, Room 903, 80 Fifth Avenue, N.Y., N.Y. 10011.

National Institute for Human Relations, 180 North Michigan Avenue, Chicago, Ill. 60601.

National Organization for Non-Parents, Box 10495, Baltimore, Md. 21209.

National Sex Forum (Multi Media Resource Center), 1523 Franklin Street, San Francisco, Ca. 94109.

Planned Parenthood Federation of America, Inc., 810 7th Avenue, N.Y., N.Y. 10019.

Planned Parenthood—World Population, 810 Seventh Avenue, N.Y., N.Y. 10019.

Population Council, 245 Park Avenue, N.Y., N.Y. 10017.

Population Institute, 110 Maryland Avenue, N.E., Washington, D.C. 20002.

Program in Human Sexuality, University of Minnesota Medical School, Mayo Building-842, Minneapolis, Minn. 55455.

Reproductive Biology Research Foundation (Masters and Johnson), 4910 Forest Park Boulevard, St. Louis, Mo. 63108.

Religious Coalition for Abortion Rights, 100 Maryland Avenue, N.E., Washington, D.C. 20002.

Resource Center on Sex Roles in Education, National Foundation for the Improvement of Education, 1156 15th Street, N.W., Washington, D.C. 20005.

Sex Information and Education Council of the U.S. (SIECUS), 137-155 N. Franklin, Hempstead, L.I., N.Y. 11550.

Society for the Scientific Study of Sex, Inc., 12 East 41st Street, N.Y., N.Y. 10017.

Synagogue Council of America, Committee on the Family, 235 Fifth Avenue, N.Y., N.Y. 10016.

Zero Population Growth, 1346 Connecticut Avenue, N.W., Washington, D.C. 20036.

II. BASIC READING GUIDE

1. GENERAL

Brecher, Edward. *The Sex Researchers*. Boston: Little Brown, 1969 (cloth); rev. ed. New York: New American Library, 1971 (paper).

Broderick, C. and Jessie Bernard, eds. *The Individual, Sex and Society, A SIECUS Handbook for Teachers and Counselors*. Baltimore, Md.: Johns Hopkins University Press, 1969.

Butler, Robert and Myrna Lewis. *Sex After Sixty*. New York: McGraw-Hill, 1975.

Comfort, Alex. *The Joy of Sex, a Gourmet Guide to Lovemaking*. New York: Crown, 1972 (cloth); Simon and Schuster, 1974 (paper).

———. *More Joy*. New York: Crown, 1974 (cloth); Simon & Schuster, 1974 (paper).

Ford, Clellan S. and Frank H. Beach. *Patterns of Sexual Behavior*. New York: Harper & Row, 1951 (cloth); Harper & Row, 1970 (paper).

Gagnon, John H. *Human Sexualities*. Chicago: Scott, Foresman & Co., 1977.

Hegeler, Inge and Sten. *Living is Loving*. New York: Stein and Day, 1973.

Hettlinger, Richard. *Human Sexuality: A Psychosocial Perspective*. Belmont, Ca.: Wadsworth, 1975.

Hunt, Morton. *Sexual Behavior in the 1970's*. Chicago: Playboy Press, 1974.

Katchadourian, Herant A. and Donald T. Lunde. *Fundamentals of Human Sexuality*. 2nd. ed. New York: Holt, Rinehart and Winston, 1975.

Kirkendall, Lester and Robert Whitehurst, eds. *The New Sexual Revolution*. Buffalo, N.Y.: Prometheus Books, 1971.

Masters, William and Virginia Johnson. *Human Sexual Response*. Boston: Little, Brown, 1966.

McCary, James L. *Human Sexuality*. 2nd. ed. New York: van Nostrand, 1973.

———. *Sexual Myths and Fallacies*. New York: Schocken, 1971.

Mead, Margaret. *Male and Female*. New York: Wm. Morrow, 1975; New Amer. Library, 1974 (paper).

Money, John and Anke Ehrhardt. *Man and Woman, Boy and Girl*. Baltimore, Md.: Johns Hopkins University Press, 1972.

Money, John and Patricia Tucker. *Sexual Signatures*. Boston: Little, Brown, 1975.

Oakley, Ann. *Sex, Gender and Society*. New York: Harper & Row, 1972.

Rubin, Isador. *Sexual Life After Sixty*. London: Allen and Unwin, 1969.

Schofield, Michael. *Sexual Behavior of Young People*. Boston: Little, Brown, 1965.

Sex Information and Education Council of the United States (SIECUS). *Sexuality and Man*. New York: Charles Scribner's Sons, 1970.

Stoller, Robert J. *Sex and Gender: On the Development of Masculinity and Femininity*. New York: Science House, 1968.

Zubin, Joseph and John Money, eds. *Contemporary Sexual Behavior: Critical Issues in the 1970s*. Baltimore, Md.: Johns Hopkins University Press, 1973.

2. MALE SEXUALITY

The Diagram Group. *Man's Body, an Owner's Manual*. New York: Paddington Press, 1976 (paper); New York: Bantam, 1977 (paper).

Feigen-Fasteau, Marc. *The Male Machine*. New York: McGraw-Hill, 1974.

Kinsey, Alfred C. et al. *Sexual Behavior in the Human Male*. Philadelphia: Saunders, 1948.

Plack, Joseph and Jack Sawyer. *Men and Masculinity*. Englewood Cliffs, N.J.: Prentice-Hall, 1974.

Pomeroy, Wardell B. *Boys and Sex*. New York: Dell, 1971.

Steinmann, Anne and David Fox. *The Male Dilemma*. New York: Jason Ronson, 1974.

3. FEMALE SEXUALITY

Barbach, Lonnie G. *For Yourself: The Fulfillment of Female Sexuality*. New York: Doubleday, 1975.

Boston Women's Health Book Collective. *Our Bodies, Ourselves*. 2nd ed. New York: Simon and Schuster, 1976.

The Diagram Group. *Woman's Body, an Owner's Manual*. New York: Bantam, 1977.

Dodson, Betty. *Liberating Masturbation: A Meditation on Self-Love*. New York: Bodysex Designs, Box 1933 N.Y., N.Y. 10001, 1974.

Fisher, Seymour. *The Female Orgasm: Psychology, Physiology, Fantasy*. New York: Basic Books, 1973.

Friday, Nancy. *My Secret Garden: Women's Sexual Fantasies*. New York: Trident, 1973.

———. *Forbidden Flowers, More Women's Fantasies*. New York: Trident, 1974.

Greer, Germaine. *The Female Eunuch*. New York: McGraw-Hill, 1971 (cloth); New York: Bantam, 1972 (paper).

Hite, Shere. *The Hite Report*. New York: Macmillan, 1976 (cloth); New York: Dell, 1977 (paper).

Kinsey, Alfred C. et al. *Sexual Behavior in the Human Female*. Philadelphia: Saunders, 1953; Pocket Books (paper).

Kline-Graber, Georgia and Benjamin Graber. *Woman's Orgasm: A Guide to Sexual Satisfaction*. New York: Bobbs Merrill, 1975.

Lowry, Thomas P. and Thea Snyder Lowry. *The Clitoris*. St. Louis: Warren H. Green, 1976.

Millett, Kate. *Sexual Politics*. New York: Avon, 1971.

Pomeroy, Wardell B. *Girls and Sex*. New York: Dell, 1969.

Sherfey, Mary Jane. *The Nature and Evolution of Female Sexuality*. New York: Random House, 1972.

Smith, Carolyn, Toni Ayres and Maggi Rubenstein. *Getting in Touch: Self-Sexuality for Women*. San Francisco: Multi Media, 1973.

4. HUMAN REPRODUCTION

Boston Women's Health Book Collective. *Our Bodies, Ourselves*. 2nd ed. New York: Simon and Schuster, 1976.

Calderone, Mary, ed. *Manual of Family Planning and Contraceptive Practice*. Baltimore, Md.: Williams & Wilkins, 1970.

Demarest, Robert and John Sciarra. *Conception, Birth and Contraception*. 2nd ed. New York: McGraw-Hill, 1969.

Dickinson, Robert L. *An Atlas of Human Sexual Anatomy*. 2nd ed. Baltimore, Md.: Williams & Wilkins, 1949.

Ehrlich, Paul A. *The Population Bomb*. New York: Ballantine Books, 1968.

Finch, B. E. and H. Green. *Contraception Through the Ages*. Springfield, Ill.: C. C. Thomas, 1963.

Hatcher, Robert A. et al. *Contraceptive Technology 1976-1977*. 8th rev. ed. New York: Irvington-John Wiley & Sons, 1976.

Shapiro, Howard I. *The Birth Control Book*. New York: St. Martin's Press, 1977.

5. SEXUAL PROBLEMS AND THERAPIES

Agel, Jerome, ed. *The Radical Therapist*. New York: Ballantine Books, 1971.

Annon, Jack S. *The Behavioral Treatment of Sexual Problems*. 2 vols. Honolulu: Enabling Systems, 1974.

Belliveau, Fred and Lin Richter. *Understanding Human Sexual Inadequacy*. New York: Bantam, 1970.

Bernstein, D. A. and T. D. Borkovec. *Progressive Relaxation Training: A Manual for the Helping Professions*. Champaign, Ill.: Research Press, 1973.

Blank, Joani. *Good Vibrations: The Complete Woman's Guide to Vibrators*. Burlingame, Cal.: Down There Press, P.O. Box 2086, 1976.

Brecher, Edward and Ruth. *An Analysis of Human Sexual Response*. New York: Signet, 1969.

De la Cruz, F. and Gerald D. LaVeck. *Human Sexuality and the Mentally Retarded*. New York: Bruner/Mazel, 1973.

Dowing, George, *The Massage Book*. New York: Random House, 1973.

Feinbloom, Deborah. *Transvestites and Transsexuals*. New York: Delacorte Press, 1976.

Green, Richard. *Sexual Identity Conflict in Children and Adults*. New York: Basic Books, 1974.

———. *Human Sexuality: A Health Practitioner's Text*. Baltimore, Md.: Williams & Wilkins, 1975.

Inkeles, Gordon and Murray Todris. *The Art of Sensual Massage*. San Francisco: Straight Arrow Books, 1971.

Kaplan, Helen S. *The New Sex Therapy*. New York: Bruner/Mazel, 1974.

———. *The Illustrated Manual of Sex Therapy*. New York: Quadrangle, 1975.

Lehrman, Nat. *Masters and Johnson Explained*. Chicago: Playboy Press, 1970; 2nd ed. 1976.

Masters, William and Virginia E. Johnson. *Human Sexual Inadequacy*. Boston: Little, Brown, 1970.

McIlvenna, Ted. *When You Don't Make It*. San Francisco: Multi Media, 1973.

McIlvenna, Ted and Herb Vandervoort. *You Can Last Longer*. San Francisco: Multi Media, 1973.

Mezzei, George. *Good Vibrations: The Vibrator Owner's Manual of Relaxation, Therapy, and Sensual Pleasure*. New York: Hawthorne, 1977.

Money, John and Richard Green, eds. *Transsexualism and Sex Reassignment*. Baltimore, Md.: Johns Hopkins University Press, 1969.

Montagu, Ashley. *Touching, The Human Significance of Skin*. New York: Columbia University Press, 1971 (cloth); New York: Harper & Row, 1972 (paper).

Mooney, Thomas O., Theodore M. Cole and Richard Chilgren. *Sexual Options for Paraplegics and Quadriplegics*. Boston: Little, Brown, 1975.

National Sex Forum. *SAR Guide for a Better Sex Life*. San Francisco: National Sex Forum, 1975.

Rosenberg, Jack. *Total Orgasm: Advanced Techniques for Increasing Sexual Pleasure.* New York: Random House Bookworks, 1973.

Rimm, D. C. and J. C. Masters. *Behavior Therapy: Techniques and Empirical Findings.* New York: Academic Press, 1974.

Stoller, Robert J. *Perversion, The Erotic Form of Hatred.* New York: Pantheon, 1975.

Young, Constance. *Self Massage.* New York: Bantam, 1973.

6. HOMOSEXUALITY

Abbott, Sidney and Barbara Love. *Sappho was a Right-on Woman: A Liberated View of Lesbianism.* New York: Stein and Day, 1972.

Altmann, Dennis. *Homosexual: Oppression and Liberation.* New York: Avon, 1973.

Churchill, Wainwright. *Homosexual Behavior Among Males, A Cross-Cultural and Cross-Species Investigation.* New York: Hawthorn, 1967 (cloth); New York: Prentice-Hall, 1971 (paper).

Gearhart, Sally and William Johnson. *Loving Women/Loving Men: Gay Liberation and the Church.* San Francisco: Glide, 1974.

Hartman, William and Marilyn Fithian. *Treatment of Sexual Dysfunction.* Long Beach, Calif.: Center for Marital and Sexual Studies, 1972.

Hoffman, Martin, *The Gay World: Male Homosexuality and the Social Creation of Evil.* New York: Basic Books, 1968.

Humphreys, Laud. *Tearoom Trade: Impersonal Sex in Public Places.* Chicago: Aldine, 1970.

Karlen, Arno. *Sexuality and Homosexuality.* New York: Norton, 1971.

Katz, Jonathan, *Gay American History.* New York: T. Y. Crowell, 1976.

Martin, Del and Phyllis Lyon. *Lesbian/Woman.* New York: Bantam, 1972.

———. *Lesbian Love and Liberation.* San Francisco: Multi Media, 1973.

McNeill, John J., S. J. *The Church and the Homosexual.* Mission, Ks.: Sheed Andrews & McMeel, 1976.

Perry, Troy. *The Lord is My Shepherd and He knows I'm Gay.* Los Angeles: Nash, 1972.

Rowse, A. L. *Homosexuals in History.* New York: Macmillan, 1977.

Tripp, C. A. *The Homosexual Matrix.* New York: McGraw-Hill, 1975.

Weinberg, Martin S. and Colin J. Williams. *Male Homosexuals: Their Problems and Adaptions.* New York: Oxford University Press, 1974.

Weinberg, George. *Society and the Healthy Homosexual.* New York: Doubleday, 1973.

7. SOCIAL ISSUES

Adams, Paul et al. *Children's Rights: Toward the Liberation of the Child.* New York: Praeger, 1971.

Barnett, Walter, *Sexual Freedom and the Constitution: An Inquiry into the Constitutionality of Repressive Sex Laws.* Albuquerque, N.M.: University of New Mexico Press, 1973.

Bell, Robert R. and M. Gordon. *The Social Dimension of Human Sexuality.* Boston: Little, Brown, 1970.

Benjamin, Harry and R. E. L. Masters. *Prostitution and Morality.* New York: Julian Press, 1964.

Bernard, Jessie. *The Future of Marriage.* New York: Bantam, 1973.

Brownmiller, Susan. *Against Our Will: Men, Women and Rape.* New York: Simon and Schuster, 1975.

Calderone, Mary S. *Sexuality and Human Values.* New York: Association Press, 1975.

Commission on Obscenity and Pornography. *The Report of the Commission on Obscenity and Pornography.* New York: Bantam, 1970.

Constantine, Larry and Joan. *Group Marriage.* New York: Collier, 1973.

Day, Beth. *Sexual Life Between Black and White: The Roots of Racism.* New York: Apollo Edition, 1974.

Francoeur, Anna and Robert. *Hot and Cool Sex: Cultures in Conflict.* New York: Harcourt Brace Jovanovich, 1974.

Frankfort, Ellen. *Vaginal Politics.* New York: Quadrangle, 1972.

Gagnon, John H. and William Simon, eds. *The Sexual Scene.* 2nd ed. New Brunswick, N.J.: Transaction Books, 1973.

Gebhard, Paul et al. *Sex Offenders.* New York: Harper & Row, 1965.

Gochros, Harvey and Jean, eds. *The Sexually Oppressed.* New York: Association Press, 1977.

Gochros, Harvey and LeRoy Schultz. *Human Sexuality and Social Work.* New York: Association Press, 1972.

Guyon, Rene, *The Ethics of Sexual Acts.* New York: Knopf, 1934, 1958.

———. *Sexual Freedom.* New York: Knopf, 1950.

Hernton, C. *Sex and Racism in America.* New York: Grove Press, 1965.

Laing, R. D. *The Politics of the Family.* New York: Pantheon, 1971.

Martin, Del. *Battered Wives.* San Francisco: Glide, 1976.

Morrison, Eleanor and Mila Price. *Values in Human Sexuality.* New York: Hart, 1975.

Poland, Jefferson Fuck and Valerie Alison. *Records of the San Francisco Sexual Freedom League.* New York: Olympia Press, 1971.

Ramey, James. *Intimate Friendships.* Englewood Cliffs, N.J.: Prentice-Hall, 1975.

Reiss, Ira. *The Social Context of Premarital Permissiveness.* New York: Holt, Rinehart & Winston, 1967.

Schur, Edwin M. *Crimes without Victims: Deviant Behavior and Public Policy.* Englewood Cliffs, N.J.: Prentice-Hall, 1965.

Smith, James and Lynn. *Beyond Monogamy.* Baltimore, Md.: Johns Hopkins University Press, 1974.

The Wolfenden Report (on homosexual offenses and prostitution). New York: Stein and Day, 1963.

8. HISTORY AND CULTURE

Brinton, Crane. *History of Western Morals.* New York: Harcourt Brace, 1959.

Bullough, Vern L. *Sexual Variants in Society and History.* New York: Wiley, 1976.

Cole, William Graham. *Sex and Love in the Bible.* New York: Association Press, 1959.

Danielsson, Bengt. *Love in the South Seas.* New York: Reynal, 1956.

De Rougemont, Denis. *Love in the Western World.* New York: Pantheon, 1956.

Edwards, Allan, *The Cradle of Erotica.* New York: Lancer, 1962.

Ellis, Havelock. *Studies in the Psychology of Sex.* 2 vols. New York: Random House, 1942.

Epstein, L. M. *Sex Laws and Customs in Judaism.* rev. ed. New York: Ktav, 1968.

Fielding, William, J. *Strange Customs of Courtship and Marriage*. London: Souvenir Press, 1961.

Forberg, Friedrich Karl. *Manual of Classical Erotology*. New York: Grove Press, 1966.

Freud, Sigmund, *Civilization and Its Discontents*. Strachey, James, ed. and tr., New York: Norton, 1962 (paper and cloth).

————. *The Future of an Illusion*. Strachey, James, ed. New York: Norton, 1975 (paper).

————. *Totem and Taboo*. Strachey, James, tr. New York: Norton, 1952 (cloth and paper).

Fromm, Erich. *Sigmund Freud's Mission*. New York: Grove, 1963.

Grimes, Alan P. *The Puritan Ethic and Woman Suffrage*. New York: Oxford University Press, 1967.

Haller, John S. and Robin M. Haller. *The Physician and Sexuality in Victorian America*. Urbana: Univ. of Illinois Press, 1974.

Hare, E. H. "Masturbatory Insanity: The History of an Idea," *Journal of Mental Science*, 452 (1962) pp. 2-25.

Himes, Norman E. *Medical History of Contraception*. New York: Schocken, 1970.

Horkheimer, Max. "Authority and the Family," *Critical Theory*. New York: Seabury, 1972.

Hyde, H. M. *A History of Pornography*. New York: Dell, 1969.

Jones, Ernest. *The Life and Work of Sigmund Freud*. 3 vols. New York: Basic Books, 1953.

Kennedy, David M. *Birth Control in America: The Career of Margaret Sanger*. New Haven, Conn.: Yale, 1970.

Kronhausen, Eberhard and Phyllis. *Erotic Fantasies*. New York: Grove Press, 1969.

————. *Erotic Art*. 2 vols. New York: Grove Press, 1970.

————. *The Sex People*. Chicago: Playboy Press, 1975.

Lewisohn, Richard. *A History of Sexual Customs*. New York: Bell, 1956.

Licht, Hans. *Sexual Life in Ancient Greece*. New York: Barnes & Noble, 1972.

Loth, D. *The Erotic in Literature*. New York: Macfadden, 1962.

Malinowski, Bronislaw. *The Sexual Life of Savages in North-Western Melanesia*. New York: Harcourt Brace Jovanovich, 1962 (pap.).

Marcus, Steven. *The Other Victorians*. rev. ed. New York: Basic Books, 1974.

Marcuse, Herbert. *Eros and Civilization*. Boston: Beacon, 1974 (paper).

Mead, Margaret. *Coming of Age in Samoa*. New York: Morrow, 1929.

————. *Sex and Temperament in Three Primitive Societies*. New York: Morrow, 1935.

————. *Male and Female*. New York: Wm. Morrow, 1975.

Meyer, Johann Jakob. *Sexual Life in Ancient India*. New York: Barnes & Noble, 1953.

Montagu, Ashley. *Sex, Man, and Society*. New York: Putnam, 1969.

Morris, Desmond. *Intimate Behavior*. New York: Bantam, 1973.

Murstein, Bernard I. *Love, Sex and Marriage Through the Ages*. New York: Springer, 1974.

Noonan, J.T. Jr. *Contraception: A History of Its Treatment by the Catholic Theologians and Canonists*. New York: New American Library, 1967.

Patai, Raphael. *Sex and Family in the Bible and the Middle East*. New York: Doubleday, 1959.

Reiche, Reimut. *Sexuality and Class Struggle*. New York: Praeger, 1971.

Schneider, Michael. *Neurosis and Civilization*. New York: Seabury, 1975.

Scott, George R. *Curious Customs of Sex and Marriage*. London: Torchstream, 1953.

Szasz, Thomas S. *The Manufacture of Madness*. New York: Harper & Row, 1970 (cloth); New York: Dell, 1971 (paper).

Vatsayana. *The Kama Sutra*. New York: Dutton, 1964.

Young, Wayland. *Eros Denied*. New York: Grove Press, 1964.

INDEX

Nature as ideology, 339–43
Naturrecht and menschliche Würde (Bloch), 343*n*
Nayar people, 402
Nero, 440
Netherlands
    Napoleonic Code in, 350
    questing in, 419
    woman's suffrage in, 305
New England, legal model of conformity and deviance in, 350
New York Society for the Suppression of Vice, 370, 473
New Zealand, woman's suffrage in, 305
Nicolson, Harold, 421
Night-courting, 419
Nightrunning, 419
Non-monogamous marriage, 420–21
Nonspecific urethritis, 121
North Carolina, law on "crime against nature" in, 361
Norway
    legal model of conformity and deviance in, 351–52
    nightrunning in, 419
Noyes, John Humphrey, 413, 421
Nuclear family, 423, 424, 427–31
Nuer people, 402
Nursing, 87

Obscenity and lewdness
    private, 369–71
    public, 356–57
Oedipus complex, 134–35
Okyo, Maruyama, 443
Older women, sexual response in, 59
Omai, 283
On Liberty (Mill), 485
On the Subjection of Women (Mill), 302
Onania, or the Heinous Sin of Self-Pollution and All Its Frightful Consequences in Both Sexes, Considered with Spiritual and Physical Advice (Bekker), 185
Onanism, or a Treatise Upon the Disorders Produced by Masturbation (Tissot), 186
Oneida community, 413, 421
Oogenesis, 67
Open marriage, 419
Oral character, 135
Oral intercourse
    heterosexual, 197, 203–9
    homosexual, 239–41
Oral phase, 134
Orgasm
    female, 58–59
    male, 35–36
    overemphasis on, 252–53
    during sleep, 188–89
Origin of the Family, Private Property and the State, The (Engels), 402
Osmond, Humphrey, 398
Ovaries, 45–46

Ovulation, preparation for, 48
Oxford English Dictionary, 125

Painful sexual intercourse
    in men, 114
    in women, 114–15
Pandering, 363
Pankhurst, Emmeline, 302
Parental marriage, 420
Patriarchy, 291–95
Patterns of Sexual Behavior (Ford and Beach), 136, 465
Paul, St., 294, 321, 348
Pederasty, 234–35
Pedophilia, 273
Penis, 27–29
    uncircumcized, 28
Performance, sexual, 131
Pericles, 293
Permissive marriage, 418
Phallic phase, 134–35
Philip, Landgrave of Hesse, 414
Philip of Macedonia, 233
Philippa of Hainault, 299
Philippe IV, King of France, 361, 362
Physical problems, 109–21
"Pill, the," 101
Pimping, 363
Pinel, Philippe, 380, 381
Planned Parenthood Federation of America, 105–6, 476, 477, 480, 481
Plateau
    in female sexual response, 58
    in male sexual response, 35
Plato, 332, 403, 462
Pleasure Bond, The (Masters and Johnson), 136
Pleasure principle, 134
Pleasure seeking, 129–32
Poe, Edgar Allan, 397
Poitiers, Diane de, 299
Politics (Aristotle), 184
Polyandry, 405
Polygamy, 405, 420
    Mormon, 413, 414, 420
Polygyny, 405
Polynesia
    adolescence in, 160
    marriage in, 413–14, 419
    models of conformity and deviance in, 330–31
Polytheism, 333
Pomeroy, Wardell B., 469
Popper, Karl, 343*n*
Population explosion, 483
Pornography, 370–71
Portugal
    divorce in, 414
    Napoleonic Code in, 350
Possession, demonic, 374–75, 377–81
Précieuses Ridicules, Les (Molière), 300
Pregnancy, 72–77
    false, 76

first trimester of, 74
    problems and complications during, 75–76
    second trimester of, 75
    sexual intercourse during, 76–77
    signs of, 73–74
    third trimester of, 75
Pregnancy, Birth and Abortion (Institute for Sex Research), 469
Premature birth, 76
Premature ejaculation, 254–55, 260–62
Prevention of venereal disease, 117–19
Primary sexual characteristics, 9–13
    female, 11, 13
    male, 9–10, 12
Prisoners, sexual oppression of, 458–59
Private lewdness and obscenity, U.S. laws on, 369–71
Prophylactics, 92–95
Prostate gland, 32
Prostitution, U.S. laws on, 363–66
Protestant churches, models of conformity and deviance of, 323–25
Protestant Reformation
    English, 349
    natural law and, 334–35
Psychiatric models of conformity and deviance, 373–400
    critique of, 394–97
    cross-cultural perspectives of, 384–86
    historical background of, 376–83
    implications of, 390–94
    new, 397–400
Psychoactive drugs, 394
Psychoanalysis
    contemporary European, 384
    nonmedical character of, 389, 397
Psychoanalytic theory
    of instincts, 129–30
    Oedipus complex in, 134–35
    See also Freud, Sigmund
Psychological Review, 131
Psychopathia Sexualis (Kaan), 382
Psychopathia Sexualis (Krafft-Ebing), 140, 382, 464
Psychosurgery, 392–94
Puberty, physical changes of, 162–64
Public bathing, 436–37
Public lewdness and obscenity, U.S. laws on, 356–57
Punalua, 419
Puritan Act (1650), 349
Puritans, 324
    legal model of conformity and deviance of, 349–50

Quarternary marriage, 418
Questing, 419

Ramayana, 329
Rape, 274
    U.S. laws on, 354–55
Rarotonga, royal incest in, 331

PICTURE CREDITS

In addition to those listed on page iv, the author wishes to acknowledge the following sources for pictures:

74 Carnegie Embryological Collection, University of California, Davis
222, top Bildarchiv Preussischer Kulturbesitz, Berlin
222, center Bildarchiv Preussischer Kulturbesitz, Berlin
222, bottom Hirmer Fotoarchiv, München
223, top Ajit Moorkerjee
223, bottom The National Sex Forum
224 The National Sex Forum
225 The National Sex Forum
226–27 The National Sex Forum
235 Bildarchiv Preussischer Kulturbesitz, Berlin
237 Musée du Petit Palais, Paris
247 Bildarchiv Foto Marburg
275 Phototrends
289, top left The New York Historical Society
289, top right New York Public Library Picture Collection
289, bottom left & right The Mansell Collection
292, top National Gallery
292, bottom The National Sex Forum
300, top The Granger Collection
300, center The Granger Collection
300, bottom The Granger Collection
301, top New York Public Library Picture Collection
303, top The Granger Collection
303, center The Granger Collection
303, bottom The Granger Collection
304, top New York Public Library Picture Collection
304, center Vassar College Library
304, bottom The Granger Collection
320 New York Public Library Picture Collection
323 Koninklijk Museum, Antwerp
326 New York Public Library Picture Collection
327 Ajit Moorkerjee
329 The National Sex Forum
330 Institute for Sex Research, Bloomington, Indiana
331 Staatliches Museum für Volkerkunde, München

345, top Bildarchiv Preussischer Kulturbesitz, Berlin
345, center New York Public Library Picture Collection
345, bottom New York Public Library Picture Collection
360, top Alinari—Scala
360, center Alinari—Scala
360, bottom Museo del Prado, Madrid
365, top Bildarchiv d. Österreichischen Nationalbibliothek, Vienna
365, center Bildarchiv d. Österreichischen Nationalbibliothek, Vienna
365, bottom The Granger Collection
368, center New York Public Library Picture Collection
368, bottom Bildarchiv d. Österreichischen Nationalbibliothek, Vienna
373 Museum of Fine Arts, Boston
379, right Historia-Photo, Bad Sachsa, West Germany
380, top Trustees of Sir John Sloane's Museum, London
380, bottom The Bettmann Archive
411, top Rijksmuseum, Amsterdam
411, bottom New York Public Library Picture Collection
413 Culver Pictures
424, top Hans Kluber, Familienbild, Kunstmuseum, Basel
424, center Historical Society of Pennsylvania
428 Staatliches Museum für Volkerkunde, München
429 New York Public Library Picture Collection
436, top Bildarchiv Preussischer Kulturbesitz, Berlin
436, bottom Graphische Sammlung Albertina, Vienna
437, top Hans Bock d.Ae., Das Bad zu Leuk, Kunstmuseum, Basel
439, above Historia-Photo, Bad Sachsa, West Germany

439, above left *Eros*
443, top Musée d'Art Ancien, Bruxelles
443, bottom The National Sex Forum
448–49 *The Granger Collection:*
  Sappho
  Sophocles
  Plato
  Alexander the Great
  Richard I
  Leonardo da Vinci
  Montezuma II
  James VI of Scotland
  von Humboldt
  Gogol
  Whitman
  Alger
  Saint-Saëns
  Tchaikovsky
  McDonald
  Rimbaud
  Proust
Culver Pictures:
  Julius Caesar
  Edward II
  Michaelangelo
  Henry III
Wide World:
  Gide
  Maugham
  Stein
  Keynes
  Nicolson
Embassy of Spain, Washington, D.C.:
  Garcia Lorca
Patrick Burns/New York Times Pictures:
  Auden
466 The Granger Collection
467, top *Sexology* Magazine
467, bottom Wide World
468 The Granger Collection
469 Wide World
473 The Granger Collection
475 Wide World
476 The Granger Collection
489 *The Hymn Book of the Anglican Church of Canada and the United Church of Canada*